2003

The Jossey-Bass Health Series brings together the most current information and ideas in health care from the leaders in the field. Titles from the Jossey-Bass Health Series include these essential health care resources:

Changing the U.S. Health Care System

Changing the U.S. Health Care System

Key Issues in Health Services, Policy, and Management

Second Edition

Ronald M. Andersen, Thomas H. Rice,
Gerald F. Kominski

Foreword by Abdelmonem A. Afifi

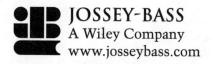

JOSSEY-BASS
A Wiley Company
www.josseybass.com

Published by

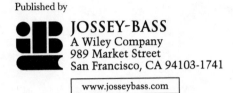

JOSSEY-BASS
A Wiley Company
989 Market Street
San Francisco, CA 94103-1741

www.josseybass.com

Jossey-Bass books and products are available through most bookstores. To contact Jossey-Bass
directly, call (888) 378-2537, fax to (800) 605-2665, or visit our website at www.josseybass.com.

Substantial discounts on bulk quantities of Jossey-Bass books are available to corporations,
professional associations, and other organizations. For details and discount information, contact
the special sales department at Jossey-Bass.

We at Jossey-Bass strive to use the most environmentally sensitive paper stocks available to us. Our
publications are printed on acid-free recycled stock whenever possible, and our paper always meets or
exceeds minimum GPO and EPA requirements.

Library of Congress Cataloging-in-Publication Data

Changing the U.S. health care system: key issues in health services, policy, and management/[edited by]
Ronald M. Andersen, Thomas H. Rice, Gerald F. Kominski.—2nd ed.
    p. cm. — (Jossey-Bass health series)
  Includes bibliographical references and index.
  ISBN 0-7879-5404-7 (hbk. : alk.paper)
    1. Health care reform—United States. 2. Medical policy—United States. 3. Medical care—United
States. I. Andersen, Ronald. II. Rice, Thomas H. III. Kominski, Gerald F. IV. Series.

RA395.A3 C478 2001
362.1'0973—dc21   00-050675

SECOND EDITION
HB Printing 10 9 8 7 6 5 4 3 2

CONTENTS

PART ONE: ACCESS TO HEALTH CARE   1

FIGURES AND TABLES

Figures

Tables

FOREWORD

The book you hold in your hand is a gift. With his wife, Audrey, the late Samuel J. Tibbitts gave a generous gift to the Department of Health Services in the UCLA School of Public Health to commission a study of key issues in health policy and management challenging the American health care system. The leadership, scholarship, and charity that Sam exhibited in making this gift typified his life in a number of ways.

Sam changed the health care system in California and the nation, perhaps in more ways than anyone else of his generation. After receiving a B.S. in public health from the University of California, Los Angeles, in 1949 and an M.S. in public health and hospital administration from the University of California, Berkeley, in 1950, he pioneered the development of integrated health care delivery and financing systems, a career course that culminated in the 1988 creation of the nonprofit UniHealth America, where he was chairman of the board until his death in 1994.

Along the way, Sam founded and chaired both PacifiCare Health Systems, one of the first major health maintenance organizations, and American Health Care Systems, a group of thirty-two hospital systems across the country that organized the nation's first preferred provider system, PPO Alliance. Both a leader and a scholar, he served as chairman of the board of trustees of the American Hospital Association and published more than one hundred articles. Sensing the need to establish a corporate conscience in a changing health care environment, he was founding chairman of the Guiding Principles for Hospitals, the first program to delineate ethical and quality principles in the industry.

Even while entering the twilight of a long and storied career, his concern for the future of health care remained. For that reason, he invested in the school that had nurtured him and asked the faculty to address afresh the crucial issues of cost, quality, and access to health care that now challenge the future of the United States.

The chapter authors in this volume, commissioned to guide us into an uncertain future, are gifted scholars. As former dean and continuing professor of biostatistics for the UCLA School of Public Health, I have known them well and followed their research closely. Also, as a public health educator, I am keenly aware of the multidisciplinary nature of our field. To understand public health as a whole, one must have a basic level of knowledge of each of its core disciplines.[1] But to gain a deeper understanding of public health in the United States, one needs a firm grasp of the issues facing the country in health care policy and management. Because of the complexity of these issues, discussions have been scattered in a multitude of references. To achieve Sam Tibbitts's vision, the editors sought to gather, in a single book, "a comprehensive, yet readable" account of these issues. I believe that they succeeded remarkably in the first edition, published in 1996, and in their efforts to update those issues in this new edition.

This book also accomplishes its initial self-prescribed task: "to examine where we are in achieving our country's health goals" following the defeat of President Clinton's comprehensive health care reform by the Congress in 1994—now updated to the new millennium with the second edition.

As anticipated by Sam, the book begins with addressing three key components of health care policy: improving access, controlling costs, and ensuring quality. As noted in Chapter Two, access to health care has always been a focus in the health care reform debate, and concludes that "the United States cannot escape the need for fundamental reforms that will extend coverage to its entire population." Cost, an element in the trade-off against adequate access and better quality, not only is the center of the ensuing debate in Congress but will continue to be a focus in health care policy making for the foreseeable future. Chapter Four explores various ways of containing health care costs and emphasizes the need for better data in order to make sensible policy decisions about alternative types of health care reform. Chapter Six examines the measurement of health outcomes and health-related quality of life (HRQL), concluding that we need "careful and appropriate inclusion of HRQL outcomes in traditional health services."

A number of subsequent chapters are devoted to segments of the population with special needs for health care. Subjects include long-term care for the elderly, providing services for the growing HIV/AIDS community, multidisciplinary coordination of the fragmented child health care system, improving access to primary health care for low income women, and increasing services to the growing homeless population. Various authors advance proposals that might improve the prognosis for these vulnerable populations.

The last portion of the volume contains discussions of the fundamental challenges facing health care researchers, policy makers, and managers at the turn of the century. A very basic challenge addressed in this area is to determine the appropriate role of competitive markets versus the regulatory role of government. Based on the experience of the managed care market in California, it was noted that increased price competition leads to reduced access for the uninsured. Despite some instances in which governmental regulation appeared to be successful in controlling expenditures and improving or maintaining access, no conclusion was drawn as to which approach should be adopted. Rather, we are presented with several research questions that require further investigation—an indication of the high degree of complexity of this topic.

The last five chapters proceed to deal with a variety of issues, starting with Medicare reform, from the role of preventive health care to the role of public health agencies in delivering personal health services, and from the continuing issue of medical malpractice liability to the ethics of public health and health care services. The collective message sent to the reader is clear: the time for health care reform is ripe, and effective research in this area is urgently needed to support this fundamental change.

This comprehensive account of important issues facing the nation in health policy and management is a valuable asset for health care policy researchers and analysts, as well as managers of health care services, providers, and practitioners. Moreover, students in health care policy and management or related fields will appreciate it as a guideline to many subject areas in the health care today. Finally, I believe that this book can serve as a readable guide to health care professionals and policy makers on health care reform during the next decade.

In the final analysis, health itself is a gift. I commend this volume to you, sharing the hope of Sam and Audrey Tibbitts, that training and discourse shall result, leading to innovations in policy and management that enable the blessings of health to be shared by all.

Abdelmonem A. Afifi
Former dean and professor of biostatistics
UCLA School of Public Health
Los Angeles, California
October 2000

Note

1. Afifi, A. A., and Breslow, L. "The Maturing Paradigm of Public Health." *Annual Review of Public Health*, 1994, *15*, 223–235.

ACKNOWLEDGMENTS

The authors of this volume met their obligations effectively and much more expediently than we had expected. Their rewards for substantial contributions to the revised edition were largely the intangible ones of providing service to the students and practitioners of health services policy and research.

Charles Doran, administrative specialist for the Department of Health Services UCLA School of Public Health, expanded his good efforts for the first edition, taking sole responsibility this time for organizing the efforts of the authors, formatting their work, and facilitating communication with our publisher, Jossey-Bass.

Jeanne Black, in addition to co-authoring a chapter, did a splendid job of editing another chapter under great stress and time pressure.

Finally, Andy Pasternack, senior editor, health at Jossey-Bass, urged us to undertake this revision and provided high-quality publishing support to complete the task.

October 2000
Los Angeles

Ronald M. Andersen
Thomas H. Rice
Gerald F. Kominski

The Authors

Ronald M. Andersen is Fred W. and Pamela K. Wasserman Professor and chair of the Department of Health Services at the UCLA School of Public Health, and a professor in the UCLA Department of Sociology. Previously he was a professor at the University of Chicago, serving for ten years as director of the Center for Health Administration Studies and the Graduate Program in Health Administration. He has studied access to medical care for his entire professional career of thirty-five years. He developed the Behavioral Model of Health Services Use that is extensively recognized nationally and internationally as a framework for utilization and cost studies of general populations as well as special studies of minorities, low-income persons, children, women, the elderly, the homeless, and people with HIV. He is a fellow of the Institute of Medicine and a recipient of the American Sociological Association's Leo G. Reeder award for distinguished service to medical sociology, the Academy for Health Services Research and Policy's distinguished investigator award, and the Baxter Allegiance Prize for health services research.

Thomas H. Rice is a professor in the Department of Health Services, UCLA School of Public Health. He is a health economist with a particular interest in health care cost containment, competition and regulation, health insurance, provider payment issues, and the Medicare program. From 1979 to 1983, he was a senior health economist at the Stanford Research Institute. Between 1983 and 1991, he was on the faculty at the University of North Carolina School of Public Health. He spent the 1989–90 academic year as a visiting senior analyst at the Physician Payment Review Commission. In 1988, he received the Association for Health Services Research (AHSR) Young Investigator Award, which is given to the outstanding health services researcher in the United States age thirty-five or under. In 1992, he received the Thompson Prize from the Association of University Programs in Health Administration, awarded annually to the outstanding health services researcher in the country age forty or under. In 1998, he received the AHSR Article of the Year Award. He served as editor of the journal *Medical Care Research and Review* from 1994 to 2000.

Gerald F. Kominski is an associate professor in the Department of Health Services, UCLA School of Public Health, and associate director of the UCLA Center for Health Policy Research. He has conducted a number of studies examining the impact of Medicare payment policies and the determinants of health care costs and utilization. Prior to joining the UCLA faculty, he worked on Medicare hospital payment issues as a staff member at the Prospective Payment Assessment Commission (ProPAC) in Washington, D.C. His current research focuses on using risk-adjusted outcome measures to improve inpatient quality of care.

Emily K. Abel is a professor in the Department of Health Services, UCLA School of Public Health, where she teaches courses titled Aging and Long-Term Care; Women, Health, and Aging: Policy Issues; and History of Public Health. Her publications on family care for disabled people include *Hearts of Wisdom: American Women Caring for Kin, 1850–1940; Who Cares for the Elderly? Public Policy and the Experiences of Adult Daughters;* and several articles in *The Gerontologist, Research on Aging,* and the *Journal of Aging Studies.*

John L. Adams is the head of the statistical consulting service at RAND. His current work focuses on improved quantitative methods in quality assessment. His interests include statistical methods for profiling managed care organizations and provider groups. With Elizabeth McGlynn, he has worked with Ford, General Motors, DaimlerChrysler, and the United Auto Workers over the past three years to develop a coordinated strategy for reporting on health plan performance to employees and retirees of the big three automobile manufacturers. He is currently involved in developing a quality measurement system for cancer care and validating patient self-reports of quality of care.

Lisa Arangua is a research analyst in the Department of Family Medicine, UCLA School of Medicine. She has been on the research staff at UC DATA at the

University of California, Berkeley, where she evaluated health and welfare programs for the state and federal government.

Jeanne T. Black is a research associate in the UCLA Center for Health Policy Research and a doctoral student in health services research in the Department of Health Services, UCLA School of Public Health, where she is the recipient of an Agency for Healthcare Research and Quality fellowship. She has extensive experience in strategic planning and management of health services organizations. She was formerly associate director of the Health Policy Institute at the University of Pittsburgh Graduate School of Public Health and has conducted research on employer-sponsored health insurance. She received her master of management degree from the Kellogg Graduate School of Management at Northwestern University in 1977.

Lester Breslow, M.D., has served as president of the American Public Health Association and as California's state director of public health. A member of the faculty of the UCLA School of Public Health since 1968, he served as dean from 1972 to 1980 and is currently an emeritus professor. He has been a member of the Institute of Medicine, National Academy of Sciences since 1975 and was founding editor of the *Annual Review of Public Health* from 1978 to 1990.

Robert H. Brook, M.D., is a vice president at RAND and director of the RAND Health Program. He is a professor of medicine and health services at the UCLA schools of Medicine and Public Health. He was head of the Health and Quality Group on the RAND Health Insurance Experiment, co-principal investigator of the Health Services Utilization Study, which developed a method for assessing appropriateness, and co-principal investigator of the national study assessing the impact of DRGs on quality and outcomes of acute hospital care.

E. Richard Brown is the director of the UCLA Center for Health Policy Research, and a professor in the departments of Community Health Sciences and Health Services at the UCLA School of Public Health. He has studied and written extensively about a range of issues and policies that affect the access to health care for disadvantaged populations. He has served as president of the American Public Health Association, as a member of several National Academy of Science study committees, and as a senior consultant to the President's Task Force on National Health Care Reform.

William S. Comanor is professor and director of the Research Program in Pharmaceutical Economics and Policy, Department of Health Services, UCLA School of

Public Health. He is also a professor of economics at the University of California, Santa Barbara. Between 1978 and 1980, he served as chief economist and director at the Bureau of Economics at the Federal Trade Commission in Washington, D.C. He also served as a member of the advisory board for the Office of Technology Assessment study of pharmaceutical research and development.

William E. Cunningham is an associate professor of medicine and public health at UCLA. He is the author of numerous manuscripts on access to medical care, case management, and health outcomes for persons with AIDS and is currently involved in several research projects addressing access to medical care and outcomes for persons with AIDS. He was co-leader of the research team investigating access to medical care in the HIV Costs and Services Utilization Study (HCSUS).

Pamela L. Davidson earned her doctorate from the UCLA Department of Health Services. Her research interests are in geographic variation in access, health outcomes and quality of life, evaluation research, and management and organization development for health care professionals. She has extensive project management experience, directing numerous research projects, and holding management and administrative positions in various organizations. Currently, she is a senior research scientist at the UCLA Center for Health Policy Research and adjunct assistant professor at the UCLA Department of Health Services. Before returning to UCLA, she spent several years as program chair and assistant professor at Chapman University's Health Systems and Health Administration programs, teaching graduate students, administering the education programs, and conducting educational research.

Susan L. Ettner is an associate professor in the Division of General Internal Medicine and Health Services Research at the UCLA School of Medicine and the Department of Health Services in the UCLA School of Public Health. She obtained her Ph.D. in economics at MIT in 1991 and served on the faculty in the Department of Health Care Policy at Harvard Medical School until joining the UCLA faculty in 1999. Her research interests include the economics of mental health and substance abuse; reciprocity in the relationship between health and labor market outcomes; insurance markets and managed care; and chronic disability, postacute, and long-term care.

Jonathan E. Fielding, M.D., is a professor of health services and pediatrics in the UCLA schools of Public Health and Medicine and co-director of the UCLA Center for Healthier Children, Families, and Communities. He is also director of public health and health officer for the county of Los Angeles. His other involvements are as founding co-director of the UCLA Center for Health Enhancement, Education, and Research; founding member of the U.S. Preventive Services Task Force, vice chair of the U.S. Community Preventive Services Task Force, and commissioner of public health for the commonwealth of Massachusetts.

Patricia A. Ganz, M.D., is a professor in the UCLA schools of Public Health and Medicine. She also serves as director of the Division of Cancer Prevention and Control Research in the UCLA Jonsson Comprehensive Cancer Center. She has been instrumental in incorporating quality-of-life assessment into cancer clinical trials, and she chaired a National Cancer Institute workshop on this topic in 1990. Her current work focuses on quality-of-care research in cancer. In 1999, she was named an American Cancer Society Professor of Clinical Research, recognizing her research on patient-focused outcomes. She serves as associate editor of the *Journal of Clinical Oncology* and the *Journal of the National Cancer Institute.*

Lillian Gelberg, M.D., is associate professor of family medicine in the UCLA School of Medicine. She is a health services researcher and family physician who conducts community-based research on health, access to care, and quality of care of the homeless and other vulnerable populations. She has studied homeless adults living in shelters and outdoor areas, and the health and use of health services among homeless and low-income housed patients. She is an alumna of the Robert Wood Johnson Foundation Clinical Scholars Program and is currently a Robert Wood Johnson Foundation Generalist Physician Faculty Scholar. She graduated with an M.D. from Harvard Medical School and completed her internship and residency at Montefiore Hospital in the Bronx.

Denise R. Globe is an assistant professor in the Department of Pharmaceutical Economics and Policy at the University of Southern California. She earned her doctorate in health services research at UCLA in 1998, specializing in finance. She has fifteen years of experience in the health care industry, focusing on quantitative policy research, with experience in disease management, including the outcomes of care, process of care, and financing and delivery of care.

Neal Halfon is professor of pediatrics in the School of Medicine, professor of community health sciences in the School of Public Health at UCLA, and a consultant in the RAND Health Program. He directs the UCLA Center for Healthier Children, Families, and Communities; the Child and Family Health Program in the School of Public Health; and the federally funded Maternal and Child Health Bureau's National Center for Infancy and Early Childhood Health Policy. His primary research interests include provision of developmental services to young children, access to care for poor children, and health services for children with special health care needs, particularly children in the foster care system.

Moira Inkelas is an adjunct assistant professor at the UCLA School of Public Health. Her research activities include evaluation of policies for financing health care for vulnerable populations, and the impact of managed care incentives on access, costs, and quality of care for children with special health needs. She received her M.P.H. degree from UCLA and her Ph.D. in policy analysis from RAND Graduate School.

Charles Lewis, M.D., is a graduate of Harvard Medical School. He received a doctorate of science degree from the University of Cincinnati. He is professor of medicine, public health, and nursing at UCLA. In 1972, he became chief of the Division of General Internal Medicine and Health Services Research. He is a member of the Institute of Medicine of the National Academy of Science. He has served as a commissioner for the Joint Commission on Accreditation of Healthcare Organizations since 1990. He is currently director of the Center for Health Promotion and Disease Prevention at UCLA, a joint effort of the schools of Public Health and Medicine.

Mark S. Litwin, M.D. is an associate professor in the UCLA schools of Public Health and Medicine. He trained in urological surgery at Harvard Medical School's Brigham and Women's Hospital and spent two years as a Robert Wood Johnson Clinical Scholar at UCLA and RAND. His primary research interests include medical outcome assessment, health-related quality of life, patient preferences, resource utilization in urological care, physician payment systems, and urological oncology with particular interest in prostate cancer.

Elizabeth A. McGlynn is the director of the Center for Research on Quality in Health Care at RAND Health. She is a nationally known expert on quality measurement. She has directed the RAND development of a comprehensive system for quality assessment that can be used in managed care, medical group, and community settings. She has worked with Ford, General Motors, DaimlerChrysler, and the United Auto Workers to develop a coordinated strategy for reporting on health plan performance to their employees and retirees. She directed a related project for the Health Care Financing Administration to develop a reporting strategy for Medicare beneficiaries enrolled in managed care.

Glenn Melnick is the Blue Cross of California Chair in Health Care Finance and professor at the USC School of Policy, Planning, and Development. He joined the faculty of the former USC School of Public Administration in 1996. Previously, he served on the faculty at the UCLA School of Public Health, as a consultant at RAND, and as an expert witness to the Federal Trade Commission. He received his Ph.D. at the University of Michigan in urban and regional planning and health economics. He is currently director of the Center for Health Care Finance, Policy, and Management in the USC School of Policy, Planning, and Development.

David M. Mosen is a research associate and outcomes analyst at the Intermountain Health Care Institute for Health Care Delivery Research. He received his Ph.D. from the Department of Health Services, UCLA School of Public Health in 1997. He wrote his dissertation using data from a study of hospitalized HIV patients in the greater Los Angeles area, examining the relationship of access to health care and long-term survival. While at UCLA, he was a recipient of a University of California AIDS Research Program (UARP) fellowship.

Nadereh Pourat is an adjunct assistant professor of health services at the UCLA School of Public Health and senior researcher at the UCLA Center for Health Policy Research. She has studied access to and utilization of health services in a variety of settings, with particular focus on the elderly and underserved populations. Her research includes the study of long-term care use among white and minority elderly, issues facing the elderly within managed care, the effects of culture on elders' use of services, and disparity in supplemental coverage of Medicare beneficiaries. She received her Ph.D. in health services from UCLA in 1995.

Ruth Roemer is adjunct professor emerita, Department of Health Services, UCLA School of Public Health, and a past president (1987) of the American Public Health Association. As a consultant to the World Health Organization on health legislation, she has worked on nursing education and regulation, legislation on human resources for health, use of fluorides for dental health, and tobacco control. Among her publications is *Legislative Action to Combat the World Tobacco Epidemic,* a monograph published by WHO in 1982, with a second edition in 1993. In 1989 she was awarded the WHO Medal on Tobacco or Health and in 1991 the American Public Health Association's Sedgwick Memorial Medal for distinguished service and advancement of public health knowledge and practice.

Mark A. Schuster, M.D., is an assistant professor of pediatrics and health services at UCLA and a senior natural scientist at RAND. He is the director of the UCLA/RAND Center for Adolescent Health Promotion, a prevention research center funded by the CDC. His research focuses on adolescent sexuality and risk prevention, the role of parents in child and adolescent development, child and adolescent quality of care, worksite health promotion, and children of HIV-infected adults. He received his M.D. and MPP from Harvard in 1998 and his Ph.D. in policy analysis at the RAND Graduate School in 1994.

Stuart O. Schweitzer is professor of health services in the UCLA School of Public Health and associate director of the UCLA Research Program in Pharmaceutical Economics and Policy. He has been on the research staff of the Urban Institute in Washington, D.C., and at the National Institutes of Health. In 1980, he was in charge of health policy development for President Carter's Commission for a National Agenda for the Eighties. He has held visiting appointments at Oxford University; CREDES and ESSEC in Paris; and the universities of Ferrara and Bologna, in Italy.

Beatriz M. Solís is director of culture and linguistic services for the L.A. Care Health Plan. Prior to working at L.A. Care, she was a research associate and project manager with the Center for Health Policy Research. She is currently a doctoral student in the School of Public Health at UCLA, where she also earned her master's degree. She has worked on research topics such as HIV/AIDS and the impact on women of color, access to health care for women, and welfare reform. She has co-authored articles and reports on these topics.

Pamela Stefanowicz was a doctoral candidate in the Department of Health Services, UCLA School of Public Health. While a graduate student, she conducted research for her dissertation, "Home Care for the Frail Elderly: The Process of Delivering and Receiving Care."

Pauline Vaillancourt Rosenau is an associate professor at the School of Public Health, University of Texas Health Science Center at Houston. Her Ph.D. was awarded by the Political Science Department of UC Berkeley in 1972, and she received her MPH degree in 1992 from UCLA. She was a professor at the University of Quebec in Montreal for nearly two decades before joining the School of Public Health in 1993. She is a member of the editorial board of *Social Science Quarterly* and *Medical Care Research and Review*. She edited *Public/Private Policy Partnerships* and *Health Reform in the Nineties.*

Steven P. Wallace is associate professor of public health in the UCLA Department of Community Health Sciences, associate director of the UCLA Center for Health Policy Research, and co-director of the California Geriatric Education Center's Health and Aging Faculty Development Program. He has published widely on access to long-term care for racial and ethnic minorities and is also researching the impact of managed care on access to health care for elders of color. He was a Fulbright Scholar in Santiago, Chile, in 2000–01, where he studied equity and access to health care for the elderly under Chile's partially privatized national health care system.

David L. Wood, M.D., completed residencies in pediatrics and preventive medicine and a federally funded research fellowship at RAND; he became a faculty member of the UCLA School of Medicine, as well as a member of the Ahmanson Department of Pediatrics, Cedars-Sinai Medical Center in Los Angeles and senior social scientist at RAND. His research, conducted in collaboration with RAND scientists, has focused on the health status and the quality of health services among high-risk and disadvantaged child and family populations. He is currently associate medical director for clinical outcomes management for the twenty-two Shriners hospitals for children in North America.

Roberta Wyn is an associate director at the UCLA Center for Health Policy Research. She has conducted research in several health care policy areas, with a particular focus on access to health insurance coverage and health care for women, ethnic populations, and lower-income populations. Her most recent research has focused on differences in access to care across urban areas and changes in health insurance coverage for low-income women.

To the late Samuel J. Tibbitts and to Audrey Tibbitts, whose
generosity made this work possible

And to our departed friend and colleague Milton F. Roemer,
contributor to the first edition of this work and
preeminent scholar of health services systems

INTRODUCTION AND OVERVIEW

Ronald M. Andersen, Thomas H. Rice, and
Gerald F. Kominski

As we enter the twenty-first century, the U.S. health care system continues to face several significant challenges. Despite one of the longest economic expansions in U.S. history, the number of uninsured individuals continued to grow through the 1990s and now totals almost forty-two million. Meanwhile, managed care has become the dominant form of health care delivery. Although managed care may have contributed to slower growth in health care costs for several years, high-cost technology and the aging population are once again causing higher growth in national health expenditures. Furthermore, both employers and consumers are growing increasingly disenchanted with managed care because it has not substantially improved the quality or efficiency of the U.S. health care system.

These challenges and pressures for change are tempered by a political environment fundamentally opposed to comprehensive change. The defeat of comprehensive health reform in the early 1990s shaped the directions for changing the U.S. health care system for the remainder of the decade. In particular, as the 1990s progressed, the polarized political climate made it clear that:

- Many, if not most, of the problems we face in ensuring access to affordable, high-quality health care would have to be dealt with incrementally rather than through comprehensive reform

- Greater reliance would be placed on private markets rather than additional governmental regulations

These conditions remain as true today as they were when the first edition of this book was published in 1996. Thus, for the foreseeable future, the goals of improving access, ensuring quality, and controlling costs will continue to be addressed through private market initiatives or through enactment of piecemeal legislation.

This edition follows the general format of the first edition. Our goal is to take a comprehensive and careful look at current issues in health care policy and management. To carry this out, we have assembled a group of talented and experienced researchers and asked them to take stock of the past, present, and future in their particular areas of expertise. For a specific topic, we asked the authors of each chapter to present the most current research and policy issues pertaining to it, summarize existing empirical research on the topic, and discuss research and management strategies that can be used to address current problems. Because of continuous change in the health care system since the first edition was published, we asked authors of chapters that were in this second edition to emphasize recent developments in their areas of expertise. Further, to make the second edition even more comprehensive, we have added entirely new chapters on public information and quality, mental health services, and Medicare reform.

This book continues to aim at providing, in a single source, a comprehensive yet readable account of the issues facing the United States in health care policy and management. We expect it to continue benefiting a variety of audiences:

- Students specializing in health care policy and management, or in other fields, who will benefit from having a thorough and up-to-date review of the literature in many subject areas in the health care field
- Health services researchers and policy analysts, who will find it useful to have ready access to the state of the art in research, as well as analysis of policy options relevant to many aspects of the health care market
- Health care managers, who will benefit from having a single source of information on how to promote quality and better health outcomes while controlling expenditures
- Practitioners and providers, especially doctors and nurses, who will find special issues of interest addressed in various chapters

Organization and Summary of the Volume

The volume is divided into five parts. Each contains two or more chapters relevant to that particular topic. We begin with discussion of the three key components of health care policy: access (Chapters One and Two), costs (Chapters Three through Five), and quality (Chapters Six through Eight). These chapters look at measurement and trends, as well as policy options.

Beginning with Chapter Nine, in Part Four we turn to matters of special populations, with individual chapters on long-term care and the elderly, AIDS, children's health, mental health, women's health, and the homeless.

The final part, Chapters Fifteen through Twenty, concerns proposals for reform; you will find chapters on managed care, Medicare, the role of prevention, public and personal health, medical malpractice, and ethical issues in public health and health services management. Let us briefly summarize some of the key material contained in these twenty chapters.

Access to Health Care

It is particularly appropriate to start with the topic of access, since concerns about it were largely responsible for instigating the health care reform debate. Consequently, access was also the major casualty. The United States holds the dubious distinction of being the only developed country that does not ensure access to health care through guaranteed coverage. Furthermore, many analysts—ourselves included—believe that one of the major barriers to controlling health care costs is exactly this lack of universal coverage. This is not only because it makes it difficult for poor and sick people to seek preventive care but also because it fragments the financing system, requiring the existence of an expensive safety net as well as aggravating the problem of cost shifting.

Chapter One, by Ronald M. Andersen and Pamela L. Davidson, offers a comprehensive examination of access to health care. The authors argue that understanding access is the key to understanding the health policy because the access framework predicts and measures health service use; this understanding can be used to promote social justice and promote health outcomes as well. The chapter explains the multiple dimensions of access using a revised version of the behavioral model that emphasizes contextual as well as individual determinants of health services utilization. The chapter explains exactly how access can be measured, and it presents data on the levels of access and trends in the United States. A number of trends that emerge from this analysis. First, although an increasing number of people are being covered by Medicaid, there has been a decline in the number covered by private insurance in the last fifteen years and an overall increase in the proportion without any health insurance coverage. Second, low-income and black populations appear to have achieved equity of access according to gross measures of hospital and physician utilization but continue to lag considerably in receipt of dental care. Third, equity has certainly not been achieved according to health insurance coverage; the proportion of uninsured is 50 percent higher for blacks and more than twice as high for Hispanics and the low-income population compared to the uninsured rate for non-Hispanic whites.

Chapter Two, by E. Richard Brown, follows this tack by examining alternative public policies for achieving greater health care coverage in the United States. After providing a historical perspective on why so much of the population remains uninsured, the author discusses the successes and failures of Medicare, Medicaid, and the new State Children's Health Insurance Program (SCHIP), with regard to extending access to affordable, high-quality coverage for their beneficiaries. The chapter discusses the pros and cons of alternative policy options to extend coverage through the private sector, including consideration of small-group and individual health insurance reform, employer mandates, purchasing cooperatives, and subsidies for small-group and individual coverage. It also discusses alternatives to expand public coverage through incremental changes in Medicaid as well as universal coverage through social insurance, with a focus on the political barriers that have prevented the United States from achieving universal coverage. In spite of these barriers, the author concludes that the United States cannot escape the need for fundamental reforms that extend coverage to its entire population.

Costs

Health care costs were controlled rather well in the United States in the mid- and late 1990s, although they still far exceed those of other developed countries. In spite (or perhaps because) of this recent success on the cost front, more Americans lack insurance coverage, and concerns about overall quality have been accentuated by the sharp increase in the use of strict managed care techniques to control utilization. It is the trade-off between costs on the one hand and access and quality on the other that will continues to generate the major tension in health care policy for the foreseeable future.

Chapter Three, by Thomas H. Rice, focuses on measuring health care costs and presenting their trends. With regard to measurement, the chapter distinguishes between expenditures and costs, focusing thereafter on the more easily measured concept of expenditures. It also discusses the advantages and disadvantages of various measures of alternative health care prices and expenditures, and the reliability of the data sources that are used to measure expenditures in the United States and throughout the world. A number of tables present trends in actual expenditures; noteworthy is a recent decline in the rate of growth of expenditures in the United States, although the nation still devotes far more of its income to health care than do other countries. The chapter also discusses the need for better data in the United States, concluding that requiring private insurers to collect and release data on expenditures is essential for making sensible policy decisions about alternative types of health care reform. As a lead-in to Chapter Four, Rice concludes with a discussion of the reasons that cost control is important and is likely to be in the forefront of health policy for years to come.

Chapter Four, by Thomas H. Rice and Gerald F. Kominski, focuses on alternative ways of containing health care costs. It begins by developing a conceptual framework that divides cost-containment methods into two categories, based on fee-for-service or capitation. Within fee-for-service, strategies fall into one of three groups: price controls, volume controls, and expenditure controls. Most of the remainder of the chapter reviews the literature and experiences, both in the United States and in other developed countries, regarding the success and failure of the many strategies that have been employed to contain costs, including hospital rate-setting programs, diagnosis-related groups, certificate-of-need programs, utilization review, technology controls, physician fee controls, practice guidelines, expenditure controls, health maintenance organizations, and managed competition. Although no conclusions are warranted about the best way to control costs, the chapter indicates that it is important to regularly assess experience—domestic and international—in light of the successes and failures of both market and government strategies to control health care costs.

Chapter Five, by Stuart O. Schweitzer and William S. Comanor, examines a particular aspect of health care costs: pharmaceuticals. The cost of pharmaceuticals has been an important policy issue for decades, with concern among many consumer advocates that they are too high and should be controlled, despite the fact that recently pharmaceuticals have increased less quickly than most other components of health care costs. The authors analyze the causes of increasing pharmaceutical costs, by critiquing studies conducted by others and then by conducting their own review of drug prices and expenditures over time in the United States and in other countries, adjusting for improvements in quality. They also review the many public policies that have been employed to control these costs, which have been aimed at consumers, physicians, and manufacturers. Although the authors do not reach any definitive conclusion about which policy levers work best, they are particularly concerned whether success can be achieved without sacrificing the vitality and viability of the industry, whose hallmark is a large investment in R and D for new products.

Quality

There is little question that establishing and preserving quality in health care has become the leading issue for health care managers. With tremendous competitive pressures to control health care costs, managers are faced with the task of formulating financial incentives and other mechanisms that help ensure a high-quality, cost-effective product for patients. The advent of health care report cards and the wider dissemination of information on health care quality, especially over the Internet, symbolize consumers' need for easily digestible information as to the relative quality of their alternative insurance choices. This interest is paralleled on the research front, where a great deal of effort is being expended to produce reliable measures of health care outcomes.

Chapter Six, by Patricia A. Ganz and Mark S. Litwin, examines the measurement of health outcomes and quality of life. After providing an historical perspective on the health outcomes movement, the authors present an overview of the concept of health-related quality of life (HRQL), which focuses on the patient's own perception of health and the ability to function as a result of health status or disease experience. Much of the remainder of the chapter is devoted to the challenging goal of measuring HRQL and to presenting health services research studies that have attempted to measure HRQL. An important conclusion is that patients are most concerned not with prolonging their lives per se, but rather with improving the quality of their remaining years. Therefore, the authors argue, consumers are anxious to have information about the HRQL impact of new treatments. What is needed is careful and appropriate inclusion of HRQL outcomes in traditional health services.

Chapter Seven, by Elizabeth A. McGlynn and Robert H. Brook, focuses on ensuring quality of care. The chapter begins by considering criteria for selecting topics for quality assessment. Next, it presents a conceptual framework useful for organizing evaluations of quality. The definitions, methods, and state of the art in assessing the structure, process, and outcomes of care are then discussed. The bottom line to this chapter is that scientifically sound methods exist for assessing quality and that these must be employed systematically in the future to guard against deterioration in quality that might otherwise occur as an unintended result of organizational and financial changes in the health services system.

Elizabeth A. McGlynn and John L. Adams observe in Chapter Eight that routine public reports on the quality of health care are being demanded because of changes in the organization and financing of care. In the unrestricted choice model characterized by fee-for-service, individual providers were accountable for ensuring delivery of high-quality health care. However, as third parties began to use financial incentives to control costs and restrict choices, the perception (if not the reality) was that the physician could no longer act solely in the patient's interest. We have moved from assuming that adequate mechanisms of accountability existed in the health system to demanding proof that various levels within the health system are accountable for the decisions that are made regarding resource allocation. Routine reports to the public on the quality of health care are one response to concerns about accountability. This chapter describes the type of information that is currently being publicly released; it then discusses some of the methodological issues that arise in producing information for public release and summarizes what is known regarding use of information about quality when it comes to choice for consumers. The authors conclude that the evidence on use of report cards by various audiences—consumers, purchasers, providers—suggests that the information is not widely used and appears to have only a small effect on performance. However, it is premature to declare this experiment a failure. Increased attention to the methods that are used to construct report cards, better use of communication techniques that are known to be effective, and more formal evaluations of such efforts are required before we have the information necessary to draw conclusions about the utility of public reporting.

Special Populations

The problems of access, cost, and quality have varied historically for segments of the U.S. population because of their special needs and how the health care system has responded to those needs. It is likely that the nature of the problems faced by different groups will continue to change, given major alterations in the way health services are organized and financed. All of the authors in Chapters Nine through Fourteen have suggestions for health services research and policy implementation that might improve the prognosis for these vulnerable populations.

Chapter Nine, by Steven P. Wallace, Emily K. Abel, Pamela Stefanowicz, and Nadereh Pourat, is a comprehensive overview of the long-term care system as a response to the rapidly increasing number of elderly in the United States and their needs for treatment of chronic and disabling illness. This chapter reviews the recent literature on long-term care, showing how financial considerations have framed the dominant policy debates and research agenda. It contains up-to-date information on nursing homes, the range of community-based care, informal long-term care, and workers in the long-term care system. The authors emphasize that long-term care includes social as well as medical services, is provided overwhelmingly by family and friends, and is financed primarily by Medicaid and out-of-pocket payments. After documenting that the driving force in policy and research in long-term care for the past twenty years has been cost containment and efficiency, the authors identify as the most critical policy and research question how to offer adequate, high-quality, long-term services to a growing and diverse older population. Policy makers frequently view nursing homes as low-cost alternatives to hospitals and consider community services and family care as less expensive substitutes for nursing homes, to the neglect of quality-of-life issues. The chapter concludes that the limited financial resources of many older persons—especially racial and ethnic minorities, widows, and the working class—create a need for a universal, Medicare type of social insurance.

In Chapter Ten, David M. Mosen, Denise R. Globe, and William E. Cunningham argue that the characteristics of HIV/AIDS—contagious, chronically disabling, fatal, and of epidemic proportions—increasingly force health care policy makers and managers to reevaluate the organization, delivery, and financing of health services for the HIV population. The authors state that more than seventy million individuals worldwide are living with HIV, including nine hundred thousand U.S. residents. The authors review what is known, and what research needs to be done, concerning the changing epidemiology and treatment of AIDS, including the use of new and expensive antiretroviral drugs; measures of access, cost, and quality; and the range of services needed to treat AIDS (including not only formal medical services but also prevention, psychosocial services, and community-based health and social services). They discuss the increasing challenges in offering and paying for services as the HIV/AIDS epidemic expanded from its initial geographic epicenters of Caucasian homosexual men to a much broader community of socially and economically disadvantaged populations, among them women, children, adolescents, and minority groups.

Chapter Eleven, by Neal Halfon, Moira Inkelas, David L. Wood, and Mark A. Schuster, examines the key issues underlying the incongruity between the needs of children and families, and the current and evolving structure of the health services organization in the United States. The authors review the health needs of children and families by examining children's unique vulnerabilities, current health risks and conditions, and service needs. Next, they describe the characteristics of the health care system that influence children's access to care and the overall efficiency of health care for children. They find the organization of services to be disjointed, with multiple financial and structural barriers to children's receipt of care, despite recent enactment of the federally supported State Children's Health Insurance Program. They note that the movement to manage care to rationalize delivery of personal medical services may substantially improve children's access to basic medical care, but many of their health needs—especially for complex medical or socially based health problems—may not be adequately addressed. The authors conclude that adequate response to the health care needs of at-risk children requires greater effort to expand coverage for the uninsured, especially enrolling eligible children in current programs and developing multidisciplinary coordination that integrates the fragmented child health system.

Chapter Twelve, by Susan L. Ettner, examines mental health services, with emphasis on public policy toward their use. She notes the substantial access barriers facing those with mental health problems; only about one-third of the 21 percent of the population with diagnosable mental or substance abuse disorders receive treatment in a given year. After giving an overview of the mental health service system in the United States, the author grapples with a number of difficult issues, including the stigma associated with mental illness, lack of use of appropriately trained mental health providers, and gaps in both public and private insurance coverage for mental health conditions. She notes that several population groups—the elderly, children, minorities, and those living in rural areas—tend to underuse mental health services in relation to their needs. The chapter concludes with a discussion of several actions that can be taken by federal and state governments to improve the mental health care system: supporting safety-net providers such as public hospitals, tailoring mental health benefits to meet the needs of publicly insured patients, and requiring that all insurers offer mental health benefits at parity with other medical services.

Chapter Thirteen, by Roberta Wyn and Beatriz M. Solís, examines how women's health status, socioeconomic status, and multiple role responsibilities interface with their access to and use of services. Although women and men share the same need for affordable, accessible, and quality care, there are specific health concerns and patterns of use unique to women that are often overlooked. Many health conditions are particular to women, occur with greater frequency among women, or have different consequences for women than for men. The chapter examines the adequacy of women's access to health insurance coverage and the ability of that coverage to protect against the costs of health services; it explores how health insurance coverage affects women's access to care and looks beyond financial barriers to other aspects of the health care system that influence access. Women have lower uninsured rates and higher utilization rates than men, but the authors call attention to women's more limited health insurance options and the large discrepancy in rate of coverage and health care use among women according to income, education, and ethnicity. They also document women's differential access to procedures and outcomes after they gain access to the system. The authors conclude that particular consideration of low-income women is required in formulating new health policy regarding financing of services. They have the lowest rate of screening for certain clinical preventive services, have the poorest health status, and are most vulnerable to the effects of cost. However, unintended effects of welfare reform legislation may make it even harder for low-income women to obtain health insurance coverage. Medicaid enrollment is declining after a decade of growth, attributable in large measure to welfare reform legislation.

In Chapter Fourteen, Lillian Gelberg and Lisa Arangua describe the sociodemographic characteristics of homeless adults and children as well as their health status, risk factors for illness, barriers to care, quality of care, and current medical programs available to homeless individuals. They note that homelessness has reached crisis proportions, with estimates of up to 3.5 million currently homeless, heterogeneous persons including families, runaway youths, the physically and mentally ill, and substance abusers. The homeless population experiences high rates of acute and chronic illness but has limited access to medical care as reflected by high inpatient utilization and low ambulatory service use relative to their high level of need. The medical care they do receive is limited in terms of availability, continuity, and comprehensiveness. The authors find the homeless particularly vulnerable in the policy arena because of the absence of strong advocates, tendencies by the public to accept large-scale homelessness as inevitable, and commonly held beliefs that the homeless are responsible for their status. Still, their plight could be improved by stabilizing funding for health care, funding respite care, medical education reform, and more affordable housing options. They conclude that the best way to help the homeless is for the United States to address more fundamental issues concerning alleviation of poverty.

Directions for Change

The defeat of comprehensive health care reform at the national level in the early 1990s has created a unique opportunity to reexamine the goals of health care reform and the methods for achieving those goals in a political environment that remains strongly polarized over the need for such reform. Health services research has clearly played an influential role in developing policy options at the local, state, and national levels during the past two decades. What significant contributions will health services researchers make during the next decade? The remainder of this volume addresses some of the fundamental challenges facing health care researchers, policy makers, and managers as we enter the twenty-first century.

Perhaps the most basic challenge involves determining the appropriate role of the market versus the role of the government in addressing issues of access, cost, and quality. Chapters Fifteen and Sixteen deal directly with the research evidence and policy issues related to the predominant form of private health care delivery (managed care) and the pressures facing the largest government insurance program, Medicare.

Chapter Fifteen, by Gerald F. Kominski and Glenn Melnick, evaluates the role of managed care and price competition in controlling health care costs. The chapter describes the various models of managed care that have evolved from the traditional model of prepaid group practice. It then summarizes the growth in managed care during the past three decades and the factors that have contributed to its growth. The authors argue that because California is considered to be the most mature managed care market in the country, it can serve as a laboratory to inform policy makers on what might be expected in other parts of the country as managed care expands nationally. The introduction of price competition among California hospitals, beginning in 1982, had a dramatic effect on hospitals in highly competitive markets by the end of the 1980s. Hospitals in the most-competitive markets had significantly lower growth in their revenue compared to hospitals in the least-competitive markets. As managed care continues to grow rapidly in private markets and in the Medicare and Medicaid programs, important issues require further investigation. They conclude that along with additional research on the impact of managed care on costs, prices, and expenditures, further work is necessary on the implications for quality and access of a competitive system.

Chapter Sixteen, by Jeanne T. Black and Gerald F. Kominski, examines the federal government's largest health insurance program–Medicare–and the challenges facing the program's future. They review the political conditions leading to enactment of Medicare, which was widely viewed as a compromise on the road to national health insurance when it was enacted in 1965. Thirty-five years later, Medicare faces several significant challenges—notably ongoing cost increases and a rapidly expanding eligible population—that threaten its public support. These challenges have led to recent proposals to transform Medicare from a defined-benefit to a defined-contribution program, in which the government makes a fixed contribution on behalf of beneficiaries. The authors examine the expected implications of such a transformation and conclude that defined-contribution health benefits should become more prevalent in the private market before moving Medicare away from its founding principles. Until then, incremental expansion of benefits and additional subsidies to low-income beneficiaries are likely to reduce existing disparity within the program.

Chapter Seventeen, by Charles Lewis, discusses the role of preventive health services and reasserts the continuing value of these services in maintaining individual and population health. The author focuses on three major questions: What is preventable? How can barriers to application of effective treatments be overcome? And what value does society place on prevention? After discussing the recent history of prevention, the author applies these questions to case studies dealing with the worldwide HIV/AIDS epidemic, cardiopulmonary diseases attributable to cigarette smoking, and deaths due to gun shot wounds. Although there are scientifically valid preventive interventions in each case, values (confounded with economic interests) are the primary obstacles to successful prevention of tobacco and firearm-related deaths.

In Chapter Eighteen, Lester Breslow and Jonathan E. Fielding reexamine the significant role of public health agencies in delivering personal health services in the United States. They find that these agencies have a vital interest in health care delivery because a substantial portion of the population has inadequate access to services or unstable health benefits. Public health has traditionally been directed toward ensuring a safe environment and addressing the behavioral influences on health. Access to quality personal health services provided by the public health system, they argue, is also an important determinant of health. The ability of public health agencies to perform all their core public health functions, however, requires greater commitment to public health and health promotion.

Chapter Nineteen, by Ruth Roemer, deals with the continuing issue of medical malpractice liability. The author first raises the politically sensitive issue of whether patients should be able to sue their managed care plans. She then steps back and explores the history of malpractice insurance crises in the 1970s and 1980s, state legislative responses, and the impact of those responses. The chapter then addresses the major potential reforms to the tort system, including alternative dispute resolution, enterprise liability, no-fault insurance, and medical accident compensation. Reviewing U.S. and international experience with these options, the author concludes that despite the soundness of the no-fault approach, political realities seem to mitigate against adoption of this alternative. Instead, the climate may be favorable for rationalizing our handling of medical injury compensation by adopting an administrative system that is more equitable and less costly than the tort system.

Chapter Twenty, by Pauline Vaillancourt Rosenau and Ruth Roemer, deals with the ethics of public health and health care services. The cardinal principles of medical ethics—autonomy, beneficence, and justice—also apply in public health ethics, but in a somewhat altered form. The authors contrast these principles as they are usually applied in medical ethics, where individual rights and autonomy prevail, with a broader social perspective in which individual rights may be subsumed by considerations of social welfare. At a time when we continue moving toward market-based solutions, the authors present a framework for reexamining some of the ethical and social issues related to resource development, economic support, organization, management, delivery, and quality of care. Ethical issues in public health and health services management are likely to become increasingly complex in the future. The authors conclude, however, that even in the absence of agreement on ethical assumptions and in the face of diversity and complexity that prohibit easy compromise, mechanisms for resolving ethical dilemmas in public health do exist.

Conclusion

We have asked the chapter authors in this volume to explore what health services research has to tell us about making fundamental changes to ensure access to affordable high-quality health care. We think that as an informed reader, you will find the authors have met the dual challenge of, first, presenting comprehensive reviews of key policy and management issues regarding problems of access, cost, and quality and, second, serving special populations and assessing strategies for reform. Unfortunately, neither the authors of this volume nor any other possible set of authors, for that matter, have answers for all the major challenges facing our health care system, but you will find that they delineate the critical questions clearly and propose a number of informed, innovative solutions.

Changing the U.S. Health Care System

PART ONE

ACCESS TO HEALTH CARE

CHAPTER ONE

IMPROVING ACCESS TO CARE IN AMERICA

Individual and Contextual Indicators

Ronald M. Andersen and Pamela L. Davidson

The purpose of this chapter is to present basic trends as well as research and policy issues related to health care access. We define *access* as actual use of personal health services and everything that facilitates or impedes their use. It is the link between health services systems and the populations they serve. Access means not only getting to service but also getting to the right services at the right time to promote improved health outcomes. Conceptualizing and measuring access is the key to understanding and making health policy in a number of ways: (1) predicting *use* of health services, (2) promoting social *justice,* and (3) improving *effectiveness* and *efficiency* of health service delivery.

The chapter presents a conceptual framework for understanding the multiple dimensions of access to medical care. The various types of access are considered and related to their policy purposes. Examples of key access measures are given and trend data are used to track changes that have occurred over time in these access indicators. The chapter addresses the questions, Is access improving or declining in the United States? For whom? According to what measures? It concludes by discussing future access indicators and research directions.

Understanding Access to Health Care

This section proposes a conceptual framework based on a behavioral model of health services use that emphasizes contextual as well as individual determinants of access to medical care. Also reviewed are the dimensions of access defined according to components of the framework and how access might be improved for each dimension.

Conceptual Framework

Compared to the framework presented in the first edition of this volume, the version shown in Figure 1.1 stresses that improving access to care is best accomplished by focusing on contextual as well as individual determinants.[1] By *contextual* we point to the circumstances and environment of health care access. Context includes health organization and provider-related factors as well as community characteristics.[2] Contextual factors are measured at some aggregate rather than at the individual level. These aggregate levels range from units as small as the family to those as large as a national health care system. In between are workgroups, provider organizations, health plans, local communities, and metropolitan statistical areas. Individuals are related to these aggregate units through either membership (family, workgroup, provider institutions, health plan) or residence (community, metropolitan area, national health system).

The model shown in Figure 1.1 suggests that the major components of contextual characteristics are divided in the same way as individual characteristics determining access: (1) existing conditions that *predispose* people to use or not use services even though these conditions are not directly responsible for use, (2) *enabling* conditions that facilitate or impede the use of services, and (3) *need* or conditions recognized by laypeople or health care providers as requiring medical treatment.[3] The model shown in Figure 1.1 emphasizes contextual factors in recognition of the importance of community, the structure and process of providing care,[4] and the realities of a managed care environment.[5] Still, the ultimate focus of the model remains on health behaviors of *individuals* (especially their use of health services) and resulting outcomes regarding their health and satisfaction with services.

We now turn to brief consideration of each major component of the model shown in Figure 1.1.

Contextual Predisposing Characteristics. *Demographic* characteristics include the age, gender, and marital status composition of a community. Thus, a community populated primarily by older persons might well have a different mix of

FIGURE 1.1.   A BEHAVIORAL MODEL OF HEALTH SERVICES USE INCLUDING CONTEXTUAL
AND INDIVIDUAL CHARACTERISTICS.

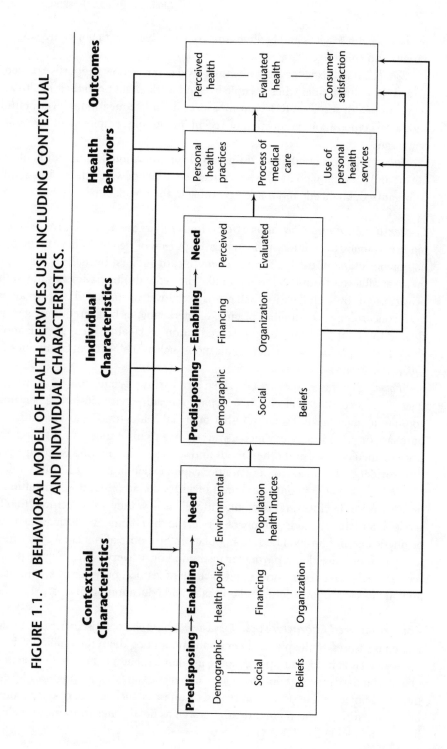

available health services and facilities than one in which the majority are younger parents and children.

Social characteristics at the contextual level describe how supportive or detrimental the communities where people live and work might be to their health and access to health services. Relevant measures include educational levels, ethnic and racial composition, proportion of recent immigrants, employment levels, and crime rates.

Beliefs refer to underlying community or organizational values and cultural norms and prevailing political perspectives regarding how health services should be organized, financed, and made accessible to the population.

Contextual Enabling Characteristics. *Health policies* are authoritative decisions made pertaining to health or influencing the pursuit of health.[6] They can be public policies made in the legislative, executive, or judicial branches of government, at all levels from local to national. They can also be policies made in the private sector by such decision makers as executives of managed care organizations concerning product lines, pricing, or marketing, or by accrediting agencies such as the Joint Commission on Accreditation of Health Care Organizations (JCAHO) or quality assessment organizations such as the National Committee for Quality Assurance (NCQA).

Financing characteristics are described by an array of contextual measures that suggest resources potentially available to pay for health services, including per capita community income, and wealth. Other financial characteristics are incentives to purchase or provide services such as rate of health insurance coverage, relative price of medical care and other goods and services, and method of compensating providers. Also included here are per capita expenditures for health services.

Organization at the contextual level includes the amount and distribution of health services facilities and personnel as well as how they are structured to offer services. Structure includes supply of services in the community such as the ratios of physicians and hospital beds to population. Structure also includes how medical care is organized in a particular institution or delivery system where people receive care, such as office hours and location of service, provider mix, utilization and quality control oversight, and outreach and education programs.

Contextual Need Characteristics. *Environmental need* characteristics include health-related measures of the physical environment, among them the quality of housing, water, and air (for example, residing in counties that met national ambient air quality standards throughout the year).[7] Other measures suggesting how healthy the environment might be are injury and death rates, such as rate of occupational injury and disease and related deaths as well as death rates from motor vehicle injuries, homicides, and firearms.

Population health indices are more general indicators of community health that may or may not be associated with the physical environment. These indices include general and condition-specific rates of mortality (for example, infant mortality; age-adjusted mortality; and mortality rates for heart disease, cancer, stroke, HIV); morbidity (incidence of preventable childhood communicable diseases and AIDS, and prevalence of cancer, hypertension, and untreated dental caries); and disability (disability days due to acute conditions and limitation of activity due to chronic conditions).

The arrows in Figure 1.1 leading from the contextual characteristics indicate that they can influence health behaviors and outcomes in multiple ways. They can work through individual characteristics—for example, when increased generosity of a state Medicaid program leads to previously uninsured low-income children being covered by health insurance and subsequent increase in their use of health services. Contextual characteristics can also influence health behaviors and outcomes directly, over and above their influence through individual characteristics, as when presence of community health clinics in a metropolitan statistical area leads to increased use of primary care services by low-income persons independent of personal income or other individual characteristics. Understanding the nature of contextual influences on access to care presents many analytic challenges,[8] but it may permit important new insights into how to improve access to care.

Individual Predisposing Characteristics. *Demographic factors* such as age and gender of the individual represent biological imperatives suggesting the likelihood that people will need health services.[9]

Social factors determine the status of a person in the community as well as his or her ability to cope with presenting problems and command resources to deal with those problems. Traditional measures include an individual's education, occupation, and ethnicity. Expanded measures might include people's social network and social interactions that can facilitate or impede access to services.[10]

Health beliefs are attitudes, values, and knowledge people have about health and health services that can influence their subsequent perception of need and use of health services.

Individual Enabling Characteristics. *Financing* of health services for the individual involves the income and wealth available to the individual to pay for services. Financing also includes the effective price of health care to the patient, determined by having insurance and cost-sharing requirements.

Organization of health services for the individual describes whether or not the individual has a regular source of care and the nature of that source (private doctor, community clinic, emergency room). It also includes means of transportation and reported travel time to, and waiting time for, care.

Individual Need Characteristics. *Perceived need* is how people view their own general health and functional state. Also included here is how they experience, and emotionally respond to, symptoms of illness, pain, and worry about their health condition (is a condition judged of sufficient importance and magnitude to seek professional help?). Perceived need is largely a social phenomenon that, when appropriately modeled, should itself be largely explainable by social characteristics (such as ethnicity or education) and health beliefs (health attitudes, knowledge about health care, and so on).

Evaluated need represents professional judgment and objective measurement about a patient's physical status and need for medical care (blood pressure readings, temperature, blood cell count, as well as diagnoses and prognoses for particular conditions the patient experiences). Of course, evaluated need is not simply, or even primarily, a valid and reliable measure from biological science. It also has a social component and varies with the changing state of the art and science of medicine, clinical guidelines and protocols, and prevailing practice patterns, as well as the training and competency of the professional expert doing the assessment.

Logical expectations of the model are that perceived need helps us better understand the care-seeking process and adherence to a medical regimen, while evaluated need is more closely related to the kind and amount of treatment that is given after a patient has presented to a medical care provider.

Health Behaviors. *Personal health practices* are behaviors by the individual that influence health status. They include diet and nutrition, exercise, stress reduction, alcohol and tobacco use, self-care, and adherence to medical regimens.

The *process of medical care* is the behavior of providers interacting with patients in the process of care delivery.[11] General process measures might relate to patient counseling and education, test ordering, prescribing patterns, and quality of provider-patient communication. Process measures might also describe the specifics of caregiving for particular conditions, such as whether a provider checks a CD4 cell count in a person with HIV disease or reviews the patient's record of home glucose monitoring in a diabetic.

Use of personal health services is the essential component of health behaviors in a comprehensive model of access to care. The purpose of the original behavioral model was to predict health services use, measured rather broadly as units of physician ambulatory care, hospital inpatient services, and dental care visits. We hypothesized that predisposing, enabling, and need factors would have differential ability to explain use depending on what type of service was examined.[12] Hospital services used in response to more serious problems and conditions would be primarily explained by need and demographic characteristics, while dental services (considered more discretionary) would likely be explained by social conditions, health beliefs, and enabling resources.

We expected all the components of the model to explain ambulatory physician use because the conditions stimulating care seeking would generally be viewed as less serious and demanding than those resulting in inpatient care, but more serious than those leading to dental care. More specific measures of health services use are now being employed to describe a particular medical condition or type of service or practitioner, or are linked in an episode of illness to examine continuity of care.[13] For example, a longitudinal study of rheumatoid arthritis patients could measure visits to various types of provider, treatment used, level of patient compliance with treatment, and associated changes in functional status and pain over time.

Although specific measures are, in many ways, likely to be more informative, the more global ones (number of physician visits, self-rated general health status) still have a role to play. Global measures are needed comprehensive indicators of the overall effects of policy changes over time.

Outcomes. One kind of result or outcome of health behavior and contextual and individual characteristics is an individual's or patient's *perceived health* status. This depends on many factors in addition to the use of personal health services, including all of the contextual factors as well as an individual's demographic and social characteristics, health beliefs, and personal health practices. Perceived health status indicates the extent to which a person can live a functional, comfortable, and pain-free existence. Measures include reports of general perceived health status, symptoms of illness, and disability.

Evaluated health status is dependent on the judgment of the professional, based on established clinical standards and state-of-the-art practices. Measures include tests of patient physiology and function as well as diagnosis and prognosis regarding their condition.

Outcome measures of perceived and evaluated heath may appear suspiciously like perceived and evaluated need measures. Indeed, they are. The ultimate outcome validation of improved access is to reduce individual needs previously measured and evaluated.

Consumer satisfaction is how individuals feel about the health care they receive. It can be judged by patient ratings of waiting time, travel time, communication with providers, and technical care received. From a health plan perspective, an ultimate outcome measure of patient satisfaction in this era of managed care might be whether or not enrollees choose to switch plans.[14]

Central to the model shown in Figure 1.1 is feedback, depicted by the arrows from outcomes to health behaviors, individual characteristics, and contextual characteristics. Feedback allows insights about how access might come to be improved. For example, outcomes might influence contextual characteristics, as illustrated by Karen Davis, president of the Commonwealth Foundation.[15] Davis noted that the continued failure of our health services system to provide access to care, particularly for vulnerable populations, as well as the generally low level of satisfaction of the public with the health services system leads her to conclude that our health care system needs to be fundamentally changed. Such conclusions, drawn by enough influential persons, as well as dissatisfaction on the part of the public can ultimately lead to contextual changes in the health policy of the country and subsequent reforms in financing and organizing health services with the intent to improve access to care.

Feedback, of course, can occur at the community or institutional level as well as at the national level. Certainly there are expectations that feedback to health care institutions from JCAHO or NCQA might result in contextual changes in the institutions' organization of care and processes of care for their patients.

Defining and Improving Dimensions of Access to Care

We have long considered access to care to be a relatively complex multidimensional phenomenon, and deemed the behavioral model to be a tool to help us to define and differentiate these dimensions. In this section, we review these dimensions of access in terms of the components of the model and suggest how access to care might be "improved" according to each dimension (see Figure 1.2).

Potential Access. Potential access is indicated by the enabling variables of the model at both the contextual and individual levels. More enabling resources constitute the means for use and increase the likelihood that it will take place.

Realized Access. Realized access is the actual use of services. Realized access indicators include utilization of physician, hospital, and other health services.

Historically, the United States experienced improving trends in access to health care as measured by increasing health services utilization rates. Access to health services was considered an end goal of policy change. Potential access measures were used as indicators of increasing access to medical care services. Realized access measures were used to monitor and evaluate policies to influence health services use. Policies were implemented in the 1950s and 1960s to increase the number of physicians, to supply hospital beds in rural communities, and to create federal programs to increase access (including Medicare and Medicaid legislation).

The U.S. health care system evolved from decision making grounded in altruism through increasing the access and supply of resources to a position of caution and financial prudence.[16] The predominant focus on increasing medical care utilization shifted in the 1970s to concern for health care cost containment

FIGURE 1.2.   THE POLICY PURPOSES OF ACCESS MEASURES.

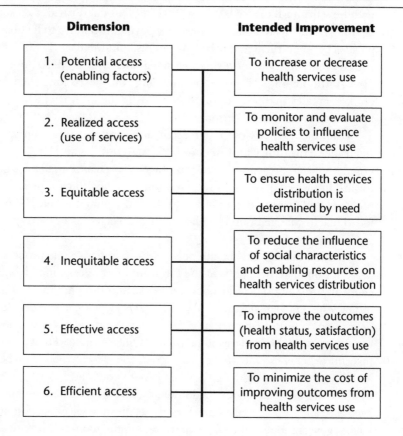

Dimension	Intended Improvement
1. Potential access (enabling factors)	To increase or decrease health services use
2. Realized access (use of services)	To monitor and evaluate policies to influence health services use
3. Equitable access	To ensure health services distribution is determined by need
4. Inequitable access	To reduce the influence of social characteristics and enabling resources on health services distribution
5. Effective access	To improve the outcomes (health status, satisfaction) from health services use
6. Efficient access	To minimize the cost of improving outcomes from health services use

and creation of mechanisms to limit access to health care, including HMO legislation, coinsurance, deductibles, utilization review, and the genesis of managed care. In the 1980s and early 1990s, managed care, competing with fee-for-service organizations, enjoyed double-digit growth in profit margins.[17] However, in recent years its growth has slowed, and managed care organizations have come under increased scrutiny regarding whether they limit needed services for their enrollees. (See the discussion of managed care and its impact on access to care in the later section on trends.)

The Balanced Budget Act of 1997 (BBA) is an example of a recent policy designed to limit health services utilization. Developed as a strategy for extending Medicare solvency at least through 2007, the fiscal impact of BBA implementation is being felt by beneficiaries and health plans alike. Medicare beneficiaries are facing reduced choice in plans thanks to health plan reactions to the

BBA. Almost one hundred HMOs either reduced their service areas or completely withdrew from Medicare by early 1999.[18] Plans cited various reasons for withdrawing from selected market areas: low payments relative to fee-for-service, disparities between rural and urban payments, and the like. By 2007 beneficiaries will pay more for benefits owing to gradual increases in Medicare Part B premiums. Additionally, policy options are being considered for beneficiaries to pay an even greater share of out-of-pocket costs in the future, which will be particularly burdensome for low-income seniors.[19]

Examples of policies to increase health services utilization are the Health Insurance Portability and Accountability Act of 1996 (HIPAA) and the proposed Medicare prescription drug coverage. Viewed as a small but significant step toward improved access to and renewability of health care benefits in employment-related group health plans and the individual market, HIPAA allows an individual to change insurers without being subjected to a new waiting period for preexisting conditions.[20]

Another incremental health policy reform initiative, the proposed Medicare prescription drug benefit, is at the forefront of congressional debate. Pharmaceuticals are a major out-of-pocket expense and threaten the financial security of lower-income beneficiaries, but policy makers would have to decide who should bear these costs and whether subsidies could be extended to assist lower-income beneficiaries.[21] The Congressional Budget Office estimated that adding the pharmaceutical benefit to the Medicare program could cost $136 billion between 2002 and 2009.[22] Others estimate the drug benefit could add 7–20 percent per year to Medicare program costs.[23] Additionally, several risks have been identified for Medicare and its potential contractors: those affecting selection, cost management, having government as a business partner, existing competitive advantages, and national price controls.[24] The proposed Medicare prescription drug coverage would expand utilization of pharmaceuticals for seniors, but the long-term cost implications need to be carefully weighed.

Equitable Access. Equitable (as well as inequitable) access is defined according to what determinants (age, ethnicity, insurance status, or symptoms) of realized access are dominant in predicting utilization. Equity is in the eye of the beholder. Value judgments about which components of the model should explain utilization in an equitable health care system are crucial to the definition. Traditionally, *equitable access* has been defined as occurring when demographic (age and gender) and, especially, need variables account for most of the variance in utilization.[25]

Inequitable Access. Inequitable access occurs when social characteristics and enabling resources, such as ethnicity or income, determine who gets medical care.

The social justice movement, dominant in the 1960s and early 1970s with the passage of Medicare and Medicaid, sought to ensure that health services distribution was determined by need and to reduce the influence of social characteristics and enabling resources on health services distribution.

Equity of access to medical care is the value judgment that the system is deemed fair or equitable if need-based criteria, rather than enabling resources (such as insurance coverage or income), are the main determinants of whether or not—or how much—care is sought. Subgroup disparities in use of health services (say, according to race or ethnicity, or health insurance coverage) would be minimized in a fair and equitable system, while underlying need for preventive or illness-related health care would be the principal factor determining utilization.

Policies to improve social justice include the Children's Health Insurance Program and the Federal Safety Net Initiative. A $48 billion federal action in the form of the State Children's Health Insurance Program (SCHIP) stimulated virtually every state to expand coverage for low-income children.[26] Prior to the enactment of SCHIP, little progress had been made in more than fifteen years to reduce the size of the uninsured population of children.[27] Attracting children into these programs depends on ease of enrollment, cost-sharing requirements, whether programs are packaged in such a way to reduce stigma, the effectiveness of outreach efforts, and overcoming administrative barriers.[28]

But is SCHIP an effective and efficient policy intervention for improving health care access for children's safety-net resources?[29] Lave and colleagues conducted evaluation research to determine the impact of SCHIP on improving access to health care and other aspects of children's and families' lives. Results indicated that twelve months following enrollment 99 percent (baseline was 89 percent) of children had a usual source of medical care, 85 percent (baseline was 60 percent) had a regular dentist, and unmet need or delayed care in the past six months decreased to 16 percent (baseline was 57 percent) after one year. Additionally, parents reported that having health insurance for children reduced family stress, enabled the children to obtain the care they needed, and eased family burdens, producing an overall positive impact for children and their families.[30]

Other policies promoting social justice have been created to support safety-net providers who care for uninsured and underinsured persons.[31] The institutional safety-net system consists of a patchwork of hospitals, community clinics, and programs whose nature varies dramatically across the country. But financing for safety-net institutions has always been tenuous and subject to changing politics, available resources, and public policies.[32]

Many are concerned that the viability of the safety net may be threatened because of changes occurring in federal, state, and local policies (Medicaid managed care, welfare reform initiatives, redirection of funds intended for disproportionate-share hospitals or uncompensated pools), increased competition in the health care delivery system, and closings or mergers of not-for-profit and public hospitals.[33]

Financing the care for the uninsured in a managed care environment and preserving safety-net providers for communities that remain unattractive to the managed care industry are among the most challenging policy considerations for health care reform.[34]

Effective Access. The cost-containment movement became more sophisticated in the late 1980s and 1990s. The next generation of health services research transitioned to measuring the impact of health services utilization on health outcomes. Accordingly, the Institute of Medicine Committee on Monitoring Access to Medical Care defined *access* as timely use of personal health services to achieve the best possible health outcomes.[35] This definition relies on use of health services and health outcomes as yardsticks for judging whether access has been achieved. The resulting measures are referred to as effective access.

Measures of effectiveness examine the relative impact of health services utilization within the context of other predisposing, enabling, need, and health-behavior variables. Predisposing variables, such as age, gender, and social support variables, can influence the patient's health status following treatment. Access to personal enabling resources (health insurance, income, regular source of care) can result in expeditious medical treatment with highly trained practitioners using state-of-the-art medical technology. Conversely, lack of enabling resources can lead to delays in seeking medical advice; and episodic, fragmented treatment with a potential negative impact on health outcomes and satisfaction with medical care.

Researchers conducting effectiveness and outcomes research have developed strategies for risk adjustment to control for the effects of medical need (severity of illness, number of symptoms, and co-morbidities) before intervention. Personal health practices (diet, exercise, stress management) and compliance with medical regimens prior and subsequent to treatment can also influence health outcomes. Analytical models used to determine the effectiveness of alternative medical treatments on health outcomes must consider the influence of these varying personal and behavioral factors, as well as contextual differences in health care delivery systems and external environment.

Efficient Access. Most recently, concerns about cost containment have been combined with those directed to improving health outcomes. The results are measures of efficient access. These measures are similar to measures of effective access with the added emphasis on measuring resources used to influence outcome.

Improvement is attained by promoting health outcomes while minimizing the resources required to attain improved outcomes. Aday, Begley, Lairson, and Slater describe efficiency as producing the combination of goods and services with the highest attainable total value, given limited resources and technology.[36] *Efficiency* is an attempt to quantify the cost-effectiveness or cost benefit of health services in assessing the extent to which finite private, public, or personal resources should be invested in assuring access to those procedures.[37]

Trends in Access to Care

In this section, trends in access are examined according to several dimensions of access. We consider changes over time in potential access (health insurance coverage), realized access (use of hospital, physician, and dental services), and equitable access (health insurance and health services use according to income and race). We also examine some key research findings concerning effective and efficient access.

Potential Access (Enabling Health Insurance)

Table 1.1 reports a critical potential access measure: health care coverage for persons under sixty-five years of age from 1984 to 1997. The uninsured proportion of the population increased from 14 percent to 17 percent in that time period. Medicaid coverage actually increased (from 7 percent to 11 percent), but the overall decline in coverage resulted from a drop in the proportion covered by private insurance, from 77 percent to 70 percent.

The proportion of population eighteen to forty-four who were uninsured increased during the 1980s and 1990s, reaching 22 percent in 1997. The proportion covered by private insurance decreased for every age group between 1984 and 1994, but overall there was no further decline from 1994 to 1997. Between 1989 and 1994 the proportion of all children covered under Medicaid increased from 14 percent to 20 percent. This increase reflected the expanded Medicaid income eligibility enacted by Congress in the mid-1980s (see Chapter Two). However, the proportion of children covered by Medicaid dropped back to 18 percent in 1997.

The results overall leave little doubt that a decline in potential access has occurred for the U.S. population since the early 1980s—particularly for people aged eighteen to forty-four—because of a decline in private health insurance coverage.

Realized Access (Utilization over Time)

Table 1.2 presents a historical perspective of personal health care use for the U.S. population from 1928–1931 to 1996. It presents trend data on realized access for three types of service: those in response to serious illness (hospital admissions), services for a combination of primary and secondary care (physician visits), and services for conditions that are rarely life threatening and generally considered

TABLE 1.1. HEALTH INSURANCE COVERAGE FOR PERSONS UNDER SIXTY-FIVE, BY AGE, RACE AND ETHNICITY, AND POVERTY LEVEL.

	Private Insurance[e]				Medicaid[e]				Not Covered[e]			
						Percentage of Population						
	1984	1989	1994	1997	1984	1989	1994	1997	1984	1989	1994	1997
Age												
Under 18	73	72	64	66	12	14	20	18	14	15	15	14
18–44	77	75	70	69	5	5	7	7	17	18	22	22
45–64	83	83	80	79	3	4	5	5	10	11	12	12
Race and ethnicity[a]												
White, non-Hispanic	82	82	77	78	4	5	7	7	12	12	14	13
Black, non-Hispanic	59	58	52	55	21	19	27	23	19	21	19	19
Hispanic, Mexico[b]	54	48	46	43	12	12	18	17	33	39	36	38
Hispanic, Puerto Rican[b]	49	46	48	47	31	28	36	31	18	23	15	19
Hispanic, Cuban[b]	72	69	64	71	5	8	10	9	22	22	26	20
Asian or Pacific Islander[c]	70	71	67	68	10	12	10	12	18	18	20	19
Percent of poverty level[a,d]												
Below 100 percent	32	27	21	23	32	37	45	42	34	35	33	33
100–149 percent	62	55	47	42	8	11	16	19	26	31	34	35
150–199 percent	78	71	66	64	3	5	6	8	17	21	25	25
200 percent or more	92	91	89	88	1	1	1	2	6	7	8	9
Total[a]	77	76	70	70	7	8	11	11	14	15	17	17

Notes: [a]Age adjusted.

[b]Persons of Hispanic origin may be white, black, or Asian or Pacific Islander.

[c]Includes persons of Hispanic and non-Hispanic origin.

[d]Poverty level is based on family income and family size, using Bureau of the Census poverty thresholds.

[e]The sum of percentages for private insurance, Medicaid, and not covered may not sum to 100 percent because other types of health insurance (Medicare, military) do not appear in the table and because persons with both private insurance and Medicaid are counted in both columns.

Source: National Center for Health Statistics. *Health United States, 1999.* Hyattsville, Md.: National Center for Health Statistics, 1999, pp. 299–300.

TABLE 1.2. PERSONAL HEALTH CARE USE BY INCOME.

	1928–1931[a]	1952–1953[a]	1963–1964[a]	1974[a]	1990[b,f]	1996[b,f,g]
Hospital admissions (per 100 persons per year)						
Low income[c]	6	12	14	19	14	15
Middle income[d]	6	12	14	14	9	8
High income[e]	8	11	11	11	7	5
Total	6	12	13	14	9	8
Physician visits (per person per year)						
Low income[c]	2.2	3.7	4.3	5.3	6.3	7.5
Middle income[d]	2.5	3.8	4.5	4.8	5.5	5.7
High income[e]	4.3	6.5	5.1	4.9	5.6	5.3
Total	2.6	4.2	4.5	4.9	5.5	5.8
Percentage seeing a dentist (within one year)						
Low income[c]	10	17	21	35	38	36
Middle income[d]	20	33	36	48	65	64
High income[e]	46	56	58	64	65	64
Total	21	34	38	49	62	61

Notes: [a]Various national surveys reported in Andersen, R., and Anderson, O. "Trends in the Use of Health Services." In H. E. Freeman, S. Levine, and L. G. Reeder (eds.), *Handbook of Medical Sociology.* (3rd ed.). Upper Saddle River, N.J.: Prentice Hall, 1979, pp. 374, 378, 379.

[b]National Center for Health Statistics. *Health United States, 1999.* Hyattsville, Md.: National Center for Health Statistics, 1999, pp. 246, 229, 242.

[c]Lowest 15–27 percent of family income distribution for 1928–1931, 1952–1953, 1963–1964, 1974. Lowest income category for 1990, 1996 for hospital admissions and physician visits. Below poverty for 1990, 1996 for percentage seeing a dentist.

[d]Middle 51–73 percent of family income distribution for 1928–1931, 1952–1953, 1963–1964, 1974. Average of middle three income categories for 1990, 1996 for hospital admissions and physician visits. At or above poverty for 1990, 1996 for percentage seeing a dentist.

[e]Highest 12–32 percent of family income distribution for 1928–1931, 1952–1953, 1963–1964, 1974. Highest income category for 1990, 1996 for hospital admissions and physician visits. At or above poverty for 1990, 1996 for percentage seeing a dentist.

[f]Estimates only for adults twenty-five years of age and older.

[g]Year is 1993 for percentage seeing a dentist.

discretionary but still have an important bearing on people's functional status and quality of life (dental visits).

The hospital admission rate for the U.S. population doubled between 1928–1931 (six admissions per one hundred persons per year) and the early 1950s (twelve admissions). A rising standard of living, the advent of voluntary health insurance, the increasing legitimacy of the modern hospital as a place to deliver babies and treat acute illness, and the requirements necessary for developing sophisticated medical technology all contributed to expanded use of the acute care hospital. Hospital admissions further increased in the 1960s and early 1970s (reaching fourteen admissions per hundred persons per year in 1974) reflecting continued growth in medical technology, private health insurance, and the advent of Medicare coverage for the elderly and Medicaid coverage for the low-income population in 1965.

However, beginning in the mid-1970s use of the acute care hospital began to decline, dropping to nine admissions per hundred population by 1990 and eight in 1996. There were also substantial decreases in average length of stay per admission during this period, from 7.1 days in 1980 to 6.2 days in 1990 and 5.1 days in 1996. Those declines accompanied increasing efforts to contain health care costs by a shift in care from the more expensive inpatient setting to less expensive outpatient settings, a shift from fee-for-service to prospective payments by Medicare, reduced coverage and benefits with increasing coinsurance and deductibles for health insurance, and a shift in certain medical technology and styles of practice that meant reduced reliance on the inpatient settings.

Contributing to the decline of inpatient volume since 1980 has been the significant growth of managed care. Managed care is a health care plan that integrates financing and delivery of health care services by using arrangements to provide services for covered individuals.[38] Plans are generally financed using capitation fees. There are significant financial incentives for members of the plan to use the health care providers associated with the plan. The plan includes formal programs for quality assurance and utilization review.

Health maintenance organizations (HMOs) and preferred provider organizations (PPOs) are primary examples of managed care. HMOs are prepaid health plans delivering comprehensive care to members through designated providers, having a fixed monthly payment for health care services, and requiring members to be in a plan for a specified period of time (usually one year). PPO health plans generally offer inpatient and outpatient services to plan members, usually at discounted rates in return for expedited claims payment. Plan members can use PPO or non-PPO health care providers; however, financial incentives are built into the benefit structure to encourage utilization of PPO providers.

In 1980 9.1 million persons were enrolled in HMOs. The number rose to 33 million in 1990 and to 81 million by 1999—a 145 percent increase in nine years.[39] PPO enrollment also increased significantly in the last decade. In 1991, 67 percent of employees with medical care benefits in private establishments of one hundred or more workers received their benefits through traditional fee-for-service arrangements, compared to 17 percent through HMOs and 16 percent through PPOs. In just six years (by 1997), the proportion had dropped to 27 percent for fee-for-service, while HMOs increased to 33 percent and PPOs increased even more, to 40 percent.[40] This growth of managed care with its emphasis on utilization review and cost containment has contributed to reduction in hospital admissions and the length of hospital stays.

Physician visits (Table 1.2), like inpatient services, increased substantially from 1928–1931 (2.6 visits per person per year) to the early 1950s (4.2 visits) and for many of the same reasons hospital admissions were increasing in this period. However, unlike hospital admissions, the number of physician visits continued to increase, reaching 4.9 visits in 1974 and 5.8 visits in 1996. In part, the continued growth of managed care, with its relative deemphasis of the inpatient setting and greater focus on outpatient settings, may account for the divergence in trends of these basic realized access measures.

Trends in dental visits (Table 1.2) for the total U.S. population paralleled those for physician visits. Twenty-one percent of the population visited a dentist in 1928–1931, and the proportion increased consistently, reaching one-half of the population in 1974. Further increases in the last twenty years resulted in 61 percent of the population visiting a dentist in 1993.

Equitable Access (Health Insurance and Use According to Income and Race)

Table 1.3 combined with Tables 1.1 and 1.2 presents health insurance coverage and personal health care use by race and income for the U.S. population for selected years. Recall that we have suggested that "equitable access" is indicated by similar levels of insurance coverage and use by various income and ethnic groups. "Inequitable access" is indicated by discrepancies in coverage and use for these groups.

Health Insurance. Table 1.1 suggests considerable inequity in insurance coverage in 1980 that continues to present time. Minorities and low-income people are, generally, least likely to have private health insurance. However, there are striking differences among minority groups regarding private health insurance coverage in 1997. Blacks (55 percent), Mexicans (43 percent), and Puerto Ricans (47 percent) are far below the national average (70 percent), but Cubans (71 percent) and

TABLE 1.3.   PERSONAL HEALTH CARE USE BY RACE OR ETHNICITY.

	1964[a]	1981–1983[b,c]	1987–1989[a,c]	1996[d]
Hospital admissions (per 100 persons per year)				
White	11	12	10	8
Black[e]	8	14	12	10
Total	11	12	10	8
Percentage seeing a physician (within one year)				
White	68	76	77	80
Black[e]	58	75	75	81
Total	67	76	77	80
Percentage seeing a dentist White, non-Hispanic[f]	45	57	62	64
Black, non-Hispanic[e,g]	22	39	43	47
Hispanic[h]	—	42	49	46
Total	43	54	59	61

Notes: [a]National Center for Health Statistics. *Health United States, 1993.* Hyattsville, Md.: National Center for Health Statistics, 1994, pp. 174, 179, 180.

[b]For hospital admissions and percentage seeing a doctor: National Center for Health Statistics. *Health United States, 1988.* Hyattsville, Md.: National Center for Health Statistics, 1989, pp. 107, 111.

[c]For percentage seeing a dentist: National Center for Health Statistics. *Health United States, 1999.* Hyattsville, Md.: National Center for Health Statistics, 1999, p. 242.

[d]National Center for Health Statistics. *Health United States, 1999.* Hyattsville, Md.: National Center for Health Statistics, 1999, pp. 246, 232, 242. Year is 1993 for percentage seeing a dentist.

[e]1964 includes all other races.

[f]1964 includes white Hispanics.

[g]1964 includes black Hispanics.

[h]Persons of Hispanic origin may be of any race.

Asian and Pacific Islanders (68 percent) are close to that national average. Medicaid compensates for some of this inequity but still leaves especially high proportions of Mexicans (38 percent) and the lowest-income groups (below 150 percent of federal poverty guidelines, 33–35 percent) uninsured in 1997.

The trends in Table 1.1 suggest a somewhat mixed picture as to whether inequities in health insurance coverage are increasing over time. Between 1984 and 1997 coverage through private health insurance declined while the proportions covered by Medicaid increased for white non-Hispanics and most minority groups. The decrease in private insurance coverage tended to be offset by an increase in Medicaid so that the proportions left uninsured for both whites and minorities were about the same in 1997 as they had been in 1984—except for Mexicans, for whom the uninsured proportion increased from 33 percent to 38 percent over this fifteen-year period, indicating increasing inequity. One reason for the increase in uninsured among Mexicans is their relatively high immigration rates into the United States during this same period. Recent immigrants are less likely to have health insurance coverage.

Trends in insurance coverage according to income level since 1984 generally suggest increased inequity (Table 1.1). Between 1984 and 1997 private health insurance coverage of the low-income groups declined considerably (with the greatest decline, from 62 percent to 42 percent, for those with incomes of 100–149 percent of poverty). There was also a decline for the highest-income group over this period, but it was much less (from 92 percent to 88 percent) as most of the highest-income group retained private health insurance coverage. Increases in Medicaid coverage compensated for decline in private insurance coverage for the lowest-income group so that the proportion uninsured was similar in 1984 (34 percent) and 1997 (33 percent). This was not the case for the lower-income groups above poverty, for whom the proportions uninsured rose considerably—from 26 percent to 35 percent for those at 100–149 percent of poverty and from 17 percent to 25 percent for those at 150–199 percent of poverty. Consequently, it appears that inequity in insurance coverage has been increasing for these lower-income groups above poverty.

Hospital Admissions. Tables 1.2 and 1.3 suggest increasing equity according to income and race for hospital admissions since use by low-income and minority groups compared to the rest of the population has grow consistently over the past seventy years.

However, such a general conclusion about improvement in equity needs to be qualified in important ways. First, the relative needs of the low-income and minority populations for acute hospital care are often much greater. Also, increased use of inpatient hospital care suggests that limited access to preventive and primary services at an earlier time might increase subsequent need for inpatient hospital services for serious acute and uncontrolled chronic disease problems.

In 1928–1931 the highest-income group had the highest admission rate (Table 1.2). By the 1950s, the rates had equalized. In subsequent years, the rates by income diverged, with the lowest-income group increasing relative to those with higher incomes so that by 1996 the lowest income had a rate (15 per hundred) three times that of the highest-income group (5 per hundred). Does this indicate that inequity exists in favor of the low-income group? Probably not. Studies taking into account the need for medical care suggest that the greater use for low-income persons can be largely accounted for by their higher rates of disease and disability.[41]

The hospital admission rate in 1964 for whites (11 per hundred) was still considerably higher than the rate for blacks (8 per hundred; Table 1.3). However, by the 1980s the rate for blacks exceeded the rate for whites, and the higher rate for blacks continued through the 1990s. The higher hospital admission rate for blacks, similar to the higher rate for low-income people, can be largely accounted for by higher level of medical need.[42] Unlike the case with blacks, hospital stays for most Hispanics continues to lag stays for non-Hispanic whites. For the period 1992–1995, the age-adjusted proportion of the population with one or more hospital stays within a year was 6.1 percent for Mexicans and 6.3 percent for Cubans, compared to 6.5 percent for non-Hispanic whites. Among major Hispanic groups, only the percent for Puerto Ricans (8.4) exceeded the non-Hispanic white rate.[43]

Physician Visits. The trends in Tables 1.2 and 1.3 also suggest increasing equity for physician visits according to income level and ethnicity. In 1928–1931 the lowest-income group averaged only one-half as many visits to the doctor (2.2 visits) as the highest-income group (4.3 visits; Table 1.2). Over time, the gap narrowed. By 1974 the lowest-income group was actually visiting a physician more than the higher-income groups, and the difference increased in the 1980s and 1990s. Again, research results suggest that the apparent excess for the low-income population can be accounted for by their greater level of medical need.[44]

Similar trends have taken place for the black population (Table 1.3), but parity with the white population in the proportion seeing a doctor did not take place until the early 1980s, and the proportion seeing a doctor has remained about the same for blacks and whites in 1996. The average number of physician contacts per year for most Hispanic groups (Mexican: 5.1, Cuban: 4.5) remained considerably below those for both blacks (6.2) and non-Hispanic whites (6.3) during the years 1992–1995. As with hospital inpatient services, the rate of use of physician visits for Puerto Ricans for physician contacts (6.4) exceeded that for other Hispanic groups.[45]

Dental Visits. Tables 1.2 and 1.3 tell a story of major inequity according to income and race in dental visit rates that existed in 1928–1931 and continue to exist into the 1990s. The proportion seeing a dentist has increased considerably for all income and racial groups. Still, by 1993 only 36 percent of the low-income group saw a dentist, compared to 64 percent of those in the higher-income groups (Table 1.2). Further, 47 percent and 46 percent of blacks and Hispanics respectively saw a dentist, compared to 64 percent of whites (Table 1.3).

Effective Access

The effectiveness-and-outcomes movement initiated in the late 1980s was in response to several major developments converging on the national scene.[46] The Health Care Financing Administration (HCFA) proposed a research program called the Effectiveness Initiative, stimulated by its need (1) to ensure quality of care for the thirty million Medicare beneficiaries, (2) to determine which medical practices worked best, and (3) to aid policy makers in allocating Medicare resources. At about the same time, an Outcomes Research Program was authorized by Congress, largely inspired by the work of John Wennberg and associates in small-area variations in the utilization and outcomes of medical interventions. A third major development stimulating the effectiveness movement stemmed from efforts led by Robert Brook and associates to determine whether medical interventions within the normal practice setting were being used appropriately. Within the same time period, the Agency for Health Care Policy and Research (AHCPR, recently renamed the Agency for Healthcare Research and Quality) was created, with responsibility for developing medical practice guidelines that represent practical application of the outcomes-and-effectiveness research movement.

Prior to the effectiveness initiative, research findings were hampered by weak study designs (that is, observational and cross-sectional) that were incapable of determining the clear direction of effects and their potential causality.[47] Most studies used mortality as the outcome variable, which was shown to be more sensitive to environmental and socioeconomic factors than medical care utilization.[48] Moreover, the appropriate risk adjustments were usually not available in mortality data sets.

The Medical Outcomes Study (MOS) was undertaken in response to these methodological limitations. The MOS sampled physicians and patients from different health care settings—that is, traditional indemnity (FFS) plan, independent practice association (IPA), or health maintenance organization (HMO)—to investigate the relationships between structure, process, and medical outcomes. Specifically, the MOS was designed to (1) determine whether variations in medical outcomes were explained by differences in the system of care (structure and process) and medical specialty; and (2) develop instruments to assess and monitor medical outcomes (clinical endpoints, functioning, perceived general health status and well-being, and satisfaction with treatment).[49] Ultimately, research results demonstrated that multiple factors—namely, patient mix, medical specialty and system of care, influence or patient outcomes, and when patient and physician characteristics are controlled, quality indicators of primary care—vary across systems of care.[50]

In more recent years, "evidence-based medicine" and "evidence-based management" have emerged from the effectiveness movement. Evidence-based medicine synthesizes research results from multiple clinical trials to help clinicians make judicious use of the best scientific evidence for decisions in patient care. In fact, the Agency for Healthcare Research and Quality (AHRQ) sponsors an Evidence-Based Practice Program comprising twelve centers nationwide. Centers conduct systematic reviews and technology assessments, perform research on improving methods of synthesizing scientific evidence and developing evidence reports and technology assessments, and extend technical assistance to other organizations in their effort to translate evidence reports and technology assessments into guidelines, performance measures, and other quality improvement tools.[51] Evidence-based management, on the other hand, is not nearly as well organized or funded as its counterpart in medicine. Nevertheless, the evidence-based management movement is in response to growing concern about managers in large health care organizations making strategic decisions based on evidence that is not systematically gathered or assessed.[52]

The demand for health services organizations to demonstrate their effectiveness in providing quality patient services will continue to grow. Federal and state governments, managed care organizations, the JCAHO, and businesses and insurers purchasing and paying for medical services have all insisted on greater accountability.[53] Evidence-based medicine and evidence-based management are two complementary approaches for achieving more effective outcomes in the health services industry.

Efficient Access

Efficiency studies have been conducted at both the contextual level (for example, national health care systems and health plans) and the individual level (consumer behavior). At the macroeconomic level, comprehensive data available on major, industrialized countries have been used to compare health services utilization, health resources and expenditures, and health outcomes. For example, the Organization for Economic Cooperation and Development (OECD) study comparing per capita health care expenditures in seven major industrialized countries found that the United States spent about 40 percent more than Canada and almost three times more than the countries with the lowest expenditures. The large expenditure gap for the United States was not offset by health outcome advantages, which raised concerns that resources were being misallocated to services with low benefit relative to cost.[54]

Efficiency analyses conducted at the level of the health plan system have been used to compare traditional indemnity plans with FFS providers to HMOs.[55] Other studies have conducted production efficiency analyses concentrating on the size and personnel mix of physician practices and other medical care delivery settings.[56] Results from these efficiency studies can be used for making managed care contract specifications to ensure that services are accessible, efficient, and effective.

Efficiency analyses focusing on consumers and providers have investigated the effects of cost sharing on health services utilization to determine the optimal combinations of cost sharing and managed care.[57]

Conclusion

Is access improving or declining in the United States? For whom? And according to what measures? Although we have documented continuing increases in some realized access measures, including physician and dental visits, inpatient hospital use has been declining for twenty-five years. However, the declining hospital use rate reflects, in part, the shift to outpatient services and greater emphasis on primary care, possibly reducing the need for acute inpatient services. A key potential access measure, health insurance, reveals that although an increasing number of people are being covered by Medicaid, there has been a decline in the number covered by private insurance in the last fifteen years and an overall increase in the proportion without any health insurance coverage.

Low-income and black populations appear to have achieved equity of access according to gross measures of hospital and physician utilization (not adjusting for their greater need for medical care) but continue to lag considerably in receipt of dental care.

Equity has certainly not been achieved according to health insurance coverage, as the proportion uninsured is 50 percent higher for blacks and more than twice as high for Hispanics and the low-income population, compared to the uninsured rate for whites. Further, numerous investigations have noted large inequities in access for low-income and minority populations regarding not having a regular source of care; not getting preventive care; delay in obtaining needed care; and higher rates of morbidity, hospitalization, and mortality that could have been avoided with appropriate access to care. Many of these documented discrepancies are increasing over time.[58]

Improving access to care can be greatly facilitated by a new generation of access models and indicators. They should stress the importance of contextual as well as individual characteristics to promote policies to improve access for defined populations.[59] They should focus on the extent to which medical care contributes to people's health. Access measures should be developed specifically for particular vulnerable population groups. These measures are especially important because of the cross-cutting needs of many of the vulnerable groups: persons with HIV/AIDS, substance abusers, migrants, homeless people, people with disabilities, and those suffering from family violence.[60]

Improving equity, effectiveness, and efficiency should be the guiding norms for research on access.[61] Among the most important areas for research are:

- Promoting successful birth outcomes—research on the relationships among medical risk factors, the content of prenatal care and birth outcomes; continued research on the increasing disparity between black and white infant mortality
- Reducing the incidence of vaccine-preventable childhood diseases—research on the relationships among race, barriers to access, and infectious disease
- Promoting functional dentition status—research to examine continuing differences in use of dental services according to income and ethnicity and the impact of these differences on functional status
- Reducing the effects of chronic diseases and prolonging life—research concerning the differences in use of high-cost discretionary care according to gender, ethnicity, income, and insurance status and whether these differences represent overuse or underuse of these services
- Reducing morbidity and pain through timely and appropriate treatment—research exploring methods to better define what constitutes timely and appropriate use of physician services during episodes of acute illness and research on factors that lead to hospitalization of people with acute diseases

Notes

1. Phillips, K. A., Morrison, K. R., Andersen, R., and Aday, L. A. "Understanding the Context of Health Care Utilization: Assessing Environmental and Provider-Related Variables in the Behavioral Model of Utilization." *Health Services Research*, 1998, *33*, 571–596.
2. Robert, S. A. "Socioeconomic Position and Health: The Independent Contribution of Community Socioeconomic Context." *Annual Review of Sociology*, 1999, *25*, 489–516.
3. Andersen, R. M. *A Behavioral Model of Families' Use of Health Services*. Research Series no. 25. Chicago: Center for Health Administration Studies, University of Chicago, 1968; and Andersen, R. M. "Revisiting the Behavioral Model and Access to Medical Care: Does It Matter?" *Journal of Health and Social Behavior*, 1995, *36*, 1–10.
4. Donabedian, A. *Exploration in Quality Assessment and Monitoring*. Vol. 1: *The Definition of Quality and Approaches to Its Assessment*. Ann Arbor, Mich.: Health Administration Press, 1980.
5. Bindman, A. B., and Gold, M. R. (eds.). "Measuring Access Through Population-Based Surveys in a Managed Care Environment: A Special Supplement to HSR." *Health Services Research*, 1998, *33*, 611–766.
6. Longest, B. B., Jr. *Health Policymaking in the United States*. (2nd ed.) Chicago: Health Administration Press, 1998.
7. National Center for Health Statistics. *Health, United States, 1999, with Health and Aging Chart Book*. Hyattsville, Md.: National Center for Health Statistics, 1999.
8. Robert (1999).

9. Hulka, B. S., and Wheat, J. R. "Patterns of Utilization: The Patient Perspective." *Medical Care*, 1985, *23*, 438–460.

10. Bass, D. M., and Noelker, L. S. "The Influence of Family Caregivers on Elders' Use of In-Home Services: An Expanded Conceptual Framework." *Journal of Health and Social Behavior*, 1987, *28*, 184–96; Guendelman, S. "Health Care Users Residing on the Mexican Border: What Factors Determine Choice of the U.S. or Mexican Health System?" *Medical Care*, 1985, *23*, 438–60; and Portes, A., Kyle, D., and Eaton, W. W. "Mental Illness and Help-Seeking Behavior Among Mariel Cuban and Haitian Refugees in South Florida." *Journal of Health and Social Behavior*, 1993, *33*, 283–98.

11. Donabedian (1980).

12. Andersen (1968).

13. Andersen (1995).

14. Cunningham, P. J., and Kohn, L. "Health Plan Switching: Choice or Circumstance?" *Health Affairs*, 2000, *19*, 158–164.

15. Davis, K. Baxter Allegiance Foundation Prize for Health Services Research, acceptance speech, June 24, 2000, Los Angeles. New York: Commonwealth Fund, 2000.

16. McManus, S. M., and Pohl, C. M. "Ethics and Financing: Overview of the U.S. Health Care System." *Journal of Health and Human Resources Administration*, 1994, *16*(3), 332–349.

17. Kenkel, P. J. "HMO Profit Outlook Begins to Brighten." *Modern Healthcare*, 1989, *19*, 98; Larkin, H. "Law and Money Spur HMO Profit Status Changes." *Hospitals*, 1989, *63*, 68–69; Coyne, J. S., and Meadows, D. M. "California HMOs May Provide National Forecast." *Healthcare Financial Management*, 1991, *45*, 36–39.

18. Harrison, S., and Kornfield, T. "Policy Implications of 1999 Plan Pullouts from Medicare+Choice." Abstract book. *Association for Health Services Research*, 1999, *16*, 285–286.

19. Gross, D. J. "Medicare Beneficiaries' Costs After BBA: Projections of Out-of-Pocket Health Spending, 1998–2007." Abstract book. *Association for Health Services Research*, 1999, *16*, 285.

20. DiSimone, R. L. "Health Insurance Reform Legislation." *Social Security Bulletin*, 1997, *60*, 18–31; Shultz, P. T., and Greenman, J. F. "Congress Advances on Health Care Reform: One Step at a Time." *Employee Relations Law Journal*, Winter 1996, *22*, 89–106.

21. Gluck, M. E. "A Medicare Prescription Drug Benefit." *Medicare Brief*, 1999, *1*, 1–13.

22. Christensen, S. and Wagner, J. "The Cost of a Medicare Prescription Drug Benefit." *Health Affairs*, 2000, *19*, 212–218.

23. Gluck, M. E. "A Medicare Prescription Drug Benefit." *Medicare Brief*, 1999, *1*, 1–13; Lillard, L. A., Rogowski, J., and Kington, R. "Insurance Coverage for Prescription Drugs: Effects on Use and Expenditures in the Medicare Population." *Medical Care*, 1999, *37*, 926–936.

24. Etheredge, L. "Purchasing Medicare Prescription Drug Benefits, a New Proposal." *Health Affairs*, 1999, *18*(4), 7–19.

25. Andersen, R. M., Kravits, J., and Anderson, O. *Equity in Health Services: Empirical Analysis in Social Policy.* Boston: Ballinger, 1975.

26. Alpha Center. "State of the States." Prepared for State Coverage Initiatives, Robert Wood Johnson Foundation, Jan. 2000.

27. Newacheck, P. W., and others. "Adolescent Health Insurance Coverage: Recent Changes and Access to Care." *Pediatrics*, 1999, *104*, 195–202.

28. Reschovsky, J. D., and Cunningham, P. J. "CHIPing away at the Problem of Uninsured Children: Why Children Lack Health Insurance and Implications for the New State Children's Health Insurance Program." Center for Studying Health System Change. [http://www.hschange.com/researcher/rr2_toc.html]; Reschovsky, J. D., and

Cunningham, P. J. "CHIPing away at the Problem of Uninsured Children." Issue Brief. *Center for Studying Health System Change*, 1998, *14*, 1–7.

29. Long, S. H., and Marquis, M. S. "Geographic Variation in Physician Visits for Uninsured Children: The Role of the Safety Net." *Journal of the American Medical Association*, 1999, *281*, 2035–2040.

30. Lave, C. R., and others. "Impact of a Children's Health Insurance Program on Newly Enrolled Children." *Journal of the American Medical Association*, 1998, *279*, 1820–1825.

31. Fishman, L. E., and Bentley, J. D. "The Evolution of Support for Safety-Net Hospitals." *Health Affairs*, 1997, *16*, 30–47; Gaskin, D. J., and Hadley, J. "Identify Urban Safety Net Hospitals and the Populations They Serve." (Abstract.) *Abstract Book, Association for Health Services Research*, 1997, *14*, 62–3.

32. Institute of Medicine. *America's Health Care Safety Net: Intact But Endangered.* Washington, D.C.: National Academy of Science, 2000.

33. Lipson, D. J., and Naierman, N. "Snapshots of Change in Fifteen Communities: Effects of Health System Changes on Safety Net Providers." *Health Affairs*, 1996, *15*, 33–48; Weissman, J. "Uncompensated Hospital Care: Will It Be There If We Need It?" *Journal of the American Medical Association*, 1996, *276*, 823–828; Gaskin and Hadley (1997), 62–63; Norton, S. A., and Lipson, D. J. "Public Policy, Market Forces, and the Viability of the Safety Net Providers." Occasional Paper no. 13. Washington, D.C.: Urban Institute, 1998; Baxter, R. J., and Feldman, R. L. "Staying in the Game: Health System Change Challenges Care for the Poor." Center for Studying Health System Change. [http://www.hschange.com/researcher/rr3_toc.html]; Institute of Medicine. *America's Health Care Safety Net: Intact But Endangered.* IOM Committee on the Changing Market, Managed Care, and the Future Viability of Safety Net Providers. Washington, D.C.: National Academy Press, 2000.

34. Lillie-Blanton, M., and Rowland, D. "Medicaid's Role in the Health Care Safety Net." (Abstract.) *AHSR and FHSR Annual Meeting Abstract Book*, 1996, *13*, 40–41.

35. Institute of Medicine (U.S.), Committee on Monitoring Access to Personal Health Care Services. *Access to Health Care in America.* (M. Millman, ed.). Washington, D.C.: National Academy Press, 1993.

36. Aday, L. A., Begley, C. E., Lairson, D. R., and Slater, C. H. *Evaluating the Health Care System: Effectiveness, Efficiency, and Equity.* (2nd ed.) Ann Arbor, Mich.: Health Administration Press, 1998.

37. Aday, L. A. "Access to What and Why? Towards a New Generation of Access Indicators." Proceedings of the Public Health Conference on Records and Statistics, DHHS Pub. No. 94214. Washington, D.C.: U.S. Government Printing Office, 1993.

38. National Center for Health Statistics (1999).

39. National Center for Health Statistics. *Health, United States, 2000, with Adolescent Health Chartbook.* Hyattsville, Md.: National Center for Health Statistics, 2000.

40. National Center for Health Statistics (2000).

41. Davis, K., and Rowland, D. "Uninsured and Underserved: Inequities in Health Care in the United States." *Milbank Quarterly*, 1983, *61*, 149–176.

42. Manton, K., Patrick, C., and Johnson, K. "Health Differentials Between Blacks and Whites: Recent Trends in Mortality and Morbidity." *Milbank Quarterly*, 1987, *65* supp. 1, 129–199.

43. Hajat, A., Lucas, J. B., and Kington, R. "Health Outcomes Among Hispanic Subgroups: United States, 1992–95." *Advance Data from Vital and Health Statistics*, no. 310. Hyattsville, Md.: National Center for Health Statistics, 2000.

44. Davis and Rowland (1983).

45. Hajat, Lucas, and Kington (2000).
46. Heithoff, K. A., and Lohr, K. N. (eds.). *Effectiveness and Outcomes in Health Care.* Washington, D.C.: National Academy Press, 1993.
47. Aday, Begley, Lairson, and Slater (1998).
48. Martini, C., Allen, J. B., Davidson, J., and Backett, E. M. "Health Indexes Sensitive to Medical Care Variation." *International Journal of Health Services,* 1977, *7,* 293–309.
49. Tarlov, A., and others. "The Medical Outcomes Study: An Application of Methods for Monitoring the Results of Medical Care." *Journal of the American Medical Association,* 1989, *262,* 925–930; Ware, J. E. "Measuring Patient Function and Well-Being: Some Lessons from the Medical Outcomes Study." In Heithoff and Lohr (1993); Kravitz, R. L., and others. "Differences in the Mix of Patients Among Medical Specialties and Systems of Care: Results from the Medical Outcomes Study." *Journal of the American Medical Association,* 1992, *267,* 1617–1623.
50. Kravitz and others (1992); Greenfield, S., and others. "Variations in Resource Utilization Among Medical Specialties and Systems of Care: Results from the Medical Outcomes Study." *Journal of the American Medical Association,* 1992, *267,* 1624–1630; Safran, D. G., Tarlov, A. R., and Rogers, W. H. "Primary Care Performance in Fee-for-Service and Prepaid Health Care Systems: Results from the Medical Outcomes Study." *Journal of the American Medical Association,* 1994, *271,* 1579–1586.
51. RAND Corporation. "Evidence Report and Evidence-Based Recommendations: Interventions That Increase the Utilization of Medicare-Funded Preventive Services for Persons Age 65 and Older." Prepared for U.S. Department of Health and Human Services, Health Care Financing Administration. (Contract no. 500-98-0281, Sept. 1998–2003.)
52. Kovner, A. R., Elton, J. J., and Billings, J. "Transforming Health Management: An Evidence-Based Approach." *Frontiers of Health Services Management,* 2000, *16*(4), 3–24.
53. White, A. W., and Wager, K. A. "The Outcomes Movement and the Role of Health Information Managers." *Topics in Health Information Management,* May 1998, *18,* 1–2.
54. Aday, Begley, Lairson, and Slater (1998).
55. Aday, Begley, Lairson, and Slater (1998); Manning, W. A., Liebowitz, A., and Goldberg, G. A. "A Controlled Trial of the Effect of a Prepaid Group Practice on Use of Services." *New England Journal of Medicine,* 1984, *310,* 1505–1510.
56. Reinhardt, E. "A Production Function for Physician Services." *Review of Economics and Statistics,* 1972, *54,* 55–66; Smith, K. R., Miller, M., and Golladay, F. L. "An Analysis of the Optimal Use of Inputs in the Production of Medical Services." *Journal of Human Resources,* 1972, *7,* 208–255; Brown, D. M. "Do Physicians Underutilize Aides?" *Journal of Human Resources,* 1988, *23,* 342–355; and Rohrer, J. E., and Rohland, B. M. "Oversight of Managed Care for Behavioral Sciences." *Journal of Public Health Management and Practice,* 1998, *4,* 96–100.
57. Shapiro, M. F., Ware, J. E., and Sherbourne, C. D. "Effects of Cost Sharing on Seeking Care for Serious and Minor Symptoms: Results of a Randomized Controlled Trial." *Annals of Internal Medicine,* 1986, *104,* 246–251; Rohrer and Rohland (1998).
58. Institute of Medicine (1993); Center for Health Economics Research. *Access to Health Care: Key Indicators for Policy.* (Prepared for the Robert Wood Johnson Foundation.) Chestnut Hill, Mass.: Center for Health Economics Research, 1993; Commonwealth Fund. *Managed Care: The Patient's Perspective: A Briefing Note—Karen Davis, President* (New York: Harkness House, 1995); Collins, K. S., Hall, A., and Neubus, C. *U.S. Minority Health: A Chartbook.* New York: Commonwealth Fund, 1999; Mayberry, R. M., and others. Racial and Ethnic Differences

in Access to Medical Care. (Prepared for the Henry J. Kaiser Family Foundation.) Atlanta: Morehouse Medical Treatment Effectiveness Center, 1999; Brown, E. R., Ojeda, V. D., Wyn, R., and Levan, R. *Racial and Ethnic Disparities in Access to Health Insurance and Health Care.* (Prepared for the Henry J. Kaiser Family Foundation.) Los Angeles: UCLA Center for Health Policy Research, 2000.

59. Bindman and Gold (1998); Docteur, E. R., Colby, D. C., and Gold, M. "Shifting the Paradigm: Monitoring Access in Medicare Managed Care." *Health Care Financing Review,* 1996, *17,* 5–21.

60. Aday, L. A. *At Risk in America: The Health and Health Care Needs of Vulnerable Populations in the United States.* San Francisco: Jossey Bass, 1993.

61. Aday, Begley, Lairson, and Slater (1998).

CHAPTER TWO

PUBLIC POLICIES TO EXTEND HEALTH CARE COVERAGE

E. Richard Brown

The United States remains alone among the economically developed countries in not providing health care coverage to its entire population. The new century began with approximately forty-four million uninsured Americans—people who have no private or public health insurance of any kind.

This chapter examines the origins and status of the American system of health care coverage and the options available to extend coverage to the uninsured. First, it describes the current state of health insurance coverage, with an examination of historical trends and the public policies that shaped the current system. The chapter concludes with a review of the major policy options to extend coverage to the remaining uninsured population.

Why is health insurance coverage important? It is the principal financial means by which people can obtain services. The importance of health insurance coverage has been shown in cross-sectional surveys that compare the access of insured and uninsured people, and in panel or longitudinal studies that examine over time the effects of losing or gaining health insurance on access and health status.[1]

The United States has repeatedly toyed with major reforms to establish a universal social insurance program to extend health care coverage to the entire population. Each time it has failed to come to grips with this issue or has adopted partial reforms, sometimes enacting programs based on a public-assistance, or welfare, approach. After these repeated failures to enact comprehensive reform, and despite the partial solutions that have been adopted, the problems of lack of coverage remain a continuing challenge to the U.S. health system and the nation's political institutions.

The Uninsured

The large and growing number of Americans who have no health care coverage continues to be one of the most compelling—and intractable—policy and political issues in the United States. In 1977, following failed attempts to enact national health insurance, twenty-seven million Americans, 13.8 percent of the nonelderly population, were uninsured (Table 2.1). A decade later, the uninsured population had grown to 17.4 percent of the nonelderly. By 1997, three years after the end of the most extensive effort to enact universal coverage, the uninsured rate had reached 18.9 percent.[2]

By 1998, more than forty-four million persons were uninsured, including eleven million children under age eighteen and nearly thirty-three million adults ages eighteen to sixty-four.[3] However, just 358,000 persons age sixty-five or over (less than 1 percent of all the uninsured) are completely uninsured, because nearly all the elderly receive at least Medicare coverage.

Because the uninsured population includes so few elderly persons, most analysts of this problem focus on the nonelderly population. Despite an historic period of economic growth, very low unemployment, and relatively stable costs for health insurance coverage, 18.3 percent of those under age sixty-five were completely uninsured in 1998 (Figure 2.1). (These data are from the Current Population Survey, conducted by the U.S. Census Bureau. These estimates, the most widely used data on health insurance coverage, may differ slightly from those cited earlier because of differences in measurement.)

TABLE 2.1.   PERCENTAGE OF NONELDERLY POPULATION WHO ARE UNINSURED, AGES 0–64, UNITED STATES, 1977, 1987, AND 1997.

1977	13.8
1987	17.4
1997	18.9

Sources: 1977 data from National Medical Care Expenditure Survey, and 1987 data from National Medical Expenditure Survey, both cited in Brown, E. R. "Access to Health Insurance in the United States." *Medical Care Review*, 1989, 46, pp. 349–385; 1997 data from Medical Expenditure Panel Survey, cited in Vistnes, J. P., and Zuvekas, S. A. *Health Insurance Status of the Civilian Noninstitutional Population: 1997.* Rockville, Md.: Agency for Health Care Policy and Research, 1999.

FIGURE 2.1.   HEALTH INSURANCE COVERAGE OF THE
NONELDERLY POPULATION, UNITED STATES, 1998.

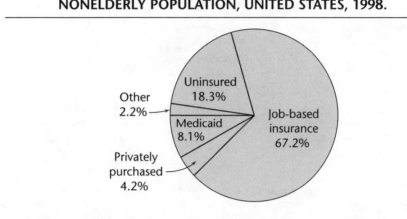

Source: Analysis of March 1999 Current Population Survey by UCLA Center for Health Policy Research.

More than eight of ten (84 percent) of the nonelderly uninsured are working adults and their children. Half (50 percent) of the uninsured are in families headed by at least one employee who works full-time all year, and another 15 percent are in families of full-time employees who work less than a full year (Figure 2.2).[4]

Three-fourths of the uninsured have low or moderate family incomes. More than half (54 percent) have incomes below 200 percent of the federal poverty level (that is, less than $34,000 for a family of four in 2000), and another fifth (18 percent) have moderate family incomes (between 200 percent and 299 percent of the poverty level; Figure 2.3). The low and moderate incomes of the uninsured mean that efforts to extend coverage to them require considerable financial assistance to make it affordable, assistance that can come only from employers or government. Only one in four uninsured have family incomes at least three times the poverty level ($51,000 for a family of four); it is unlikely that any of the uninsured below this level could afford a significant share of the costs of family coverage.

Because of their predominance in the population, 53 percent of the uninsured are non-Latino whites, but ethnic minorities have disproportionately high uninsured rates. More than one out of three nonelderly Latinos (38 percent), one in four African Americans (24 percent), and one in five Asian Americans and Pacific Islanders (22 percent) are uninsured, compared to 14 percent of non-Latino whites.[5]

Ten states have uninsured rates in excess of 20 percent of their nonelderly population, while eight states have rates below 12 percent.[6] Differences in uninsured rates across states are driven mainly by state variations in employment-based

FIGURE 2.2.   FAMILY WORK STATUS OF UNINSURED NONELDERLY
PERSONS, UNITED STATES, 1998.

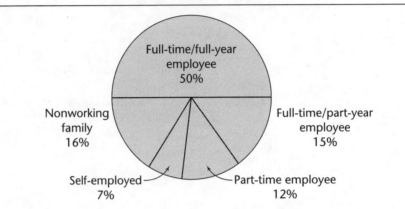

Source: Analysis of March 1999 Current Population Survey by UCLA Center for Health Policy
Research.

FIGURE 2.3.   FAMILY INCOME OF UNINSURED NONELDERLY
PERSONS, UNITED STATES, 1998.

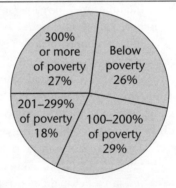

Note: Total family income relative to the federal poverty level.

Source: Analysis of March 1999 Current Population Survey by UCLA Center for Health Policy
Research.

health insurance, but they are also influenced by the generosity of each state's eligibility policy for Medicaid and other public health care insurance programs.

Private Health Insurance Coverage

In 1998, 67.2 percent of the nonelderly obtained private health insurance through their own or a family member's employment (Figure 2.1). Another 4.2 percent purchased private health insurance on their own through the nongroup market. Among all nonelderly persons with any private health insurance, 94 percent obtained it through employment. How did employment-based health insurance gain such a dominant position in the United States, despite the absence of any nationwide requirement that employers provide their workers with coverage?

From World War II through the mid-1970s, private health insurance covered a growing proportion of the American population. World War II produced several forces that encouraged expansion of private health insurance: wage-and-price controls that exempted employee benefits, cost-plus government war contracts, federal tax policies that allowed employers to deduct premiums for health plans from business revenues and allowed employees to deduct employer-paid health insurance premiums from taxable earnings, and demands from labor unions in a very tight labor market and a war-focused economy. By 1945, enrollment in hospital insurance plans had spread to 24 percent of the population, up from 10 percent in 1940. After the war, commercial insurance companies, following the early leadership of not-for-profit Blue Cross plans, pushed into the employer-sponsored health insurance market. By 1950, private hospital insurance covered 51 percent of the population; by 1962, about 70 percent of the entire population had hospital benefits and 65 percent were covered for physicians' surgical services.[7]

Private health insurance was popular among consumers of health services because it spread the risk of expensive medical conditions across a large population base, reducing the threat of personal bankruptcy in the event of serious health problems and making health services financially more accessible to the covered population. It was also popular among hospitals, physicians, and other health care providers because it created a stable base of revenues that reduced their risk of bankruptcy during recession and permitted them to expand and introduce new technologies during good years. The expansion of private health insurance coverage was the financial foundation for the rapid growth of medical care, including escalating investments in medical technology, hospitals, and specialty care.

The large proportion of the uninsured who are in working families—84 percent—underscores the less-than-universal character of employment-based health insurance. Employment-based health insurance peaked in the mid-1970s and has ebbed and flowed since that time, especially with each expansion and contraction of the economy. This dynamic is illustrated by changes in job-based insurance coverage following the recession of the early 1990s. The proportion of the nonelderly population with job-based coverage rose from 65.6 percent in 1994 (as the country was just beginning to emerge from the recession) to 67.2 percent in 1998 (as the economy boomed). But this slight growth in employment-based insurance coverage was due to more families gaining the benefits of full-time employment generated by an unprecedented period of economic growth. The booming economy did not, however, increase the proportion of employees with job-based insurance. The proportion of adults and children in families headed by a full-time, full-year employee rose from 65 percent in 1994 to 69 percent in 1998, but the proportion of persons in full-time, full-year employee families who had job-based insurance remained flat: 81.1 percent in 1994 and 80.4 percent in 1998.[8]

The lack of health insurance coverage among the working population is because many employers are not offering health benefits, some workers are not eligible for benefits when they are offered, and some workers who are offered and eligible for health benefits are not accepting them. Job-based insurance among workers fell from 63.9 percent in 1987 to 60.4 percent in 1996. Contrary to conventional wisdom, most recent studies have found little or no decline in the proportion of employers who offer health benefits to at least some of their workers (the "offer rate"), except among young workers. But there is growing evidence of a decline in eligibility for health benefits (the "eligibility rate") among employees who work less than full-time, full-year and a decline among full-time, full-year employees in acceptance of health insurance when it is offered (the "take-up rate"). Between 1987 and 1996, take-up rates have declined significantly among young workers, Hispanic workers, those with low educational attainment, and those with low wages.[9] In other studies, the decline also has been attributed to rising costs for health care services, employers requiring that an increased share of health insurance premiums be paid by the employee, and stagnant incomes for a significant part of the workforce.[10]

Although the proportion of employees who are offered health benefits does not appear to have been declining, there are large disparities in the offer rate. Small firms, especially those with fewer than twenty-five workers, are far less likely to offer their employees health benefits than are larger firms. Only 55 percent of firms with fewer than ten employees offer health benefits to any of their workers, compared to 72 percent of those with ten to twenty-four employees and 86 percent of those with twenty-five or more workers.[11] Consequently, nearly half (46 percent) of uninsured employees work in firms with fewer than twenty-five workers. But larger firms also contribute to the problem; one in four uninsured employees (28 percent) works in a firm with five hundred or more workers.[12]

The probability that a worker is offered health benefits in general depends on the labor market in which the worker is competing for a job. Those who work for small firms, in agriculture or the service sector, or for a nonunion firm are less likely to have an employer that offers health benefits. Workers whose employers do not offer health benefits to anyone working for them disproportionately are Latino, young adults, or noncitizens; they have less education, work less than full-time, and earn low wages.[13] Because they have no subsidy from their employer or the government, the low-to-moderate income of these groups makes private purchase of health insurance unaffordable.

Thus private health insurance has not served all sectors of American society. The elderly and the poor were effectively priced out of the market for private coverage even in its period of rapid growth during the 1950s and early 1960s. In 1958, while 86 percent of the upper-income third of all American families had some type of private health insurance, only 42 percent of the lower-income third had any coverage at all. Like the lower working class and the poor, the elderly were unable to obtain adequate private hospitalization coverage at a price they could afford. In 1958, only 43 percent of persons age sixty-five and over had insurance for hospital care, compared with at least two-thirds of the nonelderly population.[14] Although private health insurance dramatically reduced disparities in the use of health services related to income for the population with coverage, it remained for Medicare and Medicaid to significantly improve access for the elderly and the poor.

Medicare, Medicaid, and SCHIP

By 1960, political pressures to enact public programs to provide for the poor, especially the low-income elderly, had become irresistible.[15] The Kerr-Mills Act, enacted in that year, offered generous matching federal grants to states to encourage them to develop medical care programs for the elderly poor and the nonelderly disabled and blind. But the program was implemented unevenly by the states, with the bulk of the federal funds going to a handful of states that developed comprehensive programs. Senior citizen groups, not assuaged by this public assistance program, continued to demand health insurance under Social Security, not a welfare program.[16]

The November 1964 election gave the Democrats a landslide victory (the most lopsided popular vote in this century) and gave President Lyndon Johnson both a clear mandate for his Great Society reforms and a Democratic Congress (two-thirds in both houses) to enact them. The next year, Congress established Medicare, a social insurance program for hospital care and voluntary insurance for physician services for the elderly, and Medicaid, a public assistance program for poor people who meet "categorical" requirements. Medicare was a landmark in American health care reform because, as a contributory program that provided entitlement to health benefits without a means test, it was the first successful enactment of social insurance for health services. Medicaid also was important because of its broad potential scope of benefits and population coverage, despite its public assistance, or welfare, character that rested on means testing.

Medicare: Improving Access for the Elderly

Medicare has extended coverage to virtually all the elderly and to many blind and long-term disabled persons for a significant portion of their medical expenses. Medicare is the largest source of public financing for health care services in the United States. Persons age sixty-five and over with social security benefits are automatically entitled to receive Medicare Part A (coverage for hospital services) and to enroll in Medicare Part B (coverage for physician and other services). Part A is a mandatory program financed by a special social security tax paid by all workers and deposited in the Medicare Trust Fund, while Part B is a voluntary plan funded by beneficiary premium payments and contributions from the U.S. Treasury. In 1999, Medicare covered more than thirty-nine million beneficiaries (thirty-four million aged and five million disabled enrollees), at a cost of $213 billion.[17]

Medicare is a social insurance program. This is a very important characteristic. Like Social Security, Medicare Part A is a contributory program, which means that everyone who works contributes to it through a tax on earnings. And Medicare is an entitlement program, which means that everyone is eligible for Medicare upon reaching age sixty-five or, if younger, meeting a stringent disability test. It is *not* a means-tested welfare program; this distinction will be clearer when we discuss Medicaid.

Medicare quickly improved access to medical services, especially hospital care, for the elderly. But even under Medicare—an entitlement program with uniform benefits and standards—beneficiary access problems remain. In the program's first few years, more affluent elderly beneficiaries received more physician and hospital services than did the lower-income elderly. Similarly, white Anglo beneficiaries received more health services than did African American beneficiaries. Over time, however, both income and racial differentials were reduced. Recent studies have found that the vast majority of Medicare beneficiaries report no access problems, but some groups do encounter serious barriers. About one in seven Medicare beneficiaries do not have a usual source of care or have not seen a physician for a medical problem that warranted medical attention. Studies that examine access to specific procedures consistently find differences by race in the rate of selected diagnostic and treatment procedures performed. African American beneficiaries are less likely than Anglo beneficiaries to receive a variety of high-technology procedures.[18]

Lack of coverage for several key benefits limits the effectiveness of Medicare for many types of health service, particularly for lower-income beneficiaries. First, Medicare originally did not emphasize preventive care or early detection of life-threatening diseases, and only recently has it begun to cover screening mammograms and Pap tests. Second, Medicare still does not cover prescription medications, a problem that has been exacerbated for the elderly, among others, by rising expenditures for prescription drugs. Growing political support for adding prescription drug coverage to Medicare has pushed this issue onto the policy agenda, and it is likely that Congress will enact a coverage program in the near future. A third notable lack of coverage is for long-term care services. Medicare restricts coverage for nursing home stays and home health visits to post-hospital use of limited duration, imposing hardships on the elderly who must use extensive personal resources to pay for care or, if poor or impoverished by medical expenses, who may apply to Medicaid.

Medicare cost-sharing provisions for covered services also pose financial barriers. Premium costs, deductibles, and coinsurance, as well as physician charges resulting from "balance billing," can impose high out-of-pocket expense on the beneficiary. A high proportion of beneficiaries have supplemental coverage to offset these costs, but private "Medigap" insurance has become increasingly expensive. An estimated 16.5 percent of Medicare beneficiaries also qualify for financial assistance and supplemental benefits under their state Medicaid programs because their incomes are low.

Approximately 15 percent of Medicare beneficiaries were enrolled in managed care plans (Medicare+Choice) in January 1998, gaining such additional benefits as prescription drug coverage. In the Medicare Current Beneficiary Survey in 1996, beneficiaries enrolled in HMOs were more likely than those with fee-for-service coverage to be very satisfied with costs and all aspects of quality of care, but, paradoxically, HMO enrollees were also more likely to be very dissatisfied with provider attitudes, access to specialty care, and getting information on the phone.[19] In 2000, large numbers of HMOs pulled out of the Medicare market, jeopardizing the continuity of care for many beneficiaries.

Medicaid: Improving Access for the Poor

Medicaid was enacted in 1965 to provide coverage to poor persons who were eligible for federally supported, state-run welfare programs. These welfare programs give cash assistance to families with dependent children (formerly Aid to Families with Dependent Children, or AFDC) and to the disabled, the blind, and the elderly (SSI/SSP). Through this latter component, Medicaid assists elderly Medicare beneficiaries who could not afford the required cost sharing for Medicare or supplemental insurance. Medicaid is administered by the states under federal guidelines that require minimum standards for eligibility, benefits, and in some cases provider payments. Funding is shared between the federal government and the states, with the federal share (called the Federal Medical Assistance Percentage, or FMAP) ranging from 50 percent up to 77 percent.

In 1999, Medicaid covered an estimated forty-one million persons at a cost of $180.9 billion. Half of Medicaid beneficiaries are low-income children, about a fifth are low-income women, and the remaining quarter are low-income disabled and elderly persons. Medicaid spending is tilted toward the elderly (who in 1998 accounted for 11 percent of all recipients and averaged about $9,700 per person) and toward the disabled (who made up 18 percent of recipients and averaged about $8,600 per person, compared with children, who constitute 51 percent of all Medicaid recipients and average about $1,150 per child).[20]

There is substantial evidence that Medicaid is responsible for a significant increase in use of health services among low-income persons. In 1964, two years before the Medicaid program began operation, poor persons averaged 4.3 doctor visits per year, compared to 4.6 visits for the nonpoor. By the mid-1970s, when nearly all states were operating Medicaid programs, poor adults averaged more physician visits than nonpoor adults, and the gap between poor and nonpoor children had been reduced (though not eliminated). However, use of a greater volume of services by the poor may not necessarily indicate complete equity in access because of the poorer health status of many low-income people.[21]

Medicaid's positive effect on utilization rates of low-income persons is, of course, limited to those who are eligible for the program. Numerous studies have found that Medicaid beneficiaries, in contrast to uninsured low-income persons, use health services at a rate comparable to that of higher-income people, after adjusting for differences in health status. Among poor and near-poor persons who are sick or in poor health, those who are uninsured during the entire year use far fewer medical services than those who have Medicaid for even part of the year.[22]

Prospective studies find that loss of Medicaid coverage has an adverse impact on the health status of low-income people, especially among persons with chronic illness. Loss of Medicaid has a serious adverse impact on access to health services and on the health status of anyone with a chronic illness, such as diabetes or high blood pressure.[23]

Despite its important contributions, Medicaid's ability to improve access to medical care for the nation's low-income population has been hampered by several factors. State-level discretion in the Medicaid program has resulted in great variation across states in the population covered and the benefits provided. Federal guidelines define mandatory eligible populations and covered benefits, but they allow states considerable latitude beyond this floor. States vary markedly in their Medicaid income eligibility level for a family, which ranges from nineteen states with income eligibility below 50 percent of the federal poverty level for parents of eligible Medicaid children to ten states with income eligibility at or above 100 percent. States also differ in the benefits covered in the Medicaid program. Each state defines its own package of benefits beyond the mandatory services defined by federal Medicaid law. For example, coverage for such essential services as prescription drugs, physical therapy, occupational therapy, respiratory care services, and corrective eyeglasses are all optional. Reimbursement levels for Medicaid also vary considerably across states, contributing to differences by state in the rate of physician participation.[24]

Medicaid's limitations in covering the poor were exacerbated by budget cuts during the Reagan administration and ratcheting down by states of income limits for AFDC eligibility. As a result, Medicaid enrollees as a proportion of all poor persons declined from 51 percent in 1981 to 45 percent in 1982. Beginning in the mid-1980s, however, Congress enacted a series of expansions in Medicaid income eligibility in order to extend Medicaid's beneficial effects to more low-income pregnant women and their children. Although only 51 percent of poor children were on Medicaid in 1985, 60 percent were covered by Medicaid in 1994, an important reversal of the trend of a decade earlier.[25]

Most of this increase was aimed at ensuring financial access to pregnant women to enable them to obtain prenatal care early in pregnancy in order to improve birth outcome and the health of the infant. Congress required states to cover pregnant women up to 133 percent of the poverty level and encouraged states to voluntarily expand coverage up to 185 percent of poverty. This extension of Medicaid to a population well above the income eligibility for cash public assistance programs partially severed the historic link between Medicaid and welfare. In addition, Congress required states to increase fees for obstetric care to attract an adequate number of providers, and it appropriated other funds for enhanced perinatal care. By 1994, thirty-four states had expanded coverage of pregnant women beyond federally mandated levels, all fifty states had streamlined the eligibility process to at least some extent, and forty-four states offered Medicaid reimbursement for enhanced prenatal services. Nearly one-third of all births in the United States now are paid for by Medicaid, while other programs fund improvement in the supply and accessibility of prenatal care services and nutritional and other supports for mothers and young children.[26]

The Medicaid program's improvements in eligibility for pregnant women to meet specific public health goals is a valuable example of how public policy may be used directly to improve access. The effects of Medicaid expansion on prenatal care use and birth outcomes are inconsistent. Some studies show improvement in access to care and birth outcomes, while others do not. These findings suggest that there are multiple components to providing prenatal care that include, but go beyond, improving financial access: outreach and educational programs, case management, and supply of providers.[27]

The expansion of Medicaid coverage appeared to come to a halt with the enactment and implementation of the Personal Responsibility and Work Opportunity Reconciliation Act of 1996, better known as welfare reform. Nationally, Medicaid coverage fell from 12.5 percent of the nonelderly population overall in 1994 to 10.4 percent in 1998, but it fell even more sharply among nonworking families, from 52.8 percent in 1994 to 40.8 percent in 1998.[28] As the economy continued to improve, some families and individuals who formerly relied on Medicaid may have obtained low-wage jobs that permitted some access to health benefits, or they earned more money that enabled them to pay the employee's share of premiums. But many of these newly employed workers and their families found themselves in low-wage jobs without health benefits and joined the ranks of the uninsured. Although welfare reform promised public assistance recipients that they will receive transitional Medicaid coverage for at least a year when they leave public assistance, both advocates and analysts argue that this policy is inadequately implemented.[29]

Finally, many noncitizen families refrained from applying for Medicaid. They feared being labeled a "public charge" if they enroll themselves or their children in a means-tested program, and that this classification would be used against them if they tried to renew their visas, return to the United States from abroad, or apply for citizenship.[30] This problem is likely to be moderated by new policies, issued in May 1999 by the Immigration and Naturalization Service (INS), specifying that noncitizens will not be classified as a public charge if they or their children enroll in Medicaid (except those who receive long-term care under Medicaid). However, immigrant parents who are undocumented and fear contact with the INS are likely to continue to refrain from applying for Medicaid even for their U.S.-citizen children, who are fully eligible on the same basis as other citizens.

One important characteristic of the Medicaid program is its origin as a public assistance program. Welfare programs, even federally supported ones such as Medicaid, tend to be administered by the states, albeit under some federal regulation. Unlike Medicare, which is administered as a social insurance program by the federal government and includes the same eligibility and benefits throughout the country, the Medicaid program is administered by the states. Medicaid is in reality fifty-one programs, with variations in eligibility and benefits across all fifty states and the District of Columbia.

Many of the problems associated with Medicaid are the legacy of its welfare-based origin. Welfare programs tend to rely on stigmatizing means tests, usually conducted in welfare offices.[31] It is noteworthy that there is no stigma attached to Medicare, which is viewed as a universal entitlement, a social contract between the nation's young and old generations. Nor is there stigma associated with the tax exemption of employer-paid health insurance for largely middle- and upper-income workers, which cost the federal government about $79 billion in 1998—a health insurance subsidy program that no one calls welfare.[32] Despite Medicaid's welfare origins, expansion of eligibility in the 1980s to low-income pregnant women and children at higher income levels—nearly twice the poverty level for pregnant women and infants—loosened the connection with welfare and created the logic for 1990s policies that went further.

A second important characteristic of Medicaid is that it is an entitlement program. Although it originated as a welfare program, anyone who meets Medicaid's eligibility requirements is entitled to receive its benefits, and expenditures for these benefits thus generate a cost to the state and draw the specified federal matching payment. In this way, Medicaid differs from block grant programs, in which the federal government gives the states a maximum allocation; once a state has expended its allocation, any additional services for eligible persons become the sole fiscal responsibility of the state. This characteristic has been the nub of major conflict between liberals and conservatives, with liberals defending Medicaid as an entitlement and conservatives often proposing to turn it into a block grant—as they tried unsuccessfully to do in 1996, when welfare reform ended the entitlement of poor children and families to cash assistance.

Expanding Medicaid with Waivers and Managed Care. With the failure to enact national health care reform, many states looked to Medicaid, among other approaches, to extend coverage to their uninsured residents. Many states have expanded or otherwise modified their Medicaid programs with the aid of a waiver under section 1115 of the Social Security Act. These waivers, which must be granted by the federal Health Care Financing Administration, permit states to modify eligibility, payment methods, and other characteristics in their Medicaid programs. All of the waivers permit states to require Medicaid beneficiaries to enroll in a managed care plan, based on the expectation that managed care enables the state to slow the growth of its Medicaid expenditures and, in some cases, improve access to health services. Most of the recent waivers also extend coverage to the working poor and their families, who were not previously eligible for Medicaid, promising to use at least some of the expected savings from managed care to expand coverage to low-income uninsured persons. By 1998, 53.6 percent of all Medicaid beneficiaries were enrolled in managed care, up from 9.5 percent in 1991.[33]

By the end of 1999, fifteen states had comprehensive health care reform Medicaid waivers, including thirteen that used their waivers to expand enrollment.

Tennessee undertook the most ambitious expansion as it replaced its fee-for-service Medicaid program with TennCare, a fully capitated managed care program. By the end of 1999, TennCare had enrolled more than 1.3 million Medicaid beneficiaries in managed care, including more than 506,000 who did not fit traditional Medicaid eligibility. Altogether, these thirteen waiver states covered 1.2 million persons who would not have been eligible without the waiver.[34]

These successes not withstanding, Medicaid managed care programs raise concerns among many groups. Community health centers, a critical part of the health care safety net for the uninsured poor and Medicaid recipients, fear that they will lose current Medicaid fees, which are a major source of their funding. In 1997, Medicaid revenues represented a third of federally funded health centers' total operating revenue, matching the third of their patients who were covered by Medicaid.[35] Although many community health centers have developed contracts with managed care plans that enroll Medicaid recipients, they worry that their lost Medicaid fees will not be offset by serving patients enrolled in these plans. Without Medicaid revenues, and with declining federal grants, there is widespread concern that community health centers and other safety-net providers will not have the financial support they need to continue to serve uninsured patients. Advocates for the uninsured and low-income communities share the concerns of safety-net providers that, without Medicaid revenues, these last-resort providers will lose their financial viability, and the safety net will be shredded.

Advocates for Medicaid beneficiaries also worry that managed care will end up reducing access to health services for enrollees because capitation creates incentives for health plans and providers to reduce use of services and because enrollees are locked into their plans for at least several months. They are also concerned that Medicaid HMOs may offer poorer care than fee-for-service practice. These concerns have been reinforced by some past experience. In the 1970s, California's Medicaid beneficiaries suffered from abuses by managed care plans that marketed door-to-door with deceptive sales information, raised serious barriers to obtaining services, and often provided poor quality care. In the 1980s, Medicaid enrollees in Chicago-area HMOs experienced similar marketing abuses, failure to provide services, and quality problems.[36]

Medicaid managed care has yielded a mixed record. On some measures, such as having a regular provider, Medicaid managed care beneficiaries appear to be doing better than their fee-for-service counterparts, but managed care enrollees are more likely to report not getting needed care and more dissatisfaction with some aspects of their care. There is, however, a growing body of evidence that, overall, managed care plans offer Medicaid beneficiaries access to health services that is at least as good as in the fee-for-service Medicaid program and quality of care that is equal to or better than care in the fee-for-service program.[37] Nevertheless, there is little evidence that managed care reduces Medicaid costs— in part because most Medicaid managed care enrollees have not been the higher-cost disabled or elderly for whom substantial savings might be realized and in part because Medicaid expenditures per beneficiary had already been ratcheted down to an extremely low level in many states.

Expanding Income-Eligibility for Medicaid. States can also cover parents of children who are income-eligible for Medicaid, under the new section 1931 of the Social Security Act, which allows states considerable flexibility in setting Medicaid income eligibility for families.[38] By 2000, however, only fifteen states had used either section 1931 or an 1115 waiver to cover parents to at least 100 percent of the poverty level.[39] Other states remain well below that level.

The State Children's Health Insurance Program (SCHIP). With the collapse in 1994 of efforts to cover the entire population, many health care reform advocates joined with children's advocacy groups to expand coverage for children. They focused a great deal of attention on the fact that there were then more than eleven million uninsured children eighteen or younger in the United States, many of whom had low family incomes that were above their state's often less-than-generous Medicaid income eligibility level. Children are an appealing group to cover, both because there is wide political support for public programs that benefit children and because insuring children costs much less than insuring adults.

In 1997, Congress enacted the State Children's Health Insurance Program (SCHIP), providing funds to states to expand health insurance coverage to uninsured, low-income, and moderate-income children. Although liberals and conservatives fought over whether to make SCHIP an entitlement that expanded Medicaid or a block grant that established a separate private insurance program, in the end Congress compromised on a generous block grant that could be used by the states to do either or both.

SCHIP was generous in two ways. First, it enabled states to set income eligibility levels up to 200 percent of the federal level (in 1999, up to $22,500 for a family of two or $28,300 for a family of three) or even higher. Second, it gives states more generous matching funds than under Medicaid—30 percent higher than the state's federal Medicaid match, up to 85 percent of a state's expenditures—an incentive to induce states to implement the program quickly and vigorously. SCHIP implementation has been slow and has fallen short of early enrollment goals, but it is enrolling previously uninsured children and is likely to help slow the growth in the uninsured population.

Reforms to Expand Private Coverage

In addition to expanding the population groups covered through Medicaid and SCHIP, states have also experimented with an array of reforms aimed at expanding private coverage to the uninsured population. The collapse of national health care reform efforts has increased pressure to implement state, rather than national, solutions to rising health care costs and access problems. However, states vary in their political and economic capacity to effectively implement reforms, and they also lack the legislative authority to enact reforms that would achieve universal coverage.

The main approaches that states and the federal government have pursued to expand private coverage of the uninsured have included reform of insurance laws to increase affordability or access to coverage, creation of purchasing alliances or cooperatives, and, in a few states, passage of legislation mandating coverage. To varying degrees, these approaches build upon the existing employment-based insurance system, strengthening the connection between coverage and work.

Small Group and Individual Health Insurance Reform

Compared to larger groups, small groups and individuals face higher premiums for health insurance as a result of higher marketing and administrative costs and more difficulty in managing risk in this market. Consequently, they also face such problems as frequent jumps in premium, frequent changes in insurance carrier, and medical underwriting (that is, basing premiums on the particular group's expected use of health services).[40]

Furthermore, groups or individuals considered at highest risk often were not able to obtain any coverage. The Consolidated Omnibus Budget Reconciliation Act of 1985 (COBRA), for example, addressed this problem by requiring employers and insurers to allow employees who lost or changed their employment to keep their health insurance if they pay 102 percent of the full premium. Although this provision is useful to higher-risk persons who are very concerned about being without coverage, it does not help those who cannot afford the full costs of their health plan—the situation facing the great majority of the uninsured, and especially those who have become unemployed.

The Health Insurance Portability and Accountability Act (HIPAA) of 1996 required states to reform their individual and small-group health insurance markets. It guaranteed that individuals could buy health insurance without exclusion for a preexisting condition if they have been covered by an employer-sponsored health plan for at least eighteen months, exhaust any continuation of their employer's health benefits available through COBRA, are not eligible for any other public or private health insurance, and were uninsured no longer than two months. HIPAA also limited insurers' ability to exclude preexisting conditions and prohibited them from defining pregnancy as a preexisting condition. It prohibited employers from charging employees higher premiums according to health status or other factors related to potential usage, and it required insurers to guarantee issue and renewal of health insurance for small employers (those with two to fifty employees). HIPAA also gradually raised the tax deductibility for health insurance purchased by self-employed persons from 30 percent in 1996 to 80 percent by the year 2006.

What HIPAA did not do was limit the amount that an insurer could charge for coverage that it guaranteed. As a result, HIPAA-protected coverage is often unaffordable to individuals who need it, resulting in a negligible impact on the uninsured population. Moreover, since almost all states had already enacted some type of small-group and individual market insurance reforms,[41] HIPAA served to bring all states up to a uniform national standard, rather than dramatically change the accessibility and affordability of coverage. In sum, reforms that extend guaranteed coverage to small groups and individuals help regulate the market, but they will have limited impact in expanding coverage unless they are accompanied by some form of subsidy.

Purchasing Groups

Unlike high-risk pools that target individuals, purchasing cooperatives target small businesses. These cooperatives or alliances of small firms are designed to increase their purchasing power and lower administrative costs. Two-thirds (68 percent) of small firms that do not offer health benefits cite the high cost of coverage as a "very important" reason why they do not do so, far ahead of any other reason.[42] State-sponsored cooperatives enable small businesses to pool the risk of insurance coverage, thus lowering premium costs and improving their bargaining power in the health insurance market. National estimates from the 1997 Robert Wood Johnson Foundation Employer Health Insurance Survey suggest that about one-quarter of all businesses participate in a purchasing pool and that smaller businesses are more likely to participate. The survey also found that pools modestly increased the availability of employee choice among plans and promoted information for employees about plan quality, but pooling did not increase the accessibility or affordability of insurance for employers.[43]

Employer Mandates

The reforms that have been discussed so far create incremental change in how health services are financed and in the proportion of the uninsured population gaining access to coverage. These reforms make coverage available to employers or individuals whose high risk or small size has made it difficult for them to find coverage at rates available to other employers or individuals. Such reforms may help employers deal with the problem of rising benefit costs, but they do not make health insurance more affordable for the moderate- and low-income families and individuals who make up the majority of the uninsured.

To make health insurance more affordable to this currently uninsured population—as well as to stabilize the employment-based system for financing health insurance—there has been considerable national and state interest in requiring employers to help pay for coverage for their employees. Despite the apparent value of an employer mandate, only Hawaii has implemented this reform. The ability of states to adopt employer mandates has been thwarted by the federal Employee Retirement Income Security Act (ERISA), which exempts self-insured businesses from state insurance regulations and taxes, although it does not bar states from regulating health insurance coverage that employers purchase for their employees.[44] Nationally, up to half of all medium and large firms self-insure (that is, assume all or part of the financial risk of coverage), greatly limiting states' authority over the employer group insurance market. Hawaii is the only state that received a Congressional exemption from ERISA for its employer mandate because Hawaii enacted its mandate legislation in 1974, before ERISA itself was enacted.

Both ERISA and the political and economic implications of employer mandates have led the few other states that planned to enact mandate policies to abandon their efforts or place on hold implementation of the mandate.[45] Employer mandates have won the vehement and aggressive opposition of employers, especially interest groups representing small business. It was the inclusion of a provision that employers help pay for their workers' health insurance coverage that generated one of the most aggressive and effective lobbying campaigns against President Clinton's health care reform proposal—perhaps providing the crushing blow.

Frustrations on the Road to Universal Coverage

For at least the last half century, many Americans have found the concept of government health insurance an appealing way to cover the population.[46] Funded by taxes and administered as a universal national program by the federal government, or by a combination of federal and state governments, such a social insurance program would pay physicians, hospitals, and other health care providers, eliminating the need for private health insurance. Since 1965, Medicare has provided virtually universal coverage for the elderly, but throughout much of the twentieth century repeated efforts to enact a universal system for the entire population have consistently foundered.

Social Insurance: The Elusive Option

Social insurance systems have many advantages. Canada's single-payer system, a social insurance program that has received a great deal of attention in the United States, has been an efficient means of extending universal coverage with comprehensive health benefits. The Canadian system has many advantages that attracted Americans at the beginning of the 1990s. Canada's provincial-run national program provides universal coverage, excellent access to primary care, patients' freedom to choose their own physicians, a superior record of controlling expenditures for physicians and hospitals, lower administrative costs, lower out-of-pocket costs for patients, and less restricted clinical autonomy for physicians.[47] However, steady reductions in federal support for the provincial programs, from 50 percent in 1971 to just 23 percent in 1997, has led to lower per capita spending, a shortage of medical personnel and facilities, and increased waiting time for specialty care and surgery. The decline in federal support and its sequelae yielded a dramatic decline in popular satisfaction with the system, with the proportion of the public saying "On the whole the system works pretty well, and only minor changes are needed to make it work better" falling from 56 percent in 1988 to just 20 percent in 1998.[48]

Despite these advantages and support, social insurance proposals have not fared well in the United States since the enactment of Medicare. Although the single-payer proposals[49] introduced into Congress in the recent health care reform effort received substantial support from some unions and consumer-based organizations, they could not overcome the powerful opposition of an array of interest groups representing health care providers, insurers, and business. In November 1994, California voters rejected (by a 73–27 margin) a Canadian-style single-payer ballot initiative that had been opposed by a very well-funded campaign.

Given the particular political system of the United States, universal coverage reforms of all kinds are likely to continue to face stiff opposition, despite their demonstrated need.

Political Barriers to Universal Coverage Reform

There are many barriers to adopting policy options that would lead to universal coverage. The effort at health care reform in the early 1990s started out with massive public support, but many forces combined to sap the political momentum for change. As we entered the 1990s, nine out of ten Americans, driven by fear of losing health insurance coverage and being unable to afford the rising cost of care, told pollsters that they believed the nation's health care system needed fundamental change or complete rebuilding.[50] The same proportion of chief executive officers of Fortune 500 corporations, whose attention was focused on their rising health benefits costs, supported fundamental change or complete rebuilding of the nation's health care system.[51] Three-fourths of these corporate executives said the problems could not be solved by companies working on their own and that government must play a bigger role. The leaders of four major national business organizations jointly appealed to the Congress to "do something" about health care costs.[52]

This impressive support for comprehensive reform dissipated rapidly as opposition interest groups eroded public support and threw their impressive weight against Congressional efforts to find a consensus.[53] The Clinton administration created a cumbersome policy process to develop and promote its health care proposal, and (unlike reform opponents) the administration waged a feckless public campaign that did not mobilize grassroots support. Popular support for any specific proposal began to decline. Waning prospects for health care reform encouraged major employers to turn from policy change to other options to lower their own costs, including encouraging or forcing their employees into managed care and limiting their own costs by providing employees with a fixed contribution for health benefits.

Underlying this successful frustration of health care reform efforts is, in addition to the administration's flawed process to develop and promote the President's reform proposal, the nation's political system itself. Compared to all parliamentary democracies that have developed national health insurance systems, the U.S. political system, institutions, and culture pose significant challenges to enacting major reforms.[54]

In the United States, political power is dispersed—divided between the executive (the government), the legislative body, and the judiciary—rather than concentrated, making it more difficult for the government to push through controversial reforms. In parliamentary democracies, the government represents a majority party or coalition in the parliament, creating a greater concentration of political power and fewer opportunities for blocking legislation that the government supports.

In the United States, the government (headed by the president or a governor) gains office through a winner-take-all election that reduces the opportunity for third parties to influence policy, quite a different situation from parliamentary systems. The winner-take-all provision encourages parties to "market" themselves to the broadest part of the electorate and discourages formation of political parties with coherent policy or political commitments.

These systemic conditions make U.S. political parties weak institutions. They are organized as loose coalitions and more focused on fundraising than on policy guidance. The weakness of political parties opens the door widely to interest group influence in the policy process. The influence of interest groups has been greatly enhanced by the growing dominance of expensive television advertising in political campaigns and the dependence of parties and candidates on large donations from interest groups, corporations, and individuals with resources to give.[55] Thus, a political party that "controls" the White House and the Congress—as the Democrats did in 1993 and 1994—lacks coherence and a means of enforcing its policy platform. In parliamentary democracies, parties have more political coherence and more leverage over legislators elected as part of the party slate.

Compounding the weakness of parties, labor unions in the United States historically have played a more modest political role than they do in other industrial democracies. In most parliamentary democracies, the power of the labor-controlled party, clearly representing working families and individuals, was a critical factor in enacting national health insurance. In the United States, throughout the twentieth century and at the beginning of the current century, labor tied itself to the Democratic Party, which it influences but does not control. In contrast to labor's relatively weak role, business-oriented interest groups in the United States assert a broad and powerful influence and have repeatedly undermined or vetoed efforts to enact national health insurance.

Finally, the United States has a very ingrained political culture that supports weak government, a tradition that goes back to the very founding of this country. The United States has never developed either a strong civil service or a tradition of people looking to government to solve social problems—a different set of popular expectations than prevail in other industrial democracies.

There are additional political and economic barriers for states that try to tackle these problems outside a national framework. ERISA limits states' ability to regulate employer health and welfare benefit programs. Limited state fiscal resources create competition among constituencies and interest groups, especially when the state's fiscal condition is tight—and state residents who lack health insurance coverage tend not to be among the more influential political groups. Elected officials fear raising taxes, which would be needed to fund a health insurance subsidy, because higher taxes may encourage some businesses to move to other states or countries, and a vote for higher taxes certainly would be a weapon in a challenger's hands at the next election. Finally, many elected officials worry that generous public subsidies for health insurance coverage will attract a lot of low-income people to move to the state.

In the Twenty-First Century: Important Roles for Research and Policy

The new century brought no signs of improvement in our system of providing and paying for health care coverage. If anything, health insurance coverage appears to be continuing its long and bumpy slide. Employer-funded health insurance seems to respond to changes in the economy but otherwise shows little evidence of expansion to uninsured working families. Changes in the labor market—the decline in manufacturing, the increase in low-wage service-sector jobs, and the increasing use of temporary and part-time employment arrangements—and the decline in real (inflation-adjusted) income among working families and individuals have, over time, eroded the foundation of the nation's voluntary private health insurance system. Many employers are increasing employee contributions for health benefits, especially for family coverage, which makes the employee contribution increasingly unaffordable for low-wage workers and contributes to growing the ranks of the uninsured. In the long run, these structural changes are likely to undermine our reliance on private employment-based health insurance.

Compounding this diminishing private insurance coverage, recent declines in Medicaid coverage have offset the small gains in private insurance that resulted from improved employment in the strong economy. The growing number and proportion of the population who are completely uninsured place enormous burdens on those individuals and families, who must cope with reduced access and increased personal expense. But this problem also burdens others who help pay for whatever health services the uninsured receive; this includes employers and employees, who pay for private health insurance; and state and local taxpayers, who bear the financial burden of public hospitals and clinics for the medically indigent.

SCHIP and other modest public-sector incremental reforms help states address these problems. Taken together, SCHIP and Medicaid provide expanded federal and state resources to cover uninsured working families and (with ingenuity) individuals. The critical question is whether there is sufficient political will to maximize the use of these resources and to extend affordable coverage to the entire population for good access to quality health care.

Despite the many political challenges, there is support for government to expand and strengthen health insurance coverage. Americans express strong support for universal coverage, although support for any particular approach is thin. In an election-focused public opinion poll in 2000, seven in ten adults said the federal government should help increase the number of Americans covered by health insurance, but only 38 percent were willing to pay additional taxes for a major government program to cover all of the uninsured.[56] Nevertheless, administration and congressional proposals to use federal funds to expand coverage receive broad support, and a number of states, including some with Republican governors such as Wisconsin, have been taking significant steps to cover their uninsured residents. The path to universal coverage in the United States may well be through federal support and incentives to states to develop their own strategies to cover their entire populations.[57] It almost certainly will require a strong grassroots campaign by a broad coalition that favors it, including senior citizens groups, consumer organizations, women's organizations, people of color, and labor unions, which have recently been undergoing a revitalization and resurgence.

Health services research continues to be important to help policy makers and the public understand the impact of these trends. Health services research has played an important role in identifying gaps in insurance coverage, monitoring the effects of those gaps, and modeling the impact of reform options on coverage and costs. The devolution of responsibilities for funding and oversight of publicly financed programs enhances the importance of state- and local-level studies. In addition, studies of the effects of devolution and related policy changes on low-income populations and ethnic and racial minorities—especially studies that examine differences across states and local areas—are particularly important.

Studies of the effect of the type of insurance plan on access and on the process and quality of care become increasingly important as managed care and market-based prices dominate the health care field. The shift of both public and private purchasers to managed care exposes the gaps in knowledge about which aspects of managed care promote effective use of services and which impede appropriate use.[58]

Policy interventions are needed to shore up growing gaps in coverage. Health services research is needed to inform policy analyses and development. Whether solutions are developed at the state or the federal level, through private-sector insurance and financing or through public programs and taxes, with social insurance programs such as Medicare or means-tested programs such as Medicaid and SCHIP, the United States cannot escape the need for fundamental reforms that extend coverage to its entire population.

Notes

1. Aday, L., Andersen, R. and Fleming, G. V. *Health Care in the U.S.: Equitable for Whom?* Thousand Oaks, Calif.: Sage, 1980; Aday, L., Begley, C. E., Lairson, D. R., and Slater, C. H. *Evaluating the Health Care System: Effectiveness, Efficiency and Equity.* (2nd ed.) Chicago: Health Administration Press, 1998; Marquis, M. S., and Long, S. H. "Reconsidering the Effect of Medicaid on Health Care Services Use." *Health Services Research,* 1996, *30,* 791–808; and Lurie, N., and others. "Termination of Medi-Cal Benefits: A Follow-up Study One Year Later." *New England Journal of Medicine,* 1986, *314,* 1266–1268.
2. Measurement differences (between surveys in questions asked, and changes in questions over time within the same repeated survey) make it difficult to track rates over the years. The data reported here are from a series of surveys that were conducted by the same federal agency (the Agency for Healthcare Research and Quality, which operated under a series of names during this period) and used similar methodologies, thus increasing the comparability of the estimates during this twenty-year period.

3. Estimates in this paragraph are from the Current Population Survey, conducted by the U.S. Census Bureau.

4. Author's analysis of March 1999 Current Population Survey.

5. Author's analysis of March 1999 Current Population Survey.

6. Author's analysis of March 1999 Current Population Survey.

7. Mueller, M. S. "Private Health Insurance in 1973: A Review of Coverage, Enrollment, and Financial Experience." *Social Security Bulletin*, Feb. 1975, *38*, 21–40; Mueller, M. S. "Private Health Insurance in 1975: A Review of Coverage, Enrollment, and Financial Experience." *Social Security Bulletin*, June 1977, *40*, 3–21; Cambridge Research Institute. *Trends Affecting the U.S. Health Care System*. Washington, D.C.: Health Resources Administration, 1976.

8. Author's analysis of March 1995 and 1999 Current Population Survey.

9. Estimates for some years vary, depending on the data source. The estimates in this paragraph are from Cooper, P. F., and Steinberg Schone, B. "More Offers, Fewer Takers for Employment-Based Health Insurance: 1987 and 1996." *Health Affairs*, 1997, *16*(6), 142–149. See also Rice, T., and others. *Trends in Job-Based Health Insurance Coverage*. Los Angeles: UCLA Center for Health Policy Research, 1998; and Farber, H. S., and Levy, H. "Recent Trends in Employment-Sponsored Health Insurance Coverage: Are Bad Jobs Getting Worse?" (Working paper.) Princeton University Industrial Relations Section, July 1998.

10. Fronstin, P. "The Erosion of Employment-Based Health Insurance: Costs, Structural and Non-Structural Changes in the Economy." Paper presented at annual meeting of the American Public Health Association, Nov. 1997; U.S. General Accounting Office. *Employment-Based Health Insurance: Costs Increase and Family Coverage Decreases*. GAO/HEHS-97-35. Washington, D.C.: U.S. General Accounting Office, Feb. 1997; Kronick, R., and Gilmer, T. "Explaining the Decline in Health Insurance Coverage, 1979–1995." Unpublished paper, Oct. 1997.

11. Employer Health Benefits. *1999 Annual Survey*. Menlo Park, Calif.: Kaiser Family Foundation, and Health Research and Educational Trust, Oct. 1999.

12. Author's analysis of March 1999 Current Population Survey.

13. Author's analysis of February 1999 Current Population Survey.

14. Somers, H. W., and Somers, A. R. *Doctors, Patients and Health Insurance*. Washington, D.C.: Brookings Institution, 1961.

15. Marmor, T. R. *The Politics of Medicare*. Chicago: Aldine, 1970; Starr, P. *The Social Transformation of American Medicine*. New York: Basic Books, 1982.

16. Stevens, R., and Stevens, R. *Welfare Medicine in America: A Case Study of Medicaid*. New York: Free Press, 1974.

17. *Medicare: A Brief Summary*. Baltimore, Md.: Health Care Financing Administration Website. [www.hcfa.gov/medicare/medicare.htm]

18. Mitchell, J. B., and Khandker, R. K. "Black-White Treatment Differences in Acute Myocardial Infarction." *Health Care Financing Review*, 1995, *17*, 61–70; Davis, K. "Equal Treatment and Unequal Benefits: The Medicare Program." *Milbank Memorial Fund Quarterly/Health and Society*, 1975, *53*, 449–488; Long, S. H., and Settle, R. F. "Medicare and the Disadvantaged Elderly: Objectives and Outcomes." *Milbank Memorial Fund Quarterly/Health and Society*, 1984, *62*, 609–656; Link, C. R., Long, S. H., and Settle, R. F. *"Equity and the Utilization of Health Services by the Medicare Elderly." Journal of Human Resources*, 1982, *17*, 195–212; Physician Payment Review Commission (PPRC). *Annual Report to Congress, 1994*. Washington, D.C.: Physician Payment Review Commission, 1994; Wenneker, M. B.,

and Epstein, A. M. "Racial Inequalities in the Use of Procedures for Patients with Ischemic Heart Disease in Massachusetts." *Journal of the American Medical Association*, 1989, *261*, 253–257; McBean, A. M., and Gornick, M. "Differences by Race in the Rates of Procedures Performed in Hospitals for Medicare Beneficiaries." *Health Care Financing Review*, 1994, *15*, 77–90; Ayanian, J. Z., and others. "Acute Myocardial Infarction: Process of Care and Clinical Outcomes." *Journal of the American Medical Association*, 1993, *269*, 2642–2646.

19. *A Profile of Medicare: Chart Book*. Baltimore, Md.: Health Care Financing Administration, May 1998, Figures 15 and 52; and *1998 Data Compendium*. Baltimore. Md.: Health Care Financing Administration, Aug. 1998.

20. Medicaid: A Brief Summary. Washington, D.C.: Health Care Financing Administration Website.

21. Health Resources Administration (HRA). *Health of the Disadvantaged. Chart Book II*. DHHS Pub. No. (HRA) 80-633. Washington, D.C.: U.S. Government Printing Office, Sep. 1980; Aday, L., and Andersen, R. "Equity of Access to Medical Care: A Conceptual and Empirical Overview." In *Securing Access to Health Care: The Ethical Implications of Differences in the Availability of Health Services*. Washington, D.C.: President's Commission for the Study of Ethical Problems in Medicine and Biomedical and Behavioral Research, 1983, *3*, 19–54.

22. Berk, M. L., Schur, C. L., and Cantor, J. C. "Ability to Obtain Health Care: Recent Estimates from the Robert Wood Johnson Foundation National Access to Care Survey." *Health Affairs*, Fall 1995, *14*(3), 139–146; Schoen, C., and others. "Insurance Matters for Low Income Adults: Results from a Five State Survey." *Health Affairs*, 1997, *16*(5), 163–171; Millman, M. (ed.). *Access to Health Care in America*. Washington, D.C.: National Academy Press, Institute of Medicine, 1993; Newacheck, P. "Access to Ambulatory Care for Poor Persons." *Health Services Research*, 1988, *23*, 401–419; Wilensky, G. R., and Berk, M. L. "Health Care, the Poor, and the Role of Medicaid." *Health Affairs*, 1982, *1*, 93–100; and Kasper, J. D. "Health Status and Utilization: Differences by Medicaid Coverage and Income." *Health Care Financing Review*, Summer 1986, *7*, 1–17.

23. Lurie, N., Ward, N. B., Shapiro, M. F., and Brook, R. H. "Termination from Medi-Cal: Does It Affect Health?" *New England Journal of Medicine*, 1984, *311*, 480–484; Lurie, N., and others. "Termination of Medi-Cal Benefits: A Follow-up Study One Year Later." *New England Journal of Medicine*, 1986, *314*, 1266–1268.

24. Eligibility information from Guyer, J., and Mann, C. *Employed But Not Insured*. Washington, D.C.: Center on Budget and Policy Priorities, Feb. 1999; other information from "Medicaid: A Brief Summary." Baltimore, Md.: Health Care Financing Administration Website.

25. Rowland, D., Lyons, B., and Edwards, J. *Annual Review of Public Health*, 1988, *9*, 427–450; Rosenbaum, S., and Darnell, J. *Medicaid Section 1115 Demonstration Waivers: Approved and Proposed Activities as of November 1994*. Washington, D.C.: Kaiser Commission on the Future of Medicaid, 1994.

26. General Accounting Office. *Medicaid Prenatal Care: States Improve Access and Enhance Services, But Face New Challenges*. GAO/HEHS-94-152BR. Washington, D.C.: U.S. General Accounting Office, May 1994.

27. Loranger, L., and Lipson, D. *The Medicaid Expansions for Pregnant Women and Children*. Washington, D.C.: Alpha Center, 1995.

28. Author's analysis of March 1995 and 1999 Current Population Survey data.

29. Krebs-Carter, M., and Holahan, J. *State Strategies for Covering Uninsured Adults*. Discussion paper. Washington, D.C.: Urban Institute, Feb. 2000.

30. Perry, M. J., Stark E., and Valdez R. B. *Barriers to Medi-Cal Enrollment and Ideas for Improving Enrollment: Findings from Eight Focus Groups in California with Parents of Potentially Eligible Children.* Menlo Park, Calif.: Henry J. Kaiser Family Foundation, 1998.

31. For evidence of Medicaid's stigmatizing welfare image, see Perry, Stark and Valdez (1998).

32. U.S. Congress. *Reducing the Deficit: Spending and Revenue Options.* Washington, D.C.: Congressional Budget Office, Mar. 1997.

33. *Medicaid and Managed Care. Fact sheet.* Washington, D.C.: Kaiser Commission on Medicaid and the Uninsured, June 1999.

34. "States with Comprehensive Health Care Reform Demonstrations." Dec. 31, 1999. Washington, D.C.: Health Care Financing Administration Website.

35. Rosenbaum, S., Shin, P., Markus, A., and Darnell, J. *Health Centers' Role as Safety Net Providers for Medicaid Patients and the Uninsured.* Washington, D.C.: Kaiser Commission on Medicaid and the Uninsured, Feb. 2000.

36. General Accounting Office. *Better Controls Needed for Health Maintenance Organizations Under Medicaid in California.* B-164031. Washington, D.C.: U.S. General Accounting Office, Sept. 10, 1974; D'Onofrio, C. N., and Mullen, P. D. "Consumer Problems with Prepaid Health Plans in California." *Public Health Reports,* 1977, *92,* 121–134; General Accounting Office. *Medicaid: Oversight of Health Maintenance Organizations in the Chicago Area.* GAO/HRD-90-81. Washington, D.C.: U.S. General Accounting Office, Aug. 27, 1990.

37. Rosenbaum, Shin, Markus, and Darnell (2000); Kaiser Commission on the Future of Medicaid. *Medicaid and Managed Care: Lessons from the Literature.* Menlo Park, Calif.: Henry J. Kaiser Family Foundation, 1995; and General Accounting Office. *Medicaid: States Turn to Managed Care to Improve Access and Control Costs.* GAO/HRD-93-46. Washington, D.C.: U.S. General Accounting Office, Mar. 1993.

38. Guyer, J., and Mann, C. *Taking the Next Step: States Can Now Take Advantage of Federal Medicaid Matching Funds to Expand Health Care Coverage to Low-Income Working Parents.* Washington, D.C.: Center on Budget and Policy Priorities, Aug. 1998. See also section 1931(b)(2)(c) of the Social Security Act.

39. Krebs-Carter and Holahan (2000).

40. Thorpe, K. "Expanding Employment-Based Health Insurance: Is Small Group Reform the Answer?" *Inquiry,* 1992, *29,* 128–136.

41. Riley, T. "State Health Reform and the Role of 1115 Waivers." *Health Care Financing Review,* 1995, *16,* 139–149.

42. Employer Health Benefits. *1999 Annual Survey,* Menlo Park, Calif.: Kaiser Family Foundation, and Health Research and Educational Trust, Oct. 1999. See also Small Business Administration. *The State of Small Business: A Report of the President.* Washington, D.C.: U.S. Government Printing Office, 1987.

43. Long, S. H., and Marquis, S. M. "Pooled Purchasing: Who Are the Players?" *Health Affairs,* July–Aug. 1999, *18,* 105–111.

44. Butler, P. *ERISA Preemption Primer.* Washington, D.C.: Alpha Center, and National Academy for State Health Policy, 2000.

45. Freudenheim, M. "States Shelving Ambitious Plans on Health Care." *New York Times,* July 2, 1995, pp.1, 14.

46. Starr (1982).

47. Fuchs, V. R., and Hahn, J. S. "How Does Canada Do It? A Comparison of Expenditures for Physicians' Services in the United States and Canada." *New England Journal of Medicine,* 1990, *323,* 884–890; Evans, R. G., Lomas, J., Barer, M. L., and others. "Controlling

Health Expenditures: the Canadian Reality." *New England Journal of Medicine*, 1989, *320*, 571–577; U.S. Congressional Budget Office. *Single-Payer and All-Payer Health Insurance Systems Using Medicare's Payment Rates. CBO Staff Memorandum.* Washington, D.C.: U.S. Congressional Budget Office, Apr. 1993; Woolhandler, S., and Himmelstein, D. U. "The Deteriorating Administrative Efficiency of the U.S. Health Care System." *New England Journal of Medicine*, 1991, *324*, 1253–1258; General Accounting Office. *Canadian Health Insurance: Lessons for the United States.* GAO/HRD-91-90. Washington, D.C.: U.S. Government Accounting Office, June 1991; and Hayes, G. J., Hayes, C., and Dykstra, T. "Physicians Who Have Practiced in Both the U.S. and Canada Compare Systems." *American Journal of Public Health*, 1993, *83*, 1544–1548.

48. Iglehart, J. K. "Revisiting the Canadian Health Care System." *New England Journal of Medicine*, 2000, *342*, 2007–2012; Donelan, K., and others. "The Cost of Health System Change: Public Discontent in Five Nations." *Health Affairs*, May-June 1999, *18*, 206–216.

49. Bills introduced into the U.S. Senate by Paul Wellstone and into the House of Representatives by Jim McDermott and John Conyers to create a Canadian-style single-payer system, and the bill introduced into the House of Representatives by Pete Stark to make Medicare universally available.

50. Blendon, R. J., and Taylor, H. "Views on Health Care: Public Opinion in Three Nations." *Health Affairs*, Spring 1989, *8*, 149–157.

51. Cantor, J. C., and others. "Business Leaders' Views on American Health Care." *Health Affairs*, 1991, *10*, 98–105.

52. Rosenblatt, R. A. "Business Groups Plead for Health-Care Support." *Los Angeles Times*, Nov. 16, 1989, p. A20.

53. West, M. W., Heith, D., and Goodwin, C. "Harry and Louise Go to Washington: Political Advertising and Health Care Reform." *Journal of Health Politics, Policy and Law*, 1996, *21*, 35–68; Podhorzer, M. "Unhealthy Money: Health Reform and the 1994 Elections." *International Journal of Health Services*, 1995, *25*, 393–401; and *Well-Healed: Inside Lobbying for Health Care Reform.* Washington, D.C.: Center for Public Integrity, 1994.

54. See Weissert, C. S., and Weissert, W. G. *Governing Health: The Politics of Health Policy.* Baltimore, Md.: Johns Hopkins University Press, 1996; Skocpol, T. *Boomerang: Clinton's Health Security Effort and the Turn Against Government in U.S. Politics.* New York: Norton, 1996; Morone, J. A. *The Democratic Wish: Popular Participation and the Limits of American Government.* New York: Basic Books, 1990; Navarro, V. "Why Some Countries Have National Health Insurance, Others Have National Health Services, and the U.S. Has Neither." *Social Science and Medicine*, 1989 *28*, 887–898; Rothman, D. J. "A Century of Failure: Health Care Reform in America." *Journal of Health Politics, Policy and Law*, 1993, *18*, 271–286.

55. Corrado, A., and others (eds.). *Campaign Finance Reform: A Sourcebook.* Washington, D.C.: Brookings Institution, 1997.

56. Morin, R., and Broder, D. S. "A Health Care Muddle." *Washington Post*, July 28, 2000, p. A01; McGregor, D. "Deciphering the Polls on the Health Issue." *Congressional Quarterly Weekly Report*, 1994, *52*, 1846; Blendon, R. J., and Brodie, M. "Public Opinion and Health Policy." In T. J. Litman and L. S. Robins (eds.), *Health Politics and Policy.* (3rd ed.) Albany, N.Y.: Delmar, 1997.

57. See "The Health Security for All Americans Act" (S. 2888, 106th Congress) by Sen. Paul Wellstone (D-Minn.).

58. Bindman, A. B., and Gold, M. R. (eds.). "Measuring Access to Care Through Population-Based Surveys in a Managed Care Environment." *Health Services Research*, 1998, *3* part 2, 33.

PART TWO

COSTS OF HEALTH CARE

CHAPTER THREE

MEASURING HEALTH CARE COSTS AND TRENDS

Thomas H. Rice

In 1996, U.S. health care expenditures eclipsed the $1 trillion mark. It is difficult to fathom such a large number. To put it in perspective, suppose you lined up a trillion dollar bills end to end. They would stretch all the way to the sun![1]

This chapter focuses on how these health care expenditures are measured and then discusses the trends. It concludes with a discussion of whether health care cost control is even necessary, as a bridge to the following chapter, where particular strategies are evaluated. Although data and measurement may seem a bit pedestrian to the analyst interested in proceeding quickly to policy issues, this is an unfortunate viewpoint. Accurate data on national health care spending are necessary in order to enact appropriate health policy reforms. (A blunter reason for accurate data that may ring true to the policy analyst comes from computer programming: "garbage in, garbage out.") Once these tools are in hand, Chapter Four can analyze alternative methods of containing health care expenditures.

Measuring Health Care Expenditures

As just noted, understanding measurement is essential if one is to fully appreciate many issues that are currently in the forefront of health policy. To give one example, debate continues about whether the United States, a country that relies more heavily than others on markets in its health care system, has been as successful as other countries in controlling health expenditures during the 1990s. Resolution of this ostensibly straightforward issue would yield insights as to the potential savings or losses, if any, that might accrue if the United States adopted some aspects of other countries' organization and financing systems. But to ascertain an accurate answer to this question, it is necessary to understand how health expenditures are compiled in various countries as well as how they can be compared.[2] This section of the chapter discusses a number of key issues concerning measurement of health care expenditures.

Expenditures Versus Costs

Most policy discussions employ the term *costs* rather than *expenditures*; indeed, the next chapter also adopts this convenience. It is important to understand that the two concepts are hardly the same.

Expenditures, of course, mean how much is spent on a particular thing. As discussed in Chapter Four, in a fee-for-service system expenditures are simply the product of unit prices and the quantity of goods or services purchased. Total expenditures can then be broken down in a number of ways, such as by type of service (for example, hospital expenditures, physician expenditures) or by payer source (private insurers, Medicare, out-of-pocket).

In contrast, costs apply to the *production* process. Specifically, the term *costs* refers to the value of resources used in producing a good or service. There are two distinct definitions of cost: accounting and economic. The *accounting* definition includes only the value of the resources used in production (that is, labor and capital). The difference between the sales revenue from a good or service and the accounting cost is defined as net revenue or profit.

This differs from the *economic* definition of cost. To an economist, the term includes not only the value of resources expended in the production process but in addition a "normal" return on investment.[3] Using their definition, economists predict that in a competitive market profit levels are near zero—that is, a typically efficient producer garners only a normal rate of return on investment. The persistence of economic profit levels far above zero over a long period of time may indicate the existence of "market failure," which in turn might call for government policy intervention.

Accounting and economic profits are therefore related to each other. The latter is approximately equal to the former minus a normal rate of return on investment.[4] But both definitions of cost differ from the definition of expenditure. The distinction is shown in Figure 3.1; for simplicity, we use the economic definition of cost and compare that to the definition of expenditure. In the figure,

FIGURE 3.1.   DISTINCTION BETWEEN ACCOUNTING AND ECONOMIC PROFITS.

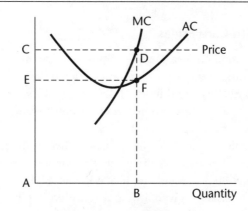

the horizontal axis shows the quantity of a particular good or service; the vertical axis, sales prices and production costs. MC refers to marginal costs—the cost of producing the last unit of output. AC is average cost of output, and Price is the selling price. Both of the cost curves include a normal rate of return on investment.

Health care *expenditures* are equal to the rectangle ABCD, which is simply the selling price multiplied by the quantity sold, AB. In contrast, economic costs are shown by a smaller rectangle, ABEF; this is average costs (AE) multiplied by the quantity sold (AB). In this example, expenditure exceeds cost by the rectangle CDEF. This implies that excess profits are being obtained by firms in the industry. Other firms therefore may be stimulated to enter the market to reap these profits, which in turn may drive down price and restore profit to a normal level. If this does not occur, then some form of government intervention may be necessary to correct market failure.

With these distinctions in mind, we can address the question of whether we should spend most of our effort analyzing health care cost or expenditure. Although both are useful, analyses of the entire health care system turn out to be considerably easier to conduct using the concept of expenditure. This is because it is extremely difficult to obtain reliable data on cost; private firms are rarely expected to report their internal cost data to any sort of governmental body. One exception is Medicare hospital costs, because such data are collected by the federal government. But for other sectors, such as physician care, pharmaceuticals, and the like (and for services that are covered by private insurers rather than Medicare and Medicaid), reliable data on costs are exceedingly difficult to obtain. The remainder of this chapter, then, focuses on measurement and trends in health care expenditure rather than cost. First, however, we discuss measuring changes in unit price.

Measuring Health Care Prices

The most common measure of health care prices in the United States is the medical care component of the Consumer Price Index (CPI). The CPI, which is published monthly by the Bureau of Labor Statistics, provides information on the *change* in prices charged to urban consumers for a variety of consumer goods and consumers.[5]

To obtain the index, the CPI begins with a common "market basket" of goods and services. The monthly price data are obtained from urban localities that represent about 80 percent of the U.S. population. To form the index, each item in the market basket is given a weight representing its relative importance in the spending patterns of urban consumers. An index is then formed that compares the change in prices in a current time period to a base period (usually 1982–1984) whose index value is set to a value of 100. For example, in 1998 the medical care component of the CPI had a value of 242.1, which means that medical care prices were two-and-a-half times what they were during the base period.

As shown later in this chapter when trends are presented, the medical care component of the CPI is further subdivided into several categories, making it possible to monitor inflation in various health related markets. The two main subcategories are medical care services and medical care commodities. Within services, there are separate indices constructed for physicians' services, dental services, eye care, other medical professionals, hospital rooms, other inpatient services, and hospital outpatient services. Within commodities, separate indices exist for prescription drugs, over-the-counter drugs and medical supplies, internal and respiratory over-the-counter drugs, and medical equipment and supplies.

There are a number of limitations to the CPI.[6] First, and perhaps most important, the CPI measures change in price, not in expenditure. It does not take into account change in the quantity of services provided, only the price.

Second, the CPI measures changes in prices, not price levels. The index cannot be used to compare difference in health care prices among parts of the country. Suppose, for example, that in 1998 the medical component of the CPI was 295 in New York City, and 270 in Los Angeles. All that one could say is that prices rose faster in New York than Los Angeles since the base year in which the index was set to 100. It cannot be concluded that health care prices necessarily are lower in Los Angeles than New York.

Third, the CPI measures the price charged, not the price received by a producer. This is a critical distinction because of the prevalence of discounts offered by providers to managed care plans such as preferred provider organizations (PPOs). In some competitive parts of the country, such as California, providers' list or billed charges are illusory; almost no one pays them. However, these prices are exactly what is measured by the CPI. What this means is that the CPI might overstate the amount of medical care inflation in certain parts of the country because, over time, the true price of care has deviated further below the billed charge.

Fourth, the CPI measures changes in price for a *fixed market basket of consumer goods.* In fact, the entire notion of the CPI is based on the existence of such an "apples to apples" comparison. By using a standard market basket of goods, it is possible to determine how price alone has changed. But this also leads to two difficulties. First, people *do* change their consumption habits over time, so the market basket being measured by the CPI may become increasingly irrelevant. The Bureau of Labor Statistics (BLS), the federal agency responsible for the index, is dealing with this problem by updating the composition of the market basket more frequently than it had previously. The second difficulty is that the CPI does not take into account change in the quality of goods and services produced—although again, BLS is currently grappling with this problem. To illustrate this issue, note that an increase in per diem hospital charges over the last twenty years is likely to be exaggerated by the CPI. Over this period, hospital rooms have become much more expensive not only from inflation but also because of enhancements in the type of service and facility available to the hospital patient. In theory, the CPI should hold these changes constant and only look at price inflation of hospital care of a given quality. This has not been the practice, however.

Fifth, the CPI measures only changes in consumers' expenditures (premiums plus out-of-pocket payments). If, as in the case of hospital care, a majority of expenditures are not paid out of pocket, then the index does not capture the majority of underlying inflation. This could bias the index figures because there has been a gradual movement away from out-of-pocket expenditure toward more employer and government payment, which is not included in the CPI.[7]

These caveats are not meant as criticism; any differently configured index would raise a host of other problems. Rather, the limitations of the CPI must simply be understood when using the index.

Measuring Expenditures

This section examines U.S. expenditures and international comparisons.

U.S. Expenditures. There are many sources of data on U.S. health expenditure; space does not permit separate discussion of each. Rather, we focus on the primary source: the national health accounts produced by the Office of the Actuary of the Health Care Financing Administration (HCFA), which is housed in the U.S. Department of Health and Human Services. Trends in these data are presented later in the chapter.

Data on U.S. national health expenditures are published regularly—usually annually—in the *Health Care Financing Review*.[8] The data for one year can be viewed best as a matrix. Each row of the matrix represents the group that spends the money, whereas each column indicates the provider of services that receives the funds.[9] (An example is presented later in the chapter, as Table 3.5.) A cell in the matrix therefore represents how much a particular payer (for example, a private insurer) spends on a specific service (say, hospital care). Because these same data are compiled annually, by comparing the matrices of several years one can calculate the rate of change in expenditure in various components of the health care sector.

When viewing the matrix, one might think that the data come from a single, consistent source. They do not. Literally dozens of sources are used to piece the matrices together. Some of the data are collected in a relatively systematic fashion, but others are not. For example, data from the Medicare program are systemically collected by HCFA through the Medicare Statistical System (MSS). One file in the MSS, the hospital insurance claims file, contains information on each beneficiary's spending for Part A (hospital) services, while the supplementary Medicare insurance file includes similar data for Part B (primarily physician) services. Although somewhat more unwieldy, Medicaid data are also collected from the states in a consistent format by HCFA.

But because there are no national data collection requirements for private insurers, other aspects of the matrices have to be pieced together from multiple data sources. Some are more systematic than others. Hospital expenditures, for example, largely come from a single source: the American Hospital Association's annual survey of hospitals. But out-of-pocket expenditures come from any number of sources: a consumer expenditures survey, conducted by the Bureau of Labor Statistics; periodic surveys of nursing homes, conducted by the National Center for Health Statistics; surveys about home health care, conducted by the Visiting Nurse Association; physician and dentist surveys, conducted by the American Medical Association and the American Dental Association; data about outpatient clinic services, collected by the Bureau of the Census; and information about Community Health Centers, collected by the Health Resources and Services Administration.[10] As discussed at the end of the chapter, the lack of a consistent data source makes it difficult to successfully administer certain types of health care reform, particularly regulatory ones such as national expenditure targets.

Over the years, there have been various revisions to the national health accounts. The most noteworthy ones, which applied to the estimates beginning in 1988, employed new data sources and produced a higher level of detail. An account of the changes made, as well as a detailed discussion of the data sources that are currently being used, can be found in the Summer 1990 issue of the *Health Care Financing Review.*[11]

There are, nevertheless, a number of problems, most of which are caused by the lack of source data:

- The accounts are unable to distinguish between some inpatient and outpatient expenditures (for example, salaried physician care counted as hospital rather than physician expenditure).
- Premium expenditures by consumers (Medicare Part B payments, private insurance premiums) are included as payment made by insurers rather than as out-of-pocket expenditure by consumers.
- Some capital expenditures are double-counted.

These and other issues, as well as recommendations for improving the accounts, are discussed in a report published by an HCFA technical advisory panel.[12]

International Comparisons. The primary source of data on international health care spending for more than two dozen developed (and some developing) countries is collected by the Organization for Economic Cooperation and Development (OECD), which is based in Paris. These data are published in periodic articles in the journal *Health Affairs.*[13] Data from the OECD database are presented later in the chapter.

The previous discussion about U.S. health expenditures focused on the lack of a consistent data source. As can be imagined, the problem of lacking consistent data is even greater when one compares data from two dozen countries. Those who compile the OECD data have attempted to make them reliable by disseminating definitions of key terms as well as common accounting principles to all member countries. Nevertheless, one must use a great deal of caution in employing the data because of differences in definition, source of data, and variation in accuracy among the countries.

Among the areas of particular concern:

- How countries distinguish between health and social services.[14] Some, for example, may classify certain domiciliary care to the elderly as health, while others might not.

- How countries distinguish between hospital and long-term care. In some countries the distinction between the two is much finer than in the United States, with more long-term care being provided in hospitals.
- Accurate conversion of numerous currencies to a common unit. This is typically done through purchasing power parities (PPPs), which are "indices that relate the prices of a market basket of goods in one country to the prices in a comparative group of countries."[15] For this reason, it is probably safer to rely on figures pertaining to the *proportion* of a country's national income devoted to health than to an absolute monetary amount.
- Underreporting of certain categories of expenditure by some countries, which is due in part to data limitations.

Schieber and Poullier, who have published the OECD data for many years, have responded to various criticisms of the data by noting that "these data have the advantage of being based on an internationally accepted functional classification; receiving direct comment and input from the statistical offices of the countries; and having methodology, sources, and underlying assumptions widely disseminated."[16]

Trends in Health Care Expenditure

This section is divided into three parts: trends in prices, U.S. expenditures, and international expenditures.

U.S. Prices

Table 3.1 presents the values for the major components of the CPI from 1975 to 1998, while Table 3.2 shows the corresponding annual rates of change.[17] Tables 3.3 and 3.4 present similar data for the items that make up the medical care component of the CPI.

Beginning with Tables 3.1 and 3.2, we see that since 1975 medical care prices have grown far faster than others in the U.S. economy. Between 1975 and 1998, they rose more than fivefold, whereas the index as a whole increased only threefold, and the other components listed grew less than threefold. The pattern is most pronounced in the early years; between 1975 and 1985 medical prices rose by 140 percent, compared to 100 percent for the CPI as a whole. The last three years shown—1995 through 1998—are a noticeable departure from the previous trends. During these three years, medical prices rose by a total of only 10 percent, not much higher than the 7 percent increase for the CPI as a whole.

TABLE 3.1. CONSUMER PRICE INDEX (CPI) FOR ALL ITEMS: UNITED STATES, SELECTED YEARS, 1976–1998.

Year	All Items	Medical Care	Food	Apparel	Housing	Energy
		Consumer Price Index				
1975	53.8	47.5	59.8	72.5	50.7	42.1
1980	82.4	74.9	86.8	90.9	81.1	86.0
1985	107.6	113.5	105.6	105.0	107.7	101.6
1990	130.7	162.8	132.4	124.1	128.5	102.1
1991	136.2	177.0	136.3	128.7	133.6	102.5
1992	140.3	190.1	137.9	131.9	137.5	103.0
1993	144.5	201.4	140.9	133.7	141.2	104.2
1994	148.2	211.0	144.9	133.4	144.8	104.6
1995	152.4	220.5	148.4	132.0	148.5	105.2
1996	156.9	228.2	153.3	131.7	152.8	110.1
1997	160.5	234.6	157.3	132.9	156.8	111.5
1998	163.0	242.1	160.7	133.0	160.4	102.9

Source: U.S. Department of Health and Human Services. *Health United States, 1993.* (DHHS publication no. PHS 94-1232.) Hyattsville, Md.: Public Health Service, U.S. Department of Health and Human Services, May 1994), p.221; and U.S. Department of Health and Human Services. *Health United States, 1999.* (DHHS publication no. PHS 99-1232.) Hyattsville, Md.: Public Health Service, U.S. Department of Health and Human Services, Sept. 1999), p.285 (modified by author).

Note: 1982–1984 = 100.

Tables 3.3 and 3.4 show the patterns within the medical care sector. The largest growth rate was for hospital, which increased almost sevenfold in 1995–1996. As mentioned earlier, however, one should be skeptical about this number because the CPI does not do a good job of accounting for the changing nature of the hospital product. What is most noteworthy, however, is the consistently low increase in nearly all medical prices between 1995 and 1998. The only line items experiencing an annual increase in excess of 4 percent were outpatient and dental services; both of these rose by only 4.5 percent annually.

U.S. Expenditures

Table 3.5 presents 1997 data on U.S. health expenditures from the U.S. national health accounts. The rows give information on the source of funds, while the columns indicate the provider of services that received the funds. Some noteworthy aspects of the data:

TABLE 3.2.   ANNUAL CHANGE IN CPI FOR ALL ITEMS: UNITED STATES, SELECTED YEARS, 1975–1998.

Year	All Items	Medical Care	Food	Apparel	Housing	Energy
		Average Annual Percentage Change				
1975–1980	8.9	9.5	7.7	4.6	9.9	15.4
1980–1985	5.5	8.7	4.0	2.9	5.8	3.4
1985–1990	4.0	7.5	4.6	3.4	3.6	0.1
1990–1991	4.2	8.7	2.9	3.7	4.0	0.4
1991–1992	3.0	7.4	1.2	2.5	2.9	0.5
1992–1993	3.0	5.9	2.2	1.4	2.7	1.2
1993–1994	2.6	4.8	2.8	−0.2	2.5	0.3
1994–1995	2.8	4.5	2.4	−1.0	2.6	0.6
1995–1996	3.0	3.5	3.3	−0.2	2.9	4.7
1996–1997	2.3	2.8	2.5	0.9	2.6	1.3
1997–1998	1.6	3.2	2.1	0.1	2.3	−7.7
1990–1995	3.1	6.3	2.3	1.2	2.9	0.6
1995–1998	2.3	3.2	2.7	0.3	2.6	−0.7

Source: U.S. Department of Health and Human Services. *Health United States, 1993.* (DHHS publication no. PHS 94-1232.) Hyattsville, Md.: Public Health Service, U.S. Department of Health and Human Services, May 1994), p.221; and U.S. Department of Health and Human Services. *Health United States, 1999.* (DHHS publication no. PHS 99-1232.) Hyattsville, Md.: Public Health Service, U.S. Department of Health and Human Services, Sept. 1999), p.285 (modified by author).

- Government expenditures account for 45 percent of total health expenditures, 78 percent of which are federal. Government pays far more of the bill for hospital care (61 percent) than physician services (32 percent).
- Although out-of-pocket costs make up, on average, 20 percent of total expenditures, this figure varies tremendously by type of service. It ranges from only 3 percent for hospital care to about 50 percent for dental services, drugs and other medical nondurables, and vision products and other medical durables.
- Private insurance pays a substantial proportion (over 30 percent) of expenditure for hospital, physician, dental, and other professional services, but relatively little (less than 15 percent) for nursing homes, home health, and vision care.

More can be learned by examining trends in U.S. expenditures over time, which are shown in Table 3.6. Between 1975 and 1996, the annual rate of change in health expenditures has typically exceeded a double-digit rate, but since 1996 it has been lower. The period 1990 through 1994 was a transition period, where the inflation rate in medical spending averaged about 8 percent. It was lower than 5 percent from 1995 to 1998.

Item and Medical Care Component	1975	1980	1985	1990	1991	1992	1993	1994	1995	1996	1997	1998
						Consumer Price Index						
CPI, all items	53.8	82.4	107.6	130.7	135.2	140.3	144.5	148.2	152.4	156.9	160.5	163.0
Less medical care	54.3	82.8	107.2	128.8	133.8	137.5	141.2	144.7	148.6	152.8	156.3	158.6
CPI, all services	48.0	77.9	109.9	139.2	146.3	152.0	157.9	163.1	168.7	174.1	179.4	184.2
All medical care	47.5	74.9	113.5	162.8	177.0	190.1	201.4	211.0	220.5	228.2	234.6	242.1
Medical care services	46.6	74.8	113.2	162.7	177.1	190.5	202.9	213.4	224.2	232.4	239.1	246.8
Professional medical services	50.8	77.9	113.5	156.1	165.7	175.8	184.7	192.5	201.0	208.3	215.4	222.2
Physician services	48.1	76.5	113.3	160.8	170.5	181.2	191.3	199.8	208.8	216.4	222.9	229.5
Dental services	53.2	78.9	114.2	155.8	167.4	178.7	188.1	197.1	206.8	216.5	226.6	236.2
Eye care	—	—	—	117.3	121.9	127.0	130.4	133.0	137.0	139.3	141.5	144.1
Services by other medical professionals	—	—	—	120.2	126.6	131.7	135.9	141.3	143.9	146.6	151.8	155.4
Hospital and related services	—	69.2	116.1	178.0	196.1	214.0	231.9	245.6	257.8	269.5	278.4	287.5
Hospital rooms	38.3	68.0	115.4	175.4	191.9	208.7	226.4	239.2	251.2	261.0	—	—
Other inpatient services	—	—	—	142.7	158.0	172.3	185.7	197.1	206.8	216.9	—	—
Outpatient services	—	—	—	138.7	153.4	168.7	184.3	195.0	204.6	215.1	224.9	233.2
Medical care commodities	53.3	75.4	115.2	163.4	176.8	188.1	195.0	200.7	204.5	210.4	215.3	221.8
Prescription drugs	51.2	42.5	120.1	181.7	199.7	214.7	223.0	230.6	235.0	242.9	249.3	258.6

(Continued)

TABLE 3.3. CPI FOR ALL ITEMS AND FOR MEDICAL CARE COMPONENTS: UNITED STATES, SELECTED YEARS, 1975–1998. (Continued)

Item and Medical Care Component	1975	1980	1985	1990	1991	1992	1993	1994	1995	1996	1997	1998
					Consumer Price Index							
Nonprescription drugs and medical supplies	—	—	—	120.6	126.3	131.2	135.5	138.1	140.5	143.1	145.4	147.7
Internal and respiratory over-the-counter drugs	51.8	74.9	112.2	146.9	152.4	158.2	163.5	165.9	167.0	170.2	173.1	175.4
Nonprescription medical equipment and supplies	—	79.2	109.6	138.0	145.0	150.9	155.9	160.0	166.3	169.1	171.5	174.9

Source: U.S. Department of Health and Human Services. *Health United States, 1993.* (DHHS publication no. PHS 94-1232.) Hyattsville, Md.: Public Health Service, U.S. Department of Health and Human Services, May 1994), p.222; and U.S. Department of Health and Human Services. *Health United States, 1999.* (DHHS publication no. PHS 99-1232.) Hyattsville, Md.: Public Health Service, U.S. Department of Health and Human Services, Sept. 1999), p. 285 (modified by author).

TABLE 3.4. AVERAGE ANNUAL CHANGE IN CPI FOR ALL ITEMS AND FOR MEDICAL CARE COMPONENTS: UNITED STATES, SELECTED YEARS, 1975–1998.

Item and Medical Care Component	1975–1980	1980–1985	1985–1990	1990–1991	1991–1992	1992–1993	1993–1994	1994–1995	1995–1996	1996–1997	1997–1998	1990–1995	1995–1998
						Average Annual Percentage Change							
CPI, all items	8.9	5.5	4.0	4.2	3.0	3.0	2.6	2.8	3.0	2.3	1.6	3.1	2.3
Less medical care	8.8	5.3	3.7	3.9	2.8	2.7	2.5	2.7	2.8	2.3	1.5	2.9	2.2
CPI, all services	10.2	7.1	4.8	5.1	3.9	3.9	3.3	3.4	3.2	3.0	2.7	3.9	3.0
All medical care	9.5	8.7	7.5	8.7	7.4	5.9	4.8	4.5	3.5	2.8	3.2	6.3	3.2
Medical care services	9.9	8.6	7.5	8.9	7.6	6.5	5.2	5.1	3.7	2.9	3.2	6.7	3.3
Professional medical services	8.9	7.8	6.6	6.1	6.1	5.1	4.2	4.4	3.6	3.4	3.2	5.2	3.4
Physician services	9.7	8.2	7.3	6.0	6.3	5.6	4.4	4.5	3.6	3.0	3.0	5.4	3.2
Dental services	8.2	7.7	6.4	7.4	6.8	5.3	4.8	4.9	4.7	4.7	4.2	5.8	4.5
Eye care	—	—	—	3.9	4.2	2.7	2.0	3.0	1.7	1.6	1.8	3.2	1.7
Services by other medical professionals	—	—	—	5.3	4.0	3.2	4.0	1.8	1.9	3.5	2.4	3.7	2.6
Hospital and related services	—	10.9	8.9	10.2	9.1	8.4	5.9	5.0	4.5	3.3	3.3	7.7	3.7
Hospital rooms	12.2	11.2	8.7	9.4	8.8	8.5	5.7	5.0	3.9	—	—	7.4	—

(Continued)

TABLE 3.4.   AVERAGE ANNUAL CHANGE IN CPI FOR ALL ITEMS AND FOR MEDICAL CARE COMPONENTS: UNITED STATES, SELECTED YEARS, 1975–1993. (Continued)

Item and Medical Care Component	1975–1980	1980–1985	1985–1990	1990–1991	1991–1992	1992–1993	1993–1994	1994–1995	1995–1996	1996–1997	1997–1998	1990–1995	1995–1998
						Average Annual Percentage Change							
Other inpatient services	—	—	—	10.7	9.1	7.8	6.1	4.9	4.8	—	—	7.7	—
Outpatient services	—	—	—	10.6	10.0	9.2	5.8	4.9	5.1	4.6	3.7	8.1	4.5
Medical care commodities	7.2	8.8	7.2	8.2	6.4	3.7	2.9	1.9	2.9	2.3	3.0	2.4	2.7
Prescription drugs	7.2	10.6	8.6	9.9	7.5	3.9	3.4	1.9	3.4	2.6	3.7	5.3	3.2
Nonprescription drugs and medical supplies	—	—	—	4.7	3.9	3.3	1.9	1.7	1.9	1.6	1.6	3.1	1.7
Internal and respiratory over-the-counter drugs	7.7	8.4	5.4	4.5	3.8	3.4	1.5	0.7	1.9	1.7	1.3	2.6	1.6
Nonprescription medical equipment and supplies	—	6.7	4.7	5.1	4.1	3.3	2.6	3.9	1.7	1.4	2.0	3.8	1.7

Source: U.S. Department of Health and Human Services. *Health United States, 1993*. (DHHS publication no. PHS 94-1232.) Hyattsville, Md.: Public Health Service, U.S. Department of Health and Human Services, May 1994, p.222; and U.S. Department of Health and Human Services. *Health United States, 1999*. (DHHS publication no. PHS 99-1232.) Hyattsville, Md.: Public Health Service, U.S. Department of Health and Human Services, Sept. 1999), p. 285 (modified by author).

TABLE 3.5. PERSONAL HEALTH CARE EXPENDITURES, BY TYPE OF EXPENDITURE AND SELECTED SOURCES OF PAYMENT, 1997.

Source of Payment	Total	Hospital Care	Physician Service	Dental Service	Other Professional Services	Home Health Care	Drugs and Other Medical Nondurables	Vision Products and Other Medical Durables	Nursing Home Care	Other Personal Care
Personal health Care expenditures	969.0	371.1	217.6	50.6	61.9	32.3	108.9	13.9	82.8	29.9
Out-of-pocket payments	187.6	12.4	34.1	23.9	24.6	7.0	53.0	6.8	25.7	—
Private health insurance	313.5	113.0	109.1	24.3	18.9	3.7	39.9	0.5	4.0	—
Other private	35.6	17.2	4.3	0.2	4.8	3.9	—	—	1.6	3.6
Government	432.4	228.4	70.1	2.3	13.6	17.7	16.0	6.6	51.4	26.3
Federal	337.3	185.6	58.4	1.3	10.8	15.4	9.2	6.4	34.5	15.6
State and local	95.1	42.8	11.7	1.0	2.8	2.3	6.8	0.1	16.9	3.6

Note: 0.0 denotes amounts less than $50 million.

Source: Braden, B. R., and others. "Natural Health Expenditures, 1997." *Health Care Financing Review,* Fall 1998, 20, 116.

TABLE 3.6. ANNUAL PERCENTAGE CHANGE IN NATIONAL HEALTH EXPENDITURES, BY SOURCE OF FUNDS: UNITED STATES, SELECTED YEARS, 1975–1993.

Year	All Health Expenditures	Private Funds	Public Funds
1975–1980	13.6	13.6	13.6
1980–1985	11.6	12.3	10.7
1985–1990	10.2	10.3	10.2
1990–1994	7.9	6.0	10.5
1994–1995	4.9	2.6	7.7
1995–1996	4.9	4.2	5.7
1996–1997	4.8	4.3	5.3

Source: U.S. Department of Health and Human Services. *Health United States, 1999.* (DHHS publication no. PHS 99-1232.) Hyattsville, Md.: Public Health Service, U.S. Department of Health and Human Services, Sept. 1999), p. 284 (modified by author).

The other noteworthy trend is the distribution of spending between public and private funds. Until 1990, the annual rate of increase was nearly identical between these two sectors, but since 1990 public expenditure increases have far outpaced private. This stems from a number of causes, most notably cost-containment efforts by private employers and managed care plans (keeping private spending lower) and expansion of the Medicaid program (raising public expenditures).

Analysts have not only studied past trends in expenditures; they have also used simulation models to project what expenditures will be in future years. One recent set of projects was computed by the Health Care Financing Administration.[18] It concluded that the proportion of gross national project accounted for by health expenditures will increase from 13.5 percent in 1997 to 16.2 percent in 2008.

In considering these figures, one should keep in mind that they often turn out to be quite off the mark. For example, in a report published in 1992, the Congressional Budget Office estimated that health expenditures would consume about 18 percent of GDP by the year 2000.[19] The more likely figure is about 14 percent.

Needless to say, accurately projecting health spending is difficult if not impossible. One problem is that, over time, the estimates can become increasingly farfetched. A recent analysis of these issues was conducted by Warshawsky, who concluded that "even the most conservative projections, which assume either robust economic growth, improved demographic trends, or some moderation in health care price inflation, foresee the health care sector consuming more than a quarter of national output by [the year] 2065. If, on the other hand, current relative price trends continue, economic growth remains anemic, demographic trends continue or worsen, or the health care sector becomes a major user of capital, [simulation models] predict that health care expenditures will comprise between a third to a half of national output."[20]

Aside from a number of technical assumptions, the problem with believing these projections is that they assume, on some level at least, a continuation of current expenditure trends. This is unlikely to be the case as health care continues to crowd out other public and private expenditures. Nevertheless, the increasing ability of new medical technologies to improve people's health, coupled with the inability of the U.S. Congress to approve health care reform containing strong cost control measures, lends credence to the belief that health expenditures will continue to grow rapidly in the years to come.

International Expenditures

Table 3.7 shows total health expenditures as a percentage of GDP in OECD countries over the period 1980–1997. The 1997 figure for the U.S., 13.5 percent, is about one-third higher than for any other country; only Germany also exceeded the 10 percent mark. Not shown in the table are per capita expenditures expressed in dollars. In 1997, the U.S. figure was about $3,925, a full 54 percent higher than the next highest (for Switzerland).[21]

The Need for Timely and Complete Data Systems

An important issue facing the United States is availability of accurate and timely data on national health care utilization rates and expenditures. The United States does not have a system in place that allows it to compute expenditures for the entire health care sector in a consistent and timely fashion. Such a data set would be extremely beneficial, and perhaps even essential, for enacting certain types of health care reform, particularly those that are regulatory in nature.

The problem, in a nutshell, is this: the U.S. government does not require private insurers to collect and release data on expenditures. Such data, if available in a consistent format, would increase the country's flexibility in adopting various types of reform.

One of the reforms discussed in the next chapter designed to control health care costs is expenditure targets, which applies to a fee-for-service system. Under such a system, unit prices are adjusted annually if utilization is above or below a designated target. To implement such a system requires timely data on health

TABLE 3.7.   TOTAL HEALTH EXPENDITURES AS A PERCENTAGE
OF GROSS DOMESTIC PRODUCT: SELECTED COUNTRIES
AND YEARS, 1990–1997.

Country	1980 in Percent	1985 in Percent	1990 in Percent	1995 in Percent	1997 in Percent
Australia	7.3	7.7	8.2	8.4	8.4
Austria	7.9	6.7	7.1	8.0	7.9
Belgium	6.6	7.4	7.6	7.9	7.6
Canada	7.3	8.4	9.2	9.7	9.0
Denmark	6.8	6.3	6.5	8.0	7.4
Finland	6.5	7.3	8.0	7.6	7.2
France	7.6	8.5	8.9	9.9	9.6
Germany	8.1	8.5	8.2	10.4	10.4
Greece	3.6	4.0	4.2	5.8	7.1
Iceland	6.2	7.3	8.0	8.2	8.0
Ireland	8.8	7.8	6.6	7.0	7.0
Italy	7.0	7.1	8.1	7.7	7.6
Japan	6.4	6.7	6.0	7.2	7.3
Luxembourg	6.2	6.1	6.6	6.7	7.1
Netherlands	7.9	7.9	8.3	8.8	8.6
New Zealand	6.0	5.3	7.0	7.3	7.7
Norway	7.0	6.6	7.8	8.0	7.5
Portugal	5.8	6.3	6.5	8.2	7.8
Spain	5.7	5.7	6.9	7.3	7.4
Sweden	9.4	9.0	8.8	8.5	8.6
Switzerland	7.3	8.1	8.4	9.6	10.1
Turkey	3.3	2.2	2.5	3.3	4.0
United Kingdom	5.6	5.9	6.0	6.9	6.7
United States	8.9	10.3	12.2	13.7	13.5

Source: U.S. Department of Health and Human Services. *Health United States, 1993.* (DHHS publication no.
PHS 94-1232.) Hyattsville, Md.: Public Health Service, U.S. Department of Health and Human Services, May
1994), p. 221; and U.S. Department of Health and Human Services. *Health United States, 1999.* (DHHS publication no. PHS 99-1232.) Hyattsville, Md.: Public Health Service, U.S. Department of Health and Human
Services, Sept. 1999), p. 283 (modified by author).

expenditures on a subnational (statewide) basis for all payers. (The current dearth of statewide data is one important impediment to enacting major health care reform.) Current data systems, however, do not support such a system, largely because private insurers and health plans are not required to compile aggregate utilization and expenditure information.

Is Cost Control Even Necessary?

This chapter has discussed how health care costs are measured and has shown recent levels and trends. The next chapter considers various methods of controlling these costs. Before doing so, however, a natural question to ask is it is even necessary to control national health expenditures.

The question is not a trivial one. If people wish to spend more on health care, and consequently less on other things, why should they be stopped—particularly when it seems increasingly clear that certain new medical devices, products, and procedures can improve the quality and length of life?

It turns out that there are several reasons cost control is important and likely to be in the forefront of health policy for years to come. First, there are significant opportunity costs associated with additional spending. A dollar spent on health cannot be spent on such other things as education, housing, or consumer goods. Cost control continues to be a major issue simply because it is imprudent to waste money in the face of so many strong consumer desires and societal needs.

Second, there are various ways in which the health care market is imperfect, which fact may lead to more spending than is desirable. Unlike other goods and services, health care services are often well insured, which insulates consumers from facing their true cost (that is, resource value). In addition, because consumer information is often poor, people may demand medical goods and services in part because of strong advertising, or because they are "induced" to do so by providers who have a pecuniary incentive to increase demand.

Third, government now pays for almost half of U.S. health care spending. Even though the United States is now going through a period of unprecedented budget surplus, the future of social programs is nevertheless worrisome, particularly for programs such as Medicare that face more recipients and fewer contributors when the baby boom generation retires.

Finally, one of the major reasons that the number of uninsured persons continues to rise in the United States is health care costs. Although more employers are offering insurance than in the past, fewer workers are purchasing it because they cannot afford the premiums.[22] This trend is likely to accelerate if health care costs start to rise again at the levels seen in the 1970s and

1980s. In summary, then, there are compelling reasons to believe not only that health care costs will remain a central policy interest but also that their control is in the national interest.

Notes

1. A dollar bill is roughly six inches, or half a foot, long. Lining up one trillion of them would therefore stretch five hundred billion feet, or more than ninety-four million miles. The sun, in contrast, is only ninety-three million miles from earth.

2. A tremendous amount of effort has gone into compiling accurate health expenditure figures across countries. For a presentation of the most recent estimates by the Organization for Economic Cooperation and Development (OECD), which has sponsored much of this work, see Anderson, G. F., and Poullier, J. "Health Spending, Access, and Outcomes." *Health Affairs,* May–June 1999, *18*(3), 179–192.

3. Miller, R. L., and Meiners, R. E. *Intermediate Microeconomics.* New York: McGraw-Hill, 1986.

4. There are other distinctions in how economists and accountants define cost. Specifically, economic profits equal an organization's cash flow minus a normal rate of return on investment. For a discussion of these issues, see Feldstein, J. P. *Health Care Economics,* New York: Wiley, 1988, pp. 451–455; and Brealey, R. A., and Myers, S. C. *Principles of Corporate Finance,* New York: McGraw-Hill, 1988, p. 264.

5. For more information on the index, including some important revisions made in 1977, see U.S. Department of Labor, Bureau of Labor Statistics. *Handbook of Methods.* BLS Bulletin no. 2285. Washington, D.C.: U.S. Department of Labor, Apr. 1988. The many components of the CPI can be obtained from the Internet at http://stat.bls.gov/cpihome.htm.

6. See Feldstein (1988), pp. 55–64, for a thorough discussion of the issue.

7. Feldstein (1988).

8. Braden, B. R. and others. "National Health Expenditures, 1997." *Health Care Financing Review,* Fall 1998, *20*, 83–126.

9. Office of National Cost Estimates. "Revisions of the National Health Accounts and Methodology." *Health Care Financing Review,* Summer 1990, *11*, 42–54.

10. Office of National Cost Estimates (1990).

11. Office of National Cost Estimates (1990).

12. Haber, S. G., and Newhouse, J. P. "Recent Revisions to and Recommendations for National Health Expenditures Accounting." *Health Care Financing Review,* Fall 1991, *13*, 111–116.

13. For the most recent article, see Anderson and Poullier (1999).

14. Schieber, G. J., and Poullier, J. "International Health Spending: Issues and Trends." *Health Affairs,* Spring 1991, *10*, 106–116.

15. Schieber and Poullier (1991), p. 108.

16. Schieber and Poullier (1991), 107.

17. The starting date of 1975 was chosen because it is well after the enactment of Medicare and Medicaid in 1965. Although price and expenditure data are available before these dates, trends would be colored by inclusion of these programs.

18. For example, see Smith, S., Heffler, S., Freeland, M., and the National Health Expenditures Projection Team. "The Next Decade of Health Spending: A New Outlook." *Health Affairs,* July–Aug. 1999, *18*, 86–96.

19. Congressional Budget Office. "Projections of National Health Expenditures." Washington, D.C.: Congressional Budget Office, Oct. 1992.

20. Warshawsky, M. J. "Projections of Health Care Expenditures as a Share of the Gross Domestic Product: Actuarial and Macroeconomic Approaches." *Health Services Research*, Aug. 1994, *29*, 293–313.

21. *Health, United States, 1999.* DHHS pub. no. (PHS) 99-1232. Hyattsville: Md., Public Health Service, Sept. 1999.

22. Cooper, P. F., and Schone, B. S. "More Offers, Fewer Takers for Employment-Based Health Insurance: 1987 and 1996." *Health Affairs,* 1997, *16*(6), 142–149.

CHAPTER FOUR

CONTAINING HEALTH CARE COSTS

Thomas H. Rice and Gerald F. Kominski

Since the publication of the first edition of this book in 1996, much has changed in the area of cost containment. At that time, we did not know whether or not health care cost increases had peaked after their record growth in the 1970s and 1980s. When this chapter was written for that edition, two studies had recently been published, predicting that U.S. health expenditures would consume 18 percent of national income by the year 2000.[1] These estimates turned out far off the mark. In actuality, the percentage of gross domestic product (GDP) spent on health care was constant, at a level of about 13.5 percent, from 1992 to 1996.[2] It is unlikely that the figure will even exceed 14 percent, much less 18 percent, when the year 2000 data become available.

Although analysts disagree about the exact reasons for this turnaround, most would argue that it does relate to the growth of managed care, particularly HMOs. By moving largely from a fee-for-service to a capitated-based system, at least for those under age sixty-five, all parties have less economic incentive to increase service volume. Furthermore, many would argue that competition between health care plans has set in motion strong forces to keep premiums, and hence total expenditures, lower than they would be otherwise.

Nevertheless, a number of forces could result in a resurgence of cost increase:

- Both hospitals and physician groups find themselves under financial strain and may need a substantial increase in payments from health plans to stay afloat.

- As a result of historically low unemployment, employers must compete for employees, and one method of doing so is through providing more comprehensive health insurance benefits.
- The so-called managed care backlash is likely to result in federal and state regulations that rein in the power of health plans, which in turn could increase costs—both through the regulatory oversight itself and by requiring plans to employ costly quality-enhancing processes.
- Rapid consolidation among providers and health plans may result in price-increasing monopolistic power.
- Mapping the human genome is likely to result in many new expensive therapies to correct genetic disorders.

Thus, although costs were successfully controlled during much of the 1990s, it is prudent to reconsider the issue of cost containment. This chapter has three purposes: to present a framework for assessing alternative cost-containment strategies, to review previous research on the success and failure of these strategies, and to suggest directions for future research that may help clarify the most effective future cost-containment options for the United States to pursue.

Framework

Before embarking on an analysis of alternative cost-containment strategies, it is useful to construct a framework that groups together similar strategies.[3] The framework developed here relies on two equations. The first applies to the fee-for-service system, and the second to capitated systems.

$$E = \sum_{j=1}^{j} (P_j Q_j)$$

$$E = \sum_{j=1}^{j} (C_j N_j)$$

where

E = total health expenditures

P = unit price for services

Q = quantity of services

C = cost of service per person

N = number of persons

j = index representing each payer

Equation one states that total expenditures are equal to the product of the price of services and the quantity of services, summed over all payers. In other words, it is the sum of P times Q for Medicare, Medicaid, Blue Cross and Blue Shield, each private insurer, and so on. In contrast, equation two is oriented toward the person, not the service. In this equation, total expenditures are simply the product of costs per person and the number of persons, again summed over all payers. Here, total expenditures would equal the number of Medicare beneficiaries times cost per beneficiary, plus the number of Blue Cross enrollees times the cost per enrollee, and so on.

The equations employ summation signs to illustrate the potential for "cost shifting." To illustrate, suppose that one payer, Medicare, successfully controls both P and Q. This clearly results in lower Medicare costs, but it does not necessarily contain systemwide health care costs. This is because hospitals and physicians might respond to Medicare's controls by trying to increase their Ps or Qs to the patients of other payers. The same thing could happen in equation two. A strong health alliance might cut a particularly good deal with a health maintenance organization (HMO), with the HMO responding by charging more to groups outside of the alliance.[4]

Our framework simply defines the determinants of health expenditures; what may be hidden is the fact that the success of alternative cost-containment strategies hinges on how they affect consumer and provider *behavior*. In equation one, for example, it might appear that a reasonable strategy for controlling expenditures would be to lower the price of services paid to physicians. However, this would not be successful if physicians responded to these price controls by inducing their patients to obtain more services (that is, P would go down, but Q would go up).

The same is true of the capitation strategies in equation two. The most obvious approach for controlling expenditures seemingly is to control costs per person. However, if this is accomplished by paying HMOs less, they may in turn respond by seeking to enroll only the healthiest people, or by lowering the quality of care that they provide.

In analyzing cost-containment strategies, then, we must be aware of the ability of providers (and others) to "game" the system to meet their own goals. Strategies that are difficult to game tend to be most successful. As an example, we argue that some hospital rate-setting programs were moderately successful in containing costs because it was difficult for hospitals to game the system by increasing admission rates and length of stay. Instead, physicians rather than hospitals made these decisions and physician payment rates were not affected by the rate-setting programs. In contrast, certificate-of-need programs were less successful in controlling costs because hospitals were able to respond to restrictions on growth in the number of beds by purchasing more equipment and engaging in other activities that were not regulated (or that were tolerated by the regulators). Thus in analyzing cost-containment strategies, we focus on how they influence provider and consumer behavior, which in turn strongly influences their ultimate success or failure.

Before we proceed any further, one other caveat is necessary. This chapter focuses on ways of containing costs, but it must be remembered that cost containment is not society's only goal with regard to health services; access and quality of care also matter. Consequently, if analysts find that a particular strategy is effective in controlling costs, they must also consider any spillover effects—such as decreased quality—that result. Only by considering both benefits and costs can we make the best policy decisions for reforming our health care system.

Analysis of Cost-Containment Strategies

This section uses the framework just presented to review evidence regarding the cost-containment potential of various fee-for-service and capitated cost-containment strategies. Although it addresses more than a dozen such strategies, still others cannot be included because of space limitations.

Fee-For-Service Options

Fee-for-service options[5] can be divided into three types, each corresponding to a term in equation one: P, Q, and E. The discussion here is divided accordingly.

Price Options. One type of cost-containment strategy that has been attempted at various times in the United States is controlling the unit price paid to the provider. On the hospital side, examples include state hospital rate-setting programs and using Diagnosis-Related Groups (DRGs). On the physician side, both the Medicare and Medicaid programs have, at various times, attempted to control their costs by freezing (or even lowering) physician payment rates. There is also some experience in this regard from Canada. More recently, Medicare and many Medicaid programs have adopted resource-based fee schedules, which are simply another form of price controls.

Before reviewing the available evidence, we believe it is useful to outline the overall advantages and disadvantages of price-control options. There appear to be two possible advantages. First, controlling price typically involves less administrative effort (and expense) than controlling the quantity of service. Rather than examining the appropriateness of every provider and every service, it is only necessary to ensure that payment rates conform to regulated amounts. Second—and related to this—price regulation tends to be less intrusive; it does not entail the type of micromanagement often encountered in the quantity-related options discussed next.

There are some disadvantages, however. First, it addresses only one component of total expenditure. As we shall see, a price-based strategy can be circumvented if providers are able to increase the quantity of service they provide. Second, these strategies can diminish the efficiency of the market. If the wrong price is chosen, the wrong quantity or mix of services may result.

Several states adopted hospital rate-setting programs in the 1970s and 1980s. These programs varied on a number of dimensions, the most important of which were whether they were voluntary or mandatory, and whether they applied to some or all payers. Most (but not all) were aimed at giving hospitals an incentive to spend less by controlling hospital charges per day.

Of the twenty-five state-level programs that were in effect by the end of the 1970s, only eight were mandatory as opposed to voluntary, and only four—in Maryland, Massachusetts, New Jersey, and New York—applied to all payers.[6] In most cases, these programs established uniform payment rates, so that public and private insurers paid the same price for the same unit of care (for example, day of care, admission, and so on). To include Medicare in their all-payer systems, these states had to apply to the Health Care Financing Administration (HCFA) for waivers exempting them from Medicare's national payment rules. In granting these waivers, HCFA specified limits on the rate of growth in total Medicare inpatient payments, or in Medicare inpatient payments per case, under the all-payer programs.[7]

Since 1985, with the exception of Maryland these states either have lost their waivers or allowed them to expire. Ironically, one factor contributing to the financial pressure for these states to abandon waivers was the implementation of the Medicare inpatient prospective payment system (PPS) in October 1983. Because payment rates during the first three years of PPS were a blend of hospital-specific and national payment amounts, these states felt pressure from their hospital associations to abandon the waivers because hospitals could increase their Medicare revenue by joining PPS.

Most research on the subject has found that it was these four programs that were most effective, with savings on the order of 10–15 percent.[8] It might seem surprising that a gross strategy the likes of limiting hospital payments per day would work, but apparently it did. This is likely because of the difficulty hospitals had in "gaming" such a system. If a hospital wants to raise more revenue under an all-payer, mandatory rate-setting program that establishes daily payment rates, it has two choices: increase the number of admissions, or increase length of stay.

But neither of these options is typically available to hospitals because these decisions are made by physicians, whose fees are not subject to these controls. Consequently, as much as a hospital might wish to raise more revenue, it might not have the ability to do so.

Implementation of the DRG-based Medicare PPS made such gaming even more difficult (although it led to its own gaming, of course). Under the DRG system, hospitals are paid a fixed amount of money for a particular diagnosis, irrespective of how much is spent on treating a particular patient.[9] Hospitals therefore cannot benefit by trying to keep patients longer. Another option for garnering more revenue is to increase the number of admissions, but this has not happened for two reasons: the physician rather than the hospital makes this decision, and hospitals have found it profitable to treat patients on an outpatient basis, which is paid for separately and outside the DRG system.

There remain two other avenues for increasing revenue under DRGs: earning more from treating Medicare patients on an outpatient basis, and shifting costs to other payers. Although Medicare outpatient costs have risen rapidly, this increase has not been sufficient to cut deeply into Medicare savings.[10] Medicare is also implementing an outpatient PPS, which further reduces the incentive to shift patients.

The same cannot be said about the shift to other payers. According to the Medicare Payment Advisory Commission (MedPAC), the Congressional commission that studies provider payment under Medicare, hospitals do resort to shifting costs onto private payers.[11] The magnitude of cost-shifting practice is shown in Table 4.1. In 1990, for example, Medicare paid hospitals less than 90 percent of the costs associated with treating program patients, and Medicaid only 80 percent. In contrast, private insurers paid hospitals about 28 percent *more* for their patients' care than it actually cost to provide. Cost shifting has decreased substantially in the last few years, mainly because Medicare has begun to pay its share of hospital costs, and Medicaid payments have improved as well. In 1998, private insurers were paying "only" 14 percent more than their patients actually cost hospitals.

Because of cost shifting, some analysts have concluded that DRGs have done little if anything to control national health care spending,[12] the evidence of substantial savings in the Medicare program notwithstanding.[13] This is not necessarily an indictment of DRGs, however. If other payers were to adopt DRGs, systemwide hospital spending might be better controlled. For example, a number of state Medicaid programs have adopted payment systems based on DRGs, but most commercial insurers have not.[14]

These conclusions about the successes and failures of hospital price controls are further supported by experience with physician controls. Most studies indicate

TABLE 4.1. HOSPITAL PAYMENT-TO-COST RATIOS, 1985–1999.

Year	Medicare	Medicaid	Charity	Private
1985	101.0	90.0	n/a	116.0
1989	91.4	75.8	19.3	121.6
1990	89.2	79.7	21.0	126.8
1991	88.4	81.6	19.6	129.7
1992	88.8	90.9	18.9	131.3
1993	89.4	93.1	19.5	129.3
1994	96.9	93.7	19.3	124.4
1995	99.3	93.8	18.0	123.9
1996	102.4	94.8	17.3	121.5
1997	103.6	95.9	14.1	117.6
1998	102.6	97.9	13.2	113.6

Source: MedPAC. "Report to Congress: Selected Medicare Issues." Washington, D.C.: Medicare Payment Advisory Commission, 2000.

limited cost savings when physician payments are frozen or reduced, because physicians respond by providing a greater quantity of services.[15] In making its projections about physician payment costs under the new Medicare fee schedule that was implemented starting in 1992, the Congressional Budget Office concluded that for every 1 percent reduction in physician fees, the volume of services would rise by 0.56 percent.[16]

Why might these physician controls be less effective than hospital controls? It is because physicians have greater ability to game the payment system. If their payment rates drop, physicians in a fee-for-service environment can attempt (and may very well succeed) in increasing the volume of services. Hospitals do not tend to have this ability. Nevertheless, physicians' ability to generate additional billing is probably limited. This is illustrated by the experience of the Canadian provinces, which have tightly controlled physician fees since the early 1970s. Although the quantity of services has risen faster in Canada than in the United States over this time period, it was not nearly enough to compensate for the lower fees.[17] In a country like the United States, where there are multiple payers, an effective way for a payer to control physician spending is to pay so little to doctors that they do not want to treat such patients. This, of course, is what has happened in many state Medicaid programs. Canadian provinces have not suffered from this problem because there is only one payer; the provinces are the only game in town.

Quantity Options. The next group of fee-for-service cost-containment strategies are those aimed at service quantity or utilization. Examples include certificate-of-need programs, technology controls, utilization review, and practice guidelines (to name just a few). Their primary advantage over price options is that they can focus on reducing waste in the system. For example, if a particular procedure is inappropriate for a patient with a given diagnosis, quantity options can focus on that problem.

There are two disadvantages. Like the price options, they only target one component of expenditure. If providers can game utilization controls by increasing prices, then the savings from these programs are diminished. Second, these strategies are often cumbersome from an administrative standpoint, involving much bureaucracy, paperwork, and undue oversight over the practice of medicine.

The earliest examples of quantity controls were certificate-of-need (CON) programs. These programs, which became commonplace in the early 1970s, were aimed at controlling expenditures by reducing the amount of hospital resources available—both beds and equipment. Typically, hospitals needed permission for proposed investment in excess of $100,000. A local board, called the health systems agency, ruled on a hospital's request for additional resources.

Many studies have been conducted on CON, and almost all reach the same conclusion: it did not succeed in saving money.[18] Although there was some effect on the number of hospital beds, capital equipment per bed rose even more quickly than before.[19] There are a number of reasons for this failure, but the fundamental one is that the entity making the decisions on the hospital's application (the local health systems agency, and ultimately the state) was not financially accountable for the increased cost associated with approving a hospital's request. In other words, why turn a hospital request down when the cost would be borne by such payers as Medicare, Blue Cross, or commercial insurers? On the contrary, board members would have every incentive to approve requests by their local hospital, since this would be viewed as helpful to their community and constituencies.

This is not to say that technology controls can't work; they probably can. However, they need to be implemented at a broader geographic level by an entity that is at risk for additional health care spending. The Canadian provinces give us such an example.

Despite claims to the contrary, there is no single Canadian health care system. Rather, each province has its own system, but all have to conform to various federal requirements if they are to receive federal contributions. One key point, often overlooked in the literature, is that provinces are 100 percent at risk for additional health care spending because annual federal contributions are fixed. Unlike the U.S. Medicaid program, where the federal government at least matches additional state spending, provinces do not receive an additional penny if they spend more on health care than anticipated.

Since provinces are also responsible for financing a host of other nonhealth programs, they must be judicious in allotting their tax revenues to health care. One way they have done this is by controlling the diffusion of medical technology. If a hospital wants to expand or purchase equipment, it needs the province's permission, and provinces have not been eager to grant requests. The United States has far more of most technologies than Canada, when measured on a per capita basis. For example, in 1996, the U.S. had 16.0 MRI units and 26.9 CT scanners per million people; Canada's figures were only 1.3 and 7.9, respectively.[20] Canadians often claim that they have achieved this by regionalizing their technologies, thereby making their system more efficient. Others contend, however, that the result is rationing. Indeed, evidence from a General Accounting Office study of Ontario shows that Canadians are subject to waiting lists for most kinds of elective surgery.[21]

Up to this point, the discussion of quantity has focused not on services but on hospital beds and technologies. Most recent efforts in the United States, however, have been aimed at particular services. This is commonly done through utilization management (UM). UM programs are normally implemented by third-party payers as a way to reduce provision of unnecessary or inappropriate services. Examples include preadmission certification of hospital stays, concurrent and retrospective review of stays, management of high-cost patients, requiring second opinions before embarking on surgery, and profiling of physicians' practices.

Evidence so far indicates these programs, particularly preadmission certification of hospital stay, may produce moderate savings.[22] The evidence on other programs, particularly second opinion for surgery, is less optimistic.[23] One issue for those who are concerned about controlling future health care costs is that UM programs are almost universal now, meaning that we may have already gained about as much in savings as can be extracted.

The wave of the future is now on developing UM for the outpatient setting, particularly through physician profiling. However, the savings potential of these programs is still largely untested. There is strong reason to believe that UM in the outpatient setting is much more difficult to implement, because of the difficulty in knowing whether a physician who is a high spender is less efficient or more profligate, or alternatively, has a more severely ill group of patients than his or her peers. Normally one tries to risk-adjust a provider's case mix, but this is difficult at the level of the individual physician, who experiences a relatively low caseload and therefore is more likely to have healthier or sicker patients as a result of random chance. The best we are likely to do—and this is now the emphasis—is to employ risk-adjustment formulas with physician groups.

The most recent UM efforts have focused on developing practice guidelines. These are written protocols that are designed to instruct physicians on what procedures are appropriate for a patient with a particular diagnosis. The guidelines are largely being developed by researchers under the auspices of the federal Agency for Healthcare Research and Quality, although some medical specialty groups are doing so as well. One intent of the guidelines is to increase quality by reducing the amount of regional variation in health care use. It has been widely documented that parts of the country have differing surgery rates for certain procedures, and that this cannot be readily explained by variation in patient health status.[24]

Development of practice guidelines is still in its formative stage, so we cannot know the extent to which they can control costs. There is reason to be skeptical, though. Just as practice guidelines could reduce resource use by physicians who offer too many services, they could just as well *increase* spending by physicians who currently provide fewer services than are recommended by the guidelines. The issue, then, is whether the guidelines are likely to prescribe a quantity of service that is greater or less than what is currently being provided. A General Accounting Office study on treatment of cancer patients gives evidence that many physicians are conducting less treatment than is suggested by the guidelines. It concluded that "20 percent of those with Hodgkin's disease, 25 percent of those with one type of lung cancer, 60 percent of those with rectum cancer, 94 percent of colon cancer patients—did *not* receive what [the National Cancer Institute] considers state-of-the-art treatments. This is especially troubling in that all these treatments have been proven to extend patients' survival in controlled experiments, many of which were concluded 10 or more years ago."[25]

Expenditure Options. The final group of fee-for-service options are those that directly target expenditure. Some examples include Medicare Volume Performance Standards, hospital global budgets, and national and subnational health budgeting. The overriding advantage of expenditure control is somewhat tautological—it directly aims at controlling health care expenditures. The extent to which this can succeed, however, depends in large measure on whether all health care spending is targeted, or just a component of total spending such as hospital or physician expenditures. The primary disadvantage is that implementing such controls may result in a less efficient health care system, which could reduce the quality of services.

The primary example of expenditure control in the United States was the implementation of Medicare Volume Performance Standards (VPS) in the early 1990s. (This was recently replaced by a similar system, called the Sustainable Growth Rate (SGR), described later.) The VPS system was part of the 1989 physician payment reforms adopted by Congress that also resulted in the new Medicare fee schedule with its resource-based relative values. Congress recognized that simply redistributing physician fees to make higher payments to primary care physicians, and lower payments to specialists, though more equitable, would not by itself control burgeoning program expenditures. This was left to the VPS system.

Under the system, each year Congress set a target rate of increase in Medicare Part B physician expenditures. If actual spending exceeded the target, the next year's physician fee update was normally reduced by that amount (although Congress could do, of course, whatever it chose when the time came). Conversely, if the growth in spending was less than the target, physicians would get more. Suppose, for example, that the target for 1997 was a 10 percent increase in spending. If actual spending increased by 12 percent, the target would have been exceeded. Most likely, this would be extracted the next time Congress updated Medicare physician fees. If physicians were due a 5 percent cost-of-living increase, they would likely be granted only 3 percent.

The SGR system was enacted as part of the Balanced Budget Act of 1997 and implemented in 1998. The main different between it and the VPS system was in setting the target expenditure rate of "sustainable growth," which was determined by four factors: the percentage change in physician input prices; the percentage change in Part B fee-for-service enrollment; the projected change in real GDP; and the percentage change in spending for physicians' services resulting from other changes in law.[26]

The VPS system (and by analogy, its successor) have been criticized as being too blunt an instrument for affecting the individual physician's behavior. Because it applies nationally, individual physicians who increased the volume of services they provided would not pay the price by experiencing a decline in their fees. This would only happen if all physicians behaved this way. But if a physician does not increase his or her volume and other physicians do, then the first physician suffers—volume (Q) does not climb, but the fee (P) falls as a result of the behavior of other physicians. The system may therefore contain a "perverse" incentive to increase the volume of services—which is exactly what it is supposed to prevent. One way to improve the incentives is to target smaller groups of physicians, by having separate targets for each specialty, state, or state-specialty combination.[27]

Fortunately, this type of behavior does not appear to have transpired. The volume of services, by and large, has been approximately equal to the target.[28] One possible explanation—which has not been confirmed by researchers—is that physicians could be moving more of their practices toward privately insured patients, because private insurer fees are far higher than Medicare's.

To find an example of expenditure controls applied to the hospital level, we must again look to Canada. In each of the provinces, hospitals are paid an annual global budget, which is negotiated between the provinces and each individual hospital. If a hospital exceeds its budget, there is no guarantee that it will be compensated.

Hospital global budgets seem to have worked in the sense that hospital spending in Canada has risen much less quickly than in the United States.[29]

The primary way in which this has been achieved is that Canadian hospitals now have only about half as many nonphysician personnel as do their U.S. counterparts.[30] (Capital expenditures have also been controlled, but for different reasons, since they are not included in the global budgets.) One perverse effect is that Canadian hospitals seem to prefer long-staying patients who might belong in nursing homes, because these patients occupy a bed but use few other resources. Another fear is that the lack of resources is diminishing the quality of care in Canadian hospitals. What little available evidence there is indicates, however, that inpatient outcomes appear to be similar in the two countries.[31]

The two strategies—Medicare VPS/SGR and hospital global budgets—do not constitute a comprehensive cost-control policy because they are aimed at only one component of health care expenditure. A broader strategy might be to target all (or most) health expenditures at the same time, through a system of national or subnational (regional) budgeting.

The typical way of controlling total expenditures in a fee-for-service system is through expenditure targets. Generally, under such a system unit prices are adjusted to ensure that targeted expenditures are met. This differs from the VPS/SGR system in two primary ways: (1) it applies to all payers, not just to Medicare; and (2) it applies to most of the health care system, not just physician payment. Although we have the most experience—both domestically and internationally—with using expenditure targets for paying physicians, it could nevertheless be applied to other services, such as hospitalization. In such a case, DRG payments per admission could be tied to meeting a particular growth in inpatient expenditure.[32]

The advantage of such a system, of course, is that it controls expenditures directly. But there are several possible disadvantages. It might result in inefficient use of resources, it could potentially harm quality, and it requires massive amounts of timely data that currently are not being produced.

With regard to efficiency in a competitive market, in the long run price is based on the cost of producing a good or service. If the price is too high, then the incentive is to overprice the good; if it is too low, the incentive is to underproduce. Under an expenditure target system, prices change not on account of demand and supply considerations, but rather how closely total expenditures conform to a target. The good news is that prices tend to fall when quantity is too high, so it might be argued that the system is self-correcting. The bad news is that there is no assurance that health care inputs will be used efficiently by producers when the market mechanism is circumvented. Even more troubling is the possibility that the mix of services produced is not based on what consumers would like to buy.

This touches on the second potential problem: quality. Suppose that Congress set an austere budget level, necessitating a subsequent decline in unit prices. This might dissuade providers from delivering necessary services for fear that they would exceed the expenditure target, which in turn could result in diminished quality. Because adequate data systems do not yet exist for monitoring quality, there is a strong possibility that it would be sacrificed in favor of controlling expenditures.

Finally, there is the data problem. To make expenditure targets work in a fee-for-service system, it is necessary to have up-to-date information about the quantity of services provided to all patients. It is through this information that total expenditures are tallied, and updates are made to provider prices. In the United States, however, we have no formal mechanism for obtaining timely utilization and expenditure data for privately insured patients or for publicly insured patients in managed care.[33] It would take several years to develop such a system, but the process has not yet even started. Thus, the fee-for-service method that has the greatest likelihood of controlling cost also perhaps suffers from the most shortcomings. This illustrates that there are indeed no easy answers for controlling cost under a fee-for-service system.

Capitation Options

Equation two showed that three things are necessary to control expenditures under a capitated system: control of costs per person (C), the number of persons (N), and shifting costs between payers. This section focuses on the first component; cost shifting has already been addressed, and controlling the number of persons (say, by denying eligibility for coverage)—although clearly a cost-containment strategy— is inconsistent with the notion of health care reform.

This section discusses two overlapping strategies for controlling costs under a capitated system: HMOs and managed competition. The treatment is short because these strategies are dealt with in more detail in Chapter Fifteen.

HMOs. Unlike its efforts with many so-called competitive strategies, the United States has much experience with HMOs. They have been a part of the U.S. health care system for decades and growing so rapidly that now most of the working-age population is enrolled in them or in their cousins, point-of-service (POS) plans.[34]

HMOs are given an incentive to control costs by the fact that they are paid on a capitation basis. That is, they receive a fixed payment to provide an enrollee's care for a specific length of time, and this payment is unrelated to how much the HMO actually spends. Thus, if it spends less by being more efficient (say, not hospitalizing unnecessarily), then it gets to keep more money. But how much the HMO charges in premiums is kept in check by competitive pressures; if it charges too much in premiums, fewer people are likely to enroll.

Much of the early evidence on HMOs through the 1970s focused on group and staff-model HMOs; it indicated that they could yield substantial savings—as much as 30–40 percent over fee-for-service.[35] A savings rate on that order is now viewed as somewhat optimistic. HMOs do save money, but it is difficult to know how much. On the one hand, when comparing HMOs and fee-for-service the savings of the former are exaggerated by the fact that HMOs experience a favorable selection of patients.[36] That is, healthier people are more likely to join HMOs, and this fact is partly responsible for their savings. On the other hand, HMOs probably save more than is directly attributable to them because competition between HMOs and fee-for-service plans has undoubtedly resulted in the latter reducing their costs.

Whatever savings they generate, HMOs by themselves are probably insufficient to solve long-term problems in rising health care costs. One reason is that they are subject to the same forces that raise the costs of fee-for-service medicine—overall growth in input costs and the development and diffusion of expensive medical technologies. Even less evidence is available on how HMOs affect the quality of care provided. One comprehensive review of the literature found equal numbers of studies reporting better and worse quality of care in HMOs than in fee-for-service.[37]

Managed Competition. Analysts have recognized for years that pure competition is unlikely to work well in the health care sector. There are many reasons for this; two are detailed here. First, the health care market is a complicated one, with people having relatively poor information about their alternatives and the implications (for their health and their pocketbooks) of making these choices. A second is biased selection; insurers may compete for the healthiest people, leaving sicker people with no source of insurance.

Advocates of managed competition believe that the marketplace can be trusted in the health care sector only if the players conform to certain rules.[38] To facilitate consumer understanding, health plans should be required to provide specific minimum benefits, or in some proposals conform to standardized benefits. The latter aids consumers in comparison shopping between alternative plans. Furthermore, certain practices on the part of insurers, such as "cherry picking" the healthiest people, charging unaffordably high premiums to unhealthy individuals and groups, and denying coverage for preexisting conditions, are to be prohibited. To make consumers think twice before purchasing extravagant insurance policies, employers would make a defined contribution based on the lowest-cost premium in the market. Some proposals also tax health plans that are more expensive than the cheapest approved plan in an area. All of this is to be carried out through consortiums called health insurance purchasing cooperatives, or health alliances.

There is no way to know whether managed competition can succeed in controlling health care costs; it has never been tried on a wide scale. Some elements of managed competition have been adopted voluntarily, however, and many people claim that much of the success in controlling costs in the 1990s was the result of health plans competing against each other. It must be recognized, however, that Medicare was also successful in controlling costs over this period even outside of its HMO sector, so we are not yet in a position to draw a strong conclusion about the ability of managed competition to control cost.

Future Research Issues in Cost Containment

Before addressing future research issues, it is necessary to ask a more basic question: Are health care costs in the United States too high? Unfortunately, it is impossible to know the answer to this question. To answer it, we would have to know the benefits (both tangible and intangible) that we derive from health care services, and compare them to the benefits and costs of alternative uses of our resources. The necessary information is not available to make such macro-level comparison and probably never will be.

There are, nevertheless, good reasons for ongoing research on methods to contain U.S. health care costs. First, the fact that other countries spend so much less per capita raises the possibility that there may be effective cost-control options available. Second, it is a truism that every dollar spent on health means that there is a dollar less to spend on other goods and services that the country and its citizens may want. Third, and related to this, there are strong reasons to believe that the availability of new and effective medical technologies (such as gene therapy) will result in an even greater jump in spending. It would seem prudent that we understand what options are available to control these and other costs, before health care spending absorbs even more of our national income.

If continued research on cost-containment methods is appropriate, the next question is which areas of inquiry are most fruitful. On the domestic front, there should be continued study of the effects of competition on health care costs. Various parts of the country are experimenting with competitively driven cost-containment strategies; research should continue on which of these approaches are most effective in controlling costs without harming quality and access. In this regard, federally sanctioned state demonstration projects are extremely desirable because they allow researchers to assess whether particular methods work on a large-scale basis. In addition, research on a particular component of a competitive approach (say, a risk-adjustment formula) should continue so that the tools are available to implement selective competitive reforms if there is the political will to do so.

Regulatory approaches should be studied as well. Empirical evidence from previous and current use of price controls in the United States indicates that they are effective in controlling expenditures, improving or maintaining access, and reducing or eliminating cost shifting when applied to all payers. Nevertheless, a deep distrust of increased government intervention into the health care market poses a substantial barrier to expanded use of price controls or global budgets. Thus, some types of approach (for instance, single-payer) will be difficult to test in the United States, even on a small scale. For this reason, more research on how other countries have implemented cost containment using regulatory approaches—and the effects of these approaches—is warranted.

Since the late 1980s, there has been a movement toward more funded research in the areas of medical effectiveness and clinical outcomes. Infusion of more federal monies into this branch of health services research has been widely viewed as a valuable investment because of the dearth of information on which medical interventions work best. It is hoped, however, that this recent emphasis on outcomes research does not diminish the importance of general health services research, which seeks to address some of the larger concerns discussed in this chapter.

Notes

1. Congressional Budget Office. *Projects of National Health Expenditures.* Washington, D.C.: Congressional Budget Office, Oct. 1992; and Sally, T., and others. "Projections of National Health Expenditures Through the Year 2000." *Health Care Financing Review,* Fall 1991, *13,* 1–27.
2. Cowan, C. A., and others. "National Health Expenditures, 1998." *Health Care Financing Review,* Winter 1999, *21,* 165–210.
3. The framework presented in this chapter is new but draws on somewhat different ones that Rice has published previously. See Rice, T. "An Evaluation of Alternative Policies for Controlling Health Care Costs." In J. A. Meyer and S. Silow-Carroll (eds.), *Building Blocks for Change: How Health Care Reform Affects Our Future.* Washington, D.C.: Economic and Social Research Institute, 1993, pp. 19–41; and Rice, T. "Containing Health Care Costs in the United States." *Medical Care Review,* Spring 1992, *49,* 19–65.
4. There is some evidence to indicate that this has happened in the California public employees' health benefit plan, CalPERS. See Service Employees International Union. "The CalPERS Experience and Managed Competition." Washington, D.C.: Service Employees International Union, Mar. 1993.
5. This discussion draws upon Rice's previous work (see note 3).
6. Ashby, J. L., Jr. "The Impact of Hospital Regulatory Programs on Per Capita Costs, Utilization, and Capital Investment." *Inquiry,* Spring 1984, *21,* 45–59.
7. Davis, K., Anderson, G. F., Rowland, D., and Steinberg, E. P. *Health Care Cost Containment.* Baltimore: Johns Hopkins University Press, 1990.
8. See Robinson, J. C., and Luft, H. S. "Competition, Regulation, and Hospital Costs: 1982–1986." *Journal of the American Medical Association,* Nov. 11, 1988, *260,* 2676–681; and Thorpe, K. E. "Does All-Payer Rate Setting Work? The Case of the New York Prospective Hospital Reimbursement Methodology." *Journal of Health Politics, Policy, and Law,* Fall 1987, *12,* 391–408.

9. So-called outlier payments are made for patients who become much more expensive than the typical patient with that diagnosis. Even with the formula, hospitals usually lose money on long-staying patients. Thus, there is little or no incentive on the part of the hospital to keep patients for a very long time just so that they can reap outlier payments.

10. Chulis, G. S. "Assessing Medicare's Prospective Payment System for Hospitals." *Medical Care Review,* 1991, *48,* 167–206.

11. Prospective Payment Assessment Commission (ProPAC). *Optional Hospital Payment Rates.* Congressional Report C-92-03. Washington, D.C.: ProPAC, 1992.

12. Chulis (1991).

13. Russell, L. B., and Manning, C. L. "The Effect of Prospective Payment on Medicare Expenditures." *New England Journal of Medicine,* Feb. 16, 1989, *320,* 439–444.

14. Carter, G. M., Jacobson, P. D., Kominski, G. F., and Perry, M. J. "Use of Diagnosis-Related Groups by Non-Medicare Payers." *Health Care Financing Review,* Winter 1994, *16,* 127-158.

15. For a review of early evidence from several natural experiments, see Gabel, J., and Rice, T. "Reducing Public Expenditures for Physician Services: The Price of Paying Less." *Journal of Health Politics, Policy, and Law,* 1985, *9,* 595–609.

16. Christensen, S. "Volume Responses to Exogenous Changes in Medicare's Payment Policies." *Health Services Research,* Apr. 1992, *27,* 65–79.

17. Barer, M. L., Evans, R. G., and Labelle, R. J. "Fee Controls as Cost Controls: Tales from the Frozen North." *Milbank Quarterly,* 1988, *66,* 1–64.

18. Steinwald, B., and Sloan, F. A. "Regulatory Approaches to Hospital Cost Containment: A Synthesis of the Empirical Evidence." In M. A. Olson (ed.), A New Approach to the Economics of Health Care. Washington, D.C.: American Enterprise Institute for Public Policy Research, 1981.

19. Another effect was that hospitals increased the purchase of equipment that cost less than the CON threshold (e.g., $100,000), and sometimes split the costs of more expensive equipment in order to circumvent the regulations.

20. Andersen, G. F., and Poullier, J. "Health Spending, Access, and Outcomes: Trends in Industrialized Countries." *Health Affairs,* 1999, *18*(3), 178–192.

21. U.S. General Accounting Office. *Canadian Health Insurance: Lessons for the United States.* Pub. no. HRD-91-90. Washington, D.C.: General Accounting Office, June 1991.

22. There is a perception among employees (or employee benefit managers) that management of high-cost patients can result in very large savings, because only the most costly patients are targeted. (See Gabel, J., and others. *Trends in Managed Care.* Washington, D.C.: Health Insurance Association of America, Feb. 1989.) But this has never been verified with claims data.

23. Lindsey, P. A., and Newhouse, J. P. "The Cost and Value of Second Surgical Opinion Programs: A Critical Review of the Literature." *Journal of Health Politics, Policy, and Law,* Fall 1990, *15,* 543–570.

24. This research was originally conducted by John Wennberg and his colleagues. For a review of the literature through the mid-1980s, see Paul-Shaheen, P., Clark, J. D., and Williams, D. "Small Area Analysis: A Review and Analysis of the North American Literature." *Journal of Health Politics, Policy, and Law,* Winter 1987, *12,* 741–809.

25. U.S. General Accounting Office. *Cancer Treatment, 1975-1985: The Use of Breakthrough Treatments for Seven Types of Cancer.* Pub no. PEMD-88-12BR. Washington, D.C.: General Accounting Office, 1988, p. 4.

26. Medicare Payment Advisory Commission (MEDPAC). *Report to Congress: Medicare Payment Policy.* Washington, D.C.: MEDPAC, Mar. 2000.

27. See Rice, T., and Bernstein, J. "Volume Performance Standards: Can They Control Growth in Medicare Services?" *Milbank Quarterly,* 1990, *68,* 295-319; and Marquis, M. S., and Kominski, G. F. "Alternative Volume Performance Standards for Medicare Physicians' Services." *Milbank Quarterly,* 1994, *72,* 329–357.

28. Physician Payment Review Commission. *Annual Report to Congress.* Washington, D.C.: Physician Payment Review Commission, 1993.

29. OECD Secretariat. "Health Care Expenditure and Other Data." *Health Care Financing Review,* 1989 Annual Supplement, *11,* 111–194.

30. Newhouse, J. P., Anderson, G., and Roos, L. L. "Hospital Spending in the United States and Canada: A Comparison." *Health Affairs,* Winter 1988, *7,* 6–24; Detsky, A. A., Stacey, S. R., and Bombardier, C. "The Effectiveness of a Regulatory Strategy in Containing Hospital Costs: The Ontario Experience, 1967-1981." *New England Journal of Medicine,* July 1983, *309,* 151–159.

31. Roos, L. L., and others. "Health and Surgical Outcomes in Canada and the United States." *Health Affairs,* Summer 1992, *11,* 56–72.

32. Marquis and Kominski (1994).

33. Kominski, G. Commentary on Zuckerman, S., Norton, S. A., and Verrilli, D. "Price Controls and Medicare Spending: Assessing the Volume Offset Assumption." *Medical Care Research and Review,* Dec. 1998, *55,* 479–483.

34. Point-of-service plans are like HMOs in that the health plan receives a capitation amount for providing services. Typically, enrollees must be referred by a primary care physician before receiving hospital or specialty care. The main difference is that under POS, patients can go to providers outside of the network, but usually only by paying a sizable co-payment (say, 40 percent of costs).

35. Luft, H. S. *Health Maintenance Organizations: Dimensions of Performance.* New York: Wiley, 1981; Manning, W. G., and others. "A Controlled Trial of the Effect of a Prepaid Group Practice on Use of Services." *New England Journal of Medicine,* June 7, 1984, *310,* 1505–1510.

36. Miller, R. H., and Luft, H. S. "Managed Care Plan Performance Since 1980: A Literature Analysis." *Journal of the American Medical Association,* 1994, *271,* 1512–1519.

37. Miller, R. H., and Luft, H. S. "Does Managed Care Lead to Better or Worse Quality of Care?" *Health Affairs,* 1997, *16*(5), 7–25.

38. This is the theme of the writings of Alain Enthoven. See, for example, Enthoven, A. C. "The History and Principles of Managed Competition." *Health Affairs,* 1993 Supplement, *12,* 24–48.

CHAPTER FIVE

PHARMACEUTICAL PRICES AND EXPENDITURES

Stuart O. Schweitzer and William S. Comanor

The press frequently reports on the difficulties people have in paying for prescription drugs. An article in the *New York Times* states, "Perhaps no issue touches as many lives as the cost of medication, which is why it is consuming the political landscape this year."[1] The author continues: "Prescription drugs are now the fastest-growing part of the nation's health care bill." An article in the *Wall Street Journal* noted substantial increases in pharmaceutical spending during 1997 and 1998 and stated that over the two year period, "insurers and health maintenance organizations spent 16.8 percent more on prescription drugs."[2]

These observations are hardly new. Pharmaceutical prices have been a matter of concern for nearly half a century. Our political leaders frequently comment on the increasing prices of new pharmaceuticals and deplore their consequences, particularly for elderly consumers who require large quantities of drugs and must often pay for them from their own resources. In 1961, the Kefauver Committee of the U.S. Senate produced a report on drug prices,[3] following an extensive set of hearings. Thirty years later, the same theme was repeated in 1993 hearings before the Senate Special Committee on Aging. The committee chairman, David Pryor, stated: "Millions of older Americans go to bed at night wondering if they will be able to afford their medications. . . . New drugs are selling in the United States at prices which are simply staggering. Unless I have read from the wrong economics textbook, this appears to be market failure at its worst. . . . Where the market has not, will not, or cannot work, we must take prudent actions to assure that drugs are priced reasonably." [4]

Despite major changes in the U.S. health care system since the 1950s public discourse regarding the pharmaceutical industry has remained fairly constant. The issue of pharmaceutical costs is long-standing. The purpose of this chapter is to discuss the issue's underlying causes and consider some possible solutions.

Unfortunately, part of the concern over drug expenditures is misplaced because of failure to recognize that drugs are an integral component of the medical care process. In many cases drugs are a substitute for other medical care inputs, such as hospital stays and physician visits. H_2 antagonists, like Tagamet and Zantac, for example, have practically eliminated the need for ulcer surgery, while antipsychotic drugs have substantially reduced the need for mental hospital stays. For both of these drug classes, pharmaceutical expenditures rose after their introduction. Fortunately, nobody expressed concern about the problem of rising drug costs then, and the effect on overall medical care costs has been favorable.

However, not all drugs are cost-saving substitutes. Some, like the so-called clot busters used in the emergency room for a heart-attack patient, are complements, making other services more efficient and improving outcomes. Although these drugs have also fueled rising pharmaceutical expenditures, few would deny their value in increasing the quality of health outcomes. Thus, drugs can be both substitutes and complements to other health care inputs.

The concern over pharmaceutical costs is heightened by lack of clarity about the nature of the problem. Spending on any good or service is a function of both price and quantity. Is the problem of rising drug expenditures due to the rising quantity of pharmaceuticals that are consumed? Or is it due to rising prices? The answers are complicated by the role played by rapid technological innovation in this industry, which leads to frequent replacement of older products by newer ones. Newer products are often more expensive than the older ones, so that expenditures may rise because of displacement—even if prices of all drugs, new and old, and the number of prescriptions were to remain constant.

To understand rising drug costs, we first review trends in drug expenditure in the United States. Next we look at U.S. drug prices, considering first a series of issues that make measuring drug prices especially difficult. We then look at the evidence on whether U.S. drug prices are higher than those in other countries. We also examine the intertemporal relationship between price increases and quality changes to determine whether pharmaceutical prices have increased after correcting for therapeutic improvements. Then, we describe the factors determining drug prices in the United States. Of particular importance are the roles of therapeutic advance and competition. Finally, we discuss a series of policy options for containing pharmaceutical expenditures. Some of these are directed at consumers, some at physicians, and still others at manufacturers. Current efforts to control pharmaceutical costs are a blend of all three approaches.

The Problem of Drug Expenditures

The share of pharmaceuticals and other components of the U.S. health care system from 1960 through 1997 is shown in Figure 5.1.

During this period of nearly forty years, the proportion of total health expenditures devoted to pharmaceuticals has actually declined. In 1997 its share was just under 10 percent, down by one-third from its 1960 share of over 15 percent.[5] Of course, the decline in pharmaceutical share was not due to falling drug expenditures; instead, it resulted from a far larger rise in expenditures on other health services. The pharmaceutical share is greater than that of nursing homes and dental services, but the drug sector is clearly not a dominant source of health services expenditure.

We turn next to the question of price change in pharmaceuticals. Data on consumer prices and the Consumer Price Index (CPI) and its constituent parts

FIGURE 5.1.   SHARE OF NATIONAL HEALTH EXPENDITURES BY TYPE, 1960–1997.

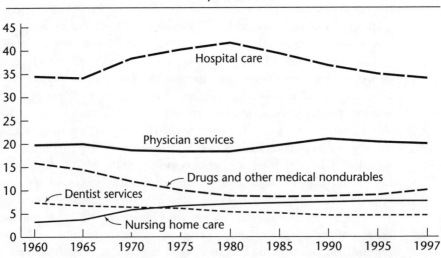

Source: Department of Health and Human Services. *Health United States, 1999.* Washington, D.C.: U.S. Government Printing Office, 2000.

(including pharmaceuticals and other health services) are calculated and published by the Bureau of Labor Statistics. Although there are various problems with these data, which we discuss in this chapter, it is still useful to review the reported trends in these statistics since they generally indicate maximum price increases.

Figure 5.2 shows time series data on the rate of increase in the overall ("all-item") CPI figures, the overall medical care component of the CPI, and CPI trends for the hospital, physician, dentist, and drug components. The data shown are the annual rate of price change for the year prior to the date on the graph.

The data show that the rate of price increase of health care exceeded that of the overall CPI for the entire period, but that the rate of increase of pharmaceuticals is similar to that of the other health care components. Prior to 1980, the rate of increase of drugs was below that of other components, but since then it has been above most of the components (although below the rate of change in hospital prices during the period for which data are available).[6]

If pharmaceuticals constitute only a small portion of overall health care expenditures, and if price increases have been relatively similar to other components for many years, what is the reason behind the continued public and Congressional concern over drug prices?

FIGURE 5.2. ANNUAL PERCENT CHANGE IN CPI FROM PREVIOUS YEAR, 1970–1998.

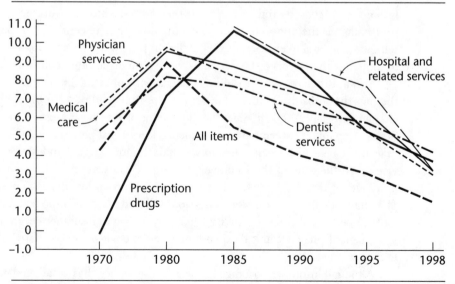

Source: Health United States 1999.

One answer to this query is that utilization has risen sharply, in part a result of the country's aging population. Furthermore, drugs can do more things today than in the past, so they are prescribed more frequently. Direct-to-consumer advertising may also have led to increased consumption. As a result of all of these factors, we observe that the number of prescriptions filled per year has risen dramatically, from 1.9 billion in 1993 to 2.5 billion in 1998.[7] Within some common therapeutic categories, the rise in quantity is even more dramatic. The number of antidepressant prescriptions filled increased by 111 percent during this period, and that for cholesterol-lowering drugs rose by 162 percent. For oral antihistamines, the increase was fully 500 percent.[8]

Another response is that there is a fundamental difference between pharmaceuticals and other health service components. Most health care purchases are exclusively *services*, but pharmaceuticals have both *service* and *manufactured* components. The service role applies to the research and development behind all pharmaceutical products and also to the professional dispensing of the drug. But the drug itself is a manufactured product, and most drugs are manufactured on a very large scale, taking advantage of economies of scale in the manufacturing process. The cost of manufacturing a drug constitutes less than half of the total cost.[9] As the price charged for the pharmaceutical is much higher than production cost, it would be possible to reduce the price substantially and still cover the cost.[10] To be sure, high pharmaceutical margins cover high research and marketing costs that accompany the continued introduction of new drugs. At the same time, these are costs that generally have already been paid, and consumers may not see a link between the purchased product and what they are asked to pay. Further obscuring this linkage is the apparent willingness of most pharmaceutical companies to sell the same or similar drugs at very different prices, whether through discounts to some health insurers or health plans, or to patients in other countries.

Still another reason for public concern with pharmaceutical prices lies in the fact that most insurance plans cover less than 100 percent of the patient charges for drugs. Although more than four-fifths of health care costs in the United States are paid by government or private insurers, third-party coverage for pharmaceuticals has historically been lower than that of hospital and physician services.[11] At the time of the Kefauver hearings, there was virtually no insurance coverage for drugs. In 1961, private insurance paid for less than 0.5 percent of pharmaceutical expenses. Consumers paid directly (as out-of-pocket payment) for 95.5 percent of drug costs.[12] By 1995, private health insurance covered nearly 40 percent of pharmaceutical expenditures, and the out-of-pocket share had fallen to 39.5 percent.[13]

Although insurance coverage for health care services has broadened in recent years, pharmaceutical coverage still lags behind the other segments of the medical care sector. In 1992, patients paid directly for 28 percent of their pharmaceutical expenses, but at the same time the out-of-pocket share for hospital and physician charges was only 5 and 18 percent respectively.[14] The higher share of pharmaceutical expenditures paid directly implies that consumers are less sheltered from the burden of paying for drugs than for other services, making pharmaceutical prices more visible to consumers.

For the elderly, the problem of substantial drug expenditure is more complicated. As we have noted, the universal health insurer for the elderly is the Medicare program. But Medicare does not cover outpatient drugs. However, approximately two-thirds of seniors either qualify for Medicaid coverage (which covers outpatient drugs) or have private health insurance as a supplement to Medicare coverage. Only about one-third of the elderly rely on Medicare alone and thus must pay fully out of pocket for their pharmaceuticals. Furthermore, cost sharing is increasingly being implemented in Medicare supplemental policies. Coinsurance and deductibles are frequently linked to the type of drug used to fill a prescription. For example, a prescription filled with a generic product may require only a $5 co-payment, while the co-payment for a brand product might be $20.

It is striking that insurance coverage for drugs is far greater today than it was in the late 1950s, at the time of the Kefauver hearings, yet the public demand for government assistance is unchanged. One explanation may be that drugs have become both more costly and more essential over time. Another factor may be the disparity in coverage among segments of the population. Some people are covered relatively well by private insurance, while others find drug coverage to be meager, and still others have no insurance coverage for drugs at all.

Interpreting Pharmaceutical Price Data

Various reports, both public and private, have described rapidly rising drug prices. A 1992 report by the U.S. General Accounting Office observed that "during the 1980s, prescription drug prices increased by almost three times the rate of general inflation and certain drugs increased in price by over 100 percent in five years."[15] This report reviewed price data for a sample of widely used prescription drugs, and concluded: "Prices for nearly all 29 drug products increased more than the percentage changes for all three consumer price indexes for the six year period ending December 31, 1991. The maximum price increase for each product during this period generally exceeded 100 percent, with some prices increasing by 200 to 300 percent. . . . During this same period, the CPI for all items increased by 26.2 percent, the CPI for medical care by 56.3 percent, and the CPI for prescription drugs by 67 percent."[16]

Unfortunately, these observations of the price of pharmaceutical products are incomplete. Since the adoption of the 1984 law facilitating approval of generic drugs upon a branded drug's patent expiration, the importance of generics in the pharmaceutical marketplace has exploded. By 1998, fully 47 percent of pharmaceuticals dispensed, in terms of physical units, were for the generic product, up from 40 percent as recently as 1993.[17] Thus, nearly half of all drugs consumed in the United States are products for which there is little suggestion that high price is a problem.

The Effect of Generic Products on Price

Not only are generic products priced substantially below their branded counterparts, but generic prices have declined over time. For most products, the share of total sales represented by generics for the particular molecule greatly expands following patent expiration. Griliches and Cockburn observe that within two years of a branded drug's patent expiration, its market share of product revenue generally falls by 50 percent.[18] If this picture is even broadly correct, then the increasing role of generic products in the pharmaceutical market has surely led to a declining average price for most products (including both the branded and generic versions) following patent expiration and the entry of generic producers. Our first question therefore is how the influence of generic entry, leading generally to a price decline, relates to the claim that pharmaceutical prices have sharply increased.

To resolve this issue, one first needs to decide whether the generic version of a drug should be considered the same "product" as its branded counterpart. Throughout most of the recent past, the Bureau of Labor Statistics (BLS) has assumed that a branded product is inherently different from the generic version.[19] It notes that both patients and physicians frequently react differently to the two types of product despite their bio-equivalence. As a result, the BLS has treated these products as distinct entities and reported their price changes independently. Thus, it has not incorporated the increasing use of generic products into its reported price series.[20]

In contrast, one could accept the implicit judgment of the Food and Drug Administration (FDA) that generic and branded versions of the same molecule are identical, and then produce a price series for the incumbent and entrants according to their relative output levels. When this procedure is carried out for individual products, we observe that average prices have typically declined.[21]

However, one cannot say that the FDA position is entirely correct and the BLS position is entirely wrong, because a substantial number of buyers do in fact treat these products as different. In their study of these issues, Griliches and Cockburn seek to account for these differences and, as might be expected, report price series that lie between the two extreme assumptions.[22] For the most part, their price series constructed for individual drugs show some decline in price after introduction of generics, although less than for the series based entirely on the assumption that branded and generic versions represent the same product.

Launch Prices and Drug Price Changes

In addition to the question of generic substitutability, there is also the effect of pricing strategies during the years following product introduction. Two strategies are used: "skimming" and "penetration." The former is setting a high introductory price and reducing it over time, while the latter is the reverse, where a low introductory price is set but prices rise over time. Clearly, prices set for the same pharmaceutical products show a declining trend where skimming strategies are commonly used, but an increasing trend with penetration strategies. There is evidence that both types of strategy are found in this industry. Skimming is typically applied to drugs representing a major therapeutic advance, while penetration is commonly used for imitative products.[23] As a result, one is likely to find rising drug prices when more imitative products are introduced, but declining prices when more innovative products are seen. Therefore, rising prices may be a consequence of low (penetration) launch prices, while more moderate price trends may result from high (skimming) launch prices.

Drug Prices and Quality Improvement

Brand-name pharmaceutical products compete with their generic substitutes, but also among themselves. Even though one drug may be therapeutically similar to the other drugs in its particular therapeutic category, it may differ in terms of side effects and adverse interaction profiles; higher prices can frequently be explained by this type of improvement.[24] Thus, the price increase for a new product reflects product improvement, while the price for an older product may actually decline.

To investigate this issue, Berndt and his colleagues estimated a series of hedonic regression equations in which several attributes were used as proxies for relative quality of various products. These measures largely reflected individual side effects. Through this technique, the authors were able to measure price trends while holding quality level constant. For the years between 1980 and 1996, and dealing only with antidepressant drugs, they report average rate of price increase under three scenarios: price increases measured without accounting for generics or quality change, 7.11 percent; price increases including generics but without incorporating the improved quality of new products, 4.73 percent; and price increases incorporating both effects, 4.33 percent. Although the former correction was far more significant throughout the entire period that they studied, they observed that there were particular years where the quality change associated with a new product was a more important factor than the increasing role of generics.[25]

Measuring Drug Prices When New Drugs Replace Old Drugs

The BLS computes the overall CPI as well as its constituent parts as a Laspeyres index, which compares the cost of a given bundle of goods (often referred to as the "market basket") purchased at current prices to the cost of that same quantity purchased at base-year prices.[26] This market basket, however, must be adjusted periodically to reflect current expenditure patterns; otherwise the index has progressively less relationship to the actual goods purchased by consumers. With regard to health care, newer treatments for old problems, such as coronary artery disease or renal failure, have totally replaced techniques in use only a few years ago. In many cases there are new therapies available for problems that were previously untreatable. If new and improved drugs replace older ones, but at a higher price, the appropriate price index should account for quality improvement as well as price increase. When price statistics fail to account adequately for quality improvement, a measure of price change is biased upward.

The method used by the BLS for measuring price change is designed to track prices for a fixed market basket, or one that changes slowly. When items in the market basket change through shifts in consumer demand, the BLS uses a "linking" technique through which the price index of a new market basket replaces the index for an older one. For example, when a new product, such as a more powerful antihypertensive drug, replaces an established but less-expensive one, price indices with the old and the new product are each calculated, and the new index (with the higher-priced product) is scaled downward to equal the older one. The index including the new item then replaces the prior index in future calculations. No attempt is made to assess whether an improved drug is more or less expensive than would be justified by the quality change represented by its introduction. The price index merely tracks the prices of all items in the market basket and then recalculates the price index when a new product is included.

Failure to capture the effect of quality change is especially serious for pharmaceuticals, where the turnover of products is rapid and new products frequently are improved versions of older ones, with greater efficacy, fewer side effects, or a more convenient regimen. The question of whether an increase in drug price exceeds, falls behind, or accurately reflects a change in quality is left unanswered.

Prices and Margins: The Difference Between Wholesale and Retail Prices

Before concluding this discussion of pharmaceutical price measurement, the important distinction between the price set by the pharmaceutical manufacturer and what is ultimately paid by the consumer must be noted. The difference between these two prices is the distribution margin, which includes the cost and profit of both the dispensing pharmacy as well as the wholesaler, if one is involved in distributing the product. In many discussions of the cost of pharmaceuticals, there is the implicit assumption that distribution margin is constant across products so that whatever price is charged by the manufacturer is passed on to the consumer, with merely a fixed amount added to cover distribution cost.

However, this picture is not generally accurate in the United States. Steiner, in particular, has pointed to "the inverse association between the margins of manufacturers and [those of] retailers."[27] His study offers empirical evidence on this relationship as well as the reasons for its presence. Salehi and Schweitzer[28] found that this relationship applies to pharmaceuticals. Branded pharmaceuticals, which typically embody a high manufacturing margin, have lower distribution margins, while generic products with lower margins at the manufacturing stage have much higher distribution margins. As a result, price differences between branded and generic products are greater at the manufacturing stage of production than at retail.

International Price Comparisons

International comparisons of drug prices have also contributed to public concern that drug prices are excessive in the United States. For example, the Congressional General Accounting Office (GAO) has published studies comparing U.S. drug prices with those in the United Kingdom and Canada.[29] These reports suggest that prices for the same branded products are generally higher in the United States than elsewhere. Even so, the GAO studies are subject to the same conceptual and methodological problems that we have already discussed.

Most important, the GAO studies fail to account for generic substitution in any comprehensive way. Thus, although their comparison of relative prices for a particular branded drug may be correct, they do not necessarily reflect differences in the actual price facing the consumer since the generic is typically more important in the United States than elsewhere. As we noted above, the share of the market accounted for by generic drugs in the United States has grown substantially and is now nearly one-half of all drug units (doses) sold.[30] Therefore, merely comparing the prices of specific branded products, without including in the analysis the presence of generic products, gives a misleading picture of the relative cost to the consumer from filling a doctor's prescription.

For example, suppose that half of U.S. prescriptions for cimetidine are filled by the generic version, the price of which is $104 per hundred, while the price of the branded product, Tagamet, is $167. The average price is $135.50. Suppose further that the price of Tagamet in Canada is $150, and the generic price is $100. But if the generic version's market share is only 20 percent in Canada, the average price there is $140, which is higher than the average U.S. price, even though the price of both products is lower in Canada.

Another problem with the GAO approach is that it relies on wholesale price, which does not account for the many discounts and rebates present in the United States. Even if these prices accurately described the charge to a pharmacy for a cash customer, they will not in general reflect the transaction price to other classes of buyers, who in fact constitute the largest segment of demand. This factor is important to the extent that discounting is more widespread in the United States than in Britain or Canada.

Finally, the GAO studies failed to deal with varying drug consumption patterns in the three countries studied. Not only are drugs used differently in each country but even the same drugs are taken in a number of forms and dosages.[31] The GAO approach side-stepped the entire question and considered a narrower one: Are wholesale prices higher in the United States than in Britain or Canada for the specific items that are major-selling American drugs? This approach may well compare the price of a highly popular U.S. product with those of less commonly used products in other countries.

In response to the GAO reports, Danzon and Chao carried out a more complete analysis of international drug price comparison.[32] They included all drugs sold in each of nine countries, incorporating over-the-counter drugs, which substitute for prescribed drugs; and use data on average transaction prices at the manufacturer level. The authors found that price differences between countries depend greatly on how the comparison is framed, particularly which country's quantity weights are used to construct the price index. Comparisons also differ depending on whether one compares price per gram of active ingredient or price per "standard unit" (for example, per capsule or milliliter of liquid). Although by most measures average U.S. drug prices did exceed those in most other countries, this result did not always apply, and it did not include the more significant role played by generic products in the United States.

The Determination of Drug Prices

We now turn to the causative factors that determine pharmaceutical prices. The research and development costs required to introduce a new drug are substantial—frequently in the hundreds of millions of dollars per drug. These costs include not only direct expenditure on research and testing, but also the time cost incurred, resulting from the substantial difference between when the outlay is made and when revenues are received. Part of this lag is the time spent waiting for the FDA to approve a new product. Furthermore, these outlays are typically made before a single prescription is filled. As a result, they represent a classic example of sunk costs, which do not vary with output. R and D costs, like those for fixed plant and equipment, have already been spent before the product is sold, so they cannot influence the actual market price. Whether these costs are high or low, the optimal price charged by the pharmaceutical company is the same.

Similarly, most marketing costs are incurred in the early years of a product's life cycle and for the purpose of introducing it to the medical community. Like research costs, they do not generally vary with output and therefore also represent sunk costs. The only variable costs in this industry therefore lie at the manufacturing stage. For large research-intensive companies, however, production costs are generally less than half of the value of the product.[33] Marginal costs for most drugs are quite low and thereby explain little about the price that is charged.

Research and development, marketing, and manufacturing costs are all factors that reflect conditions on the supply side of the market. None of them has a major impact on pharmaceutical prices. Instead, prices depend predominantly on demand-side considerations. The price charged for a pharmaceutical is determined largely by how valuable it is to consumers and what the consumer is willing to pay for it. The critical factor is "willingness to pay," which in turn depends on various considerations. In this section, we consider the relevant factors and review some available evidence on their importance.

Therapeutic Advance

The demand-side factor most important in determining the price of a pharmaceutical is its therapeutic advance as compared with products already on the market. Doctors and patients are willing to pay a larger amount for a medically improved product as compared to one without a substantial therapeutic advance. With increased willingness to pay, the seller can set a higher price without driving customers away.

To explore the importance of this factor, Lu and Comanor examined the price premium for new products as compared to the prices of their existing rivals.[34] The results are given in Table 5.1 for new products used for both acute and chronic conditions.

These data show that the launch prices of drugs that embody an important therapeutic gain are about two and a half times greater than those of existing substitutes; a drug with moderate gain is priced about one and one-half times greater, and a product with little or no therapeutic advance is generally priced at or about the same level as existing products.

Competitive Forces

When a new product is introduced—whether it embodies a small or large therapeutic advance—there are typically existing products used for the same or similar indications. These alternate products are those which physicians would prescribe in the absence of the new product and are thereby the rival products with which a new one must compete. Note that this concept of relevant market, resting on specific therapeutic indications, is far narrower than the conventional classification of a therapeutic category. Those classifications, such as antibiotics or hypertensives, are so broad that they include pharmaceuticals with dissimilar indications and actions, and hence products that do not actually compete with one another.

When there are alternative products available for the same or similar indications, the prescribing physician must select among rival drugs. The physician and the patients' willingness to pay for specific drugs are then influenced by any price differences that may exist. In this case, the seller can seek to increase sales by cutting the price; the more rival products there are competing in a market, the

TABLE 5.1. PRICES FOR NEW PHARMACEUTICALS RELATIVE TO THOSE OF EXISTING DRUGS.

FDA Designation of Therapeutic Advance	Ratio of Median Price of New Drugs to Existing Drugs	
	Acute	Chronic
Important therapeutic advance	2.97	2.29
Modest therapeutic advance	1.72	1.19
Little or no therapeutic advance	1.22	0.94

Source: Lu, Z. J., and Comanor, W. S. "Strategic Pricing of New Pharmaceuticals." *Review of Economics and Statistics*, Feb. 1998, p. 116.

more price cutting actually occurs. The Lu and Comanor study found that the launch price is substantially lower when there are more branded rivals in direct competition; subsequent price changes are lower as well. Despite common disdain for imitative products,[35] they play the essential role of promoting more competitive behavior and leading to lower final prices. New imitative products are an important competitive factor in the pharmaceutical marketplace.

Generic pharmaceuticals also have an important impact on market competition and price level. Generic producers typically start production after the relevant patent has expired. They do so by gaining FDA approval of an Abbreviated New Drug Application (ANDA), which merely requires demonstrating bioequivalence to the original product. The prices set by generic producers are much lower than those charged by the original developer of the product, as they compete largely by price. Moreover, the price of a generic product is also affected by the number of sellers. As their numbers increase, price competition becomes more vigorous, and prices decline below the level found when there is only a single entrant. A study of anti-infectives found that the largest price effects occurred when the fourth and fifth generic firms entered. Average prices per prescription declined from nearly $30 with two or three sellers to roughly $17 with the presence of a fourth rival, and then to $9.25 when a fifth firm entered.[36]

These reported declines in average price took place despite the fact that the price charged for the original branded product is typically *increased,* not reduced, when entry occurs.[37] The original manufacturer does not typically compete on the basis of price with generic entrants but rather finds it more profitable to concentrate on the segment of the market that includes brand-loyal customers. These are physicians and patients who know a particular brand and prefer it, so they continue to use it despite the presence of a lower-priced substitute. When generic manufacturers enter production, the price differential expands as the price charged for the original branded product increases.

Buyer Characteristics

Another major factor affecting consumers' willingness to pay for particular drugs is the mechanism by which payments are made. For uninsured patients who purchase pharmaceuticals much as they do other consumer goods, demand may be fairly price-elastic. The buyer is limited to the prescribed product, but he or she can sometimes influence prescribing decisions by calling attention to the prices of alternate products. Where generic versions of the drug are available, the patient may also ask the pharmacist to substitute it for the branded product. The patient always has the option of not filling the prescription, which occurs in a large number of cases.[38] For all of these reasons, producers may encounter substantial price resistance if they set the price much above the anticipated value.

On the other hand, this resistance is attenuated if the buyer has substantial insurance coverage. In that case, the out-of-pocket cost of a prescribed pharmaceutical may be minimal or quite low, and the economic reason to limit one's purchase is removed. Demand conditions thus depend on the conduct of managed care organizations and other third-party payers, and also on the nature of the contractual agreements that govern their payments.

Where payers simply agree to cover the pharmaceutical costs of insured patients, perhaps with a deductible and coinsurance provision, demand becomes less price-elastic. Judgment as to which product is prescribed is made exclusively by the physician, whose decision may depend on marketing and other idiosyncratic factors, and is not likely to be constrained by the patient's economic circumstances. The more inelastic consumer demand is, the higher the product price will be. Increased insurance coverage of pharmaceuticals would then lead directly to higher prices.

There are other circumstances where expanded insurance coverage may lead to more-elastic demand conditions such that there is a shift "from patient-driven to payer-driven competition."[39] The central factor here is the conduct of third-party payers. When insurance companies and HMOs institute formularies, which are restrictive lists of approved products, and indicate to both doctors and patients that they will pay only for those drugs, they gain a direct influence on prescribing decisions. Furthermore, the drug price can be a major determinant of whether or not it is included in the formulary. In these circumstances, pharmaceutical coverage leads to more-elastic demand, rather than less-elastic. Of critical importance is whether a third-party payer can influence prescribing decisions.

Where generic products are available in the market, the conduct of third-party payers can affect prices even without influencing prescribing decisions. This is because pharmacists can substitute generics for prescribed branded drugs, and patients can be encouraged through various incentives to buy generics. In these circumstances, the price elasticity of demand for a branded drug increases (in absolute value) and the affected producer responds by setting a lower price. Although there are few empirical studies that explore these factors, the structure of demand conditions for pharmaceuticals is clearly not a simple matter and depends on the complex relationships among patients, physicians, and third-party payers. Depending on the behavior of all of these parties, demand elasticity is determined, and so then is the price set in the marketplace.

Before concluding this section, we note that insurance coverage for prescription drugs has increased over time, so there is an increasing difference between patient cost and market price. Furthermore, there has been a general shift from an overall deductible to a fixed co-payment, which means a richer insurance benefit structure for prescription drugs.[40] These factors suggest that demand conditions in pharmaceutical markets increasingly depend on the conduct of managed care providers and other third-party payers. The prices that are set depend largely on what commitments are made by these payers to offer drugs to their subscribers.

Differential Pricing

Where price depends on demand conditions, and also where there are clear distinctions among types of buyer, we expect to find variation in the prices charged to the buyers. The economist's model of price discrimination offers a clear description of this process and indicates that prices depend strongly on the relevant price elasticity of demand. Where elasticity differs among classes of consumers, final prices differ as well. There is considerable evidence that this pattern is pervasive throughout the pharmaceutical industry. Pharmaceutical companies establish a list price for each drug, but many (or most) sales are made by discounting that price—and the discount can be substantial. A survey of drug prices in one area found that the average price charged for a selection of well-known products sold to hospitals was only 19 percent of that charged to a local pharmacy.[41] Since hospital demand for specific products is likely to be more elastic than that of an individual pharmacy, which must stock a large number of products to fill individual prescriptions, hospital prices are expected to be much lower than those charged to pharmacies. Where prices are demand-driven, differences in demand elasticity are reflected in actual prices.

These discounts may also differ between individual and chain store pharmacies, and between hospitals and HMOs. A critical fact about the pharmaceutical industry is that there is no single price for an individual product even at a specific point in time; the price depends on the demand conditions presented by particular buyers.

When generic products enter the marketplace, they typically appeal more to some buyers than to others. In particular, HMOs and hospital pharmacies are likely to use generic products because they have the knowledge and expertise required to evaluate them, in contrast to individual physicians. One expects therefore that generic rivals will make greater sales to some buyers than to others. That being so, producers of brand products will respond to generic competition more strongly in some market segments than in others. By setting much lower prices where generic competition exists, but keeping prices at their original level or even higher where generic competition is less important, the sellers of many branded products have been able to maintain a large proportion of their original sales without depressing revenues excessively.

The evidence that major pharmaceutical firms have pursued this type of strategy is that they have generally maintained market share following patent expiration and generic entry. By the sixth year after patent expiration, average market share for thirty-five products between 1984 and 1987 was fully 62 percent in physical units and 85 percent in dollar sales as compared to previous levels.[42] The strategy of charging a lower price where a firm faces strenuous competition but setting a higher price where it does not has been used by many companies to maintain sales and market share. Once again, buyers' willingness-to-pay is the critical factor that determines pharmaceutical prices.

Approaches for Containing Pharmaceutical Costs

Although pharmaceutical companies have sought to maintain or expand revenues, health care consumers, providers, and insurers have looked for methods to limit drug expenditure. Here as elsewhere, buyers and sellers face opposing incentives. Some buyers have sought to reduce the quantity of drugs consumed, but most have looked for means to lower the price paid for a specific product or to redirect the patient toward a lower-priced alternative. These methods can be divided into those focused on consumer behavior, physician prescribing patterns, and manufacturer actions. At this point, we review some measures that have been used.

Patient-Focused Measures

Consumer behavior can be altered through economic incentives or education. Economic incentives typically mean cost sharing, through which patients bear more of the financial consequences of their actions by paying a larger share of drug costs. As the cost of drugs to the consumer increases, the quantity purchased declines, with patients either going without the prescribed drug or shifting to less-expensive alternatives such as generic products or over-the-counter options.

Cost sharing is sometimes criticized as being an overly blunt instrument, because it may discourage the use of necessary, as well as unnecessary, therapies. The RAND Health Insurance Experiment examined the effect of cost sharing on the consumption of prescribed drugs. Leibowitz and her colleagues reported that pharmaceutical expenditures by individuals without cost sharing were as much as 60 percent higher than for those with cost sharing.[43] The findings were similar for patients at a large HMO, although the difference was smaller.[44] A cost-sharing requirement of $1.50 per prescription reduced the number of prescriptions filled by 10.7 percent; doubling the co-payment led to an additional 10.6 percent reduction in the number of filled prescriptions. Furthermore, the authors found that consumers were more likely to reduce consumption of discretionary rather than essential drugs in response to increased cost sharing. These findings are tempered, though, by the observation that the cost per prescription rose in response to higher cost sharing. This change may have occurred because consumers purchased a greater quantity of drug per prescription, as their cost may have been related to the prescription rather than the quantity of product actually purchased.[45]

An alternative to economic incentives in dealing with consumer behavior is patient education. An example of this type of program is informing patients that generic drugs are equivalent to brand products. Another is explaining to patients that the extensive use of certain drugs, such as antibiotics, is unnecessary and may even be harmful, thereby lowering the quantity purchased. Such programs can reduce consumer demand for specific products, but they are unlikely to limit aggregate demand for pharmaceuticals to a substantial extent. Many patients still expect a prescription at the conclusion of each physician visit, and physicians respond accordingly.

Provider-Focused Measures

Despite the presence of consumer-oriented programs, most efforts at cost containment for pharmaceuticals are directed at those who make decisions on drug therapy: the physician, the hospital, and the managed care provider. Because the physician, particularly one in private practice, has few incentives to limit pharmaceutical costs, physician-directed policies are not very different from those aimed at consumers. When financial constraints are removed from the patient, they are also removed from the physician.

However, physicians are also the subject of education programs that seek to improve the quality of prescribing and reduce overall drug expenditures. These programs are present especially in HMOs or other managed care programs, and they have great potential because the pace of new-drug introduction is rapid and physicians have difficulty keeping abreast of new therapeutic options. Without such programs, the primary means for the physician to learn about new products is from pharmaceutical company marketing efforts, which are designed to increase rather than reduce spending on pharmaceuticals.

Even if the physician has few incentives to restrain costs, this is not so for an organization that actually pays for pharmaceuticals. Generic versions of drugs are generally favored, and newer, more expensive drugs often discouraged.[46] In addition, these payers may promote the shift of certain products to over-the-counter status. These drugs can then be obtained without a visit to the physician's office, and such products are typically not reimbursed. More important, hospitals, HMOs, and government reimbursement plans have long adopted formularies designed explicitly to restrict the drug choices available to physicians in order to reduce costs. These lists of approved drugs depend in principle on the relative cost and effectiveness of alternative products. Nearly all formulary programs permit exceptions, but the burden of obtaining an exemption is often great enough to discourage a physician from doing so unless he or she feels that a nonlisted drug is absolutely necessary.[47]

Formularies, however, have the potential for increasing rather than decreasing health care costs if they are so restrictive that patients are prescribed less effective drugs. Even an expensive drug is generally less costly than a physician visit or hospital episode, so using a suboptimal drugs may be penny-wise but pound-foolish. The question of whether or not a formulary lowers or raises drug or overall health care costs depends on the relative prices of the drugs included and excluded from the formulary, the number of patients who use the more expensive product when it is not necessary, and the treatment ramifications when patients are switched to a less expensive drug but need the more expensive one. Sloan, Gordon, and Cocks found that "limiting the number of drugs [through a formulary] appears to have been a very good idea for gastrointestinal disease patients and for those with asthma, but a bad one for coronary diseases [sic] patients."[48] In the latter case, total medical costs actually increased with the adoption of the formulary. Other studies have also shown that Medicaid formularies are not effective in either lowering drug expenditures or reducing overall health care costs.[49] Apparently, formularies have not been able to discourage consumption of expensive drugs whose use is unnecessary, while allowing such use when appropriate.

Manufacturer-Focused Measures

A more direct approach to cost containment is exercising a payer's monopsony power to limit the price charged by a pharmaceutical manufacturer for its product. These actions are frequently adopted by governments that provide coverage for pharmaceuticals in their national program. Increasingly, foreign governments or insurance funds have sought to reduce drug prices as a means of cost control. In most countries, the question is not whether to fix prices, but how to do so, and in particular how to set prices without removing the incentive to develop new and improved pharmaceuticals. A typical response is to permit use of a product and reimburse the cost in accordance with its relative therapeutic benefit. Note that, ideally, this objective leads to the same price as that set in a competitive market. Regulatory objectives are thereby similar to those enforced by competitive markets.

Australia has progressed further than other countries in attempting to calculate the cost-effectiveness of new drugs and setting reimbursement prices accordingly.[50] Canada uses this model at the national level as well. Britain, on the other hand, incorporates the profitability of the pharmaceutical company into its calculation of the National Health Service price for new products.

Similarly, managed care programs in the United States frequently determine the prices they pay for pharmaceuticals purchased on behalf of their patients in accordance with the perceived value of the products. For this reason, pharmaceutical manufacturers now give managed care plans studies of the cost effectiveness of a new product. As a result of managed care purchasing power, these organizations typically pay less for pharmaceuticals than do individual patients.

Advertising is often suggested as a cause of rising pharmaceutical expenditure. With the FDA's relaxation of prohibitions against direct-to-consumer (DTC) advertising, this particular marketing approach is ever more visible to the general public. The criticism of DTC advertising is that it influences prescribing and consumption decisions adversely, that is, against patient interests. Although the FDA monitors advertising carefully to guard against unsubstantiated claims, it has followed the guidance of the Federal Trade Commission in suggesting that advertising is inherently biased in favor of the sponsor's product (for any product or service) and one should not expect any other behavior on the part of advertisers. Firms are therefore permitted to present information that is favorable to their cause, and leave it to other producers to do the same for their competing products. If there is a need for unbiased information on competing products, it should be provided separately. In the field of pharmaceuticals, for example, there are already a number of independent newsletters, some directed to physicians and others to patients, comparing alternative therapies. The potential of the World Wide Web to increase this sort of information is also enormous.

The most serious question raised in any discussion of drug cost containment is whether success can be achieved without sacrificing the vitality and viability of the industry, whose hallmark is large investment in R and D for new products. If cost containment is pursued too severely, does it diminish the return from innovation to an extent that lower spending levels on research and development ensue? Or are returns already sufficiently high that little is lost? It is obvious that some trade-off exists between cost containment and research spending, but little is known about the terms of this trade-off and thereby little about how much reduced spending on pharmaceutical R and D might result from particular cost-reducing strategies. More research is needed before we can reach a firm conclusion on this matter.

Conclusions and Directions for Future Research

Recent trends in pharmaceutical prices can be considered from various vantage points. That the prices of the most advanced drugs have increased over time is certainly correct, although this result turns largely on the increasing benefits of new products. Furthermore, this result is especially applicable if a branded product is considered to be different from and perhaps superior to a generic counterpart. On the other hand, prices for products of the same quality have tended to decline over time. Since inflation represents a price change for the same or a similar set of products, one cannot conclude from recent experience that we have seen pharmaceutical price inflation. What has occurred instead is that the price of newer products, especially brand versions, has increased substantially, even while the price of competing products and generic alternatives has declined.

Our picture of drug price control is a mixed one. The share of health expenditures devoted to pharmaceuticals is relatively low, and there is a history of moderate price increase, though with some acceleration in recent years. Furthermore, there have been rapid changes recently in the market for drugs, with increasing importance for provider-driven rather than patient-driven competition. These changes have a growing impact on both the average rate of price increase and the pattern of price dispersion for pharmaceuticals. The increased segmentation of pharmaceutical markets on the basis of insurance coverage also means that the average price level conveys less information about what is actually taking place. Traditional measures of price change are inadequate and tend to inflate the reported rate of increase; also, international comparisons yield inconclusive results.

A critical policy issue for the cost of pharmaceuticals is whether uniform pharmaceutical prices should be mandated according to the class of customer. If this type of proposal were enacted, either through legislation or judicial decisions, pricing practices would change sharply. Berndt has pointed out that under these conditions the vigor of competition in many pharmaceutical markets would diminish sharply, and we could expect higher overall prices.[51] This type of policy change would increase the cost of pharmaceuticals.

This overview of the major factors determining the cost of pharmaceuticals illustrates three important areas where additional information would assist policy analysts. The first is the need to understand better the relationship between drug price and quality level. Preliminary data show that price is positively affected by a drug's therapeutic advance, but the extent of this relationship is not well studied. The question is especially important because of our present inability to account for quality improvement in measures of pharmaceutical price increase.

Second, we know little about how the quality level of a drug is determined. Until recently, the FDA assigned a three-level quality improvement score to each drug for which marketing approval was sought. The designation was crude at best and sometimes contradicted by the marketplace. However, the FDA currently does not make even these designations, and there is no agreed-upon measure of the extent of therapeutic improvement in new drugs.

Third, we need better understanding of the degree of competition in pharmaceutical markets. This factor is especially critical, for we are now observing another wave of consolidation in the industry. Better understanding of the appropriate breadth of a pharmaceutical market is needed. How much rivalry is there within therapeutic categories (or across them)? Understanding how pharmaceutical markets are structured and interact is essential to creating appropriate public policy for this industry.

Notes

1. Stolberg, S. G. "A Drug Plan Sounds Great, But Who Gets to Set Prices?" *New York Times,* July 9, 2000, Sect. 4, p. 1.
2. *Wall Street Journal,* June 29, 1999, p. B4.
3. U.S. Senate. *Administered Drug Prices: Report of the Committee on the Judiciary, U.S. Senate, Made by Its Subcommittee on Antitrust and Monopoly.* Washington, D.C.: U.S. Government Printing Office, 1961.
4. U.S. Senate. *Hearings Before the Special Committee on Aging, Nov. 16, 1993.* Washington, D.C.: U.S. Government Printing Office, 1994, p. 3.
5. Department of Health and Human Services. *Health United States, 1999.* Washington, D.C.: U.S. Government Printing Office, 2000.
6. Department of Health and Human Services (2000).
7. National Institute for Health Care Management. "Issue Brief: Factors Affecting Growth of Prescription Drugs Expenditures." Washington, D.C.: National Institute for Health Care Management, July 1999.
8. National Institute for Health Care Management (1999).
9. Comanor, W. S., and Schweitzer, S. O. "Pharmaceuticals." In W. Adams and J. W. Brock (eds.), *Structure of American Industry.* (9th ed.) Upper Saddle River, N.J.: Prentice Hall, 1995.
10. Comanor and Schweitzer (1994).
11. Health Insurance Institute of America. "Source Book of Health Insurance Data, 1993." Prepared for National Center for Health Statistics. *National Health Expenditure Survey, 1996.* Washington, D.C.: National Center for Health Statistics, 1996.
13. National Center for Health Statistics (1996).
14. Health Insurance Institute of America (1993).
15. U.S. General Accounting Office. *Prescription Drugs Changes in Prices for Selected Drugs.* GAO/HRD-92-128. Washington, D.C.: U.S. General Accounting Office, 1992, p. 1.
16. U.S. General Accounting Office (1992), p. 2.
17. National Institute for Health Care Management (1999).

18. Griliches, Z., and Cockburn, I. M. "Generics and New Goods in the Pharmaceutical Price Indexes." *American Economic Review,* Dec. 1994.

19. Griliches and Cockburn (1994).

20. In May 1996, the Bureau of Labor Statistics announced that it was changing its procedures for constructing the Price Index for pharmaceuticals and would henceforth use linking procedures that treated generics and their branded counterparts as perfect substitutes. However, these changes are sufficiently recent that we cannot determine their impact on reported price series at the current time.

21. Griliches and Cockburn (1994).

22. Griliches and Cockburn (1994).

23. Lu, Z. J., and Comanor, W. S. "Strategic Pricing of New Pharmaceuticals." *Review of Economics and Statistics,* Feb. 1998, pp. 108–118.

24. Lu and Comanor (1998).

25. Griliches, Z., and Cockburn, I. M. "Generics and New Goods in Pharmaceutical Price Indexes." *American Economic Review,* 1994, *84,* 1213–1232.

26. Feldstein, P. J. *Health Care Economics.* (4th ed.) Albany, N.Y.: Delmar, 1993.

27. Steiner, L. R. "The Inverse Association Between the Margins of Manufacturers and Retailers." *Review of Industrial Organization,* Dec. 1993, *8,* 717–740.

28. Salehi, H., and Schweitzer, S. "Economic Aspects of Drug Substitution." *Health Care Financing Review,* Spring 1985, *6*(5), 59–68.

29. U.S. Congress, Government Accounting Office. *Prescription Drugs: Companies Typically Charge More in the United States Than in Canada.* GAO/HRD-92-110. Washington, D.C.: U.S. Government Accounting Office, Sep. 30, 1992; and *Prescription Drugs: Companies Typically Charge More in the United States Than in the United Kingdom.* GAO/HEHS-94-29, Jan. 12, 1994.

30. National Institute for Health Care Management (1999).

31. Payer, L. *Medicine and Culture: Varieties of Treatment in the United States, England, West Germany, and France.* New York: Penguin, 1988.

32. Danzon, P., and Chao, L. "Across/National Price Differences for Pharmaceuticals: How Large, and Why?" *Journal of Health Economics,* 2000, *19,* 159–195.

33. Comanor and Schweitzer (1994).

34. Lu and Comanor (1998).

35. Kessler D. "Therapeutic Class Wars: Drug Promotion in a Competitive Marketplace." *New England Journal of Medicine,* Nov. 17, 1994, *331,* 1350–1353.

36. Wiggins, S. N., and Maness, R. "Price Competition in Pharmaceutical Markets." Unpublished paper, UCLA Program in Pharmaceutical Economics and Policy, Oct. 1993.

37. Frank, R., and Salkever, D. "Pricing Patent Loss and the Market for Pharmaceuticals." *Southern Economic Journal,* Oct. 1992, *50,* 165–179.

38. Cooper, J. K., Love, D. W., and Raffoul, P. R. "Intentional Prescription Nonadherence (Noncompliance) by the Elderly." *American Geriatrics Society,* 1982, *30,* 329; and Clark, L. T. "Improving Compliance and Increasing Control of Hypertension: Needs of Special Hypertensive Populations." *American Heart Journal,* 1991, *121,* 664.

39. Dranove, D., Shanley, M., and White, W. D. "Price and Concentration in Hospital Markets: The Switch from Patient-Driven to Payer-Driven Competition." *Journal of Law and Economics,* Apr. 1993, *36,* 179–204.

40. Dranove, Shanley, and White (1993).

41. *Los Angeles Times,* Jan. 30, 1994.

42. U.S. Congress, Office of Technology Assessment. "Pharmaceutical R&D: Costs, Risks and Rewards." OTA-H-522. Washington, D.C.: U.S. Government Printing Office, Feb. 1993.

43. Leibowitz, A., Manning, W. G., and Newhouse, J. P. "The Demand for Prescription Drugs as a Function of Cost-Sharing." *Social Science and Medicine,* 1985, *21,* p. 1063.

44. Harris, B. L., Stergachis, A., and Ried, L. D. "The Effect of Drug Co-Payments on Utilization and Cost of Pharmaceuticals in a Health Maintenance Organization." *Medical Care,* 1990, *28*(10), 907–917.

45. Harris, Stergachis, and Ried (1990).

46. Harris, Stergachis, and Ried (1990).

47. Grabowski, H. G., Schweitzer, S. O., and Shiota, S. R. "The Medicaid Drug Lag: Adoption of New Drugs by State Medicaid Formularies." *Pharmacoeconomics,* 1992, *1* (supp), 32–40.

48. Sloan, F. A., Gordon, G., and Cocks, D. L. "Do Hospital Drug Formularies Reduce Spending on Hospital Services?" *Medical Care,* 1993, *31*(10), 851–867.

49. Schweitzer, S. O., and Shiota, S. R. "Access and Cost Implications of State Limitations on Medicaid Reimbursement for Pharmaceuticals." *Annual Review of Public Health,* 1992, *13,* 399–410; Moore, W. J., and Newman, R. J. "Drug Formulary Restrictions as a Cost-Containment Policy in Medicaid Programs." *Journal of Law and Economics,* Apr. 1993, *36,* 71–97.

50. U.S. Congress, Office of Technology Assessment (1993).

51. Berndt, E. R. *Uniform Pharmaceutical Pricing: An Economic Analysis.* Washington, D.C.: American Enterprise Institute, 1994.

PART THREE

QUALITY OF HEALTH CARE

CHAPTER SIX

MEASURING OUTCOMES AND HEALTH-RELATED QUALITY OF LIFE

Patricia A. Ganz and Mark S. Litwin

In the first of a six-part series on the quality of health care that appeared in the *New England Journal of Medicine* in 1996, David Blumenthal culled several definitions to support his premise that medical outcomes are a critical component of quality.[1] He noted that one of the earliest attempts to define quality had come from the American Medical Association, which in the mid-1980s stated that high-quality care was that "which consistently contributes to the improvement or maintenance of quality and/or duration of life."[2] He went on to note that the Institute of Medicine had held in the 1990s that quality consists of the "degree to which health services for individuals and populations increase the likelihood of desired health outcomes."[3] Blumenthal contended that the most important new development in our current understanding of medical outcomes was the recognition that it is patients who define which outcomes are most important and whether or not they have been achieved. "Using psychometric techniques," he argued, "researchers have developed better measures of patients' evaluations of the results of care, thus allowing patients' views to be assessed with greater scientific accuracy."[4]

Blumenthal's emphasis on quality of life in the context of quality of care underscored a body of research that grew rapidly through the 1990s. The tools for quality-of-life measurement became more refined, allowing sophisticated analysis of patients' perceived outcomes in a variety of illnesses. Today, health-related quality of life (HRQL) is studied in a variety of subjects throughout the stages of life[5] and in the community.[6]

This work has largely been built on a stage set by Paul Ellwood in his 1988 Shattuck lecture,[7] in which he advocated using a technology of patient experience, drawing on a common patient-understood language of health outcomes. He proposed that "outcomes management would draw on four already rapidly maturing techniques. First, it would place greater reliance on standards and guidelines that physicians can use in selecting appropriate interventions. Second, it would routinely and systematically measure the functioning and well-being of patients, along with disease-specific clinical outcomes, at appropriate time intervals. Third, it would pool clinical and outcome data on a massive scale. Fourth, it would analyze and disseminate results from the segment of the data base most appropriate to the concerns of each decision maker."

Later, Ellwood went on to say that "the centerpiece and unifying ingredient of outcomes management is the tracking and measurement of function and well-being or quality of life. Although this sounds like a hopelessly optimistic undertaking, I believe that we already have the ability to obtain crucial, reliable data on quality of life at minimal cost and inconvenience."[8]

Ellwood's support for the active inclusion of quality-of-life data as a key component of outcomes management lends important support for the advancement of this field; however, more than a decade later this form of outcome assessment is still in its adolescence. Despite its appeal, quality-of-life data must be collected prospectively and cannot be retrieved from the administrative databases that are commonly used by health services researchers. During the past decade, patient-rated assessments of HRQL have been included more frequently in research and clinical settings, and we are now on the verge of seeing some results.

Definition, Conceptualization, and Measurement of Quality of Life

Great energy has traditionally been expended by clinicians and other health care professionals attempting to lengthen the duration of survival in patients with various chronic diseases.[9] During the last few decades, dramatic advances in diagnosis, management, and overall understanding of the mechanisms of human disease have refined the treatment approaches to many medical conditions such that patients are now living longer with their disease. This is particularly true in oncology, where some patients live for years after their initial diagnosis.[10]

Historically, evaluation of the success of medical therapies has focused on specific clinical parameters and survival. However, the recent surge of interest in patient-centered endpoints has generated great support for the medical-outcomes movement. Not only clinicians but also payers and managers have become interested in assessing outcomes to begin to measure quality of care. Indeed, some would argue that the thrust of the outcomes movement stems largely from outside the biomedical establishment, as clinicians are held ever more accountable to external authorities. To understand better how medical outcomes fit into the framework of health services research, it is necessary to focus on assessing quality of care.

In the well-known Donabedian model,[11] health care quality is examined in three parts: structure, process, and outcomes of care.

Structure of care refers to how medical and other services are organized in a particular institution or delivery system. It may include such diverse variables as specialty mix in a multiphysician medical group, access to timely radiological files in a hospital, availability of pharmacy services in a hospice program, or convenience of parking at an outpatient surgery center. It may also involve as factors nonmedical support services such as coordination of care, social work, home care, daily assistance for the disabled, or clothing and housing for the socially disadvantaged.

Process of care refers to the content of the medical and psychological interactions between patient and provider. It may include variables such as whether or not a blood culture is ordered for a baby with a fever, the nature of the treatment prescribed for a patient with abdominal pain, how much compassion a doctor demonstrates when presenting a negative diagnosis with a patient, how many times a psychologist interrupts a client during a session, or whether a nurse regularly turns a bedridden patient to prevent bedsores.

Outcomes of care refer to specific indicators of what happens to the patient once care has been rendered. This may include clinical variables, such as blood sugar level in a diabetic, blood pressure measurement in a hypertensive, abnormal chest X ray during treatment for pneumonia, kidney function after transplantation, or pain after treatment for cancer. It may also include complications of treatment, such as bleeding after colonoscopic biopsy, allergic reaction to an antibiotic or injection of iodinated contrast material, graft occlusion after cardiac bypass surgery, infant mortality following emergency Cesarean delivery, or hospital death rate.

Outcomes of care may also include health-related quality of life, another variable commonly studied in the field of medical outcomes research. The general concept of quality of life encompasses a wide range of human experience: access to the daily necessities of life such as food and shelter, intrapersonal and interpersonal response to life events, and activities associated with professional fulfillment and personal happiness.[12] A subcomponent of overall quality of life relates to health, so HRQL focuses on the patient's own perception of health and the ability to function as a result of health status or disease experience. The World Health Organization defines *health* as a "state of complete physical, mental, and social well-being and not merely the absence of disease."[13] Since disease may affect both quantity and quality of life, the various components of well-being must be addressed when treating patients. In the Donabedian framework, health-related quality of life is considered an important outcome variable. Figure 6.1 presents a framework described by Patrick and Bergner for the theoretical relationships among HRQL concepts, disease, the environment, and prognosis.[14]

Although quantity of life is relatively easy to assess (as survival or disease-free interval, in days, months, years), measuring quality of life presents more challenges, primarily because it is less familiar to most clinicians and researchers. Proper measurement of such variables is often quite costly. To quantify what is essentially a subjective or qualitative phenomenon, the principles of psychometric test theory are applied.[15] This discipline introduces the theoretical underpinning for the science of survey research. Typically, HRQL data are collected with self-administered questionnaires, called instruments. These instruments contain questions, or items, that are organized into scales. Each scale measures a different aspect, or domain, of HRQL. Some scales comprise dozens of items, while others may include only one or two items.

HRQL instruments may be general or disease-specific. General HRQL domains address the essential or common components of overall well-being, while

FIGURE 6.1.   CONCEPTUALIZATION OF HRQL.

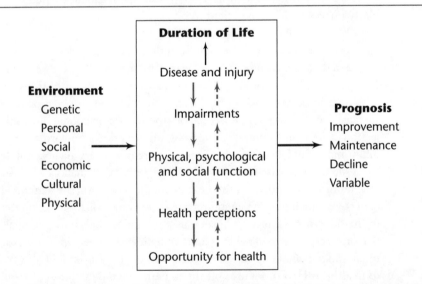

Source: Adapted from Patrick, D., and Bergner, M. "Measurement of Health Studies in the 1990s." *Annual Review of Public Health,* 1990, *11*, p. 174.

disease-specific domains focus on the impact of particular organic dysfunctions that affect HRQL.[16] Generic HRQL instruments typically address general health perceptions; sense of overall well-being; and function in the physical, emotional, and social domains. Disease-specific HRQL instruments focus on special or directly relevant domains, such as anxiety about cancer recurrence, dizziness from antihypertensive medications, or suicidal thoughts during depression therapy.

Many HRQL instruments are available. There are psychologists, sociologists, and statisticians who devote their entire professional careers to the activity of developing and validating these instruments. At least one medical journal, *Quality of Life Research*, is dedicated exclusively to presenting this research. Hence, an abundance of literature exists on general HRQL, and a significant body of work has been published on HRQL in patients with various conditions.[17]

Approaches to Measuring HRQL

The Southwest Oncology Group (SWOG) has described six principles for HRQL research in cancer clinical trials (though these principles can be applied to other clinical or research settings). Here are their recommendations:[18]

1. Always measure physical functioning, emotional functioning, symptoms, and global quality of life separately.
2. Include measures of social functioning and additional protocol-specific measures if resources permit.
3. Use patient-based questionnaires.
4. Use categorical rather than visual analog scales.
5. Select brief questionnaires, not interviews.
6. Select HRQL measures with published psychometric properties.

Using the SWOG guidelines, one can confidently select a set of instruments to assess HRQL in clinical trials involving longitudinal or cross-sectional studies of patients with malignant or benign conditions. Resources are scarce in any clinical trial, but this setting is always the best for outcomes measurement. Nonetheless, HRQL data collection is labor-intensive; hence, when planning clinical trial budgets the investigator must be aware that including HRQL may be expensive. The more instruments that are selected, the richer the potential database; however, it is important to remain parsimonious in instrument selection, choosing only the relevant domains of HRQL.

Some single instruments are multidimensional, but the SWOG investigators have proposed a "battery approach," in which the various components of HRQL are measured with different scales to ensure that each domain receives adequate attention. Ideally, the instruments should be self-administered by the patient, independent of interviewers; at times, though, a patient may need assistance in completing a questionnaire.

Self-assessment of HRQL frees patient responses from interviewer bias. Although many instruments use visual analog scales, many quality-of-life researchers believe that items with specific response sets from which to choose, such as Likert scales, produce more accurate information that is easier to interpret.[19] Longer instruments can provide greater precision, but they also increase the chance that patients will tire of the exercise and not give reliable or valid answers. This is particularly true in the multicenter clinical trial setting. Hence, shorter instruments are generally preferable when obtaining HRQL measurements under such circumstances. In general, it is easier and more efficient to use established instruments that have already undergone psychometric validation.

HRQL data collected using published instruments allow the researcher to compare the study results to data from other samples or diverse populations with various chronic diseases. Nevertheless, sometimes it is necessary to develop new questionnaire items to ensure that a particular concept is adequately evaluated. Under such circumstances, new scales can be tested for reliability and validity during the course of data collection.

Psychometric Validation of HRQL Instruments

Developing and validating new instruments and scales is a long and arduous process. It is not undertaken lightly. Simply drawing up a list of questions that seem appropriate is fraught with potential traps and pitfalls. Two important characteristics to assess in new instruments are reliability and validity. Reliability is the term used to indicate that a test instrument measures the same thing on repeated testing. Validity indicates the extent to which the instrument measures what it is intended to measure. Validity is complex and may be estimated by criterion validity (in which the test instrument is compared to a "gold standard" measure) or by construct validity (through which components of the test instrument are highly correlated with other instruments that measure similar content areas). Reliability and validity should be established before using an instrument; therefore it is preferable to use established HRQL instruments if they are available and conceptually appropriate.

When scales and instruments are developed, they are first pilot tested to ensure that the target population can understand and complete them with ease. Pilot testing reveals problems that might otherwise go unrecognized by researchers. For example, many terms that are commonly used by medical professionals are poorly understood by patients. This may result in missing data if patients leave questions blank. Furthermore, since older patients may have poor eyesight, pilot testing in this group often identifies easily corrected visual barriers such as type size and page layout. In addition, self-administered instruments with complicated skip patterns ("If you answered yes to item 16b, continue with item 16c; if you answered no to item 16b, skip to item 19a") may be too confusing for even the most competent patients to follow. This, too, can result in missing data and introduce difficulties in the analysis. Pilot testing is a necessary and valuable part of instrument development. It serves as a reality check for scale developers.

Caveats on Collecting HRQL Data

Once an instrument is thoroughly pilot tested and found to be reliable and valid, it must be administered in a manner that minimizes bias. Quality-of-life data cannot and should not be collected from patients directly by the treating health care provider. Patients often favor socially desirable responses under such circumstances.[20] This introduces measurement error. No matter how objective the treating clinician may claim to be, it is impossible for him or her to collect objective and unbiased outcome data through direct questioning. Variations in phrasing, inflection, eye contact, rapport, mood, and other factors are difficult or impossible to eliminate. Data must be gathered by disinterested third parties using established psychometric scales and instruments.

Future Directions in Applying HRQL Assessment

There is a need for basic descriptive information on the HRQL of differing patient groups, simply from an epidemiological perspective. Characterizing the fundamental elements of HRQL for these individuals requires studying their health perceptions and how their daily activities are affected by their general health and their specific illness. Physical and emotional well-being form the cornerstone of this approach, but research must also extend to issues such as eating and sleeping habits, anxiety and fatigue, depression, rapport with the clinician, presence of a spouse or partner, and social interactions. Characterization of all domains must address not only the actual functions but also the relative importance of these issues to patients.

Beyond the descriptive analysis, HRQL outcomes must be compared in patients undergoing different types of therapy for the same condition. From the perspective of health policy, both general and disease-specific HRQL should be measured to facilitate comparison among common diseases or conditions. HRQL outcomes may also be correlated with medical variables such as co-morbidity;

or sociodemographic variables such as age, race, gender, education, income, insurance status, geographic region, and access to health care. In this context, HRQL may be linked with many factors other than the traditional medical ones.

Research initiatives must rely on using established HRQL instruments with accepted psychometric characteristics, and independent data collection procedures. The basic science of measurement of HRQL is now well established[21] and is being widely adopted. However, integration of HRQL among other health services outcomes is still in its infancy. Indeed, the potential value of these methods in health management organizations has yet to be fully realized. This affords a unique opportunity for simultaneous, coordinated introduction of such measurement techniques in both the clinical and administrative spheres.

Quality-Adjusted Life Years

One popular technique used to evaluate new or established therapies is cost-effectiveness analysis. It is performed by developing a probability model of the possible medical outcomes of interventions for a given condition. For each outcome in the model, expenses are identified and the results are compared, typically as cost per year of life saved.[22] Years of life saved, or life-years, are calculated for a population, not for individuals.[23]

For example, if one treatment produces on average six years of survival with HRQL at a low level, and an alternative treatment produces on average three years of survival with HRQL at a relatively high level, then the duration of survival must be adjusted for these differences before the two treatments can be compared. Hence, before the final analysis, life-years are adjusted for HRQL to account for whatever health states may result from various treatments. These are called quality-adjusted life years (QALYs). That is, one patient who survives a given disease for ten years with 50 percent impairment in HRQL (scoring 50 of 100 potential points on an HRQL scale) would be said to have gained 5.0 QALYs; another patient who survives for only eight years but experiences just 20 percent impairment in HRQL (scoring 80 of 100 points on the HRQL scale) would be said to have gained 6.4 QALYs. Using QALYs, investigators can incorporate quality and quantity of life into the same equation. By using QALYs, researchers recognize that a year of time spent in one health state is not necessarily equivalent to the same year spent in another health state. Because medical treatments for the same illness may produce various health states, it is important to adjust for these differences.

The primary appeal of these approaches to summarizing the quality of various health states is their simplicity. By using QALYs, clinicians, managers, payers, and investigators can compare outcomes and health services utilization among individuals or populations with a uniform unit of measurement that is easily quantified. However, these approaches raise important ethical concerns for the physician providing care to an individual patient.[24] Although a wide range of variables contribute to the physician's recommendations for treatment (or no treatment), there is nothing more relevant to decision making than the patient's own assessment of quality of life. Even if a treatment may be life saving, ethical principles suggest that the patient's preference regarding treatment must be respected. If the patient feels that his or her quality of life is so poor that no treatment would make it better, then we must respect the patient's wishes.

Feedback to Patients

To give better information to patients facing such decisions, it is important to have HRQL outcome data on individual treatments to facilitate clinical decision making. Specific examples of currently available information include the finding that HRQL is better when chemotherapy is given continuously rather than intermittently in women with advanced breast cancer,[25] or that the HRQL of women receiving breast conservation treatment is no different than for women undergoing mastectomy.[26] In addition, new information has recently become available to understand HRQL in men treated for localized prostate cancer.[27] However, there are limited data of this type. We need to expand our database on HRQL outcomes to improve information for managers, payers, health care executives, and policy makers involved in the process of distributing limited health care resources, as well as to physicians and patients involved in clinical decision making.

Contributions from the Literature

In this section, we review seminal research in health services where HRQL methods were developed or incorporated as important outcomes. Although this section is not exhaustive, we present an historical framework for research in this area.

Alameda County Human Population Laboratory Studies

Three decades ago, Lester Breslow and colleagues recruited a probability sample of adults from Alameda County, California, to examine the health status and well-being of a community. This research program conceptualized health in broader terms than the traditional categories of disability and disease. Their work drew heavily on the World Health Organization (WHO) definition of health to guide their assessment of the population, focusing on the physical, emotional, and social dimensions of well-being.[28] Although they examined some social indicators (such as employment, income, and marital status) in their study sample, the focus of their work was on the self-reported evaluation of the three dimensions of well-being (physical, mental, and social) identified in the WHO definition of health. The measurement methods available at the time were less developed psychometrically than now, but the investigators consistently demonstrated the reliability and validity of their self-report surveys[29] and were able to evaluate these three dimensions of health. They established the feasibility of asking people about their HRQL and demonstrated equal response rates to personal interview, telephone, and mailed questionnaires as strategies for data collection. Further, they showed that data from the three administration strategies were nearly interchangeable.

In addition to the conceptually and methodologically pioneering work of this group, this research program made several critical observations:

- Those who were employed were healthier than those who were out of work or retired.[30]
- Separated persons were less healthy than those in other marital-status groups.[31]
- There is a positive association between physical health status and mental health status, independent of sex, age, or income adequacy.[32]
- There is a positive association between socioeconomic status and mental health.[33]
- Certain common health habits (hours of sleep, exercise, abstention from alcohol and tobacco, and so on) are positively related to physical health status,[34] and these personal health habits are inversely related to subsequent mortality[35] and disability.[36]

The RAND Health Insurance Experiment

The RAND Health Insurance Experiment (HIE) was one of the first large health services research intervention trials. It was conceived in the early 1970s at a time when there was considerable discussion about national health insurance reform and new approaches to limiting the rapidly expanding health care budget.[37] The HIE randomly assigned 2,005 families (3,958 individuals between fourteen and sixty-one years of age) to health insurance plans that provided free care, varying degrees of co-payment, or care through a health maintenance organization.[38] In addition to examining the cost of care and utilization of services, this comprehensively designed study looked at a number of important health outcomes, including physiological measures (for example, blood pressure, far vision), health habits (smoking, weight, cholesterol level), and self-reported measures of health status (physical functioning, role functioning, mental health, social contacts, health perceptions). The requirement for reliable and valid measures of health status in the RAND HIE led to one of the most extensive explorations of the conceptualization of health and the methodologies required for measuring HRQL.

Although it is not possible in this chapter to examine all of the advances in measurement of HRQL that were developed as part of the RAND HIE, a few key concepts and measures should be described. The methodological aspects of this work were spearheaded by John E. Ware, Jr., and are best captured in a paper published in 1984.[39] Ware noted that the "attention of society, government and health care providers has broadened beyond survival and biomedical status into the areas of behavioral and psychosocial outcomes. There also seems to be a shift in the objectives of health care toward more socially relevant health and quality-of-life outcomes and increased awareness of the interest in the psychological and economic costs of disease and disability."[40] He also noted the methodological advances that made it possible to have patients evaluate these matters through self-report measures.

Ware carefully clarifies that "quality of life encompasses personal health status and other factors such as family life, finances, housing and jobs," such aspects being the content of much of the social indicators research movement; however, not all of these factors are expected to be influenced by the health care system.[41] Therefore, he suggests that it is more important to consider the concept of health status as separate from the larger arena of quality of life, with health representing proper functioning and well-being (hearkening back to the WHO definition of health).[42] In this explication of a framework for measurement of health-related quality of life, Ware identifies the dimensions seen in Figure 6.2: the disease, personal functioning, psychological distress and well-being, general health perceptions, and social and role functioning.[43]

Using this framework, the RAND investigators developed a number of large questionnaire batteries to examine each dimension of HRQL. These questionnaires were developed specifically for the HIE, were tested and validated as part of the HIE, and were then used as critical outcome measures. Detailed descriptions of these measures are available as separate reports prepared through the RAND Corporation, and also through many publications.

One of the most widely used measures is the Mental Health Inventory (MHI), described by Veit and Ware in 1983.[44] In contrast to existing psychological measures designed to diagnose mental illness, the MHI was developed to look at psychological distress and well-being in the general population. Ware and associates drew heavily on existing measures of well-being in developing the MHI. However, they performed much additional work to conceptualize the issues of importance to this domain of HRQL and were careful to separate mental health from physical health. What resulted was a 38-item index of mental health that

FIGURE 6.2.   FRAMEWORK FOR MEASURING HEALTH STATUS.

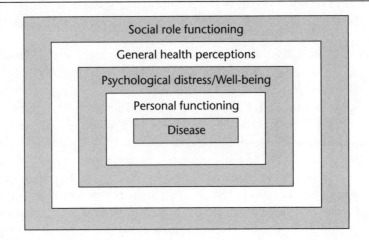

Source: Adapted from Ware, J. E., Jr. "Conceptualizing Disease Impact and Treatment Outcomes." *Cancer,* 1984, *53* Supplement, p. 2317.

could be separated into two main constructs: (1) psychological distress (anxiety, depression, loss of behavioral or emotional control) and (2) psychological well-being (general positive affect, emotional ties). Elegant psychometric evaluation of this measure was completed as part of the HIE.[45]

There are many important legacies from the RAND Health Insurance Experiment. From the point of view of quality-of-life research, conceptualizing HRQL as a key outcome of health care is critical. In addition, the HIE developed many reliable and valid tools for measuring the dimensions of health-related quality of life. However, in addition to the tools themselves, data from this study also constitute important reference points for the relative value of specific changes in scores. That is to say, what does a change in quality-of-life score mean? Data on life events captured in the RAND HIE in relation to change scores for the measures of health-related quality of life provide intervention-based validity for the quality-of-life scores. The reader is referred to a review by Testa and Nackley[46] for an excellent discussion of this issue.

The Medical Outcomes Study

The Medical Outcomes Study (MOS) is another example of a major health services research study that in its design and conceptualization included health-related quality of life as a key outcome of care[47] (see Table 6.1). Many of the key

TABLE 6.1. CONCEPTUAL FRAMEWORK FOR THE MEDICAL OUTCOMES STUDY.

Structure of Care	Process of Care	Outcomes
System Characteristics Organization Specialty mix Financial incentives Workload Access and convenience *Provider Characteristics* Age Gender Specialty training Economic incentives Beliefs and attitudes Preferences Job satisfaction *Patient Characteristics* Age Gender Diagnosis or condition Severity Co-morbid conditions Health habits Beliefs and attitudes Preferences	*Technical Style* Visits Medications Referrals Test ordering Hospitalizations Expenditures Continuity of care Coordination *Interpersonal Style* Interpersonal manner Patient participation Counseling Communication level	*Clinical End Points* Symptoms and signs Laboratory values Death *Functional Status* Physical Mental Social Role *General Well-Being* Health perceptions Energy and fatigue Pain Life satisfaction *Satisfaction with Care* Access Convenience Financial coverage Quality General

Source: Adapted from Tarlov, A. R., and others. "The Medical Outcomes Study: An Application of Methods for Monitoring the Results of Medical Care." *Journal of the American Medical Association,* 1989, *262,* p. 926.

investigators for this study had been involved in the RAND HIE. Again, Ware and colleagues at RAND were central figures in developing the health outcome measures for the MOS. Thus, it is not surprising that the measures of functional status, health, and well-being draw heavily on the prior measures developed for the Health Insurance Experiment.[48]

The self-report measures of HRQL used in the MOS were quite lengthy.[49] However, one of the major methodological advances from this project was the realization that shorter measures might be as effective as the lengthier measures traditionally used in this type of research. Longer measures lead to added precision, but they also increase the burden on the respondent and the likelihood of missing data. Furthermore, they are too cumbersome for most clinical settings. An additional conceptual breakthrough was developing a generic HRQL tool that could facilitate comparing common diseases across specific dimensions of HRQL.

Noteworthy results from this research include development of the MOS short form, first published as a 20-item questionnaire[50] and later an expanded version known as the MOS Short Form 36 or the RAND 36-Item Health Survey 1.0.[51] The short forms of the MOS instruments are being widely used in a variety of research and clinical settings to examine health outcomes of care.[52] Furthermore, these measures are being translated for use in multinational studies as well as national studies that include diverse populations.[53]

Although very promising, there are limitations to using the MOS in quality-of-life research, because of the multiple scale or dimension scores, rather than a global score. Work is ongoing to address this issue.[54] In recent years, the goal of parsimony in instrument selection has generated interest in an even shorter form of the MOS instrument, known as the SF-12.[55] This 12-item questionnaire summarizes HRQL in two domains: the mental component summary and the physical component summary. Although there is some sacrifice in richness of the data, the shorter version has useful summary scales and obviates the need to present HRQL in the eight separate domains of the SF-36. When selecting HRQL instruments, investigators are well-advised to consult http://www.qlmed.org, an outstanding source of information on new and existing HRQL measurement tools for a variety of clinical conditions. In addition, investigators are directed to the work of M. Staquet and colleagues, who recently proposed uniform guidelines for the reporting of HRQL data from clinical trials.[56]

Efficacy Studies

Quality of life has long been an implied outcome of treatment for a variety of common, chronic medical conditions. For a disease such as rheumatoid arthritis, the subjective assessment of response to anti-inflammatory agents (pain relief, increased mobility) has been critical in evaluating new treatments.[57] In the case of antihypertensive treatments, side effects from medication may interfere with compliance and affect successful control of this clinically silent condition.[58] Cancer treatments are another area where quality-of-life outcomes are salient.[59]

Randomized clinical trials of treatment efficacy are the most compelling studies in which quality-of-life measures have been used. The studies that have been most successful included adequate resources to collect extensive quality-of-life data, and they used a comprehensive battery of instruments. Recently, there has been a move toward more abbreviated quality-of-life outcome measures for integration into large multicenter trials.[60] In these situations, the burden on respondents and staff is an important consideration. It is hoped that these shorter forms will be equally sensitive to measuring difference in quality-of-life outcomes. Many studies are under way currently, and results should be forthcoming in the next few years.

Two examples of the use of quality-of-life measures in efficacy studies illustrate the added value of this outcome to standard endpoints. In 1986, Bombardier and colleagues reported on the results of a randomized, double-blind, multicenter trial in which auranofin (an oral gold salt preparation) was compared to placebo in patients with classic or definite rheumatoid arthritis.[61] Treatment was administered over a six-month period during which there was serial evaluation of traditional clinical endpoints (number of tender and swollen joints, grip strength, fifty-foot walk time, duration of morning stiffness) along with administration of an extensive battery of questionnaires designed to assess HRQL (function, pain, global impression, utility, depression, health perception). This trial demonstrated that auranofin therapy was superior to placebo using standard clinical measures, which was confirmed by similar results among the array of HRQL measures. The authors comment that although objective clinical benefits were modest in the auranofin treated group (for instance, reduction in the number of tender and swollen joints), there were meaningful improvements in patients' performance and other outcomes valued in daily life as measured by the HRQL assessments.[62]

This was an important study from the perspective of HRQL assessment, since a variety of independent instruments were used to measure the components of HRQL. For example, three instruments were used to assess functional status. Although each measure had a slightly different emphasis, the direction of change on each instrument and the comparative results in the two treatment groups were similar. Further evaluation is necessary to determine which instruments are most sensitive in detecting treatment effects.[63]

In 1986, Croog and colleagues[64] reported the results of a randomized trial that was designed specifically to address the impact of antihypertensive therapy on quality of life. In the opening paragraph of their paper, the authors say that "physicians who are successful in controlling blood pressure may be unaware of the negative effect that antihypertensive drugs can have on the quality of life on the physical state, emotional well-being, sexual and social functioning, and cognitive acuity of their patients."[65] Furthermore, they note that patients may believe that the side effects of antihypertensive medications are so serious that they become noncompliant, with resulting lack of therapeutic efficacy.[66]

In this multicenter, randomized, double-blind clinical trial, men with mild to moderate essential hypertension were evaluated for the effects of captopril, methyldopa, and propranolol on the quality of life and control of blood pressure. Since all three drugs had been shown to be effective in controlling hypertension, the major question of interest was related to their effects on HRQL. An important additional goal was to evaluate selected measures for their ability to discriminate the effects of the three medications on the HRQL of patients with hypertension.

In this study, HRQL was defined conceptually in five domains: sense of well-being and satisfaction with life, physical state, emotional state, intellectual functioning, and ability to perform in social roles and the degree of satisfaction from these roles.[67] An extensive battery of previously validated measures, as well as some newly created scales, were administered to patients by trained interviewers at a baseline assessment and twenty-four weeks later.

A number of changes in HRQL were observed within each group at twenty-four weeks. Patients treated with captopril had significant improvement in general well-being (anxiety, positive well-being, and vitality), as well as improvement in work performance and in cognitive functioning,[68] with other HRQL scales remaining unchanged. In contrast, patients receiving methyldopa showed no significant improvement except in cognitive functioning, and they had significant worsening in measures of depression, work performance, sexual dysfunction, physical symptoms, and life satisfaction.[69] Patients receiving propanolol in this study experienced improvement in cognitive functioning and social participation but experienced increased sexual dysfunction and physical symptoms.[70]

The degree of change between treatment groups was compared using multivariate analysis. This evaluation revealed significant differences between the captopril and methyldopa groups, and the captopril and propanolol groups, but not between the methyldopa and propanolol groups.[71] The authors observed that there was significantly more worsening or no change in general well-being, physical symptoms, and sexual dysfunction for those patients taking methyldopa or propanolol as compared to patients receiving captopril.[72]

The large sample sizes in this trial allowed detection of very small but significant changes in HRQL, as evaluated by a wide range of measures. Are these differences clinically relevant? The authors support the clinical importance of their findings with two comments. Most of the patients who withdrew from the trial before the second HRQL assessment did so because of adverse effects on HRQL (determined through an exit interview). Secondly, other studies have indicated that even a change of 0.15 SD on scales similar to those used in this study were associated with being laid off or fired from a job, or were predictive of using mental health services.[73] Thus, although the effect size detected in these studies was relatively small, it was related to clinically meaningful events and could thus be interpreted as showing an important change in quality of life.

Perhaps the most important aspect of this study was the observation that different antihypertensive medications vary in their impact on a number of aspects of HRQL, and that this effect can be successfully evaluated through using currently available psychosocial measures.[74] The rigorous design of the study, as well as use of standardized measures, should encourage similar evaluation of other cardiovascular drugs that may have differing effects on HRQL but similar patterns of efficacy. Beyond the research applications of HRQL assessment, the HRQL profile of various antihypertensive medications may be useful for the practicing clinician to individualize therapy and promote optimal adherence to the recommended regimen.

These two examples demonstrate the importance of evaluating quality-of-life endpoints in efficacy studies because they amount to an additional outcome that includes the patient perspective. This is most important in therapeutic situations where the toxicity of treatment is high and the benefits may be few. Quality-of-life assessment has been widely adopted by the pharmaceutical industry as a component of the drug approval process.[75] These assessments are also an expanding part of large clinical treatment trials for patients with cancer and AIDS. We are still in the early phases of experience with HRQL as an outcome in such large-scale and long-term trials.

Effectiveness Research

The newest aspect of health services research is in the area of effectiveness. Certain clinical topics do not lend themselves to randomized clinical trials because of ethical concerns, inability to control adequately for contravening factors, and various other reasons. In these clinical areas, consensus has arisen that descriptive studies are most appropriate to improve our understanding. These studies primarily address effectiveness. In contrast to controlled clinical trials that examine efficacy, effectiveness research studies the outcomes of treatment as they are actually practiced in clinical settings. To this end, in the 1990s the Agency for Health Care Policy and Research (now known as the Agency for Healthcare Research and Quality) funded a number of patient outcome research teams (PORT) to investigate common medical treatments and procedures.[76] Although this research effort has emphasized literature review of efficacy studies, as well as examination of practice variations using administrative databases, it has also been an opportunity to collect quality-of-life outcome data from patients undergoing various procedures. The PORTs have not conducted clinical trials; hence their primary contribution has been in shaping the clinical effectiveness and outcomes literature. In the future, we can expect valuable HRQL data from this research.[77]

Future Research and Policy Issues

A great deal of work remains in order to operationalize research in outcomes and HRQL to inform health policy in the United States.

Incorporating HRQL Endpoints

How can HRQL endpoints be effectively incorporated in research, clinical care, and policy decisions?

Several workshops among health services researchers[78] sponsored through the NIH and NCI[79] have emphasized the need for incorporating HRQL endpoints into research and clinical care settings. The technologies, although not yet perfect, are much more accessible and feasible than just a short time ago. Scannable, user-friendly instruments are available, and normative databases are being developed rapidly. Health care consumers and providers would like access to such information.

As has been emphasized by several prominent health services researchers,[80] it is the patient outcome that must drive our policy decisions. Prolonged survival with poor quality of life may not be desirable to patients. Consumers are anxious to have information about the HRQL impact of new treatments. If there is uncertainty about the efficacy or effectiveness of a treatment or choices among treatments, then HRQL endpoints will take on paramount importance.

Only through a concerted effort to collect primary HRQL data can this outcome be considered as a primary endpoint. All studies of efficacy and effectiveness must include patient-rated measures of HRQL whenever there is a potential quality-of-life question. Common core measures should be shared across studies so that relevant comparisons can be made. However, we must not fail to ask critical questions related to new therapies, to better understand their relevance to patients. For enough data to materialize, these measures of HRQL must be considered routine and not exceptional. The additional costs of data collection should be borne by funding agencies, insurers, and providers so that the value of new tests or procedures can be fully evaluated.

HRQL Endpoints and Changing Health Policy

Are HRQL endpoints sufficient to force a change in health policy?

In asking whether HRQL outcomes are sufficient to force changes in health policy, we must consider the reliability and validity of currently available HRQL tools. In addition, we must ask whether statistically significant changes in evaluating HRQL are clinically significant. To obtain more precise evaluation of the quality of our tools, it is necessary to reference or calibrate our HRQL instruments against known outcomes of clinical importance to patients, purchasers of health care, and health care providers. For this work to proceed, we must invest in collecting important clinical information along with our HRQL data. Research in HRQL needs to be supported to extrapolate effectively from the HRQL endpoint to decisions on public health policy. Short-term management applications include using HRQL endpoints and other outcomes and effectiveness research as critical measures in the quality assurance (QA) arena.

Advancing the HRQL Research Agenda

As Andersen, Davidson, and Ganz[81] have recently described, "There are symbiotic relationships between Health Services Research (HSR) and Quality of Life (QOL) studies." First, the HSR paradigm gives guidance for including structure and process in designing QOL studies. HSR suggests what leads to QOL improvement. It supplies ways to conceptualize, and relates the many important forces that contribute to, QOL in addition to specific clinical interventions. Second, QOL is an important outcome in the HSR paradigm. Early studies in HSR did not focus primarily on QOL as an outcome indicator. Health service utilization was investigated as a means to improve access to care and change the organization and delivery of care, rather than as a direct vehicle to enhance health status and QOL. Quality of life, however, is a key outcome in the emerging model of HSR.[82]

Until recently, and with the exception of a few studies already cited, HRQL has been included infrequently in traditional health services research. The expansion and development of HRQL measurement has emerged primarily from clinical research. What is needed urgently is careful and appropriate inclusion of HRQL outcomes in traditional health services research. Similarly, researchers in clinical settings who are measuring HRQL should account for the structure and process of care in designing their research and data collection. As suggested by Andersen and colleagues,[83] "This era of health care reform calls for a paradigm shift, away from the heroic and costly therapeutic measures that extend the quantity of life, to a patient or consumer-focused approach aimed at health promotion and disease prevention, using QOL measures as the ultimate criteria for success." As indicated throughout this chapter, the potential for accomplishing this goal is on the horizon.

Notes

1. Blumenthal, D. "Part 1: Quality of Care—What Is It?" *New England Journal of Medicine,* 1996, *335,* 891–894.

2. American Medical Association, Council on Medical Service. "Quality of Care." *Journal of the American Medical Association,* 1986, *256,* 1032–1034.

3. Lohr, K. N., Donaldson, M. S., and Harris-Wehling, J. "Medicare: A Strategy for Quality Assurance. Part V: Quality of Care in a Changing Health Care Environment." *QRB (Quality Review Bulletin),* 1992, *18,* 120–126.

4. Blumenthal (1996), p. 892.

5. Liao, Y., McGee, D. L., Cao, G., and Cooper, R. S. "Quality of the Last Year of Life of Older Adults: 1986 vs. 1993." *Journal of the American Medical Association,* 2000, *283,* 512–518; Wolfe, J., and others. "Symptoms and Suffering at the End of Life in Children with Cancer." *New England Journal of Medicine,* 2000, *342*(5), 326–333.

6. Centers for Disease Control and Prevention. "Community Indicators of Health-Related Quality of Life—United States, 1993–1997." (*Morbidity and Mortality Weekly Report.*) *Journal of the American Medical Association,* 2000, 283, 2097–2098.

7. Ellwood, P. M. "Shattuck Lecture. Outcomes Management: A Technology of Patient Experience." *New England Journal of Medicine,* 1988, *318,* 1549–1556.

8. Ellwood (1988), p. 155.

9. Tarlov, A. R. "The Coming Influence of a Social Sciences Perspective on Medical Education." *Academic Medicine,* 1992, *67,* 724–731.

10. Ganz, P. A. "Quality of Life and the Patient with Cancer: Individual and Policy Implications." *Cancer,* 1994, *74,* 1445–1452.

11. Donabedian, A. *The Definition of Quality and Approaches to Its Assessment.* Ann Arbor: Health Administration Press, 1980.

12. Patrick, D. L., and Erickson, P. "Assessing Health-Related Quality of Life for Clinical Decision-Making." In S. R. Walker and R. M. Rosser (eds.), *Quality of Life Assessment: Key Issues in the 1990s.* Dordrecht, Neth.: Kluwer, 1993, p. 19.

13. World Health Organization. *Constitution of the World Health Organization, Basic Documents.* Geneva: WHO, 1948.

14. Patrick, D. L., and Bergner, M. "Measurement of Health Status in the 1990s." *Annual Review of Public Health,* 1990, *11,* 165–183.

15. Tulsky, D. A. "An Introduction to Test Theory." *Oncology,* May 1990, *4,* 43–48.

16. Patrick, D. L., and Deyo, R. A. "Generic and Disease-Specific Measures in Assessing Health Status and Quality of Life." *Medical Care,* 1989, *27,* S217–S232.

17. McDowell, I., and Newell, C. *Measuring Health: A Guide to Rating Scales and Questionnaires.* New York: Oxford University Press, 1987; Patrick, D. L., and Erickson, P. *Health Status and Health Policy, Allocating Resources to Health Care.* New York: Oxford University Press, 1993; Spilker, B. (ed.). *Quality of Life Assessments in Clinical Trials.* New York: Raven Press, 1990.

18. Moinpour, C. M. "Quality of Life Assessment in Southwest Oncology Group Trials." *Oncology,* May 1990, *4,* 79–89.

19. Guyatt, G. H., Townsend, M., Berman, L. B., and Keller, J. L. "A Comparison of Likert and Visual Analogue Scales for Measuring Change in Function." *Journal of Chronic Disease,* 1987, 40, 1129–1133.

20. Tannock, I. F. "Management of Breast and Prostate Cancer: How Does Quality of Life Enter the Equation?" *Oncology,* May 1990, *4,* 149–156.

21. Guyatt, G. H., Feeny, D. H., and Patrick, D. L. "Measuring Health-Related Quality of Life." *Annals of International Medicine,* 1993, *118,* 622–629.

22. Kassirer, J. P., and Angell, M. "The Journal's Policy on Cost-Effectiveness Analysis." *New England Journal of Medicine* 1994, *331,* 669–670; Eddy, D. M. "Cost-Effectiveness Analysis: Is It Up to the Task?" *Journal of the American Medical Association,* 1992, *267,* 3342–3348; Weinstein, M. C., and Stason, W. B. "Foundations of Cost-Effectiveness Analysis for Health and Medical Practices." *New England Journal of Medicine,* 1977, *296,* 716; Shepard, D. S., and Thompson, M. S. "First Principles of Cost-Effectiveness Analysis in Health." *Public Health Reports,* 1979, *94,* 535.

23. Smith, T. J., Hillner, B. E., and Desch, C. E. "Efficacy and Cost-Effectiveness of Cancer Treatment: Rational Allocation of Resources Based on Decision Analysis." *Journal of the National Cancer Institute*, 1993, *85*, 1460–1474.

24. Dean, H. E. "Political and Ethical Implications of Using Quality of Life as an Outcome Measure." *Seminars in Oncology Nursing*, 1990, *6*, 303–308.

25. Coates, A., and others. "Improving the Quality of Life During Chemotherapy for Advanced Breast Cancer." *New England Journal of Medicine*, 1987, *317*, 1490–1495.

26. Ganz, P. A., and others. "Breast Conservation Versus Mastectomy: Is There a Difference in Psychological Adjustment or Quality of Life in the Year After Surgery?" *Cancer*, 1992, *69*, 1729–1738.

27. Litwin, M. S., and others. "Quality of Life Outcomes in Men Treated for Localized Prostate Cancer." *Journal of the American Medical Association* (forthcoming).

28. World Health Organization (1948); Breslow, L. "A Quantitative Approach to the World Health Organization Definition of Health: Physical, Mental and Social Well-Being." *International Journal of Epidemiology*, 1972, *1*, 347–355.

29. Breslow (1972).

30. Belloc, N. B., Breslow, L., and Hochstim, J. R. "Measurement of Physical Health in a General Population Survey." *American Journal of Epidemiology*, 1971, *93*, 328–336.

31. Belloc, Breslow, and Hochstim (1971).

32. Berkman, P. L. "Measurement of Mental Health in a General Population Survey." *American Journal of Epidemiology*, 1971, *94*, 105–111.

33. Berkman (1971).

34. Belloc, N. B., and Breslow, L. "Relationship of Physical Health Status and Health Practices." *Preventive Medicine*, 1972, *1*, 409–421.

35. Breslow, L., and Enstrom, J. E. "Persistence of Health Habits and Their Relationship to Mortality." *Preventive Medicine*, 1980, *9*, 469–483.

36. Breslow, L., and Breslow, N. "Health Practices and Disability: Some Evidence from Alameda County." *Preventive Medicine*, 1993, *22*, 86–95.

37. Starr, P. *The Social Transformation of American Medicine*. New York: Basic Books, 1982.

38. Brook, R. H., and others. "Does Free Care Improve Adults' Health? Results From a Randomized Controlled Trial." *New England Journal of Medicine*, 1983, 309, 1429–1434; Newhouse, J., and others. "Some Interim Results from a Controlled Trial of Cost Sharing in Health Insurance." *New England Journal of Medicine*, 1981, *305*, 1501–1507; Manning, W. R., and others. "A Controlled Trial of the Effect of a Prepaid Group Practice on Use of Services." *New England Journal of Medicine*, 1984, *310*, 1505–1510.

39. Ware, J. E., Jr. "Conceptualizing Disease Impact and Treatment Outcomes." *Cancer*, 1984, *53S*, 2316–2323.

40. Ware (1984), p. 2317.

41. Ware (1984).

42. World Health Organization (1948).

43. Ware (1984).

44. Veit, C. T., and Ware, J. E., Jr. "The Structure of Psychological Distress and Well-Being in General Populations." *Journal of Consulting and Clinical Psychology*, 1983, *51*, 730–742.

45. Veit and Ware (1983).

46. Testa, M. A., and Nackley, J. F. "Methods for Quality-of-Life Studies." *Annual Review of Public Health*, 1994, *15*, 535–559.

47. Tarlov, A. R., and others. "The Medical Outcomes Study: An Application of Methods for Monitoring the Results of Medical Care." *Journal of the American Medical Association*, 1989, *262*, 925–930.

48. Stewart, A. L., and Ware, J. E., Jr. (eds.). *Measuring Functional Status and Well-Being: The Medical Outcomes Study Approach.* Durham, N.C.: Duke University Press, 1992.

49. Stewart and Ware (1992).

50. Stewart, A. L., Hays, R. D., and Ware, J. E., Jr. "The MOS Short-Form General Health Survey: Reliability and Validity in a Patient Population." *Medical Care*, 1988, *26*, 724–735; Stewart, A. L., and others. "Functional Status and Well-Being of Patients with Chronic Conditions: Results from the Medical Outcomes Study." *Journal of the American Medical Association*, 1989, *262*, 907–913.

51. Ware, J. E., Jr., and Sherbourne, C. D. "The MOS 36-Item Short-Form Health Survey (SF-36). I. Conceptual Framework and Item Selection." *Medical Care*, 1992, *30*, 473–483; Hays, R. D., Sherbourne, C. D., and Mazel, R. M. "The Rand 36-Item Health Survey 1.0." *Health Economics*, 1993, *2*, 217–227.

52. Meyer, K. B., and others. "Monitoring Dialysis Patients' Health Status." *American Journal of Kidney Diseases*, 1994, *24*, 267–279; Jacobson, A. M., DeGroot, M., and Samson, J. A., "The Evaluation of Two Measures of Quality of Life in Patients with Type I and Type II Diabetes." *Diabetes Care*, 1994, *17*, 267–274; Jette, D. U., and Downing, J. "Health Status of Individuals Entering a Cardiac Rehabilitation Program as Measured by the Medical Outcomes Study 36-Item Short-Form Survey (SF-36)." *Physical Therapy*, 1994, *74*, 521–527.

53. Aaronson, N. K., and others. "International Quality of Life Assessment (IQOLA) Project." *Quality of Life Research*, 1992, 1, 349–351.

54. Ware, J. E., Jr., personal communication, Los Angeles, 1999.

55. Potts, M. K., Mazzuca, S. A., and Brandt, K. D. "Views of Patients and Physicians Regarding the Importance of Various Aspects of Arthritis Treatment: Correlations with Health Status and Patient Satisfaction." *Patient Education and Counseling*, 1986, *8*, 125–134; Ware, J. E., Jr., Kosinski, M., and Keller, S. D. *SF-12: How to Score the SF-12 Physical and Mental Health Summary Scales.* Boston: Health Institute, New England Medical Center, 1995.

56. Staquet, M., Berzon, R., Osoba, D., and Machin, D. "Guidelines for Reporting Results of Quality of Life Assessments in Clinical Trials." *Quality of Life Research*, 1996, *5*, 496–502.

57. Potts, Mazzuca, and Brandt (1986).

58. Croog, S. H., and others. "The Effects of Antihypertensive Therapy on the Quality of Life." *New England Journal of Medicine*, 1986, *314*, 1657–1664; Testa, M. A., and others. "Quality of Life and Antihypertensive Therapy in Men." *New England Journal of Medicine*, 1993, *328*, 907–913.

59. Coates, Gebski, and Bishop (1987); Ganz and others (1992); Litwin, M. S., and others. "Quality of Life Outcomes in Men Treated for Localized Prostate Cancer." *Journal of the American Medical Association*, 1995, *273*, 129–135.

60. Moinpour (1990).

61. Bombardier, C., and others. "Auranofin Therapy and Quality of Life in Patients with Rheumatoid Arthritis." *American Journal of Medicine*, 1986, *81*, 565–578.

62. Potts, Mazzuca, and Brandt (1986).

63. Potts, Mazzuca, and Brandt (1986).

64. Croog and others (1986).

65. Croog and others (1986).

66. Croog and others (1986).

67. Croog and others (1986).

68. Croog and others (1986).

69. Croog and others (1986).

70. Croog and others (1986).

71. Croog and others (1986).

72. Croog and others (1986).

73. Croog and others (1986).

74. Croog and others (1986).

75. Testa and others (1993); Bombardier and others (1986); Johnson, J. R., and Temple, R. "Food and Drug Administration Requirements for Approval of New Anticancer Drugs." *Cancer Treatment Reports*, 1985, *69*, 1155–1157.

76. Heithoff, K. A., and Lohr, K. N. "Effectiveness and Outcomes in Health Care." In *Proceedings of an Invitational Conference by the Institute of Medicine, Division of Health Care Services.* Washington, D.C.: National Academy Press, 1990.

77. Goldberg, H. I., and Cummings, M. A. (eds.). "Conducting Medical Effectiveness Research: A Report from the Inter-Port Work Groups." *Medical Care* (Supplement), 1994, *32*, JS1–JS110.

78. Lohr, K. N. (ed.). "Advances in Health Status Assessment: Conference Proceedings." *Medical Care*, 1989, *27*, S1ff; Lohr, K. N. (ed.). "Advances in Health Status Assessment: Fostering the Application of Health Status Measures in Clinical Settings." (Conference proceedings.) *Medical Care*, 1992, *30*, MS1–MS294.

79. Nagfield, S. G., and Hailey, B. J. "Quality of Life Assessment in Cancer Clinical Trials." (Report of workshop on quality of life research in clinical trials, July 16–17, 1990.) Bethesda, Md.: Public Health Service, NIH, U.S. Dept. of Health and Human Services, 1991; Furberg, C. D., and Schattinga, J. A. "Quality of Life Assessment: Practice, Problems, Promise." *Proceedings of workshop, Oct. 15–17, 1990.* Bethesda, Md.: Public Health Service, NIH, U.S. Dept. of Health and Human Services, 1991.

80. Ellwood (1988).

81. Andersen, R. M., Davidson, P. L., and Ganz, P. A. "Symbiotic Relationships of Quality of Life Health Services, Research and Other Health Research." *Quality of Life Research*, 1994, *3*, 365–373.

82. Andersen, Davidson, and Ganz (1994).

83. Andersen, Davidson, and Ganz (1994).

CHAPTER SEVEN

EVALUATING THE QUALITY OF CARE

Elizabeth A. McGlynn and Robert H. Brook

The fundamental goal of the U.S. health care system is to provide the mix of health services that optimizes the overall health of the population. The key to achieving this goal is to ensure that we continuously strive to improve the quality of health services. The Institute of Medicine has defined quality of care as "the degree to which health services for individuals and populations increase the likelihood of desired health outcomes and are consistent with current professional knowledge."[1]

The main purpose of this chapter is to review various methods for assessing quality of care and to summarize some of what is known about the current level of quality in the United States. We begin by considering criteria for selecting topics for quality assessment. Next, we present a conceptual framework useful for organizing evaluation of quality. The definitions, methods, and state of the art in assessing the structure, process, and outcomes of care are then discussed.

The bottom line to this chapter is that scientifically sound methods exist for assessing quality and that they must be employed systematically in the future to guard against deterioration in quality that might otherwise occur as an unintended result of organizational and financial changes in the health services system.

Selecting Topics for Quality Assessment

It is neither feasible nor desirable to examine everything that occurs in the health care system. Quality assessment or monitoring is conducted by selectively examining dimensions of the health delivery system. There are two possible approaches to selecting topics in order to understand performance quality. The first approach is to examine the health services delivery system without reference to specific clinical problems or treatments. Much of the work that is being done by health plans and hospitals to improve quality (for example, total quality management, continuous quality improvement) examines systems issues. An example of this approach is looking at the timeliness with which laboratory test results are received by the physician who ordered the tests.

The second approach is to examine quality from a clinical perspective, focusing on specific health conditions or services and evaluating care delivered to the population of individuals who have those health problems or who require particular services. An example of this approach is examining compliance with specific standards of care, such as whether the appropriate medication is used at the right dosage to treat a person with hypertension. In addition, quality can be assessed by a single entity with the intention of improving its own quality (internal quality assessment), or quality can be compared among several similar entities and the information made available for decision making (external quality assessment). This chapter focuses more on the clinical approach than the systems approach and on external assessments more often than internal assessments. These biases reflect the authors' belief that future public expenditures on quality methods should be targeted in these two areas.

Criteria for Selecting Quality Assessment Areas

The clinical approach to external quality monitoring begins with selecting the health conditions or problems to be included. From the work of the HMO Quality of Care Consortium,[2] five criteria for selecting conditions are recommended:

1. The condition is highly prevalent or has a significant effect on mortality and morbidity in the population.

2. There is reasonable scientific evidence that efficacious or effective interventions exist to prevent a disease from developing (primary prevention); to identify and treat the disease at an early stage (secondary prevention); or to reduce impairment, disability, and suffering associated with having an illness (tertiary prevention).

3. Improving the quality of service delivery enhances the health of the population.

4. The recommended interventions are cost-effective.

5. The recommended interventions can be significantly influenced by health plans or providers.

The first criterion emphasizes that quality assessment should focus on those conditions that seriously threaten the health and well-being of the population, as opposed to conditions without serious consequences. From a logistical viewpoint, focusing on conditions that are highly prevalent increases the likelihood of identifying a sufficient number of cases for review so that there is adequate statistical power to draw conclusions.

The second criterion underscores the idea that health plans and providers should be held accountable only for those interventions that are supported by scientific studies or formal professional consensus. The health care system should not be encouraged to deliver care of uncertain benefit, and systems that have not embraced unproven practices should not be penalized. Many health services that are provided in this country do not meet these standards; some services may never be subjected to the rigorous evaluation of a randomized trial because of concerns about the ethics of withholding treatment (as would be necessary for a no-treatment control group) or offering a treatment that is believed to be less desirable (as would be necessary to test competing treatments). For these areas, we should rely on studies with less rigorous designs or on consensus opinion. Figure 7.1 shows the distribution of evidence for some common surgical procedures and one medical condition. Among articles that were included in several systematic reviews of the literature, randomized controlled trials represented only a small fraction (4–11 percent) of the available literature.[3] As scientific knowledge expands, so too will the capacity for scientifically based quality monitoring.

The third criterion suggests quality assessment should target those interventions that have a significant positive impact on the health of the population. This recognizes that one of the potential effects of quality monitoring is to shift health plan resource allocation or physician practice choices to areas that are being evaluated, as opposed to areas that are not subject to assessment. This should only occur among services for which improved quality makes a positive contribution to the overall health of the population, rather than focusing on improving services that produce only a negligible improvement in health. The greatest potential for improving health occurs with interventions that are highly efficacious or effective and that are frequently underused or misused.

The fourth criterion acknowledges that there are limited resources available for health care today; as a result, cost must be taken into account in selecting areas

FIGURE 7.1. DISTRIBUTION OF RESEARCH ARTICLES REVIEWED, BY STRENGTH OF RESEARCH DESIGN.

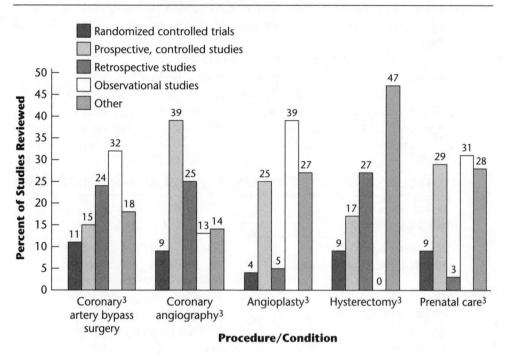

for quality assessment. There is limited information available in the literature on the cost-effectiveness of various interventions, but the criterion remains important as a framework for evaluating potential assessment areas. Within a clinical area, there may be several possible ways of evaluating quality. Among those for which positive health benefits can be shown, one should also consider whether there are differences among the interventions being evaluated in the cost-effectiveness of achieving the health benefit. If significant differences exist, the more cost-effective intervention is the preferable choice for measurement.

The final criterion affirms that only those interventions that can be significantly influenced by health plans or providers should be included. Many primary prevention campaigns (for example, seat belt use) have been most effective in a public health context rather than private. Initial survival after a myocardial infarction may be more a function of the adequacy of the trauma system in a geographic area than the quality of medical care; after admission, the focal point of responsibility shifts more clearly from the trauma system to the health plan, hospital, or provider. Some interventions may be highly dependent on patient compliance, and this may be difficult to achieve or may vary depending on the characteristics of the enrolled population. For example, return to work after a back injury may be more dependent on workers compensation benefits than the quality of care provided.

When we used these criteria with the HMO Quality of Care Consortium to select potential areas for quality-of-care assessment in managed care, we identified thirteen conditions for which measures might be developed.[4] The conditions are shown in Table 7.1. Since that time, the National Committee for Quality Assurance (NCQA) has introduced and refined a set of quality measures for man-

TABLE 7.1.   EXAMPLE OF QUALITY MEASUREMENT PRIORITIES.

Quality Area from HMO Consortium	Current HEDIS Measure
Low birthweight	Prenatal care in first trimester*
Childhood infectious diseases	Childhood immunizations Adolescent immunizations
Otitis media	None**
Childhood asthma	Appropriate medication use
Influenza	Flu shots for older adults
Breast cancer	Mammography screening
Coronary artery disease	Beta blockers after acute myocardial infarction Cholesterol control after cardiac event Control of hypertension
Lung cancer and smoking-related diseases	Advice to quit smoking
Stroke	None
Diabetes mellitus	Annual measure of glycosylated hemoglobin and control Annual measure of lipids and control Monitoring for nephropathy eye exam
Medical problems of frail elderly	Health Outcomes Survey
Hip fracture	None
Appropriateness of common medical and surgical procedures	None

Notes: *Early prenatal care may prevent low birthweight.

**A measure of appropriate prescribing for otitis media was dropped after one year because of methodological and clinical problems with the measure.

aged care plans known as the Health Plan Employer Data and Information Set (HEDIS). This is the most widely adapted system for measuring quality nationally. As Table 7.1 shows, most of the areas in which the HMO consortium recommended that measures be developed are covered in HEDIS. A few additional measures (such as cervical cancer screening, follow-up after mental health hospitalization) that were not in the HMO consortium's list are included in HEDIS.

A Conceptual Framework for Quality Assessment

A conceptual framework is a useful mechanism for defining the aspects of care that are evaluated for each condition in a quality assessment. The most commonly used conceptual framework in quality assessment is the one proposed by Avedis Donabedian.[5] He identified three dimensions of quality: structure, process, and outcomes (Figure 7.2). We organize our review of quality assessment around these three dimensions. In each section, we present a definition of the dimension of quality, discuss methods available for assessing that dimension, and summarize

FIGURE 7.2. CONCEPTUAL FRAMEWORK FOR QUALITY ASSESSMENT.

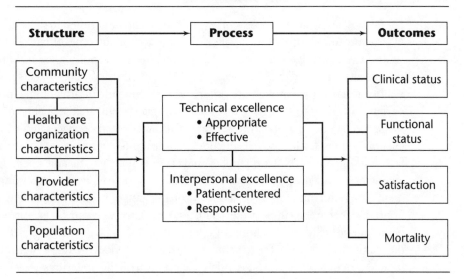

what is known about that aspect of quality of care in the U.S. health care system today.

Structural Quality

Early efforts to evaluate quality focused predominantly on structural elements, but these have garnered less attention as the field of quality measurement has improved.

Definition of Structural Quality

Structural quality refers to those stable elements of the health care delivery system in a community that facilitate or inhibit access to and provision of services. The elements include community characteristics (say, prevalence of disease), health care organization characteristics (such as number of hospital beds per capita), provider characteristics (specialty mix), and population characteristics (demographics, insurance coverage). Structural characteristics can be used to describe both the need for health care (prevalence or incidence of disease) and the capacity of the community or health care delivery system to meet those needs (availability of properly trained personnel).

Methods of Structural Quality Assessment

For purposes of quality assessment, we are particularly interested in those elements of structure that (1) predict variations in the processes or outcomes of care and (2) are subject to change. For example, the characteristics of the population residing in a community may predict differences in processes of care or outcomes. Persons without health insurance or who are otherwise economically disadvantaged may experience barriers to accessing the health service system; such barriers might be suggested by a comparatively lower rate of using necessary services among different populations. In turn, such reductions in utilization might be associated with less favorable outcomes. However, policy makers are unlikely to be able to change the characteristics of the population. The more appropriate focus for quality improvement is on reducing barriers to access, through changes in either the availability of insurance or characteristics of the health services delivery system (for example, number of public health clinics, hours of operation for other health providers). Because the relationship between the structure of the health services delivery system and the processes or outcomes of care is indirect, structural quality measures are less useful for policy makers than measures of process quality or outcomes.

Community characteristics represent the context in which the health services delivery system operates; they offer one perspective for evaluating the adequacy of the service system to respond to community needs. The prevalence of disorders in the community, for instance, may be useful in estimating specific community needs. Information about the availability of health resources may be an indicator of the potential for meeting those needs. One common measure of resource availability is the physician-to-population ratio; the general tendency is to interpret a higher ratio as representing better quality (though this is not always the case).[6] The location of the community relative to health resources is another key indicator of the ease with which residents may obtain certain services; inner-city and rural residents may have to travel further than others to obtain services. Although an evaluation of community characteristics is not generally included in quality assessment, it may be an important precursor to understanding the particular quality challenges likely to be faced in a community.

Health care organization characteristics have been evaluated in terms of the capacity of the organization to provide high-quality services. Various factors, including the quality of the physical plant and equipment, ownership, accreditation, staffing patterns, distribution of reimbursement by source of payment, organizational structure, and governance mechanisms, have been considered markers of the likelihood that an organization provides good quality of care. Most of these factors at best can be viewed as facilitating or inhibiting the likelihood of delivering good care; because these factors always appear in combination, it is difficult to evaluate the incremental effect each has on quality.

Provider characteristics have been included as explanatory factors in quality assessments, among them age (or years in practice), gender, race or ethnicity, medical school attended, location of residency training program, specialty, board certification status, job satisfaction, and method of compensation. Board certification is the professional indicator of quality; additional years of training and an examination are required to become board certified. Various specialty boards are responsible for granting board certification. Overall, about 60 percent of physicians are board certified.[7] The specialties with the highest rate (80 percent and above) of board certification include pediatric cardiology, radiology, gastroenterology, colon and rectal surgery, pulmonary disease, cardiovascular disease, allergy and immunology, medical genetics, and nuclear medicine. The specialties with the lowest rate (60 percent and below) of board certification include general practice, psychiatry, internal medicine, and general surgery.

Population characteristics may be useful in predicting the likelihood that an individual receives high-quality care. Information may be used to identify individuals who are at risk for receiving lower quality of care; in particular, organizations that provide services to individuals at high risk should be aware of the special needs of these populations. Various population characteristics have been examined: sociodemographics, insurance coverage and type, presence of co-morbid conditions, functional status, and so on.

The most common method of assessing structural quality is through organizational accreditation. Several organizations currently conduct accreditation programs. Generally accreditation requires that an on-site survey team inspect the facility and verify that the organization meets standards. The Joint Commission on the Accreditation of Healthcare Organizations accredits hospitals, health care networks, clinical laboratories, and organizations that provide home care, long-term care, behavioral health care, and ambulatory care. The National Committee for Quality Assurance (NCQA) accredits managed care organizations, managed behavioral health care organizations, credentials verification organizations, physician organization certification, and preferred provider organizations. The American Accreditation Healthcare Commission accredits utilization review programs, preferred provider organizations, and managed care organizations.

What Do We Know About Structural Quality?

Few structural factors have been found to be associated with significant variation in health outcomes, although they are frequently associated with differences in the process of care. A study of the effect of implementation of the prospective payment system on the quality of care delivered to Medicare beneficiaries, for example, found that patients who were black or from poor neighborhoods or who were admitted to rural hospitals received poorer-quality care than other Medicare patients.[8] These differences in quality, however, did not result in a higher death rate among patients who were black, Medicaid beneficiaries, or living in the poorest neighborhoods or rural areas. The same study found that higher quality of care was delivered in teaching, larger, and urban hospitals.[9] The mortality rate in the hospitals with the worst quality was 4 percentage points higher than the rate in the hospitals with the best quality. This study illustrates an important application of quality assessment for evaluating the impact of changes in public policies.

The Medical Outcomes Study found that specialty training, payment system, and practice organization had independent effects on resource utilization after controlling for differences in patient case mix.[10] Cardiologists and endocrinologists had higher utilization rates than other specialties; general internists had a somewhat higher utilization rate than family physicians. Solo practitioners and those in single specialty groups had 41 percent more hospitalizations than physicians in health maintenance organizations.

However, from a policy perspective it is important to note that variations in resource use generally have not been associated with significant differences in outcomes. A study comparing rates of hospital discharge, readmission, length of stay, and reimbursement for Medicare beneficiaries in two communities with differing resource profiles (Boston and New Haven) found significant variation in use of the hospital but no difference in mortality rate.[11] Another study comparing Massachusetts and California found no relationship between length of stay and outcomes (that is, deaths, functional status postdischarge, readmission, and patient satisfaction) for Medicare beneficiaries treated for one of six medical and surgical conditions.[12] One conclusion is that substantial reduction in utilization (and thus cost) may be possible without negative effects on health.

Socioeconomic differences (such as education, income, and race) have been shown to predict differences in utilization even when insurance coverage is similar. For example, a comparison of breast and cervical cancer screening in Ontario and the United States found that despite the availability of universal coverage in Ontario, women with less than a high school diploma and those with lower incomes were less likely to receive these two preventive services in both countries.[13] Another study examining predictors of utilization among children with special health care needs found that children who were poor, of a minority group, living with their mother or someone other than their parents, and without health insurance or a regular medical provider were more likely to experience barriers to access and to use fewer services than other children with similar needs.[14] The policy implication is that improving care for these populations may require more than just reducing financial barriers.

The structure of health insurance benefits can significantly affect utilization. In the RAND Health Insurance Experiment, the rate of cost sharing contributed to a 75 percent differential in per person expenditures between the most and least generous health plans.[15] Reduction in use of ambulatory services was greater than in use of hospital services. Despite the dramatic variance in utilization rate, there were few differences in health outcomes for the average individual. Low-income persons in the plan with no cost sharing had somewhat better control of high blood pressure, correction for vision problems, and care for dental problems compared to those in plans with cost sharing.[16] Private policy makers may have used these findings to guide development of plans with much higher cost sharing.

There is some evidence that a relationship exists between the number of procedures done by an individual physician or institution and the outcomes, with higher volume being associated with better outcomes.[17] New York state found that since the cardiac procedures reporting system was introduced, risk-adjusted mortality decreased for both high-volume and low-volume surgeons.[18] For low-volume surgeons (≤ 50 procedures annually), the risk-adjusted mortality rate declined from 7.94 percent in 1989 to 3.20 percent in 1992 (a 60 percent decrease). Among high volume surgeons (≥ 150 procedures annually), the risk-adjusted mortality rate declined by one-third, from 3.57 in 1989 to 2.36 in 1992. One of the contributing factors was that 25 percent fewer procedures were being done by low-volume surgeons in 1992 as compared with 1989. The other factors were that low-volume, high-mortality physicians stopped performing surgery in New York state and newer low-volume surgeons performed better than average. Policy makers could limit reimbursement for certain procedures to facilities and physicians with certain minimum volumes. The Pacific Business Group on Health makes information publicly available on surgical procedure volume as a means of encouraging people to go to higher-volume facilities.

Process Quality

Quality assessment done to make comparisons between organizations for consumer choice or accountability usually focuses on process quality.

Definition of Process Quality

Process quality refers to what occurs in the interaction between a patient and a provider. It is generally divided into two aspects: technical excellence and interpersonal excellence. Technical excellence means that the intervention was appropriate (that is, the health benefit to the patient exceeded the health risk by a significant margin) and that it was provided skillfully. Interpersonal excellence means that the intervention was humane and responsive to the preferences of the individual.

For purposes of quality assessment, we are primarily interested in those processes of care that are likely to produce optimal outcomes—either improvement in health or reduction in the rate of decline. The best evidence of the relationship between processes and outcomes is from randomized clinical trials because they can prove conclusively the efficacy of an intervention (the potential to produce desired outcomes under ideal circumstances). Evidence from other scientific methods, though not as conclusive, is often used to demonstrate the importance of a variety of interventions in medical care. The IOM definition of quality emphasizes this relationship between the process of service delivery and outcomes, as well as noting the role of professional consensus in defining high-quality processes.

Methods of Process Quality Assessment

We discuss four methods that have been used to evaluate the quality of medical care processes: (1) appropriateness of an intervention; (2) adherence to practice guidelines or standards of care; (3) practice profiling, and; (4) consumer ratings.

These four methods share some features, but we discuss them separately to emphasize a number of methodological considerations.

Appropriateness of Intervention. Appropriateness of intervention means that, for individuals with particular clinical and personal characteristics, the expected health benefit from doing an intervention (diagnostic or therapeutic procedure) exceeds the expected health risk by a sufficient margin so that the intervention is worth doing. RAND and UCLA have pioneered a method of assessing the appropriateness with which a variety of interventions are evaluated.[19] The basic method involves five steps.

Step One: Review the Literature. A detailed literature review is conducted to summarize what is known about the efficacy, utilization, complications, cost, and indications for the subject intervention. Where possible, outcome evidence tables are constructed for clinically homogeneous groups.

Step Two: List Indications. A preliminary list of indications is developed for the intervention that categorizes patients in terms of their symptoms, past medical history, results of previous diagnostic tests, and clinically relevant personal characteristics (such as age). The indications list is designed to be detailed enough so that patients within an indication are homogeneous with respect to the clinical appropriateness of performing a procedure; the indications are comprehensive enough so that all persons presenting for the procedure can be categorized.

Step Three: Convene a Panel to Select Indications. A nine-person multispecialty panel is assembled to assume responsibility for developing and rating the final set of indications. The panel is chosen to be diverse with respect to geographic location, practice style, and other characteristics. Both "doers" and "nondoers" of a procedure are included on the panel.

Step Four: Rate the Indications. The indications are rated using a modified Delphi process. In the first round, indications are individually rated by panelists (who have the literature review available); the panelists may also recommend changes to the structure of the indications. In the second round, the panel meets face-to-face for a discussion of the results from the first round of ratings and makes final ratings. The indications are rated from 1 to 9, where 1 means that the procedure is very inappropriate for persons within an indication and 9 means that the procedure is very appropriate for persons within an indication. The median panel rating is used to determine the appropriateness rating for each indication; a median rating of 1–3 is considered inappropriate, 4–6 is equivocal or of uncertain value, and

7–9 is appropriate. There is also a requirement that the panel have a reasonable and statistically determined level of agreement among themselves.

Step Five: Evaluate Appropriateness of Interventions. The appropriateness with which interventions are used can then be evaluated. Generally, information is abstracted from the medical record (inpatient or outpatient) because of the level of clinical detail required to assign patients to indications. An alternative approach that has been applied when appropriateness is assessed prospectively is to interview both the patient and the physician.

Observations on the Appropriateness Method. The reliability and validity of the appropriateness method has been extensively evaluated. The test-retest reliability of individual panel members' ratings and the reproducibility of overall panel ratings have been found to be comparable to the levels of common diagnostic tests.[20] The content and construct validity of ratings of appropriateness have been supported by the studies done.[21] For example, regression analysis performed on indications for patients with chronic stable angina undergoing coronary angiography demonstrated that appropriateness ratings rise as severity increases, among patients who failed medical therapy, and among patients who had positive findings on noninvasive tests.[22]

The ratings of each indication are the explicit standards by which care is evaluated. The indications can be linked to the quality of scientific evidence, and ratings can be updated as knowledge changes. It is also possible to conduct sensitivity analyses that evaluate the importance of certain factors in the indication structure with respect to determining appropriateness. For example, in our study of appropriateness of hysterectomy, we found that among women who wanted to maintain fertility, the expert panel required considerable evidence of efforts to find an alternative solution to the presenting problem before the hysterectomy was considered appropriate.[23] Because there are no national averages established for the expected appropriateness of care, most of the comparisons have been made among groups (hospitals, managed care organizations) participating in a study.[24]

Adherence to Practice Guidelines or Professional Standards. Adherence to practice guidelines or professional standards is a method of process quality assessment that evaluates the extent to which care is consistent with professional knowledge, either by examining adherence to specific practice guidelines or by evaluating whether care meets certain professional standards. The Agency for Healthcare Research and Quality (AHRQ) defines clinical practice guidelines as "systematically developed statements to assist practitioner and patient decisions about appropriate health care for specific clinical conditions."[25] Practice guidelines are often formulated graphically as decision algorithms to reflect the complexity of clinical decision making.

For a number of years, AHRQ funded the development of practice guidelines[26] and published a monograph on various methodological approaches to the development of clinical practice guidelines.[27] More recently, AHRQ has funded several Evidence-Based Practice Centers to conduct systematic reviews of the literature that can be used by others to develop practice guidelines. Today, most specialty societies develop practice guidelines in their area. The U.S. Preventive Services Task Force is one of the leading organizations developing guidelines for the use of preventive care services (for example, immunizations, Pap smears, mammograms). Because of the relative ease of evaluating adherence to preventive service standards, they represent a common basis for quality assessment. One argument that is frequently raised in objection to using the rate of adherence to preventive service recommendations as a marker of quality is the role of patient compliance in seeking such services. Despite this concern, preventive service use remains one of the leading quality indicators currently in use.

For purposes of quality assessment, it is almost always necessary to translate guidelines into review criteria by establishing operational definitions of adherence and nonadherence to the guidelines, as well as definitions for key clinical concepts employed in the guidelines. Many practice guidelines, for example, contain vague clinical terms ("mild," "moderate," "severe") that must be explicitly defined in order to evaluate whether a particular patient qualifies for a portion of the guidelines and then to assess adherence to the guideline. The performance expectation is generally 100 percent adherence to the guideline, and comparisons are made either among similar groups or compared to a benchmark.

Practice Profiling. Practice profiling is a method for comparing the patterns of cost, utilization, or quality of processes among providers.[28] The method compares practice patterns to a norm (say, the average of other physicians in the organization) or to a preestablished standard (based on a practice guideline). Profiles are generally constructed as a rate of occurrence of some process (such as office visit, service, surgical procedure, laboratory test) over a specified period of time for a defined population.[29] What distinguishes profiling from most appropriateness or guideline adherence approaches is that the review is not necessarily conducted specific to a clinical condition; rather, it may cover a broader range of practice patterns (such as hospital admission rate). Profiles can be constructed at any level in the health delivery system—nationally; regionally; or by health plan, specialty, medical group, or individual physician. Profiling is most often used to examine utilization of a variety of services, including hospital admission, ambulatory visit, laboratory test use, referral pattern, diagnostic test use, or medication prescription.

Profiling has been used for internal quality improvement and cost containment more often than for external reporting of performance. One consequence of this is that there are fewer reports in the literature about the results of profiling analysis. There are, however, a few articles that emphasize some of the critical issues that must be addressed if profiling is to be used routinely for quality assessment.[30] Perhaps the most important issue that has arisen is the need for case-mix or severity adjustment (differences in severity, prevalence of diseases, and other characteristics of the populations being compared). The methods for case-mix adjustment, particularly in the ambulatory setting, are in a developmental stage.

In addition, much of the clinical information that is typically required for case-mix adjustment cannot be found among claims data; this implies that supplemental data are required in order to make adequate adjustments. One study of referral patterns found that adjusting for the age and sex distribution of patients in a physician's panel reduced the coefficient of variation in referrals by more than 50 percent.[31] When a case-mix adjustment was applied, 75 percent of physicians identified as outliers under the age and sex adjustment method were no longer classified as outliers.

This problem is particularly important to solve for the purpose of external comparison, but even internal uses of profiling would benefit substantially from improved adjustment methods (as when physicians in a health plan are profiled). For example, the Medical Outcomes Study found that patients of cardiologists were older, had lower functional status and well-being scores, and had more chronic diagnoses than patients of general internists; patients of family practitioners were younger, had better functional status and fewer chronic conditions than patients of general internists.[32] These case-mix characteristics were associated with differences in hospitalization rate, physician visit rate, and rate of prescription drug use. Internal plan comparisons should account for these variations.

The other challenge for profiling is the problem of sample size. There is considerable interest in using profiling techniques to examine the practice patterns of individual physicians. However, one must have an adequate number of observations on each physician to determine whether the differences observed are statistically significant. Among other things, this implies that common processes (such as use of screening mammography) are more suitable for profiling than rarer processes (using adjuvant chemotherapy for breast cancer treatment). Among processes, greater aggregation is more suitable than less (using all laboratory tests versus using a single test). These issues have been pointed out even by proponents of profiling.[33]

Consumer Ratings. Consumer ratings are the most appropriate method for evaluating the interpersonal quality of care. Surveys of health plan enrollees are the most common method for eliciting information from individuals about their health care. Two types of information are generally sought: (1) reporting of events and (2) ratings of care. We discuss reporting of events (patient experience) here and ratings of care (patient satisfaction) under the outcomes section.

Consumers may be asked to report interventions such as immunizations, mammography, and cholesterol testing that are indicators for technical process quality. The National Immunization Survey, for example, tracks the rate of immunizations for children in the first two years of life. Such reporting is particularly useful if the intervention is likely to be remembered accurately by consumers and if the intervention is difficult to identify in other data sources. Consumer reports are also used for a variety of access issues, such as waiting time for an appointment or to see the doctor, distance to the nearest health facility, hours of operation, ability to see the provider one wants to see, and other similar questions regarding consumers' experiences in trying to obtain services. Consumers may also report on what the physician did during an encounter (explain options, provide requested information, counsel about health habits). Patients' ability to report on events varies with the time frame (a shorter time span produces more reliable information) and the type of event (invasive events such as surgery may be more memorable than health promotion counseling).

What Do We Know About Process Quality?

It is beyond the scope of this chapter to summarize all of the literature regarding process quality. However, we include some examples of what is known about process quality from published studies that have used one of the four methods being discussed.

Appropriateness. Figure 7.3 illustrates the results of various studies of appropriateness that have been conducted over the past ten to fifteen years.[34] Overall, the proportion of procedures judged to be inappropriate ranges from 2 percent (coronary artery bypass graft surgery or CABG, and cataract) to 32 percent (carotid endarterectomy). The proportion of procedures judged to be of uncertain clinical value ranges from 7 percent (CABG surgery) to 38 percent (percutaneous transluminal coronary angioplasty). Combining these estimates of inappropriate and uncertain care suggests that about one-third of the procedures performed in this country are of questionable health benefit relative to their risks. Although the appropriateness method has been primarily used to assess overuse of care, it can also be applied to evaluate underuse. For example, in a study done in Los Angeles county, 25 percent of patients who had indications that a CABG surgery was necessary had not received the procedure.[35]

FIGURE 7.3. PROPORTION OF PROCEDURES JUDGED TO
BE EITHER CLINICALLY INAPPROPRIATE OR OF UNCERTAIN VALUE;
SUMMARY OF SELECTED STUDIES.

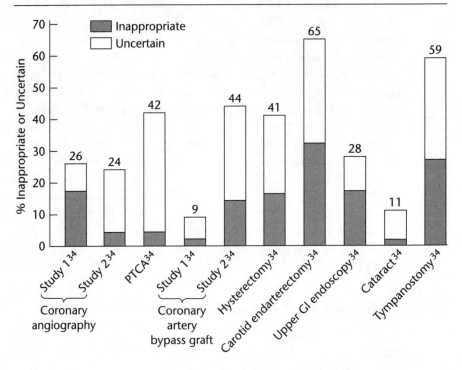

There is little evidence to suggest that a relationship exists between the rate at which procedures are done and the appropriateness of care. A study examining geographic variations in the use of coronary angiography, carotid endarterectomy, and upper gastrointestinal tract endoscopy and the appropriateness with which those procedures were used found that the rate of inappropriate use was similar among high-use and low-use sites.[36] Another study failed to find a relationship between rate of hospital admission in a community and the appropriateness of those admissions.[37] The considerably higher rate of use for coronary angiography and CABG surgery in the United States as compared to Canada were also not found to be associated with differences in the appropriateness with which the procedures were performed.[38]

We have also found little evidence to suggest that economic incentives have an influence on appropriateness. For example, in the Trent region of the United Kingdom, the proportion of inappropriate coronary angiography was similar to the rate found in the United States and varied among centers within the region.[39]

In Israel, where physicians are salaried, the proportion of inappropriate or uncertain cholecystectomy ranged from 17 percent to 36 percent.[40] The findings for managed care organizations within the United States are consistent with these international findings. The proportion of hysterectomy judged to be inappropriate among seven managed care organizations ranged from 10 percent to 27 percent. In the RAND Health Insurance Experiment, although the hospitalization rate was lower in the managed care organization as compared to fee-for-service, reductions occurred in both discretionary and nondiscretionary admissions.[41] Reduction in utilization in response to cost containment concerns may occur in ways that are not clinically sensible. For example, limitations on the number of paid prescriptions in a Medicaid program reduced the overall number of prescriptions filled by 30 percent, but these reductions occurred among effective and essential medications as well as those with limited effectiveness.[42] The lower rate of cardiac procedures found in Canada as compared to the United States is achieved almost exclusively through providing these procedures at a significantly lower rate to persons age sixty-five and older.[43] The key policy implication to be drawn from the appropriateness literature is that resource allocation strategies must incorporate clinical criteria if resources are to be spent in a way that has the greatest health benefits.

Adherence to Guidelines. Because guidelines are a relatively new phenomenon, there are few systematic studies of adherence to them. Perhaps the most important consistent finding from studies of guideline adherence is that there is substantial variability in compliance with guidelines or treatment recommendations among providers. Further, when guidelines are first promulgated, adherence tends to be fairly low overall.

A review of the effect of guidelines on clinical practice found that fifty-five of the fifty-nine evaluations reviewed detected a significant improvement in the process of care.[44] The rate of adherence reported in these studies was frequently well below 50 percent, even after implementation of the guidelines. A recent summary of the literature on quality found that 50 percent of recommended preventive services were received, 70 percent of patients received recommended acute care services, and 30 percent received contraindicated acute care. About 60 percent of patients received recommended chronic care, and 20 percent received contraindicated care.[45]

In a study of the quality of prenatal care, we examined adherence to thirty-seven process quality criteria on the basis of medical record reviews at six managed care organizations.[46] We found significant variations in compliance with the criteria among the organizations, although the rate of adherence was considerably higher than many reported in that review article. The proportion of women in each of the six health plans who received seven routine screening tests in early pregnancy ranged from 64 percent to 95 percent, with an average across all plans of 82 percent. On average, about 84 percent of these women received other routine prenatal care; the range was from 78 percent to 87 percent. The adherence to criteria covering care for specific problems encountered in pregnancy was considerably lower; overall 70 percent of women received recommended care, and the range was from 54 percent to 77 percent.

The NCQA produces an annual report on the performance of managed care organizations.[47] In 1999, performance on the eleven effectiveness-of-care measures ranged from 83.6 percent for the proportion of women receiving prenatal care in the first trimester to 40.9 percent for the proportion of persons with diabetes who received an annual eye exam. Rates of breast and cervical cancer screening were 72.2 percent and 69.9 percent, respectively. Plans that report publicly, that have been reporting for more than three years, or that are accredited tended to score higher on these measures.

Another indicator of the process quality of care is the use of best practices for certain conditions. For example, thrombolytic therapy has been shown to substantially improve the chances of survival among individuals who have suffered a myocardial infarction.[48] An evaluation of the use of thrombolytic therapy found that only about 18 percent of patients with a myocardial infarction received thrombolytic therapy, and that the proportion receiving this drug declined with age—despite evidence of increased efficacy with older persons.[49]

Similar results have been reported for use of antidepressants. Only 20–30 percent of general medical patients with depression are prescribed antidepressant medications, and 30 percent of those with prescriptions are receiving a subtherapeutic dosage.[50] Minor tranquilizers are often used to treat depression[51] despite the lack of evidence for efficacy.[52] The quality of medication use among ethnic minority patients is even lower than that found for white patients.[53] Greater attention to the use of best practices through monitoring adherence to guidelines should substantially improve the quality of health care processes.

Practice or Area Profiling. The framework for profiling comes from the literature reporting significant variations in the use of a variety of common medical and surgical procedures over the last three decades. Variations have been documented among countries, in regions of the same country, within states, and between cities in the same state or region. *The Dartmouth Atlas of Health Care* publishes national data showing rate of variation for a variety of health care procedures. The data are presented in maps that use color coding to demonstrate visually the degree of national and regional variation. Previous analyses of variations have shown, for example, that the rate of prostatectomy is 35 percent higher in the

Midwest than the West, and the hysterectomy rate is 80 percent higher in the Midwest than in the Northeast.[54] Similar results have been reported for hip and knee replacement and diagnostic procedures such as CT scan and ultrasound. A comparison of two communities in the same region found that the rates of use of a variety of common medical procedures ranged from 127 per thousand population in New Haven to 214 per thousand population in Boston.[55] The same study found that rates of use of various surgical procedures ranged from 62 per thousand in New Haven to 86 per thousand in Boston.

A study designed to illustrate the use of practice profiling as a cost-containment tool compared the patterns of resource use between physicians providing care to Medicare beneficiaries in Oregon and Florida.[56] The study found that Florida physicians used more resources on average than Oregon physicians; the results were consistent across specialties and practice types. Considerable variation within each state was found. The authors acknowledge that at the individual physician level, profiling is best used to screen for potential problems rather than draw firm conclusions.

Consumer Reports. Consumers are able to report accurately many experiences in the health service system. One study, for example, found that consumers accurately reported 80–94 percent of history and physical elements that were performed during a health examination.[57] That study found some variation by patient characteristics; elderly and less-educated consumers were less accurate in their reporting of events. Another study comparing various data-collection methods found that patients and physicians agreed 96 percent of the time on what tests had been ordered, 94 percent of the time on what treatments were discussed, and 88 percent on patient education.[58] A more recent study, however, found somewhat lower rates of agreement between audiotapes, physician notes in the medical record, and patient reports of health promotion activities (smoking, alcohol use, and blood pressure).[59] The authors concluded that, when using audiotapes as the gold standard, the medical record tends to underestimate the frequency of health promotion counseling (smoking and alcohol use), and patient reports tend to overestimate the frequency of this activity. For reporting of whether blood pressure was taken, both the medical record and patient reports are quite accurate.

The 1988 National Maternal and Infant Health Survey relied on patient reports to assess adherence to recommendations from the Public Health Service's Expert Panel on the Content of Prenatal Care. Only 56 percent of respondents indicated that they had received all six of the procedures recommended by the panel in the first two visits (blood pressure measurement, urine test, blood test, weight and height taken, pelvic examination, and pregnancy history).[60] Only 32 percent of respondents said they had received any counseling in all seven of the recommended areas (nutrition, vitamin use, smoking cessation, alcohol use, drug use, breast feeding, and maternal weight gain). This study found that women receiving care from private offices were significantly less likely to receive the full range of services than women receiving their care from publicly funded clinics.

Assessing Outcomes

Outcomes can be defined as the results of efforts to prevent, diagnose, and treat various health problems encountered by the population. Outcomes are seen by many as the bottom-line measure of the effectiveness of the health care delivery system. A wide range of potential dimensions can be included in the broad category of outcomes. In Figure 7.2, for example, we list clinical status, functional status, consumer satisfaction, and mortality to illustrate a few possible outcomes.

Clinical status refers to biological, physiological, and symptom-based aspects of health. These are the outcomes that are generally of interest to physicians because they are most directly amenable to treatment. Functional status captures multiple dimensions, including physical, mental, role, and social functioning. Assessments of functional status typically ask respondents to indicate the frequency or extent to which physical or mental disorders interfere with their ability to perform their usual activities. Functional status is of greatest interest to consumers because it represents how changes in clinical status affect their everyday life. Consumer satisfaction assesses the extent to which experiences in the health service system were consistent with expectations and were acceptable to those receiving care.

There are two key challenges in using outcome assessments for evaluating the quality of care. Both of these challenges reflect the fact that the outcomes we observe are produced through the interaction of a variety of factors both in and outside of the health service delivery system. First, to use outcomes to make externally valid comparisons among health plans or providers, adequate methods must be employed to control for differences in the severity of illness or the health profile of the populations being compared. A familiar example of an initial failure to do this was the release by the Health Care Financing Administration (HCFA) of hospital mortality data. Initially, the data were not adjusted for differences in the severity of illness for patients, and not surprisingly some of the hospitals that had the worst performance records were those serving the sickest patients (for example, hospices for the terminally ill).[61] There is still considerable controversy as to whether the severity adjustments introduced by HCFA subsequent to the initial release were adequate, but the addition of severity adjustments substantially improved the discriminant validity of the model.[62]

The second key challenge for the use of outcomes data is the issue of attribution, that is, determining the extent to which the health plan or physician that is currently being evaluated is responsible for the observed outcomes. Health outcomes are affected by a variety of factors, not all of which can be modified by the health delivery system. Because these factors may be distributed differently among populations enrolled in health plans or those seeking care from primary care physicians, these external effects must be controlled for in statistical analyses in order to understand the extent to which variations in the quality of care are contributing to the observed variations in outcomes. For interventions that take place over a long period of time (chronic disease care), outcomes observed in the current time period may be the result of actions taken (or not taken) much earlier in the course of illness, and those actions might not have been undertaken by the physicians or health plan currently responsible for treating the patient. To the extent that individuals change providers frequently, discontinuities in service may further contribute to a less-than-optimal course of treatment. Who bears the responsibility for these complex series of events remains a question open to debate.

Methods of Outcome Assessment

We consider three approaches to outcome assessment that have been used to evaluate the quality of care delivered: (1) condition-specific; (2) generic; and (3) sentinel events, or adverse outcomes.

Condition-Specific Approach. The condition-specific approach, sometimes referred to as a "tracer" condition approach, examines the outcomes for individuals who have a particular diagnosis (say, hypertension). The outcomes for condition-specific approaches may emphasize clinical status (blood pressure control for hypertension), although disease-specific measures of functional status should also be assessed (for prostate cancer, treatment assessments should include incontinence, impotence, and bowel function). The advantage of condition-specific outcome assessment from a quality perspective is that it may most closely reflect a link to the processes of care delivered. For example, if one health plan has a higher proportion of individuals with hypertension whose blood pressures are outside of the "controlled" range, one might reasonably conclude that the plan has problems in managing the disease (medication, diet, monitoring for complications). The difficulty with condition-specific approaches to quality assessment is that they require substantial investment in developing methods across a sufficiently wide range of diseases to produce a picture of the overall quality of care delivered in a health plan.

One of the things we do not know is the extent to which quality is consistent from condition to condition within a health plan. We hypothesize that even within health plans there is variability in outcomes by condition; some plans may have good outcomes for adult chronic diseases and be less successful in achieving good outcomes for chronic disease in childhood. One study of quality at the hospital level found that the relative rates of complications were similar within institutions, but there was less correlation between medical and surgical cases.[63] The other difficulty in the context of today's information systems is that one may not be able to identify individuals who have particular health problems so that population-based outcome assessments can be conducted.

Generic Approach. The generic approach examines outcomes that can be assessed on all individuals, regardless of their health problems. Mortality, general functional status, and patient satisfaction outcomes are most commonly assessed in generic approaches. The advantage to the generic approach is that it can be applied across the entire population enrolled in a health plan or seeing a particular physician. The difficulty with this approach is that research has yielded considerably less understanding of the link between what is done in the medical care system and the resulting generic outcomes of the population. There is reason to believe that other factors (education, socioeconomic status) enter into determining these outcomes. Further, the need to control for variations in severity and case mix of a population when making comparisons of generic outcomes is extremely important, and no reliable methods for doing so currently exist.

Patient satisfaction may be the most commonly evaluated generic outcome at the health plan level. Patient satisfaction measures consumers' attitudes about the quality and acceptability of care. Until recently, plans used a variety of surveys to assess satisfaction. These surveys included overall satisfaction, interpersonal communication and information giving, timeliness, intention to recommend or use the plan again, technical quality, time spent with providers, access and availability, outcomes, choice and continuity, financial aspects and billing, and physical environment.[64] Patient satisfaction is an important predictor of certain patient behaviors such as the likelihood of changing health plans[65] or physicians,[66] and compliance with recommended medical therapy.[67]

Sentinel Approach, or Adverse Events. The sentinel approach identifies some event, usually an adverse outcome, that is likely to be associated with poor quality of care and tracks the frequency with which the event occurs. Some examples of adverse outcomes are mortality, early readmission to a hospital, complications of a surgical procedure (transfusion, reoperation), nosocomial infections in the hospital, suicide, adverse drug reaction (especially drug-drug interactions), and very-low-birthweight births. Sentinel events can be useful for identifying potential problems, but it is almost always necessary to conduct further assessments to conclude whether an adverse event was "preventable" or not. The frequency with which adverse events occur affects their practicality for quality assessment. Events that occur rarely are less useful for quality monitoring because it is more difficult to determine whether differences are statistically significant.

What Do We Know About Outcomes?

As with the literature on process quality, it is beyond the scope of this chapter to summarize everything that is known about the outcomes of care. Rather, we offer examples of some of the important findings from the published literature. It should be noted that the three categories of outcomes studies—condition-specific, generic, and adverse events—are not mutually exclusive. For example, mortality is an outcome measure that can be applied in any of these contexts; however, each approach provides its own type of insight into variations in the quality of care.

Condition-Specific Outcomes. There is evidence that appropriate monitoring of outcomes can contribute to improvement in the quality and outcomes of care. Perhaps one of the leading examples of this comes from New York state's Cardiac Surgery Reporting System, administered by the New York State Department of Health. Since 1989, hospitals have voluntarily reported data to this system on all open heart surgeries. A clinical database is used to identify preoperative risk factors for CABG surgery; these factors are used to estimate risk-adjusted mortality rates (that is, predicted mortality rates) for each hospital and surgeon performing CABG in the state. Performance is evaluated by comparing the predicted rate to the actual mortality rate, and the results are made public. Since the system was implemented in 1989, the risk-adjusted mortality rate has declined from 4.17 percent to 2.45 percent—a 41 percent decrease.[68] The policy lesson is encouraging; making severity-adjusted outcomes data available to the public can lead to improved health outcomes.

When evaluating outcomes associated with a particular health plan or provider, it may be useful to examine the overall context in which changes are occurring. For example, mortality due to heart disease has been falling for the past two decades, so improvement in outcomes for heart disease might be part of a general national trend. A recent study examining changes in outcomes of acute myocardial infarction (AMI) among the elderly between 1987 and 1990 found that, in the month following the AMI, mortality decreased from 26 percent to 23 percent; mortality declined from 40 percent to 36 percent in the year following the AMI.[69] The authors indicate that only a portion of the improvement in outcomes can be attributed to changes in treatment, such as the use of thrombolytic therapy.

Condition-specific outcomes may be used to compare the results of treatment approaches or for groups of patients. One study examined the outcomes for Medicare patients undergoing lung resection for lung cancer. The authors found that perioperative mortality was 7.4 percent, survival one year postoperative was 69 percent, and two-year survival was 54 percent.[70] Survival following surgery was lower for men, older persons, and those who had pneumonectomy rather than a lesser procedure. A study examining clinical outcomes (mortality, recurrent infarctions) for men and women treated with thrombolytic therapy after an AMI found that women had worse outcomes than men; although some of the difference is attributable to baseline clinical status (women were older and had a higher prevalence of co-morbid conditions), further investigation of sex-related differences in outcome is recommended.[71]

Although mortality is one of the most common outcome measures used, it is a rather blunt instrument for examining variations in quality. Another approach is to examine variations in clinical status variables (glycemic control for diabetics, blood pressure control for hypertensives). A study of diabetes outcomes in the UK, for example, found that gender (male), years since diagnosis, and characteristics of the practice setting (larger, better equipped, dietician on team, physician specialized in diabetes treatment) were significantly related to better glycemic control.[72] Factors such as age, social class, lifestyle, attitude, satisfaction, and knowledge were not correlated with glycemic control.

Condition-specific examinations of quality can also be conducted using symptoms rather than diagnoses. A study comparing access and outcomes of care for Medicare beneficiaries enrolled in HMOs versus fee-for-service who reported having either joint pain or chest pain found that although there were differences in access to care for these patient groups (HMO enrollees with joint pain had better access to care than fee-for-service enrollees, but HMO enrollees with chest pain had somewhat less access; HMO enrollees with either symptom were less likely to see a specialists, receive follow-up care, or have their progress monitored), there were no differences in elimination of symptoms; enrollees with joint pain reported less improvement in symptoms.[73]

Condition-specific measures may also be used for evaluating the quality of comprehensive programs such as community-oriented primary care. A study examining the effectiveness of this approach for control of hypertension found that hypertensive adults treated in the community-oriented primary care model were more likely to have their hypertension under control.[74] Although improved control was greatest for men and blacks, every other age and racial group demonstrated improved outcomes in the model program as compared to other sources of care.

Generic Outcomes. A summary article examining the efficiency and effectiveness of generic occurrence screening for quality assessment concluded that this method is relatively inefficient because of high error rates; sensitivity was estimated to be 70–80 percent, but specificity ranged from 22 to 73 percent.[75] Effectiveness of the method was limited by lack of interrater reliability among peer reviewers. The authors propose that condition-specific outcome measures be used rather than generic approaches.

Functional outcomes may be used to assess the effect of a policy change. The Medicaid Demonstration Project in Hennepin County, Minnesota, randomly assigned clients with chronic mental illnesses to prepaid plans or to usual (fee-for-service) care. Some of the generic outcome measures used to evaluate the effects of prepaid care on these clients included general health status, physical functioning, social functioning, and community functioning. The authors found no consistent evidence that enrolling chronically mentally ill clients in prepaid care resulted in worse outcomes in the short run.[76]

Patient satisfaction has been used to compare systems of care, particularly HMO and indemnity insurance, but the conclusions from this work are mixed. A review of the literature on HMO performance indicates that HMO enrollees tend to be less satisfied with perceived quality of care and patient-physician interactions but more satisfied with many other aspects of their care, including financial aspects, than those in indemnity plans.[77] Results from the Medical Outcomes Study indicate that financial access was rated highest in prepaid systems. Organizational access, continuity, and accountability were rated highest in indemnity systems. Coordination and comprehensiveness were rated lowest in HMOs.[78] Another review of patient satisfaction with outpatient care indicated that, compared to patients in traditional indemnity insurance, those in HMOs were less satisfied with care overall, access to care, interpersonal aspects of care, continuity, and availability of appointments; they were more satisfied with waiting time in the physician's office and similarly satisfied with technical aspects of care.[79]

Sentinel or Adverse Events. A study examining variations among hospitals in the frequency of adverse events (defined as injuries due to medical treatment) found that primary teaching hospitals had a significantly higher rate of adverse events (4.1 percent versus 3.2 percent on average) and rural hospitals had a significantly lower rate (1 percent).[80] The proportion of adverse events that was due to negligence was lower among primary teaching (10.7 percent) and for-profit (9.5 percent) hospitals and was significantly higher among hospitals serving predominantly minority populations.

An examination of the potential for using readmission rates as an indicator of quality in the UK found that the readmission rate peaked early in the month following discharge and was considerably lower among surgical specialties as compared with medical specialties (general surgery was 4.1 percent compared with 15.1 percent for geriatric medicine).[81] Readmission patterns did vary with the age and sex of the patient, indicating that standardization for these factors is important.

Complications of care are often used as a generic indicator of adverse outcomes. One study, for instance, examined complications in trauma care to evaluate whether the adverse outcomes were the result of provider process error or a patient disease-related event. Complications were a common outcome for trauma cases, with 83 percent of patients experiencing at least one complication; however, only 27 percent of the complications were due to provider-related factors, and of those only 23 percent (or 6 percent of all complications) were judged to be a quality problem.[82] Complications of revascularization procedures (death, renal impairment, myocardial infarction) were also used to assess the quality of care delivered to Medicare patients in sixteen hospitals. The study found substantial variation in complications among the hospitals studied; risk-adjustment changed the quality ranking of hospitals performing CABG surgery but did not significantly change the quality ranking of hospitals performing angioplasty.[83] The authors conclude that if sample sizes are small, adverse outcome measures may be more sensitive than mortality alone for detecting differences in quality.

Adverse events may be used to evaluate the consequences of a policy change. When Massachusetts made health coverage available to uninsured, low-income pregnant women, there was interest in whether this would contribute to a statewide reduction in low-birthweight births. During the time period when benefits were expanded for low-income women, however, access to prenatal care declined statewide and the overall effect was that the improved access for low-income women did not result in a decrease in low-birthweight births in the state. The policy lesson here—and one that is also important for evaluation research—is that external events can sometimes overwhelm an otherwise successful experiment.[84]

A study in the twelve Veterans Administration hospitals found that lower quality of care significantly increased the risk for early hospital readmission ($p < 0.05$) for patients with diabetes, chronic obstructive lung disease, or heart failure.[85] Patients with diabetes and heart failure were at increased risk of readmission because of a failure to adhere to discharge readiness criteria. Patients with chronic obstructive lung disease were at increased risk for readmission because of poor quality workup at admission.

Conclusion

Over the next decade, as policy makers continue to struggle with mechanisms for controlling rising health care costs and the structure of the delivery system continues to change, the need to measure, monitor, and report on the quality of care will only become more important. We have demonstrated in this chapter that a variety of methods exist for systematically evaluating the quality of care.

Quality is a multidimensional topic, and efforts to understand how quality is changing with the dynamics of organization and financing in the health delivery system must include both technical and interpersonal excellence in the process of care, as well as the full range of outcomes of care—clinical, functional, satisfaction, and life-expectancy. Although the field of quality assessment stands ready to make a substantial contribution to giving purchasers of health care the information necessary to make informed choices among health plans, physicians, and hospitals, considerable methodological and logistical work remains to be done to bring quality monitoring into the mainstream of such decision making. Better methods must be developed for adjusting the results of quality assessment for differences in the severity and other characteristics of populations whose care is being evaluated. Improved techniques must be designed to effectively disseminate information on quality to various audiences.

As systems are developed to monitor and publicly report on the quality of care delivered in health plans and by different providers, more efficient methods for obtaining the data necessary to conduct these activities must be designed. An adequate quality monitoring system requires data from administrative, clinical, and consumer sources; a single data source will never be adequate to inform the multidimensional quality concerns that have been discussed in this chapter. Administrative data have been used extensively for quality assessment because of easy availability; clinically detailed assessments are not possible with administrative data. Given the importance of chronic disease for costs and quality of life, detailed clinical and consumer data must also be made available routinely for quality monitoring.

The American health care system continues to face the challenge of balancing its three competing goals: containing health care costs, improving access to care, and enhancing the quality of care. As health reform efforts continue in the private sector, at the state level, and perhaps even at the federal level, quality cannot be left behind. The incentives in current cost-containment mechanisms pose a direct challenge to quality; without an adequate system for assessing the value of the health care product, quality of care—the dimension in which this country takes greatest pride—may be severely undermined.

Notes

1. Lohr, K. N. (ed.). *Medicare: A Strategy for Quality Assurance, Vol. I.* Washington, D.C.: National Academy Press, 1990, p. 21.
2. Siu, A. L., and others. *Choosing Quality-of-Care Measures Based on the Expected Impact of Improved Quality of Care for the Major Causes of Mortality and Morbidity.* RAND publication no. JR-03. Santa Monica, Calif.: RAND, 1992.

3. Leape, L. L., and others. *Coronary Artery Bypass Graft: A Literature Review and Ratings of Appropriateness and Necessity.* RAND publication no. JRA-02. Santa Monica, Calif.: RAND, 1991; Bernstein, S. J., and others. *Coronary Angiography: A Literature Review and Ratings of Appropriateness and Necessity.* RAND publication no. JRA-03. Santa Monica, Calif.: RAND, 1992; Hilborne, L. H., and others. *Percutaneous Transluminal Coronary Angioplasty: A Literature Review and Ratings of Appropriateness and Necessity.* RAND publication no. JRA-01. Santa Monica, Calif.: RAND, 1991; Bernstein, S. J., and others. *Hysterectomy: A Literature Review and Ratings of Appropriateness.* RAND publication no. JR-04. Santa Monica, Calif.: RAND, 1992; Murata, P. J., McGlynn, E. A., Siu, A. L., and Brook, R. H. *Prenatal Care: A Literature Review and Quality Assessment Criteria.* RAND publication no. JR-05. Santa Monica, Calif.: RAND, 1992.

4. Siu and others (1992).

5. Donabedian, A. *Explorations in Quality Assessment and Monitoring.* Vol. I: *The Definition of Quality and Approaches to its Assessment.* Ann Arbor, Mich.: Health Administration Press, 1980.

6. Welch, W. P., Verrilli, D., Katz, S. J., and Latimer, E. "A Detailed Comparison of Physician Services for the Elderly in the United States and Canada." *Journal of the American Medical Association,* 1996, *275,* 1410–1416; Friedman, B., and Elixhauser, A. "The Changing Distribution of a Major Surgical Procedure Across Hospitals: Were Supply Shifts and Disequilibrium Important?" *Health Economics,* 1995, *4,* 301–314.

7. American Medical Association. *Physician Characteristics and Distribution in the U.S. 2000–2001 Edition.* Chicago: American Medical Association, 2000.

8. Kahn, K. L., and others. "Health Care for Black and Poor Hospitalized Medicare Patients." *Journal of the American Medical Association,* 1993, *271,* 1169–1174.

9. Keeler, E. B., and others. "Hospital Characteristics and Quality of Care." *Journal of the American Medical Association,* 1992, *268,* 1709–1714.

10. Greenfield, S., and others. "Variations in Resource Utilization Among Medical Specialties and Systems of Care: Results from the Medical Outcomes Study." *Journal of the American Medical Association,* 1992, 267, 1624–1630.

11. Wennberg, J. E., Freeman, J. L., Shelton, R. M., and Bubolz, T. A. "Hospital Use and Mortality Among Medicare Beneficiaries in Boston and New Haven." *New England Journal of Medicine,* 1989, *321,* 1168–1173.

12. Cleary, P. D., and others. "Variations in Length of Stay and Outcomes for Six Medical and Surgical Conditions in Massachusetts and California." *Journal of the American Medical Association,* 1991, *266,* 73–79.

13. Katz, S. J., and Hofer, T. P. "Socioeconomic Disparities in Preventive Care Persist Despite Universal Coverage: Breast and Cervical Cancer Screening in Ontario and the United States." *Journal of the American Medical Association,* 1994, *272,* 530–534.

14. Aday, L. A., and others. "Health Insurance and Utilization of Medical Care for Children with Special Health Care Needs." *Medical Care,* 1993, *31,* 1013–1026.

15. Newhouse, J. P., and Insurance Experiment Group. *Free for All? Lessons Learned from the RAND Health Insurance Experiment.* Cambridge, Mass.: Harvard University Press, 1993.

16. Brook, R. H., and others. "Does Free Care Improve Adults' Health? Results from a Randomized Controlled Trial." *New England Journal of Medicine,* 1983, *309,* 1426–1434.

17. Luft, H. S., Hunt, S. S., and Maerki, S. C. "The Volume-Outcome Relationship: Practice-Makes-Perfect or Selective-Referral Patterns?" *Health Services Research,* June 1987, *22,* 157–182.

18. Hannan, E. L., and others. "The Decline in Coronary Artery Bypass Graft Surgery Mortality in New York State: The Role of Surgeon Volume." *Journal of the American Medical Association,* 1995, *273,* 209–213.

19. Brook, R. H. "The RAND/UCLA Appropriateness Method." In K. A. McCormick, S. R. Moore, and R. A. Siegel (eds.), Clinical Practice Guideline Development: Methodology Perspectives. AHCPR publication no. 95-0009. Rockville, Md.: Agency for Health Care Policy and Research, Public Health Service, U.S. Department of Health and Human Services, Nov. 1994; Brook, R. H., and others. "A Method for the Detailed Assessment of the Appropriateness of Medical Technologies." *International Journal of Technology Assessment,* 1986, *2,* 53–63.

20. Shekelle, P. G., and others. "The Reproducibility of a Method to Identify the Overuse and Underuse of Medical Procedures." *New England Journal of Medicine,* 1998, *338,* 1888–1895.

21. Kravitz, R. L., and others. "Validity of Criteria Used for Detecting Underuse of Coronary Revascularization." *Journal of the American Medical Association,* 1995, *274,* 632–638.

22. Chassin, M. R., Kosecoff, J., and Park, R. E. "Does Inappropriate Use Explain Geographic Variations in the Use of Health Care Services? A Study of Three Procedures." *Journal of the American Medical Association,* 1987, *258,* 2533–2537; Leape, L. L., and others. Coronary Angiography: Ratings of Appropriateness and Necessity by a Canadian Panel. Publication no. MR-129-CWF/PCT. Santa Monica, Calif.: RAND, 1993.

23. Bernstein and others (1992).

24. Leape, L. L., and others. "The Appropriateness of Use of Coronary Artery Bypass Graft Surgery in New York State." *Journal of the American Medical Association,* 1993, *269,* 753–760; Bernstein, S. J., and others. "The Appropriateness of Hysterectomy: A Comparison of Care in Seven Health Plans." *Journal of the American Medical Association,* 1993, *269,* 2398–2402.

25. The definition appears in the Foreword to each of the practice guidelines. See, for example, Urinary Incontinence Guideline Panel. Urinary Incontinence in Adults: Clinical Practice Guideline. AHCPR publication no. 92-0038. Rockville, Md.: Agency for Health Care Policy and Research, Public Health Service, U.S. Department of Health and Human Services, Mar. 1992, p. iii.

26. Guidelines had been developed for a number of conditions, including acute pain management for operative or medical procedures and trauma; urinary incontinence in adults; prediction, prevention, and treatment of pressure ulcers in adults; management of functional impairment caused by cataracts in adults; detection, diagnosis, and treatment of major depression in primary care; screening, diagnosis, management, and counseling regarding sickle cell disease in newborns and infants; evaluation and management of early HIV infection; diagnosis and treatment of benign prostatic hyperplasia; management of cancer pain; diagnosis and management of unstable angina; evaluation and care of patients with left-ventricular systolic dysfunction; otitis media with effusion in young children, and acute low back problems in adults.

27. McCormick, K. A., Moore, S. R., and Siegel, R. A. (eds.). Clinical Practice Guideline Development: Methodology Perspectives. AHCPR publication no. 95-0009. Rockville, Md.: Agency for Health Care Policy and Research, Public Health Service, U.S. Department of Health and Human Services, Nov. 1994.

28. Lasker, R. D., Shapiro, D. W., and Tucker, A. M. "Realizing the Potential of Practice Pattern Profiling." *Inquiry,* 1992, *29,* 287–297.

29. Lasker, Shapiro, and Tucker (1992).

30. Welch, H. G., Miller, M. E., and Welch, W. P. "Physician Profiling: An Analysis of Inpatient Practice Patterns in Florida and Oregon." *New England Journal of Medicine,* 1994, *330,* 607–612; Salem-Schatz, S., Moore, G., Rucker, M., and Pearson, S. D. "The Case for Case-Mix Adjustment in Practice Profiling: When Good Apples Look Bad." *Journal of the*

American Medical Association, 1994, *272,* 871–874; McNeil, B. J., Pedersen, S. H., and Gatsonis,
C. "Current Issues in Profiling Quality of Care." *Inquiry,* 1992, *29,* 298–307; Lasker, Shapiro,
and Tucker (1992).

31. Salem-Schatz, Moore, Rucker, and Pearson (1994).
32. Kravitz, R. L., and others. "Differences in the Mix of Patients Among Medical Special-
    ties and Systems of Care: Results from the Medical Outcomes Study." *Journal of the Ameri-
    can Medical Association,* 1992, *267,* 1617–1623.
33. McNeil, Pedersen, and Gatsonis (1992); Welch, Miller, and Welch (1994).
34. Chassin, M. R., Kosecoff, J., Solomon, D. H., and Brook, R. H. "How Coronary Angiog-
    raphy is Used: Clinical Determinants of Appropriateness." *Journal of the American Medical
    Association,* 1987, *258,* 2543–2547; Bernstein, S. J., and others. "The Appropriateness of
    Use of Coronary Angiography in New York State." *Journal of the American Medical Associa-
    tion,* 1993, *269,* 766–769; Hilborne, L. H., and others. "The Appropriateness of Use of
    Percutaneous Transluminal Coronary Angioplasty in New York State." *Journal of the American
    Medical Association,* 1993, *269,* 761–765; Leape and others (1993); Winslow, C. M., and
    others. "The Appropriateness of Performing Coronary Artery Bypass Surgery." *Journal
    of the American Medical Association,* 1988, *260,* 505–509; Bernstein and others (1993);
    Winslow, C. M., and others. "The Appropriateness of Carotid Endarterectomy." *New
    England Journal of Medicine,* 1988, *318,* 721–727; Chassin, Kosecoff, and Park (1987);
    Tobacman, J. K., and others. "Assessment of Appropriateness of Cataract Surgery at
    Ten Academic Medical Centers in 1990." *Ophthalmology,* 1996, *103,* 207–215; Kleinman,
    L. C., Kosecoff, J., Dubois, R. W., and Brook, R. H. "The Medical Appropriateness of
    Tympanostomy Tubes Proposed for Children Younger Than 16 Years in the United States."
    Journal of the American Medical Association, 1994, *271,* 1250–1255.
35. Kravitz and others (1995).
36. Chassin, Kosecoff, and Park (1987).
37. Siu, A. L., Leibowitz, A., and Brook, R. H. "Use of the Hospital in a Randomized Trial of
    Prepaid Care." *Journal of the American Medical Association,* 1988, *259,* 1343–1346.
38. McGlynn, E. A., and others. "Comparison of the Appropriateness of Coronary Angiog-
    raphy and Coronary Artery Bypass Graft Surgery Between Canada and New York State."
    Journal of the American Medical Association, 1994, *272,* 934–940.
39. Gray, D., and others. "Clinical Practice: Audit of Coronary Angiography and Bypass
    Surgery." *Lancet,* 1990, *335,* 1317–1320.
40. Pilpel, D., and others. "Regional Differences in Appropriateness of Cholecystectomy in a
    Prepaid Health Insurance System." *Public Health Reviews,* 1992–1993, *20,* 61–74.
41. Siu, A. L., and others. "Inappropriate Use of Hospitals in a Randomized Trial of Health
    Insurance Plans." *New England Journal of Medicine,* 1986, *315,* 1259–1266.
42. Soumerai, S. M., Avorn, J., Ross-Degnan, D., and Gortmaker, S. "Payment Restrictions for
    Prescription Drugs Under Medicaid: Effects on Therapy, Cost, and Equity." *New England
    Journal of Medicine,* 1987, *317,* 550–556.
43. Anderson, G. M., and others. "Use of Coronary Artery Bypass Surgery in the United States
    and Canada." *Journal of the American Medical Association,* 1993, *269,* 1661–1666.
44. Grimshaw, J. M., and Russell, I. T. "Effect of Clinical Guidelines on Medical Practice: A Sys-
    tematic Review of Rigorous Evaluations." *Lancet,* 1993, *342,* 1317–1322.
45. Schuster, M. A., McGlynn, E. A., and Brook, R. H. "How Good Is the Quality of Health
    Care in the United States?" *Milbank Quarterly,* 1998, *76,* 517–563.
46. Murata, P. J., and others. "Quality Measures for Prenatal Care: A Comparison of Care in
    Six Health Care Plans." *Archives of Family Medicine,* 1994, *3,* 41–49.

47. National Committee for Quality Assurance. *The State of Managed Care Quality.* Washington, D.C.: NCQA, 1999.

48. Doorey, A. J., Michelson, E. L., and Topol, E. J. "Thrombolytic Therapy of Acute Myocardial Infarction: Keeping the Unfulfilled Promises." *Journal of the American Medical Association,* 1992, *268,* 3108–3114.

49. Pashos, C. L., and others. "Trends in the Use of Drug Therapies in Patients with Acute Myocardial Infarction: 1988 to 1992." *Journal of the American College of Cardiology,* 1994, *23,* 1023–1030.

50. Wells, K. B., Katon, W., Rogers, W. H., and Camp, P. "Use of Minor Tranquilizers and Antidepressant Medications by Depressed Outpatients: Results from the Medical Outcomes Study." *American Journal of Psychiatry,* 1994, *151,* 694–700; Katon, W., and others. "Adequacy and Duration of Antidepressant Treatment in Primary Care." *Medical Care,* 1992, *30,* 67–76.

51. Olfson, M., and Klerman, G. L. "Trends in the Prescription of Psychotropic Medications: The Role of Physician Specialty." *Medical Care,* 1993, *31,* 559–564; Wells, Katon, Rogers, and Camp (1994).

52. Depression Guideline Panel. *Depression in Primary Care.* Vol. 2: *Treatment of Major Depression.* Clinical Practice Guideline no. 5, AHCPR publication no. 93-0551. Rockville, Md.: Agency for Health Care Policy and Research, Public Health Service, U.S. Department of Health and Human Services, 1993.

53. Wells, Katon, Rogers, and Camp (1994).

54. Graves, E. J. "Detailed Diagnoses and Procedures, National Hospital Discharge Survey, 1990." National Center for Health Statistics, DHHS publication no. (PHS) 92-1774. *Vital Health Statistics,* 1992, vol. 13.

55. Wennberg, Freeman, Shelton, and Bubolz (1989).

56. Welch, Miller, and Welch (1994).

57. Davies, A. R., and Ware, J. E., Jr. "Involving Consumers in Quality of Care Assessment." *Health Affairs,* Spring 1988, *7,* 33–48.

58. Gerbert, B., and Hargreaves, W. A. "Measuring Physician Behavior." *Medical Care,* 1986, *24,* 838–847.

59. Wilson, A., and McDonald, P. "Comparison of Patient Questionnaire, Medical Record, and Audio Tape in Assessment of Health Promotion in General Practice Consultations." *British Medical Journal,* 1994, *309,* 1483–1485.

60. Kogan, M. D., and others. "Comparing Mothers' Reports on the Content of Prenatal Care Received with Recommended National Guidelines for Care." *Public Health Reports,* 1994, *109,* 637–646.

61. Berwick, D. M., and Wald, D. L. "Hospital Leaders' Opinions of the HCFA Mortality Data." *Journal of the American Medical Association,* 1990, *263,* 247–249.

62. Fleming, S. T., Hicks, L. L., and Bailey, R. C. "Interpreting the Health Care Financing Administration's Mortality Statistics." *Medical Care,* 1995, *33,* 186–201.

63. Iezzoni, L. I., and others. "Using Administrative Data to Screen Hospitals for High Complication Rates." *Inquiry,* 1994, *31,* 40–55.

64. Gold, M., and Woolridge, J. "Plan-Based Surveys of Satisfaction with Access and Quality of Care: Review and Critique." Paper delivered at Consumer Survey Information in a Reformed Health Care System conference, cosponsored by Agency for Health Care Policy and Research and Robert Wood Johnson Foundation, Washington, D.C., Sept. 1994.

65. Davies and Ware (1988).

66. Marquis, M. S., Davies, A. R., and Ware, J. E., Jr. "Patient Satisfaction and Change in Medical Care Provider: A Longitudinal Study." *Medical Care,* 1983, *21,* 821–829.

67. Ware, J. E., Jr., Snyder, M. K., Wright, W. R., and Davies, A. R. "Defining and Measuring Patient Satisfaction with Medical Care." *Evaluation and Program Planning*, 1983, *6*, 247–263; Sherbourne, C. D., and others. "Antecedents of Adherence to Medical Recommendations: Results from the Medical Outcomes Study." *Journal of Behavioral Medicine*, 1992, *15*, 447–468.

68. Hannan, E. L., and others. "Improving the Outcomes of Coronary Artery Bypass Surgery in New York State." *Journal of the American Medical Association*, 1994, *271*, 761–766.

69. Pashos, C. L., Newhouse, J. P., and McNeil, B. J. "Temporal Changes in the Care and Outcomes of Elderly Patients with Acute Myocardial Infarction, 1987 through 1990." *Journal of the American Medical Association*, 1993, *270*, 1832–1836.

70. Whittle, J., Steinberg, E. P., Anderson, G. F., and Herbert, R. "Use of Medicare Claims Data to Evaluate Outcomes in Elderly Patients Undergoing Lung Resection for Lung Cancer." *Chest*, 1991, 100, 729–734.

71. Becker, R. C., and others. "Comparison of Clinical Outcomes for Women and Men After Acute Myocardial Infarction." *Annals of Internal Medicine*, 1994, *120*, 638–645.

72. Pringle, M., and others. "Influences on Control in Diabetes Mellitus: Patient, Doctor, Practice, or Delivery of Care?" *British Medical Journal*, 1993, *306*, 630–634.

73. Clement, D. G., Retchin, S. M., Brown, R. S., and Stegall, M. H. "Access and Outcomes of Elderly Patients Enrolled in Managed Care." *Journal of the American Medical Association*, 1994, *271*, 1487–1492.

74. O'Connor, P. J., Wagner, E. H., and Strogatz, D. S. "Hypertension Control in a Rural Community: An Assessment of Community-Oriented Primary Care." *Journal of Family Practice*, 1990, *30*, 420–424.

75. Sanzaro, P. J., and Mills, D. H. "A Critique of the Use of Generic Screening in Quality Assessment." *Journal of the American Medical Association*, 1991, *265*, 1977–1981.

76. Lurie, N., and others. "Does Capitation Affect the Health of the Chronically Mentally Ill? Results from a Randomized Trial." *Journal of the American Medical Association*, 1992, *267*, 3300–3304.

77. Miller, R. H., and Luft, H. S. "Managed Care Plan Performance Since 1980: A Literature Analysis." *Journal of the American Medical Association*, 1994, *271*, 1512–1519.

78. Safran, D. G., Tarlov, A. R., and Rogers, W. H. "Primary Care Performance in Fee-for-Service and Prepaid Health Care Systems: Results from the Medical Outcomes Study." *Journal of the American Medical Association*, 1994, *271*, 1579–1586.

79. Barr, D. A. "The Effects of Organizational Structure on Primary Care Outcomes Under Managed Care." *Annals of Internal Medicine*, 1995, *122*, 353–359.

80. Brennan, T. A., and others. "Hospital Characteristics Associated with Adverse Events and Substandard Care." *Journal of the American Medical Association*, 1991, *265*, 3265–3269.

81. Chambers, M., and Clarke, A. "Measuring Readmission Rates," *British Medical Journal*, 1990, *301*, 1134–1136.

82. Hoyt, D. B., and others. "Analysis of Recurrent Process Errors Leading to Provider-Related Complications on an Organized Trauma Service: Directions for Care Improvement." *Journal of Trauma*, 1994, *36*, 377–384.

83. Hartz, A. J., and others. "Assessing Providers of Coronary Revascularization: A Method for Peer Review Organizations." *American Journal of Public Health*, 1992, *82*, 1631–1640.

84. Haas, J. S., Udvarhelyi, I. S., Morris, C. N., and Epstein, A. M. "The Effect of Providing Health Coverage to Poor Uninsured Pregnant Women in Massachusetts." *Journal of the American Medical Association*, 1993, *269*, 87–91.

85. Ashton, C. M., and others. "The Association Between the Quality of Inpatient Care and Early Readmission." *Annals of Internal Medicine*, 1995, *122*, 415–421.

CHAPTER EIGHT

PUBLIC RELEASE OF INFORMATION ON QUALITY

Elizabeth A. McGlynn and John L. Adams

Quality-of-care research consistently finds that a key determinant of outcomes is where and from whom an individual receives medical care. For example, Kahn and colleagues found that the mortality rate for persons admitted with a heart attack was 25 percent higher in hospitals in the lowest quartile of process quality compared to the highest quartile.[1] Performance is not always consistent, however, across patients, providers, conditions, or procedures. Health plans may do well with an employed population and less well with a low-income Medicaid population. Hospitals may provide excellent cardiac care while offering below-average labor and delivery care.

Changes in the organization and financing of care have also increased concerns about variation in quality. In the unrestricted-choice model characterized by fee-for-service, individual providers were accountable for ensuring the delivery of high-quality health care. Physicians were trusted to be effective advocates for their patients' needs. However, as third parties began to use financial incentives to control costs and restrict choices, the perception (if not the reality) was that physicians could no longer act solely in the patient's interest.

We have moved from assuming that adequate mechanisms of accountability existed in the health system to demanding proof that various levels within the health system are accountable for the decisions that are made regarding resource allocation. Such proof is being demanded by those who purchase and those who seek health care services. Through their insurance mechanisms, purchasers increasingly ask for evidence that the services they are buying are effective and necessary. Consumers are increasingly concerned about being unable to get the care they need. Both groups have cause for concern because each type of quality problem has been found in the U.S. health care system (and in other countries).[2]

Routine reports to the public on the quality of health care are one response to concerns about accountability. Public release of information on quality is intended to have two main effects: to facilitate informed choice and to stimulate quality improvement. The purpose of this chapter is to (1) describe the type of information that is currently being publicly released, (2) discuss some of the methodological issues that arise in producing information for public release, and (3) summarize what is known about the use of information on quality for consumer choice and quality improvement.

Public Information on Quality

Remarkably little information on quality is consistently available throughout the United States across all providers in the health system. Some information is available in some areas about the quality of hospitals, health plans, medical groups, and individual physicians. Table 8.1 lists the types of measures available at each level in the health system and gives some examples of organizations that have released data. This is not an exhaustive list, but one intended to demonstrate some of the options that have been tried.

Hospitals

Public information on hospital quality focuses primarily on mortality rate and accreditation status. The Health Care Financing Administration (HCFA) released information in 1986 on the mortality rate in all hospitals in the United States providing care for Medicare beneficiaries. The report was widely criticized because it did not adequately adjust for differences in the risk profile of patients being cared for in each institution.[3] In 1987, HCFA released a report that included risk-adjusted mortality rates, but concerns about the adequacy of the risk-adjustment methodology continued.

Hospital mortality rates have also been released for coronary artery bypass graft (CABG) surgery. Perhaps the leading example of this is New York state's Cardiac Reporting System, which releases risk-adjusted, in-hospital mortality rates for CABG surgery on all hospitals in New York. The Pennsylvania Health Care Cost Containment Council has also released public information on risk-adjusted,

TABLE 8.1.   ILLUSTRATION OF PUBLIC INFORMATION RELEASED BY ENTITY.

Organizational Entity	Type of Information	Examples
Hospital	Overall mortality	Health Care Financing Administration (HCFA)
	Mortality by specific procedure	New York, Pennsylvania, Pacific Business Group on Health (PBGH)
	Mortality by specific disease	California Hospital Outcomes Project, Cleveland Quality Choice
	Accreditation	Joint Commission on the Accreditation of Healthcare Organizations (JCAHO)
	Rankings by specialty area	*U.S. News & World Report*
Health plan	Process of care	NCQA (HEDIS)
	Patient experience with care	NCQA (CAHPS)
	Accreditation	NCQA
	Categorical rankings	Combined Autos/UAW Reporting System (CARS), *U.S. News & World Report*
Medical group	Process of care	PBGH
	Patient experience with care	PBGH
Physician	Mortality rate for coronary artery bypass graft surgery	New York, Pennsylvania

in-hospital mortality rates for the same surgery. An initiative is currently under way in California to release data on this procedure from hospitals that have volunteered to make data available (as compared to New York and Pennsylvania, where reporting was required). The Pacific Business Group on Health has also released data on risk-adjusted mortality rates following various transplant procedures for hospitals in California.

Hospital mortality rates have been released for specific conditions. The California Hospital Outcomes Project released information on risk-adjusted inpatient mortality for persons admitted with an acute myocardial infarction and on maternal outcomes.[4] Cleveland Quality Choice released mortality data on selected conditions, including acute myocardial infarction, congestive heart failure, obstructive airway disease, gastrointestinal hemorrhage, pneumonia, and stroke.[5]

Accreditation status represents another type of information publicly available on hospital quality. The Joint Commission on the Accreditation of Healthcare Organizations (JCAHO) is responsible for conducting hospital accreditation in the United States. Hospitals that wish to serve Medicare beneficiaries must obtain accreditation, which means that most hospitals in the United States seek it. Although there are a variety of levels of accreditation, two currently dominate: accreditation with commendation (18 percent) and accreditation with recommendations for improvement (81 percent).

In the popular press, perhaps the most familiar report card on hospitals is *U.S. News & World Report*'s annual issue on "America's Best Hospitals." The magazine examines three major aspects of performance in developing its rankings: reputation, mortality rate, and annual surveys by the American Hospital Association. Rankings are calculated for all hospitals in each of sixteen specialty areas, and the top forty-two performers in each specialty are published in the magazine. Reputation scores are based on a survey of twenty-four hundred board-certified physicians who are asked to rank the top five hospitals in the nation in their specialty (results are averaged for the most recent three years). Mortality scores are based on the ratio of observed to expected risk-adjusted mortality rates from Medicare data. The final category is composed of a variety of structural elements: whether the hospital is a member of the Council of Teaching Hospitals, availability of high-technology services, discharges, surgical volume, nurse-to-bed ratio, availability of a trauma center, discharge planning services, service mix, availability of geriatric services, and availability of gynecology services. Each of the three major components has an equal weight in determining the final ranking.

Health Plans

The National Committee for Quality Assurance (NCQA) is responsible for the widespread availability of information on the performance of managed care plans. NCQA annually produces information on selected processes of care, patient experiences with care, and accreditation. Most report cards on managed care plan performance are based primarily, or solely, on the information made public by NCQA; health plans voluntarily submit the data on which these reports are based.

Information on selected processes of care is developed by plans using standardized specifications contained in a reporting system known as the Health Plan Employer Data and Information Set (HEDIS). For HEDIS 2000, plans were asked to report on their performance in calendar year 1999 on nineteen measures of the effectiveness of care. These are shown in Table 8.2. In 1999, 247 organizations

TABLE 8.2. LISTING OF THE HEDIS 2000 EFFECTIVENESS
OF CARE MEASURES.

Area	Measure Description	Population
Preventive care	Proportion of two-year-olds who are up to date on their immunizations	Children who turn two during the reporting year
	Proportion of adolescents who are up to date on their immunizations	Children who turn thirteen during the reporting year
	Proportion of women screened for cervical cancer	Women who are twenty-one to sixty-four during reporting year
	Proportion of women screened for breast cancer	Women who are fifty-two to sixty-nine during reporting year
	Proportion of women whose first prenatal care visit was in the first trimester	Women who delivered a live infant during the reporting year
	Proportion of women who received a checkup after delivery	Women who delivered a live infant during the reporting year
	Proportion of smokers receiving advice from a physician to quit smoking	Persons who were smoking or who had recently quit during the reporting year
Diabetes care	Proportion of diabetics who had a glycosylated hemoglobin test in the past year	Persons eighteen to seventy-five years old with diabetes
	Proportion of diabetics whose glycosylated hemoglobin was greater than 9.5 percent	Persons eighteen to seventy-five years old with diabetes
	Proportion of diabetics who had a lipid profile in the past year	Persons eighteen to seventy-five years old with diabetes
	Proportion of diabetics whose LDL cholesterol was less than 130 mg/dL	Persons eighteen to seventy-five years old with diabetes
	Proportion of diabetics who had an eye exam in the past year	Persons eighteen to seventy-five years old with diabetes
	Proportion of persons who had appropriate monitoring of kidney function in the past year	Persons eighteen to seventy-five years old with diabetes
Mental health care	Proportion of persons who were hospitalized for a mental health problem who had an outpatient visit within seven and thirty days after discharge	Adults with an admission for a mental health problem

(Continued)

TABLE 8.2. LISTING OF THE HEDIS 2000 EFFECTIVENESS OF CARE MEASURES.

Area	Measure Description	Population
Mental health care	Proportion of persons who received at least three follow-up medication management visits in the first twelve weeks of treatment	Adults with depression who were receiving antidepressants
	Proportion of persons who received antidepressants continuously for twelve weeks	Adults with depression on antidepressants
	Proportion of persons who received antidepressants continuously for six months	Adults with depression on antidepressants
Heart disease care	Proportion of persons who received a beta blocker following a heart attack	Persons age thirty-five and older discharged alive following an admission for a heart attack
	Proportion of persons with known coronary disease whose LDL cholesterol was less than 130 mg/dL	Persons eighteen to seventy-five who had CABG surgery, coronary angioplasty, or a heart attack

representing 410 health plan products reported data for public release.[6] An additional 112 organizations reported data to NCQA for use in benchmarking but did not allow NCQA to release results attached to their names.

A subset of the HEDIS measures report on patients' experiences with care using a standardized survey known as the Consumer Assessments of Health Plans Survey (CAHPS).[7] The survey, developed by RAND, Harvard, and RTI under a cooperative agreement with the Agency for Healthcare Research and Quality (AHRQ), is fielded by independent vendors on behalf of participating health plans. Surveys are returned directly to the vendor, which prepares the results and sends information to NCQA. The results reported are a combination of single-item ratings (health plan, personal doctor or nurse, all health care) and multi-item composites (getting needed care, getting care quickly, courteous and helpful office staff, customer service, claims processing).

NCQA also accredits managed care plans using a set of standards that cover structural dimensions of the organization as well as indicators of performance. Starting in July 1999, part of the accreditation status for a plan is based on performance on selected HEDIS measures. Until recently, NCQA reported accreditation status as full accreditation (three years), one-year accreditation, provisional, and not accredited. Beginning in 2000, NCQA has moved to reporting accreditation in two ways. Overall accreditation status is characterized as excellent, commendable, accredited, provisional, or denied. Accreditation is also reported in consumer-oriented categories (access and service, qualified providers, staying healthy, getting better, and living with illness), using one to four stars. Both types of accreditation results are available on NCQA's Website (www.ncqa.org). Users can construct their own report card depending on the area in which they live.

A number of report cards have been constructed from NCQA data by different groups. Two are described here; one is an employer-based effort and the other is from the popular press. The Combined Autos/UAW Reporting System (CARS) was developed by RAND for the three major American automobile manufacturers (DaimlerChrysler, Ford Motor Company, and General Motors) and the United Auto Workers (UAW) to provide a consistent method for reporting on health plan performance to the employees and retirees of those organizations. Because of the interest in sending consistent messages to consumers, the work has been directed by a steering committee that includes representatives from the three automobile manufacturers, the UAW, the Greater Detroit Area Health Council (GDAHC), the State of Michigan, the U.S. Office of Personnel Management, the HCFA, the Agency for Healthcare Research and Quality, the NCQA, and the Foundation for Accountability.

The results are given to employees during open enrollment (fall for DaimlerChrysler and General Motors, winter for Ford). Scores are developed in five categories (access and service, doctor communication, staying healthy, getting better and living with illness, accreditation status) based on NCQA data using a publicly available methodology.[8] Currently, health plans receive one to five stars depending on their performance relative to all other plans with which the three automobile manufacturers and GDAHC contract. The number of stars a plan receives is based on evaluating statistically significant differences in performance compared to the median.

In the popular press, *U.S. News & World Report* also developed a method for reporting on health plan performance using data from NCQA. The most recent report was in October 1998. The methodology, developed for the magazine by the National Opinion Research Center (NORC), used twenty-eight HEDIS measures in five categories (prevention, adult access to care, member satisfaction, physician credentials, and children's access to care) to develop overall scores for 271 health plans (www.norc.uchicago.edu/new/hmo). Scores were transformed so that the best plan in the nation received a score of 100 and the worst plan received a score of 0. Plans were then assigned one to four stars according to a statistical test. The overall ratings were reported along with numeric scores (from 0–100) for each of the five categories and the plan's accreditation status (www.usnews.com/usnews/nycu/health/hmo/main1).

Medical Groups

As information on quality has become available more systematically on managed care plans, interest in having such information at the medical group level has increased. Many consumers do not understand the role health plans play in ensuring provision of high-quality care and would prefer information closer to the point of service delivery. This is particularly true in areas, such as California, where medical groups are a dominant form of physician organization and many medical groups contract with multiple health plans.

The Pacific Business Group on Health (PBGH), a coalition of large and small employers, has produced a series of report cards on fifty-one medical groups in California, and seven in Oregon and Washington. The report cards cover four major areas: preventive care service delivery, preventive care counseling, care for chronic conditions (hypertension and hypercholesterolemia), and patient satisfaction and access. The reports are based on patient survey data. Numeric scores are reported in each category along with a symbol indicating whether performance is significantly above or below average. Reports are available on a Website (www.healthscope.org) that also includes reports on health plans and hospitals in California, Oregon, and Washington.

Physicians

Consumers are probably most interested in the quality of individual physicians, but to date little information is publicly available at this level. Most of the reports at the level of the individual physician have been developed for internal use by health plans or medical groups as part of determining compensation. Risk-adjusted mortality rate following CABG surgery is available at the individual physician level in New York and Pennsylvania.

Some Methodological Issues in Performance Reporting

A number of groups are currently developing and disseminating report cards, as we have discussed. Most of these efforts are local or regional rather than national, but they reflect a shared sense that consumers want (or should want) better information about the performance of the health care system. There is some danger that, in markets with multiple report cards being made available, consumers will end up being more confused than educated. This is particularly likely because methodological choices in constructing summary scores can lead to divergent results, even when using the same data. There is likely to be some benefit to developing a national consensus on reporting strategies so that consumers become familiar with the information that is available and begin to use the information in their decision-making process. We now describe some of the choices that report card developers have to make.

Number of Measures

As the amount of information collected on quality performance has expanded, attention has shifted to how this information can be meaningfully transmitted to consumers. Both methodological and communications issues arise and interact. Cognitive psychology affords some insight into the amount of information humans can use in making a decision. Typically, five to seven "bits" of information are the maximum that can be held in short-term memory and incorporated into a single decision. This suggests that minimizing the amount of information provided facilitates use by the intended audience. However, a single number about performance (for example, overall hospital mortality or mortality following CABG surgery) may not be adequate to characterize all the important dimensions for consumers. This balancing act between enough information and yet not too much continues to be debated among those producing report cards. Making information available on the Internet may allow the best tailoring for individuals. High-level aggregate results could be displayed on the first page of a Website, and then users could seek additional detail relevant to their own circumstances on subsequent pages.

Report cards have taken numerous approaches to presentation, including giving results on individual performance measures versus summary scores for multiple measures. Some present both summary scores and individual results (for example, PBGH report cards). A review of the literature on decision making suggests strongly that the scale approach is preferable because it serves the purpose of reducing the amount of information that consumers must consider when making a decision.[9] The authors note that there is an apparent contradiction between the amount of information people can typically use in making a decision and the desire frequently expressed by consumers for more information.

A study by one of those authors yielded an interesting insight into this conflict.[10] Handicappers for horse races were given the option of selecting five to forty variables from among eighty-eight possible variables to predict the winners of horse races. Their confidence in predictions increased with the number of variables, but their accuracy did not improve. The handicappers were as accurate in predicting results with five variables as they were with forty; as the number of variables increased, the level of consistency decreased. The authors of the review article conclude that "the approach of giving consumers the maximum amount of information is not the most effective path to informed consumer choice."[11] Further, they report that in focus groups consumers "commonly respond that they find the information overwhelming and confusing and that they do not know how to bring all the pieces of information together into a decision."[12] In these focus groups, consumers were looking at report cards with about twenty measures or pieces of information (plan characteristics) on them, and in some cases as many as thirty-eight plans were included.

Credibility of Data Source

One of the challenges for public reporting is the credibility of the data source. Consumers may be suspicious of information that is produced by the entity being evaluated. Two main approaches are commonly used to enhance the credibility of the information. In some cases, a third party collects and analyzes the data. This is true for accreditation and for the consumer surveys used by NCQA (that is, CAHPS). The other approach is to audit the performance data. NCQA is now requiring that HEDIS results, based on plan analyses of their own administrative and medical record data, be audited by an outside group certified to perform this function. Auditors essentially look at both the integrity of the process used to produce the result and the reproducibility of the results in determining whether the information is accurate.

Risk Adjustment

For comparisons between entities to be fair, the data must be adequately adjusted for differences in the populations receiving services; this is known as risk adjustment. Outcome data are more likely to require risk adjustment than process measures because a larger number of factors outside the control of the organization being evaluated contribute to observed performance.[13] The reports on hospital mortality have paid the greatest attention to risk-adjustment issues.

Missing Data

In our previous work on developing reporting strategies, we have considered a number of potential solutions to handling missing data.[14] These issues are particularly important if one is developing scales (groups of measures), but some of the same issues may arise if one is reporting performance on single items. Reports based on surveys routinely face this issue because respondents may not answer all questions. One always has the option of noting nonresponse (NR) for entities that do not report on one or more measures, but it may be difficult for consumers to compare "NR" with an actual performance designation. For this reason, we prefer some type of imputation strategy. Three are summarized here.

Mean imputation takes the average value of all entities that have reported on a measure and assigns that average to entities whose results were missing for the measure. Imputing the mean value maintains the mean of the observed values and is a conservative approach that suggests that in the absence of other information we assume a plan's performance is average.

Regression imputation is a more sophisticated approach to imputing the means because it uses more information to estimate what the entity's performance might have been, given other characteristics (for example, number of enrollees or profit status) or performance on other measures. This method is likely to estimate a missing value closer to the true plan performance than simple mean imputation.

Imputing the lowest observed value is a more punitive approach to dealing with missing data in that it assigns an entity the score associated with the entity that had the worst result on the measure. This policy, used by the CARS project, is designed to encourage complete reporting by penalizing plans that fail to report.

Report cards that present summary scales must choose an imputation method. Because the method used is likely to affect the results, it would be preferable for report card developers to indicate the method they used to deal with missing data. For most report cards we looked at, it was difficult to tell which method was used.

Aggregation Issues

If a report card developer chooses to present scales, a number of other analytic issues arise in constructing the scales. Conclusions can vary with the choices in these areas.

Choosing an Organizing Framework. There are two strategies for creating a framework. The first approach, which might be called "bottom-up," starts with the individual measures that are available and creates summary categories that maximize the number of measures used. This can either be done quantitatively, using factor analysis or other methods designed to identify patterns in data, or it can be done qualitatively by obtaining expert opinion. The *U.S. News & World Report* approach to health plan performance reports used factor analysis to create categories.

The second approach, which might be called "top-down," starts with the information that potential users would like to have to make decisions and identifies measures that communicate the desired information. The Foundation for

Accountability has done considerable work in this area, which contributed to the frameworks used by NCQA and the CARS project. The methods for identifying what information the target audience wants may include surveys, focus groups, or semistructured interviews.

The bottom-up approach is more frequently associated with research or decision analysis. This approach has the advantage of trying to use all available information. Since the approach is empirically driven, another advantage is the opportunity to identify patterns in data that might otherwise escape notice. The disadvantage of this approach, particularly if done quantitatively (say, using factor analysis), is that it may produce results that are difficult to interpret and may not be valued by the intended audience. In analyzing Medicare plan performance data using factor analysis, we found some of the resulting groups impossible to interpret.[15]

The top-down approach is more audience-sensitive because it identifies attributes that are important to those making the decision. Because decision makers generally come to a task with some questions already in mind, an optimal top-down approach organizes information into categories that respond to the questions on the mind of the potential user. The disadvantage of this approach is that there may be categories of interest to decision makers for which few measures or none currently exist.

Scaling. Individual measures that are combined to create summary categories may have different means and variances. This potentially presents a problem for scaling in that it can permit some measures to have a greater (or lesser) effect on the results because of their distributional properties.

Standardization is a simple calculation, but it is frequently misunderstood owing to its similarity to related statistical calculations. The idea is to transform item scores so that entities are ranked on a comparable scale across items. This prevents an item with a large range (say 0–100) from completely dominating an item with a small range (say, 0–1).

The benefit of standardizing is that it simplifies comparing items and understanding the meaning of weights applied to those items. The standard deviation scale makes using a simple rule of thumb based on the normal distribution easy; thinking of a standard deviation increase of 1 in each item is often easier than comparing a 35-point increase on a 100-point scale with a .012 increase in the mean of a dichotomous variable.

Weights. A basic starting point in constructing new scales is to give each measure in a scale equal weight. This implies that every element of the scale is equally important in arriving at a summary assessment. For many performance measures, this assumption of equal importance is at odds with both consumer and expert assessments of the measures. In previous work, we considered six options for weighting measures within scales:[16]

1. *Equal weights.* We start with equal weights as the base case since it is the option requiring the least judgment and offers a convenient method for evaluating the effect of weights on the results. All alternative weight schemes should be compared to the results based on equal weights. Equal weights is probably the most common approach taken in current report cards.

2. *Consumer weights.* A second option would be to ask consumers to assign weights to measures. This could be done either by surveying consumers to establish standardized weights for printed publications or by establishing an interactive mechanism that allows each individual to assign weights reflecting his or her own preferences.

3. *Expert weights.* Under this approach, experts assign weights based on their assessments of the relative importance of the measured process. Importance may be determined relative to the effect on outcomes, or it may reflect expert assessments of what has been suggested as being important to consumers according to the literature. This is the approach used in the CARS report card.

4. *Population weights.* Under this approach, measures are assigned a weight that reflects the proportion of the population eligible for the service represented by the measure. Importance is established on the basis of the number of people to whom the measure might be relevant.

5. *Factor weights.* If a factor-analytic approach was used to construct the reporting framework, one could use the resulting factor weights in creating aggregate scales. This is the approach used by *U.S. News & World Report* for health plan performance.

6. *Importance weights.* This approach would adopt a particular outcome (mortality, quality-adjusted life-years) and develop weights that quantify the effect of the measures on the outcome. Values could be obtained from the literature or expert assessment.

Statistical Evaluation of Differences

The final analytic consideration for public reporting is to evaluate whether results are statistically significantly different from one another. In general, ignoring statistical significance is likely to increase misinformation. The challenge is how to present the results in a way that is interpretable by users. Given that one is committed to using statistical significance to distinguish performance, some additional analytic issues must be addressed in terms of the reference point for comparison. Performance for any one entity could be compared to:

- The average performance of all entities reporting the measure nationally
- The average performance of all entities reporting the measure in a market
- A benchmark based on actual performance (say, best result in the nation)
- A benchmark based on desired performance (best theoretical result)

There has been considerable debate about the best basis for making performance comparisons among entities. Those who favor national comparisons argue that they underscore the goal of having equal quality of care throughout the country. Those who favor using regional comparisons argue that some variation nationally is unavoidable and fundamentally people can select only from local providers. Those who favor using benchmarks (rather than relative performance) prefer to emphasize the importance of a goal rather than grading on a curve. Benchmarks can be established either by observed best practices or by reference to goals (such as Healthy People 2010). These arguments often assume that the best observed performance is suboptimal. Those favoring relative performance reporting note that choices are made relative to the available options.

The choices in this area reflect beliefs about the message that a report card is intended to deliver. First, one must consider whether quality is a relative or an absolute concept. In reality, there are very few absolutes in medicine (and by extension, in quality). Process quality, for example, in Donabedian's conceptualization incorporates both technical excellence (providing the right service competently) and interpersonal excellence (doing so humanely and with reference to the patient's preferences).[17] This suggests that there are few interventions that are clinically appropriate and acceptable to all patients all the time. Most quality measures are designed with the idea that a higher rate of performance is desirable, but unless techniques for incorporating informed patient refusal and rare clinical contraindications are factored into the measurement method, excellent quality performance should rarely reach 100 percent.

One of the policy implications of using an absolute level of performance as the metric of comparison is that entities may be encouraged to deliver care that is either clinically inappropriate or unacceptable to patients in order to raise their level of performance. Alternatively, using relative performance as a basis of comparison could fail to establish adequate incentives to improve performance. A particular concern about using relative performance is that the best observed performance may not be very good. This is not consistent with some of the data we have examined. For example, for plans contracting with the three major U.S.

automobile manufacturers, the best performance in the nation in every case exceeded the Healthy People 2000 goals.

The second consideration among the relative comparison options is whether to make national or regional comparisons. Using national standards establishes a policy of expecting equal excellence in delivery of health services nationally. For many measures, there is no strong rationale for expecting substantially different performance by region. We observe differences in the quality of care received by persons in urban and rural areas, by racial or ethnic group, by income or insurance coverage, but in most instances there is no clinical justification for these differences. The proponents of risk or case-mix adjustment suggest that these techniques be applied to quality measurement to account for differences in performance that reflect the populations served. Using national standards may provide greater incentive for quality improvement than using regional standards. This varies with the market.

The third consideration is whether to make comparisons relative to the average or best performance. Any number of cut points could be chosen within the distribution of actual plan performance. Reference to the average would seem to promote substantially less quality improvement activity than reference to the best. Using the best performance as an anchor may yield a conceptually clearer way of distinguishing the top and bottom performers.

Summary of Methodological Issues in Reporting

This section summarizes some of the methodological choices that report card developers must make when designing public reporting. Many proprietary systems may not make clear the choices they have made. In most instances, report card developers have made varying choices even while using the same basic data source. This has the potential to produce apparently different results and may contribute to consumers' confusion and subsequent unwillingness to use this information to guide choices. The main message, however, from this discussion is that there is no right or wrong way to produce public information. Since the choices made affect the results, transparency of method should be highly valued.

What Is Known About the Use of Quality Information

Relatively little is known systematically about how consumers and other target audiences for public information on quality (purchasers, providers) use the available information. The general perception, and one supported by a recent analysis of the literature, is that the information is not widely used.[18] The summary of the literature in this section relies primarily on the recent review article. One of the most interesting findings from the review was the paucity of evaluative information on this question. The reviewers found only twenty-one articles in the peer-reviewed literature that had addressed the question of use, and these studies had evaluated seven public reporting systems.

Consumer Use of Information

The evaluations of consumer use of information have been of three types: evaluating whether consumers are able to use information, asking consumers whether they used information for decision making, and examining whether patterns of utilization changed following the release of public information.

Consumers frequently are unable to understand the content of report cards.[19] Some consumers may not have the skills necessary to use comparative information in decision making. Understanding the content is a prerequisite to using the information. Additional work may be required to improve the usability of report cards. Alternatively, groups that represent consumers may be a more appropriate target for information than individual consumers.

Consumers' reporting on their use of report cards is mixed and has been evaluated in limited markets. A national survey of consumers found that most relied on family, friends, and their own doctor to make decisions about where to go for care.[20] About 40 percent of people surveyed had seen comparative information on health plans, and about one-third of those who saw the information used it (about 13 percent overall). A survey of patients who had undergone CABG surgery in one of four hospitals in Pennsylvania found that only 20 percent of patients were aware of the information on hospital mortality rates for that procedure; among those who were aware, less than 25 percent said the results influenced their choice of surgeon.[21] A study of the HCFA mortality rates found that consumers were more influenced by press reports of high-profile problems at local hospitals than by the data on risk-adjusted mortality.[22]

About half of the employees of companies in St. Louis and Denver who received health plan report cards as part of open enrollment remembered the report.[23] Among those who remembered seeing the report, 95 percent found it trustworthy, 82 percent found it helpful for learning about plan quality, 66 percent found it somewhat or very helpful in deciding whether to stay in or switch plans, and 50 percent were more confident in the decision that they made.

Few changes in utilization associated with the results of hospital report cards have been observed. A study of New York general acute hospitals found no changes in occupancy rate after release of the HCFA mortality rates.[24] A quasi-experimental study of the impact of the New York state report on mortality following CABG surgery found that hospitals and physicians with better performance experienced gains in market share and prices, although this effect diminished over time.[25]

Purchaser Use of Information

There is even less systematic information on the use of performance data by purchasers. One study that conducted interviews with large purchasers in California, New York, Ohio, and Pennsylvania found that most had HEDIS data available to them and just over half used the information to select plans with which to contract.[26] A national survey of a random sample of employers with more than two hundred employees found that larger employers were more likely to use data from NCQA than smaller employers, but that a minority (11 percent) rated the information as very important.[27]

Some important leadership in purchaser use of report cards is currently coming from the automobile manufacturers (through the CARS project) and the Office of Personnel Management (OPM) for federal employees. All three automobile manufacturers and OPM require NCQA accreditation and submission of HEDIS data as a condition of contracting. The Pacific Business Group on Health has also made performance information available to purchasers and the public in the markets in which it operates. These latter activities, however, have not been formally evaluated.

Use by Providers

Consumers and purchasers might use performance information to make choices among providers, but providers' primary use of this information is for quality improvement. Most of the peer-reviewed studies in this area have focused on the hospital report cards. NCQA has presented evidence from its recent report on managed care plan performance that public reporting may be associated with higher quality.

Two studies have been conducted on the Pennsylvania CABG surgery mortality report card. One found that whereas most cardiologists and all surgeons in the state were aware of the report, few thought that it was important or had discussed it with their patients.[28] Most were critical of the methods, particularly the adequacy of risk adjustment and the reliability of the data. A study of organizations in the state found that the information was a stimulus to development of marketing materials, provider monitoring, benchmarking, and collaborative improvement activities within the hospital.[29]

Five studies have been conducted on the New York cardiac reporting system. One study found considerably greater acceptance of the reports among physicians in New York than what was reported in Pennsylvania; 67 percent reported that they found the content very useful or somewhat useful, 22 percent said they routinely discussed the results with their patients, and 38 percent said the report had affected referral patterns.[30] A case study in a hospital that had performed poorly reported that after an initial negative reaction to the report the institution used the results productively to improve collaboration and identify sources of high mortality.[31] A survey of hospital executives found that most were knowledgeable about the methods used in the New York reports and that high-mortality hospitals were more likely to be critical of the results.[32] Outcomes appear to have improved in the state following release of the information; risk-adjusted mortality rates in the state have declined from 4.17 percent to 2.45 percent.[33] This exceeds the rate of decline nationally, but some critics suggested that this resulted from fewer high-risk procedures being done or from patients going out of state for care. In fact, a study found that fewer residents of New York went out of state for CABG surgery following the release, and the likelihood of having the surgery following a heart attack (one of the most high-risk reasons for surgery) increased.[34] The findings of studies conducted on other hospital report cards are similar.[35]

In its 1999 report on managed care quality, NCQA found that health plans submitting data for public release had a higher rate of performance than those submitting data not for public release.[36] NCQA also reported that accredited plans performed better than those that were not accredited, and plans that had been reporting for public release for three consecutive years performed better than those that had not released information in all three years.

Conclusion

Despite the high level of interest in report cards on quality performance by organizations, there are few examples available nationally. NCQA has the widest geographic reach in producing performance reports on managed care plans. California appears to be the state with the most information across levels in the health care system (health plans, hospitals, and medical groups). New York's experiment with routinely reporting risk-adjusted mortality data on one procedure has been subject to the most extensive evaluation.

Although the evidence on the use of report cards by various audiences—consumers, purchasers, providers—suggests that the information is not widely used and appears to have only a small effect on performance, it is premature to declare this experiment a failure. Studies of the rate at which innovations diffuse suggest that it takes a long time for a new approach to be widely accepted.[37] The literature on making documents useful for various audiences suggests that a key problem for many of these reports may be related to poor presentation of the information.[38] We have more information available today than we have ever had, but it reflects a small portion of the reasons people seek care—so failure to find widespread effects may be consistent with assessments of the meaningfulness of the information. Increased attention to the methods that are used to construct report cards, better use of communication techniques that are known to be effective, and more formal evaluations of such efforts are required before we have the information necessary to draw conclusions about the utility of public reporting.

Notes

1. Kahn, K. L., and others. "Measuring Quality of Care with Explicit Process Criteria Before and After Implementation of the DRG-Based Prospective Payment System." *Journal of the American Medical Association,* 1990, *264*(15), 1969–1973.

2. Schuster, M. A., McGlynn, E. A., and Brook, R. H. "How Good Is the Quality of Health Care in the United States?" *Milbank Quarterly,* 1998, *76*(4), 517–563.

3. Krakauer, H., and others. "Evaluation of the HCFA Model for the Analysis of Mortality Following Hospitalization." *Health Services Research,* 1992, *27*(3), 317–335.

4. Rainwater, J. A., Romano, P. S., and Antonius, D. M. "The California Hospital Outcomes Project." *Joint Commission Journal on Quality Improvement,* 1998, *24,* 31–39.

5. Rosenthal, G. E., Quinn, L., and Harper, D. L. "Declines in Hospital Mortality Associated with a Regional Initiative to Measure Hospital Performance." *American Journal of Medical Quality,* 1997, *12,* 103–112.

6. National Committee for Quality Assurance. *The State of Managed Care Quality.* Washington, D.C.: NCQA, 1999.

7. Crofton, C., Lubalin, J. S., and Darby, C. "Consumer Assessment of Health Plans Study (CAHPS)." (Foreword.) *Medical Care,* 1999, *37,* MS1–9.

8. Schuster and others (1998).

9. Hibbard, J. H., Slovic, P., and Jewett, J. J. "Informing Consumer Decisions in Health Care: Implications from Decision-Making Research." *Milbank Quarterly,* 1997, *75*(3), 395–414.

10. Slovic, P. "Toward Understanding and Improving Decisions." In W. C. Howell and E. A. Fleishman (eds.), *Human Performance and Productivity.* Vol. 2: *Information Processing and Decision Making.* Hillsdale, N.J.: Erlbaum 1982.

11. Hibbard, Slovic, and Jewett (1997), p. 398.

12. Hibbard, Slovic, Jewett (1997), p. 398.

13. McGlynn, E. A. "The Outcomes Utility Index: Will Outcomes Data Tell Us What We Want to Know?" *International Journal for Quality in Health Care,* 1998, *10*(6), 485–490

14. McGlynn, E. A., Adams, J., Hicks, J., and Klein, D. *Developing Health Plan Performance Reports: Responding to the BBA.* RAND publication no. DRU-2122-HCFA. Santa Monica, Calif.: RAND, 1999.

15. McGlynn and others (1999).

16. McGlynn, E. A., Adams, J., Hicks, J., and Klein, D. *Creating a Coordinated Autos/UAW Reporting System for Health Plan Performance.* RAND publication no. DRU-2123-FMC. Santa Monica, Calif.: RAND, 1999.

17. Donabedian, A. *Explorations in Quality Assessment and Monitoring.* Vol. I: *The Definition of Quality and Approaches to Its Assessment.* Ann Arbor, Mich.: Health Administration Press, 1980.

18. Marshall, M. M., Shekelle, P. G., Leatherman, S., and Brook, R. H. "The Public Release of Performance Data. What Do We Expect to Gain? A Review of the Evidence." *Journal of the American Medical Association,* 2000, *283*, 1866–1874.

19. Jewett, J. J., and Hibbard, J. H. "Comprehension of Quality Care Indicators: Differences Among Privately Insured, Publicly Insured, and Uninsured." *Health Care Financing Review,* 1996, *18*, 75–94.

20. Robinson, S., and Brodie, M. "Understanding the Quality Challenge for Health Consumers: The Kaiser/AHCPR Survey." *Joint Commission Journal on Quality Improvement,* 1997, *23,* 239–244.

21. Schneider, E. C., and Epstein, A. M. "Use of Public Performance Reports." *Journal of the American Medical Association,* 1998, *279,* 1638–1642.

22. Mennemeyer, S. T., Morrisey, M. A., and Howard, L. Z. "Death and Reputation: How Consumers Acted Upon HCFA Mortality Information." *Inquiry,* 1997, *34,* 117–128.

23. Fowles, J. B., Kind, E. A., Braun, B. L., and Knutson, D. J. "Consumer Responses to Health Plan Report Cards in Two Markets." *Medical Care,* 2000, *38,* 469–471.

24. Vladeck, B. C., Goodwin, E. J., Myers, L. P., and Sinisi, M. "Consumers and Hospital Use: The HCFA 'Death List.'" *Health Affairs,* 1988, *7,* 122–125.

25. Mukamel, D. B., and Mushlin, A. I. "Quality of Care Information Makes a Difference." *Medical Care,* 1998, *36,* 945–954.

26. Hibbard, Slovic, and Jewett (1997).

27. Gabel, J. R., and others. When Employers Choose Health Plans. Report no. 293. New York: Commonwealth Fund, 1998.

28. Schneider, E. C., and Epstein, A. M. "Influence of Cardiac-Surgery Performance Reports on Referral Practices and Access to Care." *New England Journal of Medicine,* 1996, *335,* 251–256.

29. Bentley, J. M., and Nash, D. B. "How Pennsylvania Hospitals Have Responded to Publicly Released Reports on Coronary Artery Bypass Graft Surgery." *Joint Commission Journal on Quality Improvement,* 1998, *24,* 40–49.

30. Hannan, E. L., Stone, C. C., Biddle, T. L., and DeBuono, B. A. "Public Release of Cardiac Surgery Outcomes Data in New York." *American Heart Journal,* 1997, *134,* 55–61.

31. Dziuban, S. W., McIlduff, J. B., Miller, S. J., and Dal Col, R. H. "How a New York Cardiac Surgery Program Uses Outcomes Data." *Annals of Thoracic Surgery,* 1994, 58, 1871–1876.

32. Romano, P. S., Rainwater, J. A., and Antonius, D. M. "Grading the Graders; How Hospitals in California and New York Perceive and Interpret Their Report Cards." *Medical Care,* 1999, *37,* 295–305.

33. Hannan, E. L., and others. "Improving the Outcomes of Coronary Artery Bypass Surgery in New York State." *Journal of the American Medical Association,* 1994, *271,* 761–766.

34. Peterson, E. D., and others. "The Effects of New York's Bypass Surgery Provider Profiling on Access to Care and Patient Outcomes in the Elderly." *Journal of the American College of Cardiology,* 1998, *32,* 993–999.

35. Marshall and others (2000).

36. NCQA (1999).

37. Rogers, E. M. *Diffusion of Innovations.* New York: Free Press, 1995.

38. McGlynn and others (1999).

PART FOUR

SPECIAL POPULATIONS

CHAPTER NINE

LONG-TERM CARE AND THE ELDERLY POPULATION

Steven P. Wallace, Emily K. Abel, Pamela Stefanowicz, and Nadereh Pourat

The health service needs of people in the United States have changed dramatically during the past century as a result of the shift from acute to chronic conditions and an increasing life span. In 1900, the major health problems stemmed from acute infectious diseases such as typhoid fever and smallpox. People usually recovered or died rapidly from those diseases. By midcentury, three chronic conditions alone—heart disease, cancer, and stroke—accounted for more than 50 percent of deaths; today, chronic illnesses are the predominant cause of death.[1] Reductions in acute illness have contributed to a historic increase in life expectancy, from 47 years in 1900 to 73.6 years in 1997. Because the birthrate also is falling, elderly people constitute a growing segment of the population. By 2035, when most baby boomers will have aged, one in five Americans (sixty-seven million people) will be age sixty-five or over.[2] Disabilities can affect people of any age, but the rate increases with age. Only 2.4 percent of people under sixty-five need any assistance with daily activities, compared to almost half of those eighty-five and over.[3] People with chronic illness frequently experience disability and require assistance over an extended period.

Long-term care is the set of health and social services delivered over a sustained period to people who have lost (or never acquired) some capacity for personal care; ideally, it enables recipients to live with as much independence and dignity as possible.[4] Provided in institutional, community, and home settings, long-term care encompasses an array of services ranging from high-tech care to assistance with such daily activities as walking, bathing, cooking, and managing money. The care can be furnished by paid providers (formal care) or unpaid family and friends (informal care), or by a combination of the two. Long-term care differs from most topics discussed in this volume because it includes social as well as medical services.

This chapter reviews the recent literature on long-term care, showing how financial considerations have framed the dominant policy debates and research agenda. Policy makers frequently view nursing homes as a low-cost alternative to a hospital and consider community services and family care as less expensive substitutes for a nursing home—neglecting quality-of-life issues. Both policy makers and researchers also tend to ignore the diversity among older Americans, as well as the problems faced by low-income women who serve as caregivers (whether in a paid or an unpaid capacity).

Nursing Homes

The term *nursing home* covers a variety of institutions, including skilled nursing facilities (SNFs), which offer twenty-four-hour nursing care; and residential care facilities (RCFs), which provide some personal care but no licensed nursing care. Public policy first encouraged establishment of private nursing homes in 1935, when Old Age Assistance (public aid for low-income elderly), part of the Social Security Act, specifically barred residents of public facilities (almshouses) from receiving this aid. The federal government gave funds directly for construction of nursing homes in the 1950s in an attempt to solve a hospital bed shortage and to save money by discharging hospital patients to a less-intensive level of care. Public funding of nursing homes expanded dramatically after the passage of Medicare and Medicaid in 1965, leading to rapid growth in the number of facilities. Both programs defined nursing homes as predominantly medical institutions, emphasizing the nursing over the home.[5]

At the most acute end, such policy changes as Diagnosis-Related Group (DRG) hospital reimbursement and the growth of HMOs have contributed to the growth of "subacute" care. This type of nursing home care is designed to shift care from hospitals into nursing homes, both reducing hospital costs and capturing extra Medicare reimbursement.[6] The reimbursement formula for nursing home care in general encourages for-profit enterprises; three-quarters of free-standing nursing homes now are profit-making.[7]

Although most older people assume that Medicare covers nursing home stays, it accounts for only 14 percent of total nursing home expenditures. The program pays for one hundred days of post-hospital recovery care in a nursing home; it provides no coverage for custodial care. Medicaid, by contrast, pays for custodial as well as skilled nursing care and has thus become the primary funding source. It finances 42 percent of nursing home expenditures for the elderly and represents three-quarters of the total $48.5 billion government spending on nursing homes.[8] Although about 40 percent of nursing home users enter facilities paying privately, many of them become eligible for Medicaid after "spending down" or depleting their resources. The annual cost of a nursing home stay in 1993 was $37,000, a sum that exceeded the incomes of four-fifths of elderly people.[9] Nursing home spend-down has attracted policy attention because those who spend down account for a significant proportion of Medicaid nursing home expenditures, and because the phenomenon is a demonstration of the catastrophic costs of long-term care.[10]

Nursing homes dominate long-term care spending. The rapid and unexpected rise in government expenditures for nursing homes during the 1960s and 1970s contributed to the policy focus on containing costs. Research has distinguished two types of nursing home user: (1) someone with a short stay, typical of post-hospital use; and (2) someone with a longer stays, typical of more custodial use.[11] The long-stay residents consume most nursing home funds.[12] Research in this area has been used extensively in developing private long-term care insurance.[13]

Other research has concentrated on designing, implementing, and evaluating alternative reimbursement methods.[14] Studies suggest that although various techniques, especially prospective payment, have slowed the increase in costs, they also have reduced access for Medicaid patients and limited the supply of beds below needed levels in some areas.[15] To discourage nursing homes from taking only the least disabled (and least expensive) Medicaid patients, some states have tried reimbursement formulae that pay more for the care of the most disabled. But this system may have the unintended consequence of reducing access for those needing only custodial care. One group of researchers concluded that reimbursements often reflect state budget balances and overall states resources more than the actual costs of providing nursing home care or improving quality.[16]

Although economic issues dominate research and policy, widespread concern about the treatment of nursing home residents (especially after highly publicized scandals) has kept some attention on quality-of-care issues.[17] The definition of *quality* has changed over the years. Initially, regulations defined it in terms of such "structural" features as conforming to fire and safety codes. Regulations then began to include measures of "process," such as whether a bed-bound patient is repositioned frequently enough to prevent pressure sores. Most recently, federal nursing home regulations have broadened to cover some "outcome" measures, such as change in functional status and psychosocial well-being as indicators of quality.[18]

Some researchers have shown how nursing homes can reduce accidental falls, urinary incontinence, decubitus ulcers, and use of physical restraints and psychotropic drugs.[19] Others have examined quality differences between for-profit and not-for-profit nursing homes, finding that the latter generally provide better care.[20] Studies documenting high use of chemical and physical restraints, inadequate supervision of care by physicians and professional nurses, and the poor quality of life in many institutions helped inform the federal 1987 Omnibus Budget Reconciliation Act's (OBRA) detailed language on nursing home quality. OBRA included national standards for training nursing home aides, presence of social work staff, and delivery of medical care in nursing homes,[21] but poor-quality facilities remain common.[22]

Community-Based Services

For many, long-term care conjures up the image of bedridden elderly residents in nursing homes. But most older people with functional limitations remain at home, often receiving assistance from family and friends as well as community agencies. Community-based services include adult day care, transportation, and congregate meals. Home care includes high-tech equipment, home-delivered meals, visiting nurses, home health aides with some training who can provide basic personal care such as help with bathing, and homemakers or untrained workers who assist with housecleaning and some personal care. We refer to both in-home and out-of-home services as "community-based" services in this chapter.

Public funding for community-based services remains limited. Medicare emphasizes medically oriented, postacute home care, not the ongoing social support services many people need to live independently in the community. Recipients must be homebound, under the care of a physician, and in need of part-time or intermittent skilled nursing or physical or speech therapy.[23] The way these rules was interpreted was loosened in the early 1990s, leading to rapid growth in Medicare expenditures for home health care. In reaction, Congress severely restricted reimbursements in 1997, leading to a 45 percent drop in expenditures the following year.[24] An exception to Medicare's home care restrictions is the experimental Social Health Maintenance Organizations (SHMOs), which combine the prepaid, at-risk features of regular HMOs with a modest amount of ongoing chronic care benefit. Difficulties in controlling costs, as well as the failure to coordinate acute and chronic medical services,[25] make it unlikely that SHMOs will represent a major expansion of long-term care under Medicare.

Unlike Medicare, Medicaid does not limit community-based services to postacute care. The government's concern with reducing Medicaid nursing home spending encouraged expansion of Medicaid coverage of community-based services. Legislation passed in 1981 gave states the option of applying for waivers from existing Medicaid rules in order to provide case management, personal care, respite care, and adult day care.[26] Regulations sought to ensure that such services substituted for, and cost less than, nursing home placement. Largely as a result of these waivers, Medicaid spending on community-based services doubled between 1989 and 1993. Nevertheless, 9 percent of Medicaid's $122 billion budget is spent on community-based services, compared to 24 percent on nursing homes.[27]

Two other major federal programs that fund services for elderly people in the community are Title III of the Older Americans Act (OAA) and the Social Services Block Grant (SSBG). Both have fixed annual budgets that are substantially smaller than the amount spent by Medicaid on community-based services; both programs thus sometimes run out of money before the end of the year and refuse to accept new clients. Moreover, the amount of assistance provided to each recipient tends to be even lower than that furnished by Medicaid programs.[28]

The policy focus on cost containment has shaped the direction of research on community care. A series of "channeling" demonstration projects in the early 1980s studied a range of community services in an attempt to see if funding those services could save money by keeping disabled elderly people out of nursing homes. Evaluators concluded that some highly disabled clients would not have entered institutions even without access to community services.[29] Thus, although community-based services are usually cheaper than nursing home care for a single individual, total costs tend to be higher because more persons are served by community-based care than would have been served by nursing homes. These findings, coupled with rising Medicaid costs, have stimulated research on identifying clients at imminent risk of institutionalization or those inappropriately placed in nursing homes so that community services can be targeted to them alone.[30] Drawing primarily on the Andersen model of health services utilization,[31] researchers have identified characteristics of elderly people that increase the probability of nursing home placement: advanced age, poorer health status, increased functional impairment, being white, living alone, and not owning a home.[32]

Another body of research addresses the policy concern that publicly funded care not substitute for care provided "free" by family and friends. Such a concern is based on the premise that formal (paid) and informal (unpaid) services are interchangeable and that an hour of paid care results in one less hour of care by family members. Most studies of the intersection of formal and informal services focus exclusively on allocating tasks between family caregivers and formal providers. Family members, however, typically conceptualize caregiving as a complex relationship, not simply as a set of discrete tasks. It is thus unsurprising that researchers consistently find that formal services supplement rather than supplant informal care.[33]

A similar line of research arises from the fear that large numbers of elderly people will come out of the woodwork to use new services because such community-based services as household cleaning, unlike nursing homes, are believed to lack built-in limitation on consumption. This fear, too, appears to be misdirected. Although the potential pool of clients of community-based services is vast, a critical issue for some community agencies is *recruiting* clientele, not controlling intake.[34] Some elderly people postpone assistance until they are extremely disabled in order to maintain a sense of independence.[35] Having absorbed a value system that glorifies self-sufficiency, they may be unable to rely on others even when very needy. Some elderly people also may cling to housekeeping chores as a way of separating themselves from their more severely impaired counterparts. As Alan Sager comments, "The notion of a horde of greedy old people and lazy family members anxious to soak up new public benefits appears to be more a projection by a few wealthy legislators accustomed to domestic and hotel and restaurant service than it is a realistic image of our nation's elderly citizens."[36]

Moreover, one person's "latent demand" is another's "unmet need."[37] Those who fear that the expansion of community services will open the floodgates implicitly acknowledge that the elderly are drastically underserved. Only 36 percent of the 5.6 million functionally impaired elderly people living in the community receive any formal care.[38] More than half of those with the severest disabilities receive no formal help.[39]

Policy on the quality of existing community-based care is at least fifteen years behind similar nursing home policy. Several organizations, such as the Joint Commission on the Accreditation of Health Care Organizations (JCAHO), have developed voluntary accreditation standards for some types of community care, but research is just beginning to define quality in community settings and develop a methodology for measuring it.[40]

Variations in the Need for Formal Services

As the previous two sections have shown, the research and policy focus on financial considerations has overshadowed other public health concerns such as equity, adequacy, and quality. Understanding variations by race, ethnicity, gender, and class can help identify critical research and policy issues that previously have received inadequate attention.

The elderly population is becoming increasingly African American, Latino, Native American, and Asian American. These groups constituted approximately 16 percent of the elderly population in 2000 and are expected to represent approximately 34 percent by 2050.[41] Thus, programs aimed at the types and levels of functional disability of elderly whites may become less appropriate. Elderly African Americans have the highest rate of death and functional limitation, caused in part by high rates of hypertension, diabetes, circulatory problems, and arthritis. Elderly African Americans also are more likely to rate their health as fair or poor.[42] Research on the functional disabilities of Latinos is inconsistent. Some studies show that Latinos have fewer disabilities than all other groups, some report a similar level, and some find a higher level. Older Latinos have a lower death rate than whites overall, but higher death rates from diabetes, accidents, and chronic liver disease.[43] The health status of Asian American elderly generally is similar to that of white elderly. Aggregate data, however, mask the increasing diversity within Asian American communities. Some Asian Americans groups, especially recent immigrants, have long-term care needs that differ dramatically from those of whites.[44]

Women constitute 59 percent of the elderly population and 71 percent of those eighty-five and over.[45] Women at every age experience more functional limitations than men. Women also have a disproportionate need for formal long-term care because many live by themselves. Seventy-eight percent of elderly people living alone are women; 36 percent of all elderly women and 44 percent of women seventy-five and over live alone.[46]

Class also influences the need for long-term care. Research on aging in the United States generally focuses on income (which is a point-in-time measure of cash flow) rather than class (which is a long-term position in the economic stratification system that also includes assets and occupational position). Research outside the United States suggests that class position has a direct impact on health status, independent of access to health care. A Swedish study of people eighty-five and over reported that former blue-collar workers are twice as likely as former white-collar workers to experience limitation in activities of daily living.[47] In the United States, functional limitations are highest among elderly people with relatively low income, even after controlling for age and race.[48]

Race and ethnicity, gender, and class interact, intensifying the need for long-term care and aggravating access barriers. The disability rate is highest among older African American women, being about 50 percent higher than that among older white males.[49] Those with the greatest need for long-term care have the least ability to pay for it. In 1997, elderly men's median income was $17,768, while elderly women's was $10,062. The median income for white men sixty-five and over was $15,276, two and a half times that of elderly African American and Latina women ($6,220 and $5,968, respectively).[50] Approximately 84 percent of African American elderly people enter nursing homes on Medicaid, compared to less than 44 percent of whites.[51] The term *multiple jeopardy* has been used to describe this cumulative disadvantage of age, race, gender, and class in regard to health and income.[52]

Variations in Using Long-Term Care

The elderly population is a heterogeneous group. Characteristics such as gender, race, ethnicity, and class exert a significant influence on the use of LTC services.

Gender

Women are much more likely to enter nursing homes than men; 70 percent of nursing home residents are women, and women are twice as likely as men to use a nursing home at some point in their lives.[53] The imbalance in nursing home utilization occurs not only because women have more disabilities but also because they frequently outlive their husbands and thus lack the social support needed to stay at home.[54] The cruel irony is that, after a lifetime of caring for others, many women are bereft of essential support when they are most in need. Policy makers and researchers rarely address the social and economic policies responsible for the predominance of women in nursing homes. It is unclear to what extent women also are especially likely to suffer from inadequacy of community services.

Race and Ethnicity

As early as 1980, the U.S. Commission on Civil Rights argued that racial differences in the utilization rate of nursing homes *might* indicate access barriers. In 1990, 25.8 percent of whites age eighty-five and over were in nursing homes, compared to 16.7 percent of African Americans, 11.0 percent of Latinos, and 12.1 percent of Asian Americans.[55] Differences persist even after controlling for other predictors of nursing home use.[56]

The relatively little research on the relation between race and ethnicity and use of community services is contradictory. Some studies report that minority elderly people use community-based care at the same rate as whites (or a higher rate) after controlling for need and resources.[57] Other studies find that African Americans and Latinos are less likely to use community services.[58]

Several reasons could account for the racial and ethnic differences in long-term care utilization.[59] Some studies suggest that minority elderly people are less knowledgeable than whites about the types and functions of many community-based services, others suggest that nursing homes have discriminatory admission policies, and still others suggest that health professionals are less likely to refer minority elderly people to formal services.[60] This racial and ethnic variation is typically overlooked by policy makers who design programs for the "average" elder who is white and middle class.[61]

Class

Some observers argue that social policy for older persons in the United States creates a two-class system. Low-income elderly rely on Medicaid and other poverty programs, while those who are better off benefit from tax preferences and universal programs such as Medicare. Poverty programs are the most vulnerable to cuts because their constituency lacks political and economic clout.[62]

Specific research on class factors in long-term care is sparse and primarily deals with the problems faced by Medicaid recipients. Some evidence suggests that many nursing homes discriminate against Medicaid patients. High occupancy rates (averaging 95 percent nationwide) enable nursing homes to be choosy about admissions. Because the Medicaid reimbursement rate is lower than the amount nursing homes charge private-pay residents, facilities prefer clients who can pay out of pocket.[63] Hospital discharge planners in California estimate that it is four to seven times more difficult to place Medicaid patients in nursing homes than privately-funded patients.[64]

The quality of life of Medicaid nursing home residents appears to be especially poor. Medicaid recipients tend to be relegated to institutions that, according to some measures, offer the worst-quality care.[65] Even within a facility, residents relying on Medicaid sometimes receive less care than private-pay residents. Medicaid also does not pay for "incidentals," such as laundering personal clothing or making a phone call. All such expenses must come from the $30–70 per month (varying by state) that Medicaid recipients are allowed to keep.[66]

Class also affects distribution of community-based services. Because most people who receive such care pay privately, utilization varies directly with income. Not surprisingly, people with higher incomes spend far more than others on care. Moreover, self-pay clients receive more hours of home health care than those who rely on public funds.[67] Although Medicaid increases access to community-based services, 71 percent of noninstitutionalized older persons with poverty level incomes do not receive Medicaid.[68] Other elderly people, called "tweeners," have incomes just above the poverty level and therefore do not quality for Medicaid but are too poor to pay privately for services.[69]

Recent developments have accentuated the class bias of noninstitutional care, especially home health care. First, the deregulation and cost-containment measures of the 1980s eased Medicare restrictions on proprietary home health agencies. By 1998, 56.7 percent of home health agencies were proprietary.[70] For-profit agencies seek out the best-paying (privately insured) patients, leaving other patients for nonprofit and government agencies. Second, large multihospital systems looking for a relatively inexpensive way to expand have been eager to acquire home health agencies.[71] Third, for-profit chains have expanded. Currently,

81.6 percent of the thirty-eight largest home care organizations are members of for-profit chains.[72] These changes have increased the competitiveness of the home health care system, putting agencies under growing pressure to generate revenue by focusing on the most remunerative patients and the best-paid services, thus decreasing access for those whose care is less profitable.[73] Little research has attempted to determine if the quality of care varies by type of payment or ownership or affiliation of the home health agency.

The greatest difference of class may lie in services provided outside the bounds of established organizations. Although most studies ignore the vast network of helpers recruited through ad hoc, informal arrangements, some evidence suggests that disabled elderly people rely disproportionately on this type of assistance.[74] Abel's study of fifty-one predominantly white, middle-class women caring for elderly parents found that just fifteen used services from a community agency, but twenty-eight hired helpers who were unaffiliated with formal agencies. Nine of the unaffiliated home care aides worked forty hours a week, and sixteen provided around-the-clock care.[75] The help from such workers typically is not included in government statistics; however, it constitutes a major source of assistance to the affluent that is not available to others.

Private Sector Financing Initiatives

The inequities in long-term care may become even more apparent if initiatives to rely more on private sector financing win increased support. Such initiatives take two forms. Some, such as home equity conversions and individual medical accounts, seek to promote private saving, which can then be used to finance long-term care. Others attempt to bring individuals together to pool the risks of paying for long-term care; these mechanisms include private long-term care insurance and continuing-care retirement communities.[76]

Advocates of such programs argue that the growing segment of the elderly population that is sufficiently well off to be able to pay for long-term care should not rely on limited government funds.[77] Critics charge that expansion of the private sector would sharpen the divide between rich and poor. Most private sector approaches are beyond the reach of low- and middle-income elderly people. Many elderly have neither enough equity in their homes to pay for extended long-term care nor enough income to pay for comprehensive private long-term care insurance.[78] In 1995, a policy paying $100 a day for nursing home and $50 a day for home care cost an average annual premium of $1,881 at sixty-five and $5,889 at seventy-nine.[79] Entry fees for continuing-care retirement communities can be as high as $440,000 for a two-bedroom house for a couple, with monthly fees of $4,267. Increased private financing may also dissolve whatever popular support public programs currently enjoy. Walter Leutz writes: "This could clearly lead to a two-class system of care, which would be rationalized by arguments that blame elderly victims for not insuring. It would not be uncommon to hear the argument that those who don't plan for the future don't deserve such a generous program, and so on into the all-too-familiar pattern."[80]

Informal Care

Research offers overwhelming evidence to refute the enduring myth that families abandon their elderly relatives. Shanas was one of the first scholars to show that elderly people remain in close contact with surviving kin.[81] More recent studies demonstrate that this contact translates into assistance during times of crisis. Families and friends deliver 70–80 percent of the services disabled elderly people receive.[82] A study published in 1989 concluded that seven million relatives and friends care for elderly people.[83]

Informal care continues to be allocated on the basis of gender. Women represent 72 percent of all caregivers and 77 percent of children providing care.[84] Daughters are more likely than sons to live with dependent parents and to serve as the primary caregivers.[85] Sons and daughters also assume responsibility for different tasks. Sons are more likely to assist parents with household maintenance and repairs, while daughters are far more likely to help with housework, cooking, shopping, and personal care.[86]

Research on informal care typically focuses on the burden it imposes. Studies have found that caregivers experience a range of physical, emotional, social, and financial problems. In many cases, caregiving responsibilities reignite family conflict, impose financial strain, and encroach on both paid employment and leisure activity.[87]

Despite the many reports of caregiver burden, limited assistance is available. The dominant concern of policy makers is that caregivers will unload responsibilities on the state. As a result, policy makers support social services and financial assistance for caregivers only insofar as they serve to postpone or prevent institutionalization. The major demand of many caregivers is respite services, which provide temporary relief from care.[88] Although most states have established respite programs, they tend to be grossly underfunded, able to serve a small number of families and offering very few hours of care.[89] State programs to reimburse caregivers for their services typically limit payment to those caring for patients deemed most vulnerable to institutionalization. Stringent eligibility criteria often exclude caregivers who are spouses, children over the age of eighteen, relatives who live apart from the care receivers, and relatives with income over a certain amount. The level of reimbursement tends to be low.[90]

The policy response to the conflict between wage work and care also has been limited. The Family and Medical Leave Act (FMLA), passed with widespread acclaim in 1993, covers leave of no more than twelve weeks, provides no remuneration, excludes part-time and contingent workers and those employed in small firms, and defines family narrowly. Workers who are white, middle-class, and married are most likely to be able to take advantage of the act.[91] Most state programs have similar restrictions.[92] Employer-based programs to accommodate family caregivers tend to be narrow in scope and concentrated in large businesses.[93]

Unlike respite services, financial compensation, and workplace reforms, programs enhancing the ability of caregivers to adapt to their responsibility enjoy enthusiastic support. The low cost of such programs partly explains their appeal. It is far cheaper to establish a ten-week course of lectures for caregivers than to provide them with the services of homemakers and home health aides over a period of months or even years. In addition, many caregivers attest to the benefit of such programs. Support groups alleviate the intense isolation surrounding caregiving. Educational programs that dispense information about the disease process or the new equipment dispatched to the home boost competence and confidence. Counseling services help caregivers disentangle unresolved emotional issues from the process of delivering care.[94] A major disadvantage of these programs is that they reinforce the belief that our primary goal should be to help caregivers adjust to their unavoidable burdens rather than to make care for the dependent population more just and humane.

Workers in the Long-Term Care System

Paid as well as unpaid caregivers suffer from the failure to fund long-term care adequately. Nursing homes, home health agencies, and the elderly themselves seek to save money by keeping wages low. In New York City, 99 percent of home care workers are women, 70 percent are African American, 26 percent are Latina, and almost half (46 percent) are immigrants. A high proportion are single mothers with three or four children. They typically earn less than $5,000 a year. Eighty percent cannot afford adequate housing, and 35 percent often cannot buy enough food for their families.[95] Home care work also is characterized by inadequate supervision and training and few opportunities for advancement.[96] National studies of nursing home assistants show that they receive poor wages and few benefits and in large, metropolitan areas are overwhelmingly women of color and immigrants.[97] One qualitative study found that even though most assistants took extra jobs to make ends meet, staff conversations centered "on not having enough money for rent or transportation or children's necessities."[98]

Most research on home care workers addresses the concerns of home health agencies regarding training, supervision, and especially retention of workers.[99] The high turnover rate of nursing home assistants, estimated to be 40–75 percent annually, has led to a similar focus in the nursing home literature.[100] The research focuses on factors that could be changed at the level of the individual nursing home, such as daily organization of work.[101]

Some studies report that nursing home assistants enjoy helping and caring for patients, but that rules and regulations designed to protect patients' rights, ensure quality, and promote efficiency frustrate their efforts. Racial and ethnic differences between workers, administrators, and patients further undermine positive relationships.[102] The racial, ethnic, and class composition of the home care labor force similarly creates serious problems. Many workers complain that they are treated like "maids," asked to perform tasks they consider inappropriate and demeaning. They also report that they have difficulty overcoming the distrust of some clients.[103] Overall, the challenges facing wage workers in the long-term care system receive scant attention in the research literature.

Conclusion

The rapid growth of the older population will put new strains on our long-term care system, especially when the baby boom generation reaches age eighty-five beginning around 2030. We can confidently predict that this cohort will be disproportionately widowed women with high rates of disability and poverty; many will be members of racial and ethnic minorities.

Although the priority in both policy and research is typically on cost containment, the most critical issue is how we can provide adequate and high-quality long-term care services equitably to this growing and diverse population. The limited financial resources of many older people create a need for a universal Medicare type of social insurance for long-term care. The considerable new public financing needed to establish such a system has stymied consideration of such policies in the past. Since the underlying long-term care needs will not disappear simply because public policy fails to come to terms with them, it behooves us to reform our current medical care system so that resources can be allocated to address the pressing needs of the twenty-first century.

Notes

1. McKinlay, J. B., McKinlay, S. M., and Beaglehole, R. "Trends in Death and Disease and the Contribution of Medical Measures." In H. E. Freeman and S. Levine (eds.), *Handbook of Medical Sociology*. Upper Saddle River, N.J.: Prentice Hall, 1989.

2. National Center for Health Statistics. *Health, United States, 1999, with Health and Aging Chartbook*. Hyattsville, Md.: National Center for Health Statistics, 1999; Kramarow, E., and others. *Health and Aging Chartbook. Health, United States, 1999*. Hyattsville, Md.: National Center for Health Statistics, 1999; Day, J. C. *Population Projections of the United States by Age, Sex, Race, and Hispanic Origin: 1995 to 2050*. (U.S. Bureau of the Census, Current Population Reports, P25–1130.) Washington, D.C.: U.S. Government Printing Office, 1996.

3. National Center for Health Statistics (1999); Kramarow (1999).

4. Kane, R. A., Kane, R. L., and Ladd, R. C. *The Heart of Long-Term Care*. New York: Oxford University Press, 1998.

5. Committee on Nursing Home Regulation, Institute of Medicine. *Improving the Quality of Care in Nursing Homes*. Washington, D.C.: National Academy Press, 1986.

6. Lewin-VHI, Inc. *Subacute Care: Policy Synthesis and Market Area Analysis*. Washington, D.C.: Office of the Assistant Secretary for Planning and Evaluation, U.S. Department of Health and Human Services, 1995.

7. Aaronson, W. E., Zinn, J. S., and Rosko, M. D. "Do For-Profit and Not-for-Profit Nursing Homes Behave Differently?" *Gerontologist*, Dec. 1994, *34*, 775–786.

8. U.S. Congressional Budget Office. *Projections of Expenditures for Long-Term Care Services for the Elderly*. Washington, D.C.: U.S. Congress, Mar. 1999.

9. Kane, Kane, and Ladd (1998); Reschovsky, J. D. "The Roles of Medicaid and Economic Factors in the Demand for Nursing Home Care." *Health Services Research*, 1998, *33*(4), 787–813.

10. Adams, E. K., Meiners, M. R., and Burwell, B. O. "Asset Spend-Down in Nursing Homes." *Medical Care*, Jan. 1993, *31*, 1–23.

11. Liu, K., McBride, T., and Coughlin, T. "Risk of Entering Nursing Homes for Long Versus Short Stays." *Medical Care*, 1994, *32*, 315–327.

12. Kemper, P., Spillman, B. C., and Murtaugh, C. M. "A Lifetime Perspective on Proposals for Financing Nursing Home Care." *Inquiry*, 1991, *28*, 333–344.

13. Cohen, M. A., Kumar, N., and Wallack, S. S. "Long-Term Care Insurance and Medicaid." *Health Affairs*, 1994, *13*, 127–139.

14. Schlenker, R. E. "Comparison of Medicaid Nursing Home Payment Systems." *Health Care Financing Review*, Fall 1991, *13*, 93–109.

15. Davis, M. A., Freeman, J. W., and Kirby, E. C. "Nursing Home Performance Under Case-Mix Reimbursement: Responding to Heavy-Care Incentives and Market Changes." *Health Services Research*, 1998, *33*(4), 815–834.

16. Davis, Freeman, and Kirby (1998).

17. U.S. General Accounting Office. *California Nursing Homes: Federal and State Oversight Inadequate to Protect Residents in Homes with Serious Care Violations*. GAO/T-HEHS-98-219. Washington, D.C.: U.S. General Accounting Office, 1998.

18. Hawes, C., and others. "Reliability Estimates for the Minimum Data Set for Nursing Home Resident Assessment and Care Screening (MDS)." *Gerontologist*, Apr. 1995, *35*, 172–178.

19. Starer, P., and Libow, L. S. "Medical Care of the Elderly in the Nursing Home." *Journal of General Internal Medicine*, May-June 1992, *7*, 350–362.

20. Aaronson, Zinn, and Rosko (1994).
21. Elon, R., and Pawlson, L. G. "The Impact of OBRA on Medical Practice within Nursing Facilities." *Journal of the American Geriatrics Society,* Sept. 1994, *40,* 958–963.
22. U.S. General Accounting Office (1998).
23. Health Care Financing Administration. *Medicare and You 2000.* Publication no. HCFA-10050. Baltimore: Health Care Financing Administration, U.S. Department of Health and Human Services, 1999.
24. Pear, R. "Medicare Spending for Care at Home Plunges by 45%." New York Times, Apr. 21, 2000.
25. Harrington, C., Lynch, M., and Newcomer, R. J. "Medical Services in Social Health Maintenance Organizations." *Gerontologist,* Dec. 1993, *33,* 790–800; Harrington, C., and Newcomer, R. J. "Social Health Maintenance Organizations' Service Use and Costs, 1985–89." *Health Care Financing Review,* Spring 1991, *12,* 37–52.
26. U.S. General Accounting Office. *Long-Term Care Case Management: State Experiences and Implications for Federal Policy.* GAO/HRD-93-52. Washington, D.C.: U.S. General Accounting Office, 1993.
27. U.S. Health Care Financing Administration. "Table 5. Medicaid Vendor Payments by Type of Service." [http://www.hcfa.gov/medicaid/mnatstat.htm.] Dec. 1999.
28. Wallace, S. P. "The No Care Zone: Availability, Accessibility, and Acceptability in Community-Based Long-Term Care." *Gerontologist,* 1990, *30,* 254–261; Estes, C. L., Swan, J. H., and Associates. *The Long-Term Care Crisis: Elders Trapped in the No-Care Zone.* Thousand Oaks, Calif.: Sage, 1993.
29. Weissert, W. G., Cready, C. M., and Pawelak, J. E. "The Past and Future of Home- and Community-Based Long Term Care." *Milbank Quarterly,* 1988, *66,* 309–388.
30. Safran, D. G., Graham, J. D., and Osberg, J. S. "Social Supports as a Determinant of Community-Based Care Utilization Among Rehabilitation Patients." *Health Services Research,* 1994, *28,* 729–750.
31. Andersen, R. M. "Revisiting the Behavioral Model and Access to Medical Care: Does It Matter?" *Journal of Health and Social Behavior,* Mar. 1995, *36,* 1–10.
32. Wallace, S. P., Levy-Storms, L., Kington, R. S., and Andersen, R. M. "The Persistence of Race and Ethnicity in the Use of Long-Term Care." *Journals of Gerontology, Series B, Psychological Sciences and Social Sciences,* 1998, *53*(2), S104–S112; Wallace, S. P., Levy-Storms, L., Andersen, R. M., and Kington, R. S. "The Impact by Race of Changing Long-Term Care Policy." *Journal of Aging and Social Policy,* 1997, *9*(3), 1–20.
33. Jette, A. M., Tennstedt, S., and Crawford, S. "How Does Formal and Informal Community Care Affect Nursing Home Use?" *Journals of Gerontology, Social Sciences,* Jan. 1995, *50B,* S4–S12; Spector, W. D., and Kemper, P. "Disability and Cognitive Impairment Criteria: Targeting Those Who Need the Most Home Care." *Gerontologist,* Oct. 1994, *34,* 640–651; McFall, S., and Miller, B. H. "Caregiver Burden and Nursing Home Admission of Frail Elderly Persons." *Journals of Gerontology, Social Sciences,* 1992, *47,* S73–S79.
34. Weissert, W. G. "Seven Reasons Why It Is So Difficult to Make Community-Based Long-Term Care Cost-Effective." *Health Services Research,* 1985, *20,* 423–433.
35. Wallace (1990).
36. Sager, A. "A Proposal for Promoting More Adequate Long-Term Care for the Elderly." *Gerontologist,* 1983, *23,* 13–17, p. 15.
37. See Feldblum, C. R. "Home Health Care for the Elderly: Programs, Problems, and Potentials." *Harvard Journal on Legislation,* 1985, *22,* 193–254.

38. Short, P. F., and Leon, J. *Use of Home and Community Services by Persons Ages 65 and Older with Functional Difficulties.* (National Medical Expenditure Survey Research Findings, 5, Agency for Health Care Policy and Research.) Rockville, MD: Public Health Service, 1990; Prohaska, T., Mermelstein, R., Miller, B., and Jack, S. "Functional Status and Living Arrangements." In J. F. Van Nostrand, S. E. Furner, and R. Suzman (eds.), *Health Data on Older Americans: United States, 1992.* Hyattsville, Md.: National Center for Health Statistics, 1993.

39. Agency for Health Care Policy and Research. "The Elderly with Functional Difficulties: Characteristics of Users of Home and Community Services." AHCPR publication no. 92-0112. Rockville, Md.: Public Health Service, July 1992.

40. Kane, R. A., Kane, R. L., Illston, L. H., and Eustis, N. N. "Perspectives on Home Care Quality." *Health Care Financing Review,* Fall 1994, *16,* 69–89.

41. Day (1996).

42. Blesch, K. S., and Furner, S. E. "Health of Older Black Americans." In Van Nostrand, Furner, and Suzman (1993).

43. Wallace, S. P., and Lew-Ting, C.-Y. "Getting by at Home: Community-Based Long-Term Care of Latino Elders." *Western Journal of Medicine,* Sept. 1992, *157,* 337–344.

44. Park-Tanjasiri, S., and Wallace, S. P. "Picture Imperfect: Hidden Problems Among Asian Pacific Islander Elderly." *Gerontologist,* Dec. 1995, *35,* 753–760.

45. Day (1996).

46. U.S. Census Bureau. "National Households and Families Projections, May 1996." (Public-use data file and documentation.) [http://www.census.gov/population/www/projections/nathh.html.] Dec. 1999.

47. Parker, M. G., Thorslund, M., and Lundberg, O. "Physical Function and Social Class Among Swedish Oldest Old." *Journals of Gerontology, Social Sciences,* July 1994, *49,* S196–S201.

48. House, J. S., and others. "The Social Stratification of Aging and Health." *Journal of Health and Social Behavior,* Sept. 1994, *35,* 213–234.

49. Taeuber, C. M., and Allen, J. "Women in Our Aging Society: The Demographic Outlook." In J. Allen and A. Pifer (eds.), *Women on the Front Lines: Meeting the Challenges of an Aging America.* Washington, D.C.: Urban Institute Press, 1993.

50. U.S. Census Bureau. *Money Income in the United States: 1998.* (Current Population Reports, P60–206.) Washington, D.C.: U.S. Government Printing Office, 1999.

51. Dalaker, J. *Poverty in the United States: 1998.* (U.S. Census Bureau, Current Population Reports, Series P60–207.) Washington, D.C.: U.S. Government Printing Office, 1998; Pourat, N. "Racial/Ethnic Differences in Utilization of Long-Term Care Services Among the Elderly." UMI Dissertation Services, 1995.

52. Markides, K. S. "Minority Aging." In M. W. Riley, B. B. Hess, and K. Bond (eds.), *Aging in Society: Selected Reviews of Recent Research.* Hillsdale, N.J.: Erlbaum, 1983.

53. Laditka, S. B. "Modeling Lifetime Nursing Home Use Under Assumptions of Better Health." *Journals of Gerontology, Series B: Psychological Sciences and Social Sciences,* 1998, *53*(4), S177–S187.

54. Murtaugh, C. M., Kemper, P., and Spillman, B. C. "The Risk of Nursing Home Use in Later Life." *Medical Care,* 1990, *28,* 952–962.

55. Damron-Rodriguez, J., Wallace, S. P., and Kington, R. "Service Utilization and Minority Elderly: Appropriateness, Accessibility and Acceptability." *Gerontology and Geriatrics Education,* 1994, *15,* 45–64.

56. Wallace, Levy-Storms, Kington, and Andersen (1998).

57. Miller, B., McFall, S., and Campbell, R. T. "Changes in Sources of Community Long-Term Care Among African American and White Frail Older Persons." *Journals of Gerontology, Social Sciences,* Jan. 1994, *49,* S14–S24; Wallace, S. P., Levy-Storms, L., and Ferguson, L. R. "Access to Paid In-Home Assistance Among Disabled Elderly People: Do Latinos Differ from Non-Latino Whites?" *American Journal of Public Health,* July 1995, *85,* 970–975; Mauser, E., and Miller, N. A. "A Profile of Home Health Users in 1992." *Health Care Financing Review,* 1994, *16*(1), 17–33; Wallace, S. P., Snyder, J., Walker, G., and Ingman, S. "Racial Differences Among Users of Long-Term Care: The Case of Adult Day Care." *Research on Aging,* Dec. 1992, *14,* 471–495.

58. Kemper, P. "The Use of Formal and Informal Home Care by the Disabled Elderly." *Health Services Research,* Oct. 1992, *27,* 421–451; Bass, D. M., and Noelker, L. S. "The Influence of Family Caregivers on Elders' Use of In-Home Services: An Expanded Conceptual Framework." *Journal of Health and Social Behavior,* 1987, *28,* 184–196; Wallace, S. P., Levy-Storms, L., Kington, R. S., and Andersen, R. M. "The Persistence of Race and Ethnicity in the Use of Long-Term Care." *Journals of Gerontology, Series B, Psychological Sciences and Social Sciences,* 1998, *53*(2), S104–112.

59. Barresi, C. M., and Menon, G. "Diversity in Black Family Caregiving." In Z. Harel, E. A. McKinney, and M. Williams (eds.), *Black Aged: Understanding Diversity and Service Needs.* Thousand Oaks, Calif.: Sage, in cooperation with National Council on the Aging, 1990); Spence, S. A., and Atherton, C. R. "The Black Elderly and the Social Service Delivery System: A Study of Factors Influencing the Use of Community-Based Services." *Journal of Gerontological Social Work,* 1991, *16,* 19–35.

60. Holmes, D., Teresi, J., and Holmes, M. "Differences Among Black, Hispanic, and White People in Knowledge About Long-Term Care Services." *Health Care Financing Review,* 1985, *5,* 51–67; Falcone, D., and Broyles, R. "Access to Long-Term Care: Race as a Barrier." *Journal of Health Politics, Policy, and Law,* 1995, *19,* 583–595; Wallace, S. P. "The Political Economy of Health Care for Elderly Blacks." *International Journal of Health Services,* 1990, *20,* 665–680.

61. Wallace, S. P., Enriquez-Haass, V., and Markides, K. "The Consequences of Color-Blind Health Policy for Older Racial and Ethnic Minorities." *Stanford Law and Policy Review,* 1998, *9*(2), 329–346.

62. Estes, C. L. "The Politics of Aging in America." *Aging and Society,* 1986, *6,* 121–134; Meyer, M. H. "Gender, Race, and the Distribution of Social Assistance: Medicaid Use Among the Frail Elderly." *Gender and Society,* Mar. 1994, *8,* 8–28.

63. Ettner, S. L. "Do Elderly Medicaid Patients Experience Reduced Access to Nursing Home Care?" *Journal of Health Economics,* Oct. 1993, *12,* 259–280; Buchanan, R. J., Madel, P., and Persons, D. "Medicaid Payment Policies for Nursing Home Care: A National Survey." *Health Care Financing Review,* Fall 1991, *13,* 55–72; Committee on Nursing Home Regulation (1986).

64. Lewin and Associates, Inc. "An Evaluation of the Medi-Cal Program's System for Establishing Reimbursement Rates for Nursing Homes." (Submitted to the Office of the Auditor General, State of California, 1987).

65. Rivlin, A. M., and Wiener, J. M. *Caring for the Disabled Elderly: Who Will Pay?* Washington, D.C.: Brookings Institution, 1988; Cohen, J. W., and Spector, W. D. "The Effect of Medicaid Reimbursement of Quality of Care in Nursing Homes." *Journal of Health Economics,* 1996, *15*(1), 23–48.

66. Meyer (1994); Estes, Swan, and Associates (1993).

67. Liu, K., Manton, K. G., and Liu, B. M. "Home Care Expenses for the Disabled Elderly." *Health Care Financing Review,* 1985, *7,* 51–58; Kane, N. M. "The Home Care Crisis of the Nineties." *Gerontologist,* 1989, *29,* 24–31.

68. U.S. Select Committee on Aging. *Aging America: Trends and Projections.* Washington, D.C.: U.S. Department of Health and Human Services, 1991.

69. Holden, K. C., and Smeeding, T. M. "The Poor, the Rich, and the Insecure Elderly Caught in Between." *Milbank Quarterly,* 1990, *68,* 191–219.

70. Hoechst Marion Roussel. *Managed Care Digest Series.* Kansas City, Mo.: Hoechst Marion Roussel, 1999.

71. Estes, Swan, and Associates (1993); Hoechst Marion Roussel (1999).

72. Hoechst Marion Roussel (1999).

73. Hoechst Marion Roussel (1999).

74. Wallace, Levy-Storms, Andersen, and Kington (1997).

75. Abel, E. K. *Who Cares for the Elderly? Public Policy and the Experiences of Adult Daughters.* Philadelphia: Temple University Press, 1991.

76. See Rivlin and Wiener (1988).

77. Ricardo-Campbell, R. "Aging and the Private Sector." *Generations,* Spring 1988, *12,* 19–22; Kane, Kane and Ladd (1998).

78. Leutz, W. N. "Long-Term Care for the Elderly: Public Dreams and Private Realities." *Inquiry,* 1986, *23,* 134–140.

79. U.S. General Accounting Office. Baby Boom Generation Presents Financing Challenges. GAO/T-HEHS-98-107. Washington, D.C.: U.S. General Accounting Office, 1998.

80. Leutz (1986), p. 139.

81. Shanas, E. "The Family as a Social Support System in Old Age." *Gerontologist,* 1979, *19,* 169–174.

82. See Abel (1991), pp. 3–4.

83. Stone, R. I., and Kemper, P. "Spouses and Children of Disabled Elders: How Large a Constituency for Long-Term Care Reform?" *Milbank Quarterly,* 1989, *67*(2–3), 485–506.

84. Stone, R. I., Cafferata, L., and Sangl, J. "Caregivers of the Frail Elderly: A National Profile." *Gerontologist,* 1987, *27*(5), 616–626.

85. Robinson, K. M. "Family Caregiving: Who Provides the Care, and at What Cost?" *Nursing Economics,* 1997, *15*(5), 243–247.

86. Stephens, S. A., and Christianson, J. B. *Informal Care of the Elderly.* Lexington, Mass.: Lexington, 1986.

87. See Abel (1991).

88. Montgomery, R.J.V. "Respite Care: Lessons from a Controlled Design Study." *Health Care Financing Review* (Annual Supplement), 1988, 133–138; and Wallace (1990). Respite programs take the form of either homemaker and home health services in the home or adult day care and foster care homes in the community.

89. See Hooyman, N. R., and Gonyea, J. *Feminist Perspectives on Family Care: Policies for Gender Justice.* Thousand Oaks, Calif.: Sage, 1995.

90. Burwell, B. O. "Shared Obligations: Public Policy Influences on Family Care for the Elderly." (Medicaid Program Evaluation Working Paper 2.1.) Washington, D.C.: Health Care Financing Administration, 1986.

91. Gerstel, N., and McGonagle, K. "The Limits of the Family and Medical Leave Act." Paper presented at the American Sociological Association Meeting, San Francisco, Aug. 1998.

92. Hooyman and Gonyea (1995).

93. Hooyman and Gonyea (1995).

94. Abel (1991).

95. Donovan, R. "'We Care for the Most Important People in Your Life': Home Care Workers in New York City." *Women's Studies Quarterly,* 1989, *17,* 56–65.

96. MacAdam, M. "Supply of Aides Working with the Elderly: What Do We Know from the Research?" In J. Handy and C. K. Schuerman (eds.), *Challenges and Innovations in Homecare.* San Francisco: American Society on Aging, 1994; Hayashi, R., Gibson, J. W., and Weatherley, R. A. "Working Conditions in Home Care: A Survey of Washington State's Home Care Workers." *Home Health Care Services Quarterly,* 1994, *14,* 37–48.

97. Quinlan, A. *Chronic Care Workers: Crisis Among Paid Caregivers of the Elderly.* Washington, D.C.: Older Women's League, 1988.

98. Diamond, T. *Making Gray Gold: Narratives of Nursing Home Care.* Chicago: University of Chicago Press, 1992, pp. 44–45.

99. Heard, N. L. "Recruitment and Retention of Home Care Aides: Promoting Employee Longevity." *Caring,* 1993, *12*(4), 12–15; Clinco, J. B. "The Personal Assistant: A New Option for Home Care." *Caring,* 1995, *14*(4), 65–67.

100. See Foner, N. *The Caregiving Dilemma: Work in an American Nursing Home.* Berkeley: University of California Press, 1994; Helmer, F. T., Olson, S. F., and Heim, R. I. "Strategies for Nurse Aide Job Satisfaction." *Journal of Long-Term Care Administration,* Summer 1993, *21,* 10–14; Grau, L., Chandler, B., Burton, B., and Kolditz, D. "Institutional Loyalty and Job Satisfaction Among Nurse Aides in Nursing Homes." *Journal of Aging and Health,* Feb. 1991, *3,* 47–65.

101. Bowers, B., and Becker, M. "Nurse's Aides in Nursing Homes: The Relationship between Organization and Quality." *Gerontologist,* June 1992, *32,* 360–366.

102. Foner (1994).

103. Stefanowicz, P. "Home Care for the Frail Elderly: Implications of the Worker/Client Relationship for Quality." Paper presented at the Annual Meeting of the Gerontological Society of America, Atlanta, 1994.

CHAPTER TEN

AIDS IN THE TWENTY-FIRST CENTURY

Challenges for Health Services and Public Health

David M. Mosen, Denise R. Globe,
and William E. Cunningham

The epidemic of acquired immune deficiency syndrome (AIDS) presents to the health care system myriad challenges, which have changed over time. In the 1980s and early 1990s, there were few highly effective treatments. However, recent advancements in the treatment of human immunodeficiency virus (HIV) disease now offer great hope of longer survival and better quality of life for persons with HIV disease. New treatments have demonstrated reduced morbidity and mortality associated with HIV infection.[1] But frequent side effects, the development of drug-resistant HIV, and the unknown durability of the suppressive action of antiretroviral regimens render uncertain their long-term effects on quality of life and survival.[2] Furthermore, HIV disease remains contagious, often disabling, and frequently fatal. Of particular concern is evidence of a lack of equity in the treatment of HIV disease among minorities, women, the uninsured and Medicaid insured, and heterosexual and injection drug users, compared to other groups.[3] Such challenges increasingly force health care policy makers, planners, and administrators to reevaluate the organization, delivery, and financing of AIDS health services.

Health services providers and researchers must understand the needs of people infected with HIV, as well as accessibility to care, cost of care, and quality of services. In this chapter, we cover these key issues in health services. First, important characteristics of the changing epidemiology and treatment patterns of AIDS should be understood in the context of real-life health care delivery.

Second, providers and managers need to integrate emerging data on the accessibility, costs, and quality of services in this era of more effective AIDS treatment. At the same time, the unique problems of diverse subpopulations and service systems should be addressed more rigorously. Third, these issues need to be examined not only within the arena of formal medical services but more broadly within the continuum of care, from prevention to ambulatory medical and psychosocial services and to hospital and long-term care. Fourth, the implications and research needs for policy, planning, and program administration in health services will be considered.

Developing an approach for addressing the various agendas within the context of national and local health policy for HIV, as well as other chronic diseases, is paramount. In this chapter, existing knowledge about critical issues of HIV/AIDS is discussed. The purpose is to present the necessary background for addressing the challenges of the disease and for developing health policy, planning, and program implementation. Approaches to critical policy problems are suggested, and the crucial areas for new investigation are identified to guide future HIV/AIDS health policy.

The Changing Epidemiology and Clinical Treatment of HIV/AIDS

Both the epidemiology and the clinical treatment of HIV/AIDS are changing. There are broad implications for health services.

Epidemiology

AIDS is a chronic infection, characterized by progressive failure of the immune system and development of opportunistic infections or cancers. HIV is an unusual type of virus (known as a retrovirus) that causes immune suppression leading to AIDS. Individuals infected with HIV develop antibodies within a short period of time and may exhibit no symptoms for many years. Typically, the immune system weakens gradually and the blood level of CD4 cells (a type of white blood cell known as a T-helper/inducer lymphocyte) declines from a normal level of 1,200–1,400 cells/mm^3. Persons with few CD4 cells are prone to opportunistic infections and certain cancers. Such symptoms as persistent fevers, night sweats, and weight loss begin to occur more frequently when the CD4 count drops below 500 cells/mm^3.

It is unclear whether all persons with asymptomatic HIV infection and CD4 count > 200 will eventually go on to develop AIDS; a small proportion of those infected have shown no sign of immune failure after more than a decade.[4] In addition to the CD4 count, the most powerful predictor of survival is the quantity of HIV RNA per ml of serum (known as viral load).[5] The development of AIDS has been estimated at eleven years from time of HIV infection.[6] However, with new generations of HIV treatment regimens, it is not clear how long survival can be prolonged. There is hope, however, that HIV will soon become a chronic disease like hypertension or diabetes, which are rarely fatal or disabling if timely, high-quality care is provided. New treatments, such as integrase inhibitors, fusion inhibitors, and immune modulators may be available soon, leading to additional hope and additional challenges.[7]

Worldwide, an estimated 70,930,000 individuals are living or have lived with HIV; of these, 1,800,000 adults have died of AIDS. Currently, it is estimated that about 900,000 Americans are infected with HIV, among them a growing number of women and persons of color (Table 10.1).[8] As of December 31, 1998, 688,200 people were diagnosed with AIDS, and there have been 410,800 deaths from AIDS, for a case-fatality rate of 60 percent.

For the first time since 1987, HIV is *not* on the list of the fifteen leading causes of death in the United States for 1998.[9] However, AIDS remains the leading cause of death for blacks age twenty-five to forty-four.[10] Although the overall number of annual deaths has dropped by more than 50 percent from a high of 49,897 in 1995 to 21,437 in 1997, women and people of color account for a larger proportion of AIDS-related deaths in 1997 than they did in 1995 (Table 10.2). The reduction in mortality is thought to be due to improvements in treatment, although improved health has not been the case as much for women as for men, nor for persons of color compared to whites. Further evidence of the overall improvement of the health of persons with HIV in the United States is the reduction in age-adjusted mortality rate for HIV (5.9 per hundred thousand in 1997 compared to 15.6 per hundred thousand in 1995) and the 30 percent decline in the rate of hospitalization for HIV between 1995 and 1997.[11] As we shall discuss, inequitable distribution of treatment to persons of colors, women, and other disadvantaged groups probably accounts for the corresponding disparity in health improvement for these groups.

Widely recognized risk factors for transmission of HIV include male-to-male sexual contact, male-to-female sexual contact, injection drug use (IDU), blood product exposure, and perinatal transmission from mother to infant (during pregnancy, delivery, or possibly breast feeding). Frequently, individuals are exposed through multiple infection routes, so the actual mode of HIV transmission may be unclear. A substantial portion of HIV-infected persons are unaware of their underlying HIV infection. Many cases of HIV infection remain underreported, because they may not meet the Centers for Disease Control (CDC) definition of AIDS and some states have no reporting requirements for HIV infection; the

TABLE 10.1. CUMULATIVE AIDS CASES IN THE UNITED STATES, THROUGH DECEMBER 1998.

Category	Number (688,200)	Percentage
Gender		
Male	574,783	84
Female	113,414	16
Unknown		
Ethnicity		
White, not Hispanic	304,094	44
Black, not Hispanic	251,408	37
Hispanic	124,841	18
Asian or Pacific Islander	4,974	1
American Indian or Alaska Native	1,940	0
Exposure		
Adult ($n = 679,739$)		
Men who have sex with men	326,051	48
Injection drug use	173,693	26
Men who have sex with men and inject drugs	43,640	6
Hemophilia or coagulation disorder	4,911	1
Heterosexual contact	66,490	10
Blood transfusion, blood components or tissue	8,382	1
Other or risk not reported or identified	56,572	8
Exposure		
Pediatric ($n = 8,461$)		
Hemophilia or coagulation disorder	234	3
Mother with or at risk for HIV infection	7,687	91
Blood transfusion, blood components or tissue	378	4
Other or risk not reported or identified	162	2
Residence by census area		
Metropolitan area with population > 500,000	578,010	84
Metropolitan area with 50,000 to 500,000	67,076	10
Nonmetropolitan area	39,856	6

Source: Data for this table taken from Department of Health and Human Services, Centers for Disease Control and Prevention, *HIV AIDS Surveillance Report,* 1998, *10*(2), 1–43. Data are for fifty states, the District of Columbia, and U.S. dependencies, possessions, and independent nations in free association with the United States. Includes pediatric cases under age twelve for Connecticut and Texas and under age six for Oregon.

TABLE 10.2. CHANGE IN RATE OF DEATH OF PERSONS WITH AIDS IN THE UNITED STATES, 1992 THROUGH 1997.

Category	Year						Percentage Change
	1992	1993	1994	1995	1996	1997	1995–1997
Gender							
Male	35,762	38,317	41,320	41,375	30,036	16,697	−60
Female	5,083	6,041	7,411	7,382	6,900	4,523	−39
Ethnicity							
White, not Hispanic	20,411	21,438	22,221	21,550	14,264	6,992	−68
Black, not Hispanic	13,373	15,320	17,747	18,813	15,827	10,183	−46
Hispanic	7,106	7,666	6,766	8,949	5,848	4,034	−55
Asian or Pacific Islander	270	306	40	357	278	144	−60
American Indian or Alaska Native	7	132	144	186	119	74	−60
Exposure							
Adult							
Men who have sex with men	22,791	23,634	24,919	24,369	16,523	8,348	−66
Injection drug use	10,829	12,304	13,923	14,429	11,694	7,390	−49
Men who have sex with men and inject drugs	2,783	3,072	3,382	3,321	2,488	1,349	−59
Hemophilia or coagulation disorder	353	368	370	357	264	155	−57
Heterosexual contact	3,173	4,160	5,393	6,231	5,480	3,620	−42
Blood transfusion, blood components or tissue	574	549	530	488	410	216	−56
Other or risk not reported or identified	345	271	217	165	97	68	−59
Pediatric (under thirteen years old)	423	537	576	537	424	217	−60

Residence by region							
Northeast	12,905	13,966	15,821	15,792	11,554	6,775	−57
Midwest	4,223	4,738	5,142	5,391	4,031	2,185	−59
South	13,119	14,369	16,025	16,980	13,539	8,166	−52
West	9,610	10,271	10,575	10,055	6,682	3,311	−67
U.S. dependencies, possessions, and associated nations	1,413	1,553	1,749	1,679	1,554	1,001	−40
Total	41,270	44,896	49,311	49,897	37,359	21,437	−57

Source: Data for this table taken from Department of Health and Human Services, Centers for Disease Control and Prevention, *HIV AIDS Surveillance Report,* 1998, *10*(2), 1–43. Data are for fifty states, the District of Columbia, and U.S. dependencies, possessions, and independent nations in free association with the United States. Includes pediatric cases under age twelve for Connecticut and Texas and under age six for Oregon. These numbers are point estimates adjusted for delays in the reporting of deaths but not for incomplete reporting of deaths.

accuracy of diagnosing and reporting HIV/AIDS also varies by geographic location and affected population. The growth of the HIV/AIDS epidemic is, however, in large part due to changes in the mode of transmission and the sociodemographic characteristics of the groups in which the epidemic is growing fastest.[12] Contrary to the early epidemic, the rate of increase in HIV transmission is now slower among whites and homosexuals than in communities of color and heterosexuals.

Treatment

The main type of treatment is medication to combat loss of immune function and to prevent specific disease complications. The most widely used drugs are antiretrovirals, which slow the progress of HIV infection and boost immune function. Some of the earliest developed antiretrovirals that were used to treat HIV disease were in the class of drugs known as nucleoside reverse transcriptase inhibitors, including zidovudine (ZDV/AZT), didanosine (ddI), and zalcitabine or dideoxycitidine (ddC). However, newer generations of antiretrovirals have also come into widespread use, expanding the armamentarium of treatments. In particular, protease inhibitors (PI) and nonnucleoside reverse transcriptase inhibitors (NNRTI) are frequently key ingredients, in combinations that often include three or more medications. Such combinations, or "cocktails" constitute what has become known as highly active antiretroviral therapy (HAART).

Accumulating data from clinical and pathogenesis studies support institution of combination antiretroviral therapy for patients with HIV infection and evidence of declining immune function.[13] Thus, delay in diagnosing HIV or instituting therapy is thought to represent poor access or poor quality of care. Despite gains in developing HAART medications, several problems still exist. First, HIV sometimes develops resistance to antiretroviral medication. Second, severe side effects and complications often affect people taking these medications. Third, in order for persons with HIV infection to obtain full benefit from treatment, they must withstand a variety of difficulties in adhering to treatment with a large number of pills and a complex dosing regimen for a long period of time.

Antibiotics are frequently used to prevent or treat a common pneumonia (pneumocystis carinii, or PCP) or other opportunistic infection that develops in a person with AIDS.[14] Recent research suggests that opportunistic infection prophylaxis (for example, against PCP) may be discontinued for certain patients with restored immune function as a result of receiving combination antiretroviral therapy.[15] In a study of 262 patients in the Swiss HIV Cohort Study, patients who were able to raise the CD4 level to at least 200 cells/mm^3 (through combination antiretroviral therapy) did not develop PCP or other opportunistic infection.[16]

Most clinical services are directed toward monitoring for immune function decline, development of specific HIV complications (PCP, infectious diarrhea, central nervous system infection), and reduction of treatment side effects. This monitoring involves using the full range of medical services, from physical examination to radiology and laboratory tests. Ongoing monitoring is also important because concomitant infectious diseases (such as tuberculosis and hepatitis) and metabolic complications of treatment (diabetes, lipid disorders) remain a common problem. Laboratory testing of infecting HIV specimen for resistance to various treatments has become a growing part of clinical care for HIV-infected persons.[17] In the absence of a complete cure from traditional medical treatment, many people with HIV/AIDS may also resort to alternative medicine. Alternative therapies fall into four primary groups: nonconventional drug treatment, nutrition and diet modification (vitamins, minerals, and herbs), acupuncture or chiropractic, and psychospiritual intervention. Estimates of the incidence of alternative therapy usage range from 29 percent to 42 percent of AIDS patients surveyed.[18]

Challenges of HIV/AIDS for Health Services: Access, Costs, and Quality

Investigators are beginning to shed light on important patterns in how persons with HIV/AIDS use health services. Available information on population and system characteristics and how they determine access to medical care, costs, and quality of service are important considerations. Nationally representative data from the HIV Costs and Services Utilization Study (HCSUS) are beginning to fill many critical gaps in information on these topics.

Access to Care

Access to care in HIV is often assessed by existence of regular medical care and coverage of services, as well as by an absence of delays and barriers to care.

Access to Regular Medical Care and Delays in Care. Having a regular source of medical care is recognized as important for the general population, as well as for those with various chronic diseases. Problems in access to care for persons with HIV may be reflected in the degree to which they are in regular care. The HCSUS estimated that about half (between 36 and 63 percent) of all nonmilitary, nonincarcerated adults in the contiguous United States with known or unknown HIV infection see a provider outside of an emergency room at least every six months.[19]

More than three months elapsed from the initial HIV-positive test until first medical care for HIV in nearly one-third of the HCSUS national sample of HIV-infected persons in regular care. The median duration of this delay was one year.[20] In a progressive infection such as HIV, such a lengthy delay is alarming, from a personal and a public health standpoint.[21] Opportunities for education about the disease, transmission to others, and social support may be missed during such a delay.

Public Benefits, Income, and Health Insurance. As HIV disease progresses, many persons experience disability and unemployment and rely on public entitlements and private disability programs for income maintenance and health care benefits. These include Social Security Disability Income (SSDI) and Supplemental Security Income (SSI), administered by the Social Security Administration. Medicaid and Medicare become primary payers for health care with the onset of disability and depletion of personal funds.

Overall, much of the HIV-infected population is covered by public insurance.[22] It is estimated that 29 percent of the population in care is covered by Medicaid alone and 19 percent is covered by Medicare with or without other insurance coverage. Private insurance covers 32 percent of the HIV population, while 20 percent of those with HIV disease have no health insurance coverage. Public insurance also finances the majority of HIV-related care.[23] Although public insurance covers about half of the HIV population, it accounts for 62 percent of HIV-related costs. Private insurance accounts for only 28 percent of HIV-related costs, while the uninsured account for 11 percent of HIV-related costs.[24]

Lack of private health insurance may affect the utilization pattern. For example, many states limit Medicaid coverage for the number of inpatient hospital days per year. This policy creates financial risk for providers as the average length of stay and the number of admissions are often higher for those with AIDS-related illnesses (compared to non–AIDS-related illnesses).[25] Furthermore, those with public insurance have a longer than average length of stay compared to those with private insurance. Lower use of outpatient care among those with public insurance may contribute to the longer average length of hospital stay.[26]

As with other costly chronic conditions, insurance companies have sometimes denied benefits to HIV-positive individuals based on preexisting conditions. Insurance companies sometimes require HIV antibody testing of insurance applicants and deny policies to those testing positive. Litigation has been one common avenue to resolve eligibility for health insurance benefits.[27]

Barriers to Care. Lack of insurance and underinsurance represent formidable financial barriers to treatment for HIV/AIDS.[28] Persons with HIV/AIDS are more likely than the general population to be uninsured or to have Medicaid insurance.[29] Although evidence suggests that access to care for the uninsured and Medicaid populations increased between 1996 and 1998, it still remains suboptimal.[30] Compared to those with private insurance, the uninsured and those with Medicaid are less likely to receive protease inhibitor therapy and more likely to have never received any antiretroviral medication.[31] Even among the insured, substantial disparities in access persist thanks to other barriers to care, such as competing subsistence needs. For example, HCSUS found that more than one-third of subjects went without or postponed medical care because of one or more subsistence needs; and that minorities, women, and drug users were most likely to report these problems. Going without or postponing care for one of the four subsistence needs was associated with significantly greater multivariate odds of never receiving antiretrovirals (ARVs) and having low overall access to care.[32]

Competing caregiver responsibilities may also prevent persons with HIV disease from receiving timely medical care. About 16 percent of HIV-infected patients with children delay seeking medical care, while 14 percent of those living with another HIV-positive individual also delay seeking medical care in HCSUS. Generally, women are more likely to report putting off care than men because they are more likely to be caring for someone else.[33] Thus, studies of the HCSUS sample have shown that addressing social needs may actually compete (in terms of time, energy, and money) with obtaining medical care. Other barriers may include disability from HIV/AIDS disease, loss of employment, and social stigma, resulting in the loss of private insurance coverage or moving to less generous coverage.[34] Others may be reluctant to use their private insurance because of concern about confidentiality and threat to employment.

Lack of insurance, poverty, and underuse of ambulatory services often coincide within the groups in which the epidemic is spreading most rapidly. For example, research early in the epidemic found that disadvantaged groups (minorities, women, injection drug users) often lack insurance, have difficulty with access to continuity care, and do not receive needed treatment.[35] Research conducted since the advent of HAART found that blacks, Latinos, and women continue to have trouble accessing important HIV treatment.[36] Compared to whites, blacks were more likely to have poor access to outpatient care and less likely to receive protease inhibitors.[37] In addition, female injection drug users were less likely to receive highly active antiretroviral therapy compared to homosexual men.[38]

The high costs associated with newly developed AIDS medications (not all of which are covered by insurance) may also serve as a barrier to treatment for disadvantaged groups. Studies of the diffusion of such AIDS treatments as zidovudine show that when new AIDS treatments are developed it takes time for them to diffuse through the population, and they often do so unevenly.[39]

A similar pattern has been observed in more recent studies of protease inhibitors.[40] Big gaps tend to be found between advantaged and disadvantaged groups in the use of new treatments, particularly a short time after they are introduced into the population, but the gap tends to converge over time (though not disappear).[41] One reason blacks and other disadvantaged groups have delayed access to the newest, most effective treatments may be that they are less likely to participate in clinical trials because of access barriers, mistrust, or poorer health status.[42]

Stability and continuity of care are particularly important for those with HIV infection. However, discontinuity in HIV care has been identified as a problem in obtaining appropriate access to care.[43] A cohort study in one low-socioeconomic urban population found that failure to suppress viral load with HAART was associated with higher rates of missed clinic appointments, non-white ethnicity, and drug use.[44] One potential consequence of discontinuity is greater use of the emergency department for nonemergency medical services. Inadequate access is often cited as the reason for inappropriate ER use.[45] HCSUS found that individuals with suboptimal access to care also overuse emergency room care.[46] In addition to continuity, comprehensiveness of care is important in ensuring optimal care. For example, evidence suggests that access to a broad range of services is associated with better outcomes in that poor access to comprehensive general medical care has been shown to result in poor access to needed PCP prophylaxis.[47]

Other nonfinancial barriers are language barriers, cultural competence, and illiteracy, and similar problems. For example, a recent study found that Latinos had poorer survival compared to whites, even after controlling for insurance status, socioeconomic status, and regular source of care. These findings suggest that Latinos may face access barriers related to language and culture that result in suboptimal treatment and worse outcomes.[48]

Access to care also may be related to costs of HIV care, prevention, and health outcomes. In a study of hospitalized HIV patients in Southern California, better access to comprehensive community-based services was associated with less hospitalization for HIV disease, which suggests that costs may be reduced with adequate access to care.[49] In this sample of patients, better access to general medical care was also associated with greater use of pre-hospital HIV testing and counseling.[50] Other research on persons with symptomatic HIV disease found that better access to care predicted improved health-related quality-of-life (HRQOL) outcomes.[51] Thus, augmenting access to care may prevent spread of the disease and improve outcomes without excessive costs.

Costs

The current annual expenditures to treat HIV disease are estimated to be $6.7 billion, or about $20,000 per patient per year. About 46 percent of these costs are for hospitalization, and 40 percent for medication.[52] Total pharmaceutical costs in 1997 were about $9,000 per person per year, $7,000 of which was for antiretroviral medications.[53] Since the beginning of the epidemic, the largest category of direct AIDS care costs has been for hospital utilization. However, there has been an overall reduction in hospital use, since the advent of HAART medications: 30 percent reduction in the number of hospitalizations and 40 percent reduction in the number of days hospitalized.[54]

Thus AIDS costs are not as great as feared earlier in the epidemic, and there is little reason to expect that AIDS costs will become disproportionate to other chronic diseases and threaten the financing system. The $6.7 billion in annual expenditures that HIV care consumed is less than 1 percent of the more than $700 billion spent on health care in 1996. This may be considered relatively small in relation to the 7 percent of total potential years of life lost because of HIV in the United States—an amount more than the comparable loss from pneumonia, influenza, chronic obstructive pulmonary disease, diabetes mellitus, and chronic liver disease combined.[55] However, there is preliminary evidence that costs vary greatly as a function of the population served, the type of provider, and the region of the country.

Because it is known that sicker patients cost more regardless of the disease, there is concern that much of this variation is related to the adequacy of outpatient care provided to diverse populations. Inadequate outpatient care could result in delayed initiation of HAART treatment or treatment with less effective medications and result in higher morbidity and mortality, development of preventable opportunistic infections, and rapid progression of the disease. Available data suggests that HIV/AIDS patients from groups with lower socioeconomic status and less access to care (minorities, drug users, and women) make use of costlier sources of care (such as emergency rooms and hospitals) and for longer duration, raising the concern that these variations in costs are due to variation in provider quality. Hence, the costs of HIV/AIDS care should be examined in the context of the quality of care as well.

Quality of Care

Studies of quality of care in AIDS cover underuse of needed therapy, provider experience in delivering appropriate care, patient satisfaction with and adherence to therapy, and quality of life and other outcomes.

Underuse of Therapy. The emphasis of HIV/AIDS quality-of-care assessment centers on whether those with HIV/AIDS receive appropriate clinical treatment specific to their stage of HIV disease. Despite available clinical guidelines to inform HIV providers, certain subpopulations are less likely to receive these treatments. In HCSUS, blacks and women were less likely to receive HAART therapy, compared to whites and white men respectively.[56] In addition, blacks and Hispanics were less likely to receive appropriate PCP and mycobacterium avium complex (MAC) prophylactic therapies, compared to whites.[57] Other research found that public insurance (compared to private insurance) may be associated with a poorer level of quality, or inappropriate care.[58]

Hospital and Physician Experience and Specialization. Experience in treating HIV disease is another important predictor of better-quality care. Studies have found that hospitals and staffs with greater experience in treating HIV/AIDS produce lower inpatient mortality.[59] Similarly, greater physician experience in treating HIV/AIDS also predicts longer survival.[60] Although controversial, the preponderance of evidence in AIDS indicates that the critical factor in producing better quality care is experience with a sufficient volume of patients with AIDS, rather than specialty certification in infectious disease, immunology, or oncology.[61]

Patient Satisfaction. Satisfaction is also an important indicator of the quality of care and adequacy of services for those with HIV disease. Patient dissatisfaction has been shown in the general population to predict utilization, continuity of care, switching providers, adherence to treatment, delay in obtaining treatment, and health outcomes.[62] In a study of persons with AIDS, Stein and others found that IDUs, the uninsured, and public hospital patients were less satisfied with the technical and interpersonal care they received, as well as with their access to care.[63] Similarly, in a study in Boston, blacks and drug users had lower patient satisfaction in multivariate analysis.

Adherence to Treatment. Adherence is essential for successful treatment of people with HIV because inadequate dosing of antiretroviral medication may not suppress viral replication and may allow HIV to form new genetic variants of the virus. These variants can be resistant to entire classes of drugs, rendering certain combinations of drugs ineffective. Drug-resistant strains of HIV can also be transmitted to others, creating an alarming public health threat.[64] The reasons for nonadherence are multifaceted but must be understood in order to develop effective intervention.[65] Long-term adherence to treatment with an antiretroviral regimen is critical to survival with HIV infection, but problems in adherence are commonly reported. In HCSUS, only 57 percent of those who were taking antiretroviral medication reported that they actually took all their medications as they were prescribed.[66] Blacks, Hispanics, women, and heavy alcohol and drug users were the groups least likely to adhere to treatment. Surprisingly, adherence was not necessarily worse if there are more pills to take, but it was better when the individual was aware that the medications are effective and that nonadherence could lead to viral resistance. Other factors associated with poor adherence include adverse side effects, traveling, forgetfulness, emotional distress, lack of social support, poor relationship with one's provider, low education, and low health literacy.[67]

Health-Related Quality-of-Life Outcomes. The goal of providing medical care is to improve outcomes; thus outcomes are a marker of quality of care. One important outcome of HIV care is health-related quality of life. HRQOL is increasingly recognized as an important facet of health status and health service delivery for those with HIV disease, one that comprises physical and mental functioning and well-being from the perspective of individuals. HRQOL is perhaps one of the most important health outcomes to examine in HIV disease because of the bothersome symptomatology, high mortality, and resultant need for regular and urgent medical services. Various drug treatments for HIV may also affect HRQOL differently than it affects disease progression and physiological markers of outcomes.

Both clinical trials and observational studies of HIV disease now commonly include generic measures of HRQOL outcomes to evaluate the simultaneous effects of clinical intervention, treatment side effects, and disease impact over time.[68] HRQOL measures have been shown to be associated with CD4 count, symptom severity, length of hospital stay, and disease progression (from asymptomatic HIV infection, to symptomatic infection, to AIDS).[69] The association between HRQOL and the clinical indicators of the health status of the patient supports the hope that aggressive diagnostic evaluation and targeted treatment of abnormality may improve function and the patient's sense of well-being. Although there are associations between HRQOL and clinical and utilization measures, one study found that only 12–33 percent of the variability in HRQOL was accounted for by the clinical, use, and demographic variables examined,[70] suggesting that HRQOL measures tap aspects of health that extend beyond physiological parameters. Thus HRQOL measures can be useful tools for assessing both the physical and mental health outcomes of HIV disease within inpatient and outpatient settings. Associating HRQOL and the clinical indicators of health status of the patient supports the hope that astute diagnostic evaluation and targeted treatment of abnormality may improve function and the patient's sense of well-being.

Toward a Comprehensive Continuum of Care

Persons with HIV/AIDS often present themselves to the health care delivery system in need of immediate, acute care services. However, the course of the illness is now more commonly characterized by a gradual decline in physical, cognitive, and emotional function and well-being, which may require primary care, supportive care, housing, supervised living, home health care, and hospice services.[71] Intermittent episodes of severe complications sometimes represent specific disease complications or less definitive symptoms. A longer period of relative quiescence sometimes gives way to subtle decline in functioning and loss of ability to perform usual daily activities without assistance.[72] As a result, people living with AIDS often need a wide array of personal and social services to support community-based living in the least restrictive setting.[73]

Providing a continuum of care is the ideal. What the continuum of care consists of is open to debate and is shaped by the availability of financial resources supporting various programs. In general, the continuum can encompass prevention services, public benefits and insurance counseling, primary care, dental care, mental health care, substance abuse treatment, physical and occupational therapy, coordination of long-term care, social services, and secondary and tertiary medical care. Combining medical and supportive social services may be the best approach to providing a continuum of care at the community level.

Prevention and Education

Controlling the AIDS epidemic depends on education and public health strategies to reduce high-risk behaviors. Groups with increasing incidence are targeted for intervention: men who have sex with men, IDUs, women who have partners with risk factors, adolescents, and minority ethnic groups. Education and outreach have been major approaches to risk reduction. However, controversy continues to mount around condom education in schools and needle exchange programs. Such controversy has prevented implementing programs throughout the United States. Recent research estimates that only 2.2 percent of U.S. high schools offer condom education programs, while syringe distribution is illegal in all but four states.[74]

Despite lay concerns that condom education and needle exchange programs promote increased sexual activity and injection drug use respectively, recent empirical research found no justification for these concerns.[75] Condom education programs have not been associated with increased sexual activity in adolescents. Rather, research has demonstrated that condom education programs have increased condom use among young people who choose to lead a sexually active lifestyle.[76] Similarly, rather than promote further injection drug use, needle exchange programs have reduced HIV infection by increasing the availability of clean needles for those who choose to use injection drugs.[77]

Testing and counseling services are considered vital to monitoring HIV/AIDS; however, these practices are often underused. It is estimated that fewer than 40 percent of people in the United States with HIV risk factors have been tested for HIV.[78] Confidentiality concerns affect HIV testing and care-seeking behavior.[79] A substantial proportion of untested individuals say they would be tested if their test results could not be identified.[80] Furthermore, those tested anonymously sought testing and medical care earlier in the course of HIV disease than did people tested confidentially.[81]

There are many licensed tests for clinical diagnosis of HIV infection, but the most common is the enzyme-linked immunosorbent assay (ELISA) test. The Public Health Service has provided guidelines for counseling and testing, which are felt to "help uninfected individuals initiate and sustain behavioral changes that reduce their risk of becoming infected and to assist infected individuals in avoiding affecting others."[82] Studies have shown that access to continuous medical care is associated with timely receipt of HIV testing and counseling services.[83] Thus, regular access to medical care, in addition to behavioral risk reduction, is an important factor in reducing the transmission of HIV.

Because of recent breakthroughs in antiretroviral therapy, the use of postexposure prophylaxis (PEP) as a risk-reduction method has recently been given attention. PEP is the introduction of antiretroviral therapy after possible exposure to HIV through sexual contact or injection drug use. Although the CDC recommends using PEP for health care professionals occupationally exposed to HIV, health care workers are increasingly receiving inquiries from the public about PEP following nonoccupational high-risk HIV exposure (that is, sex or injection drug use). Although somewhat limited, recent research suggests that it would be reasonable to use PEP after exposure to HIV through sex and injection drug use, but only if the probability of exposure to HIV (through sex and injection drug use) is of the same order of magnitude as percutaneous occupational exposure.[84] For individuals with continuing or low-risk exposure, more traditional state-of-the-art risk-reduction programs (for example, education and outreach) are suggested.

Notifying the partners of people with HIV, though potentially beneficial in promoting risk reduction and prevention of HIV, is not systematically used across states. Because of concern for confidentiality, most states have voluntary programs and are not required to reveal the identity of the person infected. Additionally, notification is not possible if the index case has had anonymous sex partners, and it may be inefficient in a population with a high prevalence rate of HIV infection.

Mental Health and Drug Use

In the beginning of the AIDS epidemic, many community-based organizations, such as the Shanti Foundation, were created to help with the grief associated with death and dying from AIDS. As more people with HIV became long-term survivors, mental health services and formal and informal support networks have enjoyed new importance for the individual coping with the illness.

The prevalence of psychiatric disorder (major depression, dysthymia, generalized anxiety disorder, and panic attacks) and substance abuse is disproportionately high among those with HIV disease.[85] As in the general population, psychiatric and substance abuse disorders within the HIV population may impair quality of life, adversely affect access to appropriate health care, and compromise adherence with complicated medication regimens.[86] Psychiatric and substance abuse disorders may also be associated with sexual behavior and drug-using activity that endanger others with the risk of HIV infection.[87]

Thus there is substantial need for drug and alcohol abuse treatment. Reducing substance abuse can improve HIV prevention, as well as appropriate use of services and disorders. Many HIV-infected persons need treatment for psychiatric disorder, with or without concomitant medical treatment. To the extent that mental health, substance abuse, and medical services are all needed, patients would benefit from coordination of these services, for example by sharing medical records, streamlining assessment of benefits eligibility, and providing the services in close proximity so as to reduce transportation barriers and inconvenience.

Oral Health and Dental Services

Such oral manifestations as candida, mouth ulcers, and gum disease are common in HIV disease. The occurrence of oral lesions is important for prognosis and affects quality of life. There is a broad consensus that persons with HIV should see a dentist regularly.[88] However, HCSUS findings suggest that many of these individuals do not do so.[89] Specifically, characteristics associated with lower use of dental services were not having a regular source of care, not having health insurance, lower educational attainment, female gender, and black ethnicity. The source of care also influenced dental care utilization. Patients whose usual source of care was a VA clinic were most likely to use dental services, which suggests that comprehensive delivery systems (as with the VA) may facilitate use of dental services.

HIV-infected patients have substantial dental care needs. It is estimated that 52 percent of HIV patients have a regular need for ongoing dental care; IUDs and low-income patients were more likely to perceive a need for dental care.[90]

Despite high need for dental services, dentists have not been universally receptive to caring for individuals with HIV.[91] It can be very difficult to find a dentist willing to treat an HIV patient. Dentists have seen themselves at considerable risk from HIV infection. This attitude on the part of dentists as a group may result in less disclosure by HIV patients to their dentists. One previous study found that only 53 percent of patients had told their dentist of their infection.[92] Women may be particularly at risk of poor access to dental care.[93]

Dental and medical services also have interrelated roles in managing HIV disease. Oral health problems associated with HIV are often more complicated and refractory than those in the general population and require the attention of both medical and dental personnel. Without early and adequate access to dental and medical care, periodontal disease in the immunocompromised patient can lead to life-threatening infection. HCSUS found that more than 58,000 people under treatment for HIV in the United States had unmet medical or dental needs. Unmet dental needs were more than twice as prevalent as unmet medical needs, and 11,576 people were estimated to have both unmet dental and medical needs. Those with low income were most likely to report unmet needs for both dental and medical care. Of particular policy concern, the uninsured and those insured by Medicaid without dental benefits faced more than three times the odds of unmet need for both types of care than the privately insured.[94]

Informal Social Support

Social support from family and friends has been shown to benefit HRQOL.[95] In HIV populations, the perceived availability of social support has been shown to be related to lowered hopelessness and depression and to an increased feeling of psychological well-being.[96] Social resources also influence service use. People with more social services available to them were less likely to use formal mental health services.[97] Social support can be critical in facilitating access to necessary services by helping to overcome the disruption of loss of employment and financial problems.

Formal Supportive Services

Few studies have assessed the need for supportive health-related and social services. These services have even traditionally been provided by AIDS service organizations (ASOs) such as the Gay Men's Health Care Crisis in New York, AIDS Project Los Angeles, and the San Francisco AIDS Foundation. Supportive services can include meals, food banks or pantries, residential facilities, buddies, transportation, child care, public benefits counseling, and respite care. In HCSUS, a high level of unmet need (16–40 percent) was identified for a variety of supportive services: benefits advocacy, substance abuse treatment, emotional counseling, home health care, and housing services. Unmet needs were highest for benefits advocacy, substance abuse treatment, and emotional counseling. Nonwhites had higher unmet needs for any one of five services. Compared to those who did not graduate from high school, participants with some college had less unmet need for substance abuse treatment and less unmet need for any one of the five services; and participants who were college graduates had less unmet need for emotional counseling and any unmet need. Being unstably housed was associated with higher unmet need for benefits advocacy and home health care.[98]

Caregivers

The number of persons who provide home care to people with HIV/AIDS has increased. This trend suggests the need to focus on developing more home and community-based services. In HCSUS, 21 percent of HIV-positive individuals used home care services. Use of home care services was concentrated among those with AIDS: 39.5 percent received home care, compared to 9.5 percent of those at an earlier stage of the disease.[99] It is not clear under what circumstances home care services may substitute for or complement more expensive inpatient services, although there is some evidence that this use decreases overall costs.[100] As the population with HIV changes, however, the availability of informal home care (that provided by friends and family) may decrease, threatening the adequacy of the formal home care system.

Organizing Comprehensive Care and Services

Organizing comprehensive services involves providers and managed care organizations; case management may facilitate care coordination while addressing diverse patient needs.

Providers

Up to three quarters of primary care physicians in the United States have cared for an HIV-positive patient, but national data on the distribution of current providers and the amount of care they provide are lacking. Understanding current HIV care requires understanding both the sites and types of providers. Costs, access, and quality of care depend not only on patient characteristics but also on those of the providers.

As the HIV epidemic spreads into new populations, it also is reaching new providers. Accurate assessment of present and future care requires a representative sample of all types of health care provider. Current data are limited to small numbers of institutional centers or highly identified AIDS practices, such as those involved in centrally funded research efforts. Forthcoming data on HCSUS providers will shed light on this important area.

Managed Care

HIV/AIDS treatment is offered in a growing array of settings, including those that incorporate managed care practices. The majority of Americans receive their health coverage through private insurance companies and managed care organizations, but the number of persons with AIDS covered by private plans has decreased over time.[101] Private insurers have reduced their exposure to HIV-infected persons, because of the fear of high-risk individuals and partially as a result of highly inflated estimates of the average cost of an AIDS case.[102] Thus, an individual with HIV may find it difficult to purchase an individual policy. Strategies to reduce provider risk also include tighter underwriting guidelines, use of HIV testing for enrollment, and denying insurance to those with a history of sexually transmitted disease.

Some states are experimenting with capitated arrangements and managed care as a way to provide better access to care for Medicaid recipients. In these arrangements, providers are at risk for the costs of care, creating an incentive to limit costly treatment and procedures. Very little is known about the impact on costs and quality of care when reimbursement for AIDS is capitated. Even with Medicaid's shortcomings, some have advocated for an expansion of Medicaid eligibility to address the problem of financing of care for HIV/AIDS.[103] However, the advent of managed Medicaid programs raises further questions about the adequacy of managed care or Medicaid for financing HIV/AIDS care.

The chief advantage of managed care for the HIV-infected is the potential for better delivery of comprehensive, coordinated care. Coordination of care needs to be extended to the social complexity of HIV disease, which cannot be ignored in efforts to design programs for this vulnerable population. Thus, shifting financial risk from insurers to providers presents new opportunities to improve health care—but at the same time, unfortunately, new mechanisms may restrict an HIV-infected person's opportunity to receive the highest-quality care. Inevitably, the care provided to those with HIV-infection changes under managed care, as it has for other conditions. The challenge of managed care is to develop a system to ensure efficient and high-quality care with incentives and rules to meet the needs of patients, providers, payers, and organizations in a balanced way.[104]

Case Management

Addressing problems of access, cost, and quality of HIV/AIDS care in medical and community-based settings has highlighted the importance of reducing service fragmentation and developing a more comprehensive approach to delivery. Case management has often been suggested as a strategy for coordinating care. There are many definitions of case management. Most approaches include "core activities": intake and assessment; a comprehensive, multidisciplinary care plan; referral to social and medical services; monitoring of care; modification of care plan based on current problems; and client advocacy.[105] For many, case management may offer community-based alternatives to hospitalization, which may be more cost-effective and humane. Use of home services, such as intravenous antibiotics and total parenteral nutrition, may save 30–50 percent of hospital costs.[106]

Case management has been found to contribute to longevity between HIV diagnosis and death and between first hospitalization and death.[107] Findings from the HCSUS showed that case management was associated with decreased unmet needs.[108] In longitudinal analysis, having a case manager predicted the receipt of combination antiretroviral therapy.[109]

Policy Implications and Research Needs for Management, Planning, and AIDS Policy

The HIV/AIDS epidemic has spread out from its initial geographic epicenters to much broader communities of the socially and economically disadvantaged. Concurrently, the range of medical treatments for HIV and AIDS complications has grown more effective, as well as more complex. The settings in which these treatments are administered are increasingly diverse, including those that incorporate managed care principles, such as public as well as private health maintenance organizations (HMOs). Despite these developments, public policy decisions related to HIV/AIDS have thus far relied primarily on studies that use convenience samples of the earliest affected cohort—mostly white males with male-to-male sexual contact as the identified mode of exposure. Using this information to guide public policy and other decisions concerning HIV/AIDS is potentially misguiding.

HIV/AIDS is only one of many public health problems and social issues that confront the United States as it begins the twenty-first century. The initial impetus for action has waned as the epidemic enters its third decade and the populations most affected by AIDS have changed. Within the HIV/AIDS community, allocation of scarce resources is politically charged. Should more funds be directed toward prevention, or should treatment take priority? How can research funds have the greatest impact: through a return to basic science, or expanded access to new treatments and accelerated clinical trials? What is the appropriate funding relationship between medical services and social services?

Similarly vexing questions plagued the debate about proper allocation of resources between AIDS and other diseases. Certainly, no easy answers exist for these questions, and powerful interests groups can be found on every side. A debate about priorities is healthy, but there is potential for conflict that may do a disservice to those with HIV infection. Developing partnerships and networks to effectively organize and deliver health and social services is paramount.

Health Policy Issues and Options

As HIV infection increases in communities of color and among the poor, the financial burden on public payers and health care providers inevitably grows. Reliance on Medicaid has profound implications for people with HIV/AIDS as public support for Medicaid has waned. In addition, new federal eligibility mandates of the 1990s have increased the cost of Medicaid to states. As a result, many state legislatures are searching for ways to effectively control the costs of the program. Rate setting of provider payments is one way states have attempted to control their Medicaid costs. Moving patients into managed Medicaid health plans has also become common. In many states, the reimbursement level has not kept up with inflation; Medicaid generally pays providers less than their costs of care. As providers limit the number of Medicaid patients they serve, access to care may deteriorate for those dependent on Medicaid.

Medicare currently pays for a smaller portion of AIDS expenditures than Medicaid because of the twenty-nine-month waiting period from the onset date of disability. One policy alternative is to significantly reduce or entirely eliminate this waiting period.[110] The proportion on Medicare has increased greatly since the 1990s, probably because people are living longer with the infection. The Congressional Budget Office estimated that a reduced AIDS-specific waiting period would cost the federal government $3 billion over five years, while it would generate $550 million in Medicaid savings to the states.[111] Medicare administrators may be unwilling to support another disease-specific expansion of the program, given the agency's experience with end-stage renal disease (ESRD), wherein costs have ballooned since its implementation. It is important to note that Medicare eligibility is only a partial solution for persons with AIDS because Medicare has no outpatient prescription drug benefit and most treatments for HIV disease are pharmacologically based.

Expansion of employer-based insurance is highly unlikely with the demise of the Clinton administration's 1993 Health Security Act and its employer mandate provision. Policy attention should be directed toward maintaining private health insurance for those with HIV. Some states have programs that pay private health insurance and Consolidated Omnibus Budget Reconciliation Act (COBRA) premiums for people with AIDS and other high-cost illnesses; California and New York are prominent examples. These programs represent a win-win situation for persons with AIDS and public agencies. Those with AIDS are able to remain with their current health care providers and maintain continuity of care. At the same time, public providers and payers are relieved of a substantial portion of the burden of care and treatment by shifting it to the private sector.

A large number of federal agencies and offices have responsibility for AIDS health services and health policy, among them the Department of Health and Human Services Office of HIV/AIDS policy, the White House Office of AIDS Health Policy, the Agency for Health Quality Research (AHQR), the Health Resources and Services Administration (HRSA), numerous branches of the CDC, and numerous institutes within the NIH. Better coordination is needed for the activities of these agencies and offices, and as well as the many private, state, and local organizations involved in AIDS health services and policy. Such coordination may improve the ability of these organizations to deliver HIV-related health services in an efficient and effective manner.

Ryan White CARE Act and ADAP Programs

The Ryan White Comprehensive AIDS Resource Emergency Act (CARE) was originally signed in 1990, as a federal program designed to improve the quality and availability of care for persons with HIV/AIDS and their families. Under Title I of the Care Act, covered services included a variety of medical and supportive services: primary health care, case management, home health, food services, hospice care, housing, transportation, and prevention and education services.[112] The main target population for these services were poor and uninsured populations.

Under Title I, cities qualifying for Title I funds are defined as Eligible Metropolitan Areas (EMAs). Appropriation of Title I funds are awarded by two methods: formulas (based on cumulative AIDS cases and cumulative AIDS incidence) and supplemental applications among the EMAs. These supplemental plans must include a plan for additional funds based on needs not met by the formula grants, a high incidence of AIDS, and proof of the existing commitment of area resources. In these additional applications, the needs of infants, children, women, and families are also to be addressed.

Within each EMA, the priorities for spending Title I funds must be established by HIV health services planning councils. Many EMAs have designated planning councils by expanding existing HIV-AIDS planning bodies. Examples of the representation on a planning council are housing organizations, drug treatment providers, the American National Red Cross, the United Way, the Department of Veterans Affairs, and private foundations. The CARE Act also requires that individuals with HIV/AIDS be voting members of HIV health services planning councils.

Research suggests that the CARE act has been successful in improving access to some Title I services (for example, basic medical care) for low-income populations.[113] A study of CARE and non-CARE clients in San Francisco found no differences in utilization of physician visit, hospitalization, or emergency room use, after adjusting for sociodemographic characteristics and health status.[114] However, the study also found that high unmet need existed for dental care, home health care, and alternative therapies—suggesting that further strategies are needed to increase access to care for low-income HIV-infected populations.

Pharmacy support, through the ADAP (AIDS Drug Assistance Program), is a new but increasingly important component of the CARE act.[115] Under the ADAP, uninsured and underinsured persons with HIV disease can access newly developed treatment medications (such as protease inhibitors). Although the CARE act has been successful in increasing availability of medical and nonmedical services for those with HIV disease, concern has arisen whether CARE act funding spent on newly developed medications is too high (as with HAART). Although timely use of newly developed treatment medications is important in managing HIV disease, many who use these drugs often become disabled and also need supportive services. Thus policy makers are faced with a dilemma because CARE funding spent on expensive medications may reduce funding for available supportive services, thereby possibly exacerbating unmet needs for supportive services.

Needs of Special Populations

Certain special populations deserve attention: HIV-positive women, children, adolescents, certain ethnic groups, drug-dependent individuals, and those suffering from psychiatric disorders. These groups may face additional barriers to early intervention and access to care.

Women. By the year 2000, the number of new AIDS cases reported annually in women is predicted to equal that of men.[116] AIDS is the fourth leading cause of death for twenty-to-forty-year-old women. African American and Latina women account for more than 75 percent of infected women and 80 percent of the AIDS cases reported for women in 1998.[117] The course of clinical care differs somewhat from men, as women present to the medical care system at a more advanced stage of the disease than do men and they develop some unique complications (such as cervical cancer). Women also use services differently.[118] Some studies indicate that differences between men and women in their use of services such as the emergency room and inpatient and outpatient sites may be explained by such factors as insurance status, stage of illness, and transmission risk.[119]

Obstetric and gynecological conditions and procedures may contribute substantially to the health service use of women.[120] The availability of obstetric and gynecological services, licensing and funding for trained health care providers, a shortage of obstetricians, and the limited HIV experience of health care providers with HIV-infected women may influence health service access and utilization. About 25 percent of women receiving care in the United States have dependent children under the age of eighteen.[121] The competing responsibilities of caregiving for children or other HIV-infected persons in the household often act as a barrier to receiving timely care.[122] Other gender-specific factors that may influence use include misdiagnosis or undiagnosed HIV-related conditions, sexual or domestic violence, and commercial sex work.[123]

Children. An estimated two thousand children in the country have HIV infection. As of December 1998, 1.2 percent ($n = 8,461$) of AIDS cases had been reported in children younger than thirteen; 58 percent of childhood AIDS cases are African American and 23 percent are Hispanic. Infection in children was generally acquired perinatally, and almost 91 percent had mothers with (or with known risk for) HIV infection.[124] More than one-half of mothers of perinatally infected children were IDUs or had a sexual partner who injected drugs. As many as 25 percent of children born to HIV-positive mothers are infected.[125] Although HCSUS found that only 4 percent of children of women who were HIV-positive tested positive for HIV, this figure may be considered a lower bound, since nearly half (42 percent) of HIV-positive women with children had not been tested.[126]

The costs of pediatric AIDS are higher than the costs of adult AIDS, largely because of higher hospital costs, which are estimated at about $35,000-$37,000 per year, including inpatient care, outpatient care, home health, and pharmacy service.[127] Medicaid is the primary payer for both hospital and community-based services for pediatric AIDS.[128] Contributing to the high costs are the complications of medical management owing to the absence, disability, or death of one or both parents through AIDS or drug use, urban poverty, and complex social conditions.[129]

Adolescents. AIDS is the seventh leading cause of death in people of age fifteen to twenty-four; it contributes to premature mortality of those who are supposed to be healthy and productive, and who should expect to live a normal life span. Nearly three times as many males compared to females, between the ages of fifteen and twenty-four, have been reported to have AIDS. This population is of particular concern because of the number of sexual contacts and behaviors that contribute to increased risk and likelihood of infection, although the risk is not reported for more than one-third of male adolescents and one-half of female adolescents.[130] Although adolescents are generally aware of HIV transmission and AIDS, many have misperceptions about sexual activity, drug use, and prevention measures. Despite adequate knowledge, most adolescents continue to participate in unprotected sex.[131]

Ethnic Groups. HIV/AIDS disproportionately affects certain ethnic groups; African Americans and Hispanics are most likely to be HIV-infected. Furthermore, African Americans are less likely to receive HAART than whites, for a variety of reasons (lack of insurance; lack of regular care; competing needs for food, clothing, and housing; attitudes and beliefs such as distrust of doctors). These same groups more often experience barriers to both access and outreach. Many may not be aware of the benefits of receiving early treatment. Geographic barriers to care may exist that pose access concerns. The site of care for HIV/AIDS may not be in a familiar neighborhood setting. Agencies may not be prepared to deal with the special cultural needs of racial and ethnic minorities.[132] These issues may exacerbate the vulnerability already experienced by people with HIV/AIDS in receiving the full range of health care services that are needed and available.

Drug-Dependent Individuals and Those with Psychiatric Disorders. The prevalence of drug dependence and psychiatric disorders remains disproportionately high in the HIV population. The high prevalence of these disorders in this population has important clinical and public health implications. The availability of effective, albeit complicated, treatments for HIV requires infected persons to access care, use services appropriately, and adhere strictly to medication regimens. Failure to adhere closely to treatment may facilitate development of medication-resistant viral strains that can render antiretroviral medications ineffective and increase the likelihood of transmission of a resistant strain. Psychiatric disorders, drug use, and drug dependence are likely to limit adherence to treatment as well as access to appropriate comprehensive medical and mental health care and substance abuse treatment. The high prevalence rate of these disorders points to the importance of integrating mental health and substance abuse treatment into the ongoing clinical care of persons with HIV infection.

Future Issues in HIV/AIDS Health Services Research

Ideally, policy and planning options are based on evidence of the effectiveness of treatment and an acceptable level of the costs of delivering such treatment. The completion of the landmark HCSUS study should vastly improve policy-relevant AIDS health services data. This study is providing data relevant to a wide range of issues pertinent to HIV policy, including costs and utilization, access and barriers to care, adherence, quality of life, social support services, mental health, dental health, and quality of care.

New research efforts must continue to include the changing clinical profile of the epidemic. In addition, research efforts must provide insights into national trends, such as regional variation in the pattern of HIV-related disease complication. Changes in treatment pattern and in the price of medication over time make predicting future costs even more difficult. The many nonmedical costs of HIV/AIDS should be examined (direct costs of transportation, informal support, and housing as well as indirect costs of disability days from work resulting from treatment or deteriorating health).

Studies of special populations are also needed—women, children, adolescents, IDUs, those in rural communities, and the racial and ethnic minorities who constitute a growing proportion of the HIV-infected population. Data collected on cost and use enable policy makers to compare current patterns of costs and utilization across the spectrum of HIV disease, across geographical areas, across the range of institutional and individual providers (including managed care settings), and for both the insured and the uninsured populations, as well as variations with different financing and provider arrangements.

Given that side effects are likely to be constantly associated with the medication used to treat HIV disease, further research is needed to develop and evaluate interventions to improve adherence with treatment regimens. Such research takes on greater salience with the widespread use of HAART medications. Particular populations of interest for future adherence research are those with mental disorders, substance abusers, or both.

Lack of insurance, poverty and underuse of ambulatory treatment is likely to continue within the groups in which the epidemic is spreading most rapidly. Disadvantaged groups (minorities, women, IDUs, and the poor) experience difficulty more often in obtaining access to outpatient care. In addition, they may not receive appropriate treatment, which may account for greater mortality in those populations. People with impaired access to health services often use costlier sources of medical care and use them for a longer duration. Furthermore, variation in the quality of AIDS care by geographic region, sociodemographic group, and type of provider is likely to reflect poor quality of care for certain individuals.

In view of these concerns, the important characteristics of the changing epidemiology of AIDS and clinical treatment patterns need to be continuously examined in order to address problems in access, costs, and quality. Health service delivery systems need to be developed to address the emerging needs of diverse population groups affected by HIV/AIDS. Additionally, it is important that Ryan White CARE programs also address the emerging needs of diverse population groups affected by HIV/AIDS. Neither the arena of formal medical services nor supportive services can be overlooked. Developing finance and delivery systems within the context of long-range planning and evaluation is paramount.

In this chapter, we have reviewed existing knowledge and critical gaps in information about HIV/AIDS to establish a basis for addressing the current and future challenges that HIV/AIDS present for development of relevant health policy and health and social services planning and program implementation.

Notes

1. Palella, F. J., and others. "Declining Morbidity and Mortality Among Patients with Advanced Human Immunodeficiency Virus Infection." *New England Journal of Medicine,* 1998, *338,* 853–860; Hogg, R. S., and others. "Improved Survival Among HIV-Infected Individuals Following Initiation of Antiretrovirals." *Journal of the American Medical Association,* 1998, *279,* 450–454.

2. Wainberg, M. A., and Friedland, G. "Public Health Implications of Antiretroviral Therapy and HIV Drug Resistance." *Journal of the American Medical Association,* 1998, *279,* 1977–1983; Fauci, A. S. "HIV/AIDS in 1998-Gaining the Upper Hand?" (Editorial.) *Journal of the American Medical Association,* 1998, *280,* 87–88.

3. Shapiro, M. F., and others. "Variations in the Care of HIV-Infected Adults in the United States: Results from the HIV Cost and Services Utilization Study." *Journal of the American Medical Association,* 1999, *281,* 2305–2315; Andersen, R. M., and others. "Access of Vulnerable Groups to Antiretroviral Therapy Among Persons in Care for HIV Disease in the U.S." Forthcoming; Cunningham, W. E., Markson, L. E., and others. "Prevalence and Predictors of Highly Active Antiretroviral Therapy in Persons with HIV Infection in the U.S." *Journal of AIDS,* 2000, *25*(2), 115–123.

4. Kirchhoff, F., and others. "Brief Report: Absence of Intact nef Sequences in a Long-Term Survivor with Nonprogressive HIV-1 Infection." *New England Journal of Medicine,* 1995, *332,* 228–232; Pantaleo, G., and others. "Studies in Subjects with Long-Term Nonprogressive Human Immunodeficiency Virus Infection." *New England Journal of Medicine,* 1995, *332*(4), 209–216.

5. Mellors, J. W., and others. "Prognosis in HIV-1 Infection Predicted by the Quantity of Virus in Plasma." *Science,* 1996, *272,* 1167–1170; O'Brien, W. A., and others. "Changes in Plasma HIV-1 RNA and CD4+ Lymphocyte Counts and the Risk of Progression to AIDS." *New England Journal of Medicine,* 1996, *334*(7), 426–431; O'Brien, W. A., and others, for the VA Cooperative Study Group on AIDS. "Changes in Plasma HIV RNA Levels and CD4+ Lymphocyte Counts Predict Both Response to Antiviral Therapy and Therapeutic Failure." *Annals of Internal Medicine,* 1997, *126*(12), 939–945.

6. Pantaleo and others (1995).

7. Hong, H., and others. "Identification of HIV-I Integrase Inhibitors Based on a Four-Point Pharmacophore." *Antiviral Chemistry and Chemotherapy,* 1998, *9*(6), 461–472; Bolognesi, D., Matthews, T., Kang, M. C., and Hopkins, S. "Abstract no. S16: Development and Clinical Evaluation of T-20: The First Member of a Novel Class of Anti-Retroviral Agents That Inhibit Membrane Fusion." Seventh Conference on Retroviruses and Opportunistic Infections, Foundation for Retrovirology and Human Health. San Francisco, Medical Consumer Media, 2000; Kovacs, J. A., and others. "Increases in CD4 T Lymphocytes with Intermittent Courses of Interleukin-2 in Patients with Human Immunodeficiency Virus Infection: A Preliminary Study." *New England Journal of Medicine,* 1995, *332*(9), 567–575.

8. Centers for Disease Control and Prevention, National Center for HIV, STD, and TB Prevention. "HIV/AIDS Surveillance Report, Year End Addition." (Report.) U.S. Department of Health and Human Services, 1998, pp. 1–43.

9. Martin, J., Smith, B., Matthews, M., and Ventura, S. "Births and Deaths: Preliminary Data for 1998." *National Vital Statistics Reports,* 1999, *47*(25), 1–45.

10. Hoyert, D. L., Kochanek, K. D., and Murphy, S. L. "Deaths: Final Data for 1997." *National Vital Statistics Reports,* 1999, *47*(19), 1–104.

11. Lawrence, L., and Hall, M. "1997 Summary: National Hospital Discharge Survey." *Vital and Health Statistics of the Centers for Disease Control,* 1999, *308*, 1–16.

12. Centers for Disease Control and Prevention (1998).

13. Carpenter, C.C.J., and others. "Antiretroviral Therapy for HIV Infection in 1998. Updated Recommendations of the International AIDS Society-USA Panel." *Journal of the American Medical Association,* 1998, *280*, 78–86; Carpenter, C. C., and others. "Antiretroviral Therapy in Adults: Updated Recommendations of the International AIDS Society-USA Panel." *Journal of the American Medical Association,* 2000, *283*, 381–390.

14. Pradier, C., and others. "Reducing the Incidence of Pneumocystis Carinii Pneumonia: A Persisting Challenge." *AIDS,* 1997, *11*, 832–833.

15. USPHS/ISDA Prevention of Opportunistic Infections Working Group. "1999 USPHS/ISDA Guidelines for the Prevention of Opportunistic Infections in Persons with Human Immunodeficiency Virus." *Morbidity and Mortality Weekly Report,* 1999. (Website, accessed Sept. 8, 1999.) [www.cdc.gov/mmwr/index99.htm]; Furrer, H., and others. "Discontinuation of Primary Prophylaxis Against Pneumocystis Carinii Pneumonia in HIV-1 Infected Adults Treated with Combination Antiretroviral Therapy." *New England Journal of Medicine,* 1999, *340*(17), 1301–1306.

16. Furrer and others (1999).

17. Carpenter and others (2000).

18. Abrams, D. I. "Alternative Therapies in HIV Infection." *AIDS,* 1990, *4*, 1179–1187; Greenblatt, R. M., Hollander, H., McMaster, J. R., and Henke, C. J. Polypharmacy Among Patients Attending an AIDS Clinic: Utilization of Prescribed, Unorthodox, and Investigational Treatments." *Journal of AIDS,* 1991, *4*, 136–143.

19. Bozzette, S. A., and others. "The Care of HIV-Infected Adults in the United States: Results from the HIV Cost and Services Utilization Study." *New England Journal of Medicine,* 1998, *339*(26), 1897–1904.

20. Turner, B. J., and others. "Delayed Medical Care After Diagnosis in a U.S. National Probability Sample of HIV-Infected Persons in Care." *American Journal of Medicine,* 2000, (160), 2614–2622.

21. Samet, J. H., and others. "Trillion Virion Delay: Time from Testing Positive for HIV to Presentation for Primary Care." *Archives of Internal Medicine,* 1998, *158*, 734–740.

22. Bozzette and others (1998).

23. Fleishman, J. A., and Mor, V. "Insurance Status Among People with AIDS: Relationships with Sociodemographic Characteristics and Service Use." *Inquiry,* 1993, *30,* 180–188; Goldman, D. P., and others. "The Public Burden of HIV Care." *Health Affairs,* submitted.

24. Goldman and others (submitted).

25. Buchanan, R. J., and Kricher, F. G. "Medicaid Policies for AIDS-Related Hospital Care." *Health Care Financing Review,* 1994, *15*(4), 33–41.

26. Fleishman, J. A., Hsia, D. C., and Hellinger, F. J. "Correlates of Medical Service Utilization Among People with HIV Infection." *Health Services Research: Health Services Research— Special Section on AIDS Costs and Service Utilization (ACSUS),* 1994, *29*(5), 528–581.

27. Senak, M. S. "Legal Issues Facing AIDS Patients." In K. D. Blanchet (ed.), *AIDS: A Healthcare Management Response.* Rockville, Md.: Aspen, 1988.

28. Andersen and others (forthcoming); Goldman and others (submitted); Katz, M. H., and others. "Health Insurance and Use of Medical Services by Men Infected with HIV." *Journal of Acquired Immune Deficiency Syndromes and Human Retrovirology,* 1995, *8*(1), 58–63.

29. Green, J., and Arno, P. S. "The 'Medicaidization' of AIDS: Trends in the Financing of HIV-Related Medical Care." *Journal of the American Medical Association,* 1990, *264*(10), 1261–1266.

30. Shapiro and others (1999).

31. Shapiro and others (1999).

32. Cunningham, W. E., Andersen, R. M., and others. "The Impact of Competing Needs for Basic Subsistence on Access to Medical Care for Persons with HIV Receiving Care in the United States." *Medical Care,* 1999, *37*(12), 1270–1281.

33. Stein, M. D., and others. "Delays in Seeking HIV Care Due to Competing Caregiver Responsibilities." *American Journal of Public Health,* 2000, *90*(7), 1138–1140.

34. Crawford, A. M. "Stigma Associated with AIDS: A Meta-Analysis." *Journal of Applied Social Psychology,* 1996, *26*(5), 398–416; Rotheram-Borus, M. J., Draimin, B. H., Reid, H. M., and Murphy, D. A. "The Impact of Illness Disclosure and Custody Plans on Adolescents Whose Parents Live with AIDS." *AIDS,* 1997, *11,* 1159–1164; Kass, N. E., and others. "Changes in Employment, Insurance, and Income in Relation to HIV Status and Disease Progression." *Journal of Acquired Immune Deficiency Syndrome,* 1994, *7*(1), 86–91.

35. Fleishman, Hsia, and Hellinger (1994); Stein, M., and others. "Differences in Access to Zidovudine (AZT) Among Symptomatic HIV-Infected Persons." *Journal of General Internal Medicine,* 1991, *6,* 35–40; Moore, R. D., Stanton, D., Gopalan, R., and Chaisson, R. E. "Racial Differences in the Use of Drug Therapy for HIV Disease in an Urban Community." *New England Journal of Medicine,* 1994, *330*(11), 763; Mor, V., Fleishman, J. A., Dresser, M., and Piette, J. "Variation in Health Service Use Among HIV-Infected Patients." *Medical Care,* 1992, *30*(1), 17–29.

36. Shapiro and others (1999).

37. Shapiro and others (1999); Andersen and others (forthcoming); Bing, E. G., and others. "Protease Inhibitor Use Among a Community Sample of People with HIV Disease." *Journal of Acquired Immune Deficiency Syndromes and Human Retrovirology,* 1999, *20*(5), 474–480.

38. Markson, L., and others. "Abstract no. 105: Who Receives Highly Active Antiretroviral Therapy (HAART)? Data from a Nationally Representative Sample." Sixth Conference on Retroviruses and Opportunistic Infections, Chicago, Jan. 31 to Feb. 4, 1999.

39. Crystal, S., Sambamoorthi, U., and Merzel, C. "The Diffusion of Innovation in AIDS Treatment: Zidovudine Use in Two New Jersey Cohorts." *Health Services Research,* 1995, *30*(4), 593–614.

40. Palella and others (1998); Shapiro and others (1999).

41. Cunningham, W. E., and others. "Predictors of Highly Active Antiretroviral Therapy in Persons with HIV Disease." *Journal of AIDS,* forthcoming.

42. Diaz, T., and others. "Differences in Participation in Experimental Drug Trials Among Persons with AIDS." *Journal of Acquired Immune Deficiency Syndromes and Human Retrovirology,* 1995, *10,* 562–568; Lynn, L. A. "AIDS Clinical Trials: Is There Access for All?" *Journal of General Internal Medicine,* 1997, *12,* 198–199; Stone, V. E., and others. "Race, Gender, Drug Use, and Participation in AIDS Clinical Trials." *Journal of Acquired Immune Deficiency Syndrome,* 1997, *12,* 150–157; Cunningham, W. E., Bozzette, S. A., and others. "Comparison of Quality of Life in Clinical Trial and Non-Clinical Trial HIV-Infected Cohorts." *Medical Care,* 1995, *33*(4), AS15-AS25.

43. Kissinger, P., and others. "Compliance with Public Sector HIV Medical Care." *Journal of the National Medical Association,* 1995, *87*(1), 19–24.

44. Lucas, G. M., Chaisson, R. E., and Moore, R. D. "Highly Active Antiretroviral Therapy in a Large Urban Clinic: Risk Factors for Virological Failure and Adverse Drug Reactions." *Annals of Internal Medicine,* 1999, *131*(2), 81–87; Valdez, H., and others. "Human Immunodeficiency Virus 1 Protease Inhibitors in Clinical Practice: Predictors of Virological Outcome." *Archives of Internal Medicine,* 1999, *159,* 1771–1776.

45. Schoenbaum, E. E., and Webber, M. P. "The Underrecognition of HIV Infection in Women in an Inner-City Emergency Room." *American Journal of Public Health,* 1993, *83*(3), 363–368; Markson, L. E., Houchens, R., Fanning, T. R., and Turner, B. J. "Repeated Emergency Department Use by HIV-Infected Persons: Effect of Clinic Accessibility and Expertise in HIV Care." *Journal of Acquired Immune Deficiency Syndrome,* 1998, *17*(1), 35–41; Kelen, G. D., and others. "Profile of Patients with Human Immunodeficiency Virus Infection Presenting to an Inner-City Emergency Department: Preliminary Report." *Annals of Emergency Medicine,* 1990, *19*(9), 963–969; Kelen, G. D., and others. "Human Immunodeficiency Virus Infection in Emergency Department Patients." *Journal of the American Medical Association,* 1989, *262*(4), 516–522.

46. Shapiro and others (1999).

47. Turner, B. J., and others. "Clinic HIV-Focused Features and Prevention of Pneumocystis Carinii Pneumonia." *JournalGIM,* 1998, *13,* 16–23.

48. Cunningham, W. E., and others. "The Effect of Ethnicity and Race on Long-Term Survival from Hospitalization with HIV Disease." *Journal of Health Care for Poor and Underserved,* 2000, *11*(2), 163–178; Kalichman, S. C., Ramachandran, B., and Catz, S. "Adherence to Combination Antiretroviral Therapies in HIV Patients of Low Health Literacy." *Journal of General Internal Medicine,* 1999, *14,* 267–273.

49. Cunningham W. E., and others. "Access to Community-Based Medical Services and Number of Hospitalizations Among Patients with HIV Disease: Are They Related?" *Journal of Acquired Immune Deficiency Syndrome and Retrovirology,* 1996, *13,* 341–349.

50. Mosen, D. M., and others. "Is Access to Medical Care Associated with Receipt of HIV Testing and Counseling?" *AIDS Care,* 1998, *10,* 617–628.

51. Cunningham, W. E., Hays, R. D., and others. "Access to Medical Care and Health-Related Quality of Life for Low Income, Symptomatic, HIV-Infected Individuals." *Medical Care,* 1995, *33*(7), 739–754; Cunningham, W. E., Globe, D., and Hays, R. "The Prospective Association of Physical Function with Long-Term Survival After Hospitalization for HIV Disease." *Quality of Life Research,* 1998, *7,* 584–585.

52. Bozzette and others (1998).

53. Joyce, G. "The Costs of Treating HIV/AIDS Since the Introduction of Protease Inhibitors." Paper presented at conference of the Association of Health Services Research, Chicago, June 1999.

54. Lawrence and Hall (1999).

55. Fingerhut, L. A., and Warner, M. *Injury Chartbook: Health, United States 1996–1997.* Hyattsville, Md.: National Center for Health Statistics, 1997; Pamuk, E., and others. *Socioeconomic Status and Health Chartbook: Health, United States, 1998.* Hyattsville, Md.: National Center for Health Statistics, 1998.

56. Andersen and others (forthcoming).

57. Asch, S., and others. Underuse of Primary Prophylaxis for Mycobacterium Avium Complex and Pneumocystis Carinii in a Representative Sample of HIV-Infected Patients in Care in the USA: Who Is Missing Out?" Submitted to *Lancet*, under review.

58. Bennett, C. L., and others. "Relation Between Hospital Experience and In-Hospital Mortality for Patients with AIDS-Related Pneumocystis Carinii Pneumonia: Experience from 3,126 Cases in New York City in 1987." *Journal of Acquired Immune Deficiency Syndrome*, 1992, *5*(9), 856–864.

59. Bennett and others (1992); Cunningham, W. E., Tisnado, D. M., and others. "The Effect of Hospital Experience on Hospital Mortality for Patients with AIDS in California." *American Journal of Medicine*, 1999, *107*(2), 137–143; Stone, V. E., Seage, G. R., III, Hertz, T., and Epstein, A. M. "The Relation Between Hospital Experience and Mortality for Patients with AIDS." *Journal of the American Medical Association*, 1992, *268*(19), 2655–2661; Bennett, C. L., and others. "The Relation Between Hospital Experience and In-Hospital Mortality for Patients with AIDS-Related PCP." *Journal of the American Medical Association*, 1989, *261*(20), 2975–2979.

60. Kitahata, M. M., and others. "Physicians' Experience with the Acquired Immunodeficiency Syndrome as a Factor in Patients' Survival." *New England Journal of Medicine*, 1996, *334*(11), 701–706.

61. Hecht, F. M., and others. "Optimizing Care for Persons with HIV Infection." *Annals of Internal Medicine*, 1999, *131*(2), 136–143; Lewis, C. E. "Management of Patients with HIV/AIDS. Who Should Care?" *Journal of the American Medical Association*, 1997, *278,* 1133–1134; Holmes, W. C. "Quality in HIV/AIDS Care: Specialty-Related or Experience-Related?" *Journal of General Internal Medicine*, 1997, *12,* 195–197.

62. Marquis, M. S., Ross-Davies, A., and Ware, J. E., Jr. "Patient Satisfaction and Change in Medical Care Provider: A Longitudinal Study." *Medical Care*, 1983, *21*(8), 821–829; Pascoe, G. C. "Patient Satisfaction in Primary Health Care: A Literature Review and Analysis." *Evaluation and Program Planning*, 1983, *6*, 185–210; O'Brien, M. K., Petrie, K., and Raeburn, J. "Adherence to Medication Regimens: Updating a Complex Medical Issue." *Medical Care Review*, 1992, *49*(4), 435–454; Marshall, G. N., Hays, R. D., and Mazel, R. "Health Status and Satisfaction with Health Care: Results from the Medical Outcomes Study." *Journal of Consulting and Clinical Psychology,* 1996, *64*(2), 380–390.

63. Stein, M. D., Fleishman, J., Mor, V., and Dresser, M. "Factors Associated with Patient Satisfaction Among Symptomatic HIV-Infected Persons." *Medical Care*, 1993, *31*(2), 182–188.

64. Wainberg and Friedland (1998); Hecht, F. M., and others. "Sexual Transmission of an HIV-1 Variant Resistant to Multiple Reverse-Transcriptase and Protease Inhibitors." *New England Journal of Medicine*, 1998, *339*(5), 307–311.

65. Mehta, S., Moore, R. D., and Graham, N.M.H. "Potential Factors Affecting Adherence with HIV Therapy." *AIDS*, 1997, *11*, 1665–1670.

66. Wenger, N. S., and others. "Abstract no. 98: Patient Characteristics and Attitudes Associated with Antiretroviral Adherence." Sixth Conference on Retroviruses and Opportunistic Infections, Chicago, Jan. 31 to Feb. 4, 1999.

67. Kalichman, Ramachandran, and Catz (1999); Mehta, Moore, and Graham (1997).

68. Hays, R. D., and others. "Health-Related Quality of Life in People Receiving Care for HIV Infection in the United States: Results from the HIV Cost and Services Utilization Study." *American Journal of Medicine,* revised and resubmitted; Bozzette, S. A., and others. "Derivation and Psychometric Properties of a Brief Health-Related Quality of Life Instrument for HIV Disease." *Journal of Acquired Immune Deficiency Syndromes and Human Retrovirology,* 1995, *8*(3), 253–265; Hays, R. D., and Shapiro, M. F. "An Overview of Generic Health-Related Quality of Life Measures for HIV Research." *Quality of Life Research,* 1992, *1*, 91–97; Wachtel, T., and others. "Quality of Life in Persons with Human Immunodeficiency Virus Infection: Measurement by the Medical Outcomes Study Instrument." *Annals of Internal Medicine,* 1992, *116*(2), 129–137; Wu, A., and others. "The Effect of Mode of Administration on Medical Outcomes Study: Preliminary Validation in Persons with Early HIV Infection." *Medical Care,* 1997, *8*(Supplement 1), S349–S359; Copfer, A., and others. "The Use of Two Measures of Health-Related Quality of Life in HIV-Infected Individuals: A Cross-Sectional Comparison." *Quality of Life Research,* 1996, *5*(2), 281–286; Revicki, D., Wu, A., and Murray, M. "Change in Clinical Status, Health Status, and Health Utility Outcomes in HIV-Infected Patients." *Medical Care,* 1995, *33*(4 Supplement), AS173–AS182; Stanton, D. L., and others. "Functional Status of Persons with HIV Infection in an Ambulatory Setting." *Journal of Acquired Immune Deficiency Syndromes,* 1994, *7*, 1050–1056; Wu, A., and Lamping, D. "Assessment of Quality of Life." *AIDS,* 1994, *8*(Supplement 1), S349–S359; Wu, A. W., and others. "Functional Status and Well-Being in a Placebo-Controlled Trial of Zidovudine in Early Symptomatic HIV Infection." *Journal of Acquired Immune Deficiency Syndrome,* 1993, *6*(5), 452–458.

69. Revicki, Wu, and Murray (1995); Globe, D. R., Hays, R. D., and Cunningham, W. E. "Associations of Clinical Parameters with Health-Related Quality of Life in Hospitalized Persons with HIV Disease." *AIDS Care,* 1999, *11*(1), 71–86; Wilson, I. B., and Cleary, P. D. "Clinical Predictors of Functioning in Persons with Acquired Immunodeficiency Syndrome." *Medical Care,* 1996, *34*(6), 610–623; Wu, A. W., and others. "A Health Status Questionnaire Using 30 Items from the Medical Outcome Study: Preliminary Validation in Persons with Early HIV Infection." *Medical Care,* 1991, *29*(8), 786–798; Burgess, A., and Riccio, M. "Cognitive Impairment and Dementia in HIV-1 Infection." *Clinical Neurology,* 1992, *1*(1), 155–174; Lubeck, D. P., and Fries, J. F. "Health Status Among Persons Infected with Human Immunodeficiency Virus: A Community Based Study." *Medical Care,* 1993, *31*(3), 269–276; Bozzette, S. A., Hays, R. D., Berry, S. H., and Kanouse, D. E. "A Perceived Health Index for Use in Persons with Advanced HIV Disease: Derivation, Reliability, and Validity." *Medical Care,* 1994, *32*(7), 716–731; Ganz, P. A., and others. "Describing the Health-Related Quality of Life Impact of HIV Infection: Findings from a Study Using the HIV Overview of Problems-Evaluation System (HOPES). *Quality of Life Research,* 1993, *2*(2), 109–119; Tsevat, J., and others. "Health Values of Patients Infected with Human Immunodeficiency Virus: Relationship to Mental Health and Physical Functioning." *Medical Care,* 1996, *34*(1), 44–57; Kaplan, R. M., and others. "The Quality of Well-Being Scale: Application in AIDS, Cystic Fibrosis, and Arthritis." *Medical Care,* 1989, *27*(3 Supplement), S27–S43; Wu, A. W., and others. "Quality of Life in a Placebo-Controlled Trial of Zidovudine in Patients with AIDS and AIDS-Related Complex." *Journal of Acquired Immune Deficiency Syndrome,* 1990, *3*(7), 683–690.

70. Globe, Hays, and Cunningham (1999).

71. Hays and Shapiro (1992); Hays R. D., and others. "Health Related Quality of Life in HIV Disease." *Assessment*, 1995, *2*(4), 363–380; Wu, A. W., and Rubin, H. R. "Measuring Health Status and Quality of Life in HIV and AIDS." *Psychology and Health*, 1992, *6*, 251–264.

72. Lubeck, D. P., and Fries, J. F. "Changes in Quality of Life Among Persons with HIV Infection." *Quality of Life Research*, 1992, *1*, 359–366.

73. Marx, R., Katz, M. H., Park, M. S., and Gurley, R. J. "Meeting the Service Needs of HIV-Infected Persons: Is the Ryan White Care Act Succeeding?" *Journal of Acquired Immune Deficiency Syndromes and Human Retrovirology*, 1997, *14*, 44–55; Katz, M. H., and others. "Prevalence and Predictors of Unmet Need for Supportive Services Among HIV-Infected Persons: Impact of Case Management." *Medical Care*, 2000, *38*(1), 58–69.

74. Schuster, M. A., Bell, R. M., Berry, S. H., and Kanouse, D. E. "Students' Acquisition and Use of School Condoms in a High School Condom Availability Program." *Pediatrics*, 1997, *100*, 689–694; Schuster, M. A., Bell, R. M., Berry, S. H., and Kanouse, D. E. "Impact of a High School Condom Availability Program on Sexual Activities and Behaviors." *Family Planning Perspectives*, 1998, *30*, 67–72,88; Burris, S., and others. "The Legal Strategies Used in Operating Syringe Exchange Programs in the United States." *American Journal of Public Health*, 1996, *86*, 1161–1166; Kirby, D. B., and Brown, N. L. "Condom Availability Programs in U.S. Schools." *Family Planning Perspectives*, 1996, *28*(5), 196–202.

75. Schuster, Bell, Berry, and Kanouse (1998); Longshore, D., Annon, J., and Anglin, M. D. "Long-Term Trends in Self-Reported HIV Risk Behavior: Injection Drug Users in Los Angeles, 1987 Through 1995." *Journal of Acquired Immune Deficiency Syndromes and Human Retrovirology*, 1998, *18*(1), 64–72.

76. Schuster, Bell, Berry, and Kanouse (1997); Schuster, Bell, Berry, and Kanouse (1998).

77. Heimer, R. "Syringe Exchange Programs: Lowering the Transmission of Syringe-Borne Disease and Beyond." *Public Health Report*, 1998, *113*(Supplement 1), 67–74.

78. Phillips, K. A., Coates, T. J., and Catania, J. A. "Predictors of Follow-Through on Plans to Be Tested for HIV." *American Journal of Preventive Medicine*, 1997, *13*(3), 193–198.

79. Bindman, A. B., and others. "Multistate Evaluation of Anonymous HIV Testing and Access to Medical Care." *Journal of the American Medical Association*, 1998, *280*(16), 1416–1420.

80. Phillips, Coates, and Catania (1997); Phillips, K. A., and Coates, T. J. "HIV Counseling and Testing: Research and Policy Issues." *AIDS Care*, 1995, *7*(2), 115–124.

81. Bindman and others (1998).

82. Centers for Disease Control. "Revision of the CDC Surveillance Case Definition for Acquired Immunodeficiency Syndrome." *Morbidity and Mortality Weekly Report*, 1987, *36*(supp), 1–15S.

83. Mosen and others (1998); Phillips and Coates (1995).

84. Lurie, P., and others. "Postexposure Prophylaxis After Nonoccupational HIV Exposure: Clinical, Ethical, and Policy Considerations." *Journal of the American Medical Association*, 1998, *280*(20), 1769–1773; Gerberding, J. L., and Katz, M. H. "Post-Exposure Prophylaxis for HIV." *Advances in Experimental Medicine and Biology*, 1999, *458*, 213–222.

85. Brown, G. R., and others. "Prevalence of Psychiatric Disorders in Early Stages of HIV Infection." *Psychosomatic Medicine*, 1992, *54*, 588–601; Williams, J. B., and others. "Multidisciplinary Baseline Assessment of Homosexual Men with and Without Human Immunodeficiency Virus Infection." *Archives of General Psychiatry*, 1991, *48*, 124–130; Blazer, D. G., and others. "The Prevalence and Distribution of Major Depression in a National Community Sample: The National Comorbidity Survey." *American Journal of Psychiatry*, 1994, *151*, 979–986; Kessler, R. C., and others. "Lifetime and 12-Month Prevalence of

DSM-III-R Psychiatric Disorder in the United States: Results from the National Co-morbidity Study." *Archives of General Psychiatry,* 1994, *51,* 8–19.

86. Wells, K. B., and others. "The Functioning and Well-Being of Depressed Patients: Results from the Medical Outcome Study." *Journal of the American Medical Association,* 1989, *262*(7), 914–919; Wells, K. B., and others. "Depression in General Medical Settings: Implications of Three Health Policy Studies for Consultation-Liaison Psychiatry." *Psychosomatics,* 1994, *35,* 279–296; Sherbourne, C. D., Wells, K. B., and Judd, L. L. "Functioning and Well-Being of Patients with Panic Disorder." *American Journal of Psychiatry,* 1996, *153,* 213–218.

87. Darrow, W. W., and others. "Risk Factors for Human Immunodeficiency Virus in Homosexual Men." *American Journal of Public Health,* 1987, *77,* 479–483.

88. Weinert, M., Grimes, R. M., and Lynch, D. P. "Oral Manifestations of HIV Infection." *Annals of Internal Medicine,* 1996, *125*(6), 485–496.

89. Coulter, I., and others. "Use of Dental Care by HIV Infected Medical Patients." *Journal of Dental Research,* 2000, *79*(6), 1356–1361.

90. Capilouto, E. I., Peitte, J., White, B. A., and Fleishman, J. "Perceived Need for Dental Care Among Persons Living with Acquired Immunodeficiency Syndrome." *Medical Care,* 1991, *29*(8), 745–754.

91. Gerbert, B., Maguire, B. T., and Spitzer, S. "Patients' Attitudes Toward Dentistry and AIDS." *Journal of the American Dental Association,* Nov. 1989 (Supplemental), 16S–21S; Hazelkorn, H. M. "The Reaction of Dentists to Members of Groups at Risk for AIDS." *Journal of the American Dental Association,* 1989, *119,* 611–619; May, E., Murray, K., and Blinkhorn, A. S. "AIDS and Human Immunodeficiency Virus: A Preliminary Investigation into Edinburgh General Dental Practitioner Views and Behaviors." *Health Education Research,* 1990, *5,* 321–328; Davis, M. "Dentistry and AIDS: An Ethical Opinion." *Journal of the American Dental Association,* Nov. 1989 (Supplemental), 9S–11S; Scheutz, F. "HIV Infection and Dental Care: Views and Experiences Among HIV-Seropositive Patients." *AIDS Care,* 1990, *2*(1), 37–42; Weyant, R. J., Bennett, M. E., Simon, M., and Palasisa, S. "Desire to Treat HIV-Infected Patients: Similarities and Differences Across Health Care Professions." *AIDS,* 1994, *8,* 117–125.

92. Perry, S. W., and others. "Self-Disclosure of HIV Infection to Dentists and Physicians." *Journal of the American Dental Association,* 1993, *124*(11), 51–54.

93. Shiboski, C. H., Palacio, H., Neuhaus, J. M., and Greenblatt, R. M. "Dental Care Access and Use Among HIV-Infected Women." *American Journal of Public Health,* 1999, *89*(6), 834–839.

94. Heslin, K. C., and others. "A Comparison of Unmet Needs for Dental and Medical Care Among Persons with HIV Infection Receiving Care in the U.S." *Medical Care Research and Review,* under review.

95. Donald-Sherbourne, C., Meredith, L. S., Rogers, W., and Ware, J. E., Jr. "Social Support and Stressful Life Events: Age Differences in Their Effects on Health Related Quality of Life Among the Chronically Ill." *Quality of Life Research,* 1992, *1,* 235–246.

96. Zich, J., and Temoshok, L. "Perceptions of Social Support in Men with AIDS and ARC: Relationships with Distress and Hardiness." *Journal of Applied Social Psychology,* 1987, *17*(3), 193–215; Hays, R. B., Chauncey, S., and Tobey, L. A. "The Social Support Networks of Gay Men with AIDS." *Journal of Community Psychology,* 1990, *18,* 374–385.

97. Donald-Sherbourne, C. "The Role of Social Support and Life Stress Events in Use of Mental Health Services." *Social Science and Medicine,* 1988, *27*(12), 1393–1400.

98. Katz and others (2000).

99. London, A. S., and others. "Use of Unpaid and Paid Home Care Services Among People with HIV Infection." *AIDS Care,* forthcoming.

100. Schur, C. L., and others. *Measuring Utilization and Costs of AIDS Health Care Services.* Rockville, Md.: Health Resources and Services Administration, 1992; Widman, M., Light, D. W., and Platt, J. J. "Expert Opinion on Barriers to Hospital Discharge for AIDS Patients." *AIDS and Public Policy Journal,* 1991, *5*(3), 132–136.

101. Office of Technology Assessment. "AIDS and Health Insurance: An OTA Survey (Staff Paper)." Washington, D.C.: Office of Technology Assessment, 1988.

102. Green, J., Oppenheimer, G. M., and Wintfeld, N. "The $147,000 Misunderstanding: Repercussions of Overestimating the Cost of AIDS." *Journal of Health Politics Policy and Law,* 1994, *19*(1), 69–90.

103. Makadon, H. J., Seage, G. R., III, Thorpe, K. E., and Fineberg, H. V. "Paying the Medical Cost of the HIV Epidemic: A Review of Policy Options." *Journal of Acquired Immune Deficiency Syndrome,* 1990, *3*(2), 123–133.

104. Kahn, J. G., and Smith, M. D. "Henry J. Kaiser Foundation Forum. HIV Care: A Changing Health Care System." *Journal of Acquired Immune Deficiency Syndrome,* 1995, *8,* S1–S3.

105. Mor, V., Fleishman, J. A., Allen, S. A., and Piette, J. D. *Networking AIDS Services.* Ann Arbor, Mich.: Health Administration Press, 1994.

106. Hart, J. S., and Redding, K. L. "A Physician's Perspective on the Advantage of Home Medical Care: The Other Side of Case Management." *Texas Medicine,* 1994, *90,* 50–54.

107. Sowell, R. L., and others. "Impact of Case Management on Hospital Charges of PWAs in Georgia." *Journal for the Association of Nurses in AIDS Care,* 1992, *3,* 24–31.

108. Katz and others (2000).

109. Katz and others (2000).

110. Makadon, Seage, Thorpe, and Fineberg (1990).

111. Congressional Budget Office. "Cost Estimates." HR 276, 1987.

112. Bowen, S. G, and others. "First Year of AIDS Services Delivery Under Title I of the Ryan White Care Act." *Public Health Reports,* 1992, *107*(5), 491–499; Thurman, S. L. "The Ryan White Care Act." *Journal of the Association of Nurses in AIDS Care,* 1993, *4*(4), 45–49.

113. Marx, Katz, and Gurley (1997); Marx, R., and others. "Reducing Financial Barriers to HIV-Related Medical Care: Does the Ryan White Care Act Make a Difference?" *AIDS Care,* 1998, *10*(5), 611–616.

114. Marx and others (1998).

115. Buchanan, R. J., and Smith, S. R. "State Implementation of the AIDS Drug Assistance Programs." *Health Care Finance Review,* 1998, *19*(3), 39–62.

116. Hoyert, D., Kochanek, K., and Murphy, S. "National Vital Statistics from the Centers for Disease Control and Prevention." *Center for Disease Control and Prevention (CDC),* 1997, *47*(19), 1–105; Gwinn, M., and others. "Prevalence of HIV Infection in Childbearing Women in the United States." *Journal of the American Medical Association,* 1991, *265*(13), 1704–1708.

117. Hogart, Kochanek, and Murphy (1997).

118. Hellinger, F. J. "The Use of Health Services by Women with HIV Infection." *Health Services Research,* 1993, *28*(5), 543–561; Palacio, H., and others. "Access to and Utilization of Primary Care Services Among HIV-Infected Women." *Journal of Acquired Immune Deficiency Syndromes,* 1999, *21*(4), 293–300.

119. Mor, Fleishman, Dresser, and Piette (1992).

120. Carpenter, C.C.J., and others. "Human Immunodeficiency Virus Infection in North American Women: Experience with 200 Women and a Review of the Literature." *Medicine,* 1991, *10,* 307–325.

121. Schuster, M. A., and others. "HIV-Infected Parents and Their Children in the United States." *American Journal of Public Health,* forthcoming.

122. Stein and others (2000).

123. Zierler, S., and others. "Violence Victimization After HIV Infection in a U.S. Probability Sample of Persons in HIV Primary Care." *American Journal of Public Health,* 2000, *90*(2), 208–215.

124. Hogart, Kochanek, and Murphy (1997); Scott, G. B., and Parks, W. P. *Pediatric AIDS.* Philadelphia: Lippincott, 1994; Centers for Disease Control and Prevention. *HIV/AIDS Surveillance Report, Third Quarter.* Washington, D.C.: Centers for Disease Control and Prevention, U.S. Department of Health and Human Services, 1993.

125. Centers for Disease Control and Prevention (1993).

126. Schuster and others (forthcoming).

127. Hsia, D. C., and others. "Pediatric Human Immunodeficiency Virus Infection: Recent Evidence on the Utilization and Costs of Health Services." *Archives of Pediatric Adolescent Medicine,* 1995, *149*(5), 489–496; Ball, J. K., and Thaul, S. *Pediatric AIDS-Related Discharges in a Sample of U.S. Hospitals: Demographics, Diagnoses and Resource Use.* (Publication 92-0031.) Rockville, Md.: Agency for Health Care Policy and Research, U.S. Department of Health and Human Services, 1992; Conviser, R., Arant, C. M., and Coye, M. S. "Pediatric Acquired Immunodeficiency Syndrome Hospitalizations in New Jersey." *Pediatrics,* 1991, *28,* 642–653.

128. Ball and Thaul (1992).

129. Burn, A. E., and others. "Pediatric AIDS in the United States: Epidemiological Reality Versus Government Policy." *International Journal of Health Policy,* 1991, *20,* 617–630.

130. Hogart, Kochanek, and Murphy (1997); Hein, K. "'Getting Real' About HIV in Adolescents." *American Journal of Public Health,* 1993, *83*(4), 492–494.

131. Katz, M. H., and others. "Continuing High Prevalence of HIV and Risk Behaviors Among Young Men Who Have Sex with Men: The Young Men's Survey in the San Francisco Bay Area in 1992 to 1993 and in 1994 to 1995." *Journal of Acquired Immune Deficiency Syndrome and Human Retrovirology,* 1998, *19*(2), 178–181; Koniak-Griffin, D., and Brecht, M. L. "AIDS Risks Behaviors, Knowledge, and Attitudes Among Pregnant Adolescents and Young Mothers." *Health Education and Behavior,* 1997, *24*(5), 613–624; Anderson, J. E., and others. "HIV Risk Behavior, Street Outreach, and Condom Use in Eight High-Risk Populations." *AIDS Education and Prevention,* 1996, *8*(3), 191–204; Rotheram-Borus, M. J., Koopman, C., Haignere, C., and Davies, M. "Reducing HIV Sexual Risk Behaviors Among Runaway Adolescents." *Journal of the American Medical Association,* 1991, *266*(9), 1237–1241.

132. U.S. Department of Health and Human Services. *HIV/AIDS Work Group on Health Care Issues for Hispanic Americans.* (Publication no. HRSA RD-SP-93-8.) Rockville, Md.: U.S. Department of Health and Human Services, 1991.

CHAPTER ELEVEN

HEALTH REFORM FOR CHILDREN AND FAMILIES

Neal Halfon, Moira Inkelas, David L. Wood, and Mark A. Schuster

Throughout the past century, expert panels and government commissions have highlighted the importance of certain basic principles for children's health care. Over the past decade, the Maternal and Child Health Bureau's (MCHB) Bright Futures Project has reiterated that health care for children should be comprehensive, continuous, coordinated, and accountable. Despite great technical advances and the development of important programs that have improved the health and changed the lives of many children, the system of care for children in the United States has yet to embody the principles of Bright Futures and other expert panels. Many children lack insurance and experience numerous barriers to receiving appropriate care. The medical, developmental, and environmental threats to children have changed in nature and complexity, and the system of care that has evolved to meet these changing needs is fragmented, disorganized, and difficult to navigate.

As the health care marketplace changes, attention should be directed toward how these transformations affect the availability and quality of essential child health services. The changing marketplace poses its own set of challenges, but significant changes in organization and payment of health services create new opportunities to construct a child health system more responsive to the emerging health needs of children and able to overcome deficiencies in the current system. Unfortunately, many of the design elements that should be included in a new system might not meet the narrower financial goals of a managed care organization. How can development of a child health system be supported—a system that provides home visitation for families at risk, early intervention services for children with potential developmental delay, preventive mental health services for children who have been abused and neglected, and comprehensive services to children with special medical needs? How can these and other services be ensured when they may not be profitable to the health care industry?

Whether marketplace transformations and federal and state health financing policies improve the organization of children's health services and children's overall health status depends upon the extent to which these and other questions are addressed. How do children fare under a health system restructuring driven primarily by cost considerations? How are the unique health care needs of children addressed as traditional medical services are reconfigured into managed care? Can current access barriers to comprehensive, coordinated health services be resolved? How can the principles outlined in Bright Futures guide the transformation of children's health services? By what standard should we evaluate the effectiveness of new organizational approaches to delivering child health services?

This chapter examines the key issues underlying the incongruity between the needs of children and families and the current and evolving structure of health services in the United States. We describe the unique health needs of children and the rationale for a child standard of care to ensure that emerging systems can meet these needs. Next, we examine characteristics of the U.S. health care system that influence children's access to care, including the disjointed organization of health services, and financial and structural barriers to health care. In the context of proliferating state-based initiatives and sweeping market-based reforms in the health system, we present several options for accommodating the special needs of children. Finally, we describe how emerging models of care can be modified to provide more effective, organized, and family-centered health services for children.

Special Health Needs of Children

Children's health needs and risks fundamentally differ from those of adults and thus require special consideration in structuring, organizing, and delivering health services.[1] Among the unique characteristics of childhood that have important implications for health system design are a child's developmental vulnerability, dependency, and differential patterns of morbidity and mortality.

Developmental Vulnerability

Developmental vulnerability refers to rapid and cumulative physical and emotional changes that characterize childhood, and the potential impact that illness, injury, or untoward family and social circumstances can have on a child's life-course trajectory. Physical health conditions (such as low birthweight or asthma) as well as the child's social environment (severe poverty, unstable family, environmental exposures such as lead) can harm the developmental process.[2] Several conceptual models have been used to elucidate the dynamic relationships between factors that can promote or adversely affect children's capacity to achieve their physical, emotional, and cognitive potential.[3] Studies demonstrate two phenomena: the substantial, cumulative impact of early exposures and adverse social conditions on health status throughout the life course; and the role of critical developmental periods in which early insults cause long-term consequences.[4] Research linking the impact of various risks and insults to the developmental pathways supports a broader conceptualization of health determinants and of health services.

The potential to alter the life-course trajectory is illustrated by studies that demonstrate the effectiveness of timely intervention in modifying adverse biological and social conditions that may harm a child's development. For example, cognitive development and behavioral competence at preschool age is greater when low-birthweight children receive supportive family and educational services.[5] Such studies support the notion that timely and appropriately organized services can prevent loss of developmental potential; they highlight the mutability of various risks and their life-course effects.[6]

Children's developmental vulnerability also implies that interventions must be sustained over time to appropriately address periodic, recurrent, and ongoing biological and environmental threats. For example, although comprehensive early childhood intervention programs that serve socially disadvantaged children have improved young children's cognitive abilities, postintervention exposure to ongoing social disadvantage may offset earlier gains.[7] Discontinuities in health care and interrupted eligibility for early childhood intervention programs are examples of modifiable threats to sustained developmental improvement for at-risk children.

New and Differential Morbidities

The declining prevalence in the United States of nutritional and infectious disease and the changing patterns of childhood risk have increased the prominence of other causes of morbidity and mortality.[8] Children increasingly are affected by a broad and complex array of conditions termed "new morbidities": drug and alcohol use, family and neighborhood violence, emotional disorders, learning problems, and so on. These new morbidities originate in complex family or socioeconomic conditions rather than an exclusively biological etiology and cannot be adequately addressed by traditional medical services.[9] Instead, such conditions require a continuum of comprehensive services that include multidisciplinary assessment, treatment, and rehabilitation as well as community-based prevention strategies to sustain positive outcomes.[10] Such multidisciplinary approaches often incorporate and integrate public and private sector services. For example, early intervention, family preservation, and violence prevention programs involve broad-based, multisector approaches that transcend agency and service-sector boundaries.[11]

The types and patterns of condition for children are changing, and patterns of morbidity and the manifestation of medical conditions in children fundamentally differ in their pathophysiology and treatment compared to adults.[12] Serious, chronic medical conditions are less prevalent in children and usually are related to birth or congenitally acquired conditions, rather than the degenerative conditions that affect adults. Age-specific drug metabolism, disease expression, and health status assessments differentiate children from adults. For example, in children, cardiac conditions may result from any number of distinct congenital malformations, whereas in adults, cardiac conditions are dominated by a single degenerative disorder (atherosclerotic heart disease). These differences explain why pediatric specialists are more prepared to diagnose and treat many children's chronic and severe conditions. Age-related differences in disease prevalence, expression, and management have important implications for issues such as ensuring appropriate access to care, developing age-specific quality assessment measures, guaranteeing availability of adequately trained providers, and furthering regional distribution of pediatric health professionals and services.[13]

Dependency

Children also have complex and changing dependency relationships that affect their development and their use of health services. Children depend on their parents or other caregivers to recognize and respond to their health needs, to organize their care and authorize treatment, and to comply with recommended treatment regimens. The importance of this dependency for children's access to health care is illustrated by studies comparing maternal utilization of health services with children's use of care. Studies find that maternal and child use of care is highly correlated, irrespective of the level of health status.[14] Recent reports such as those by the National Commission on Children and the Carnegie Commission on Early Childhood further address the interdependency of family and social environments and their impact upon children's health and development.[15]

Health Service Delivery for U.S. Children

Although the principle that children's health services should be organized into a comprehensive, coordinated, continuous, and accessible system of health services is broadly supported, it is not clear how evolution in the health care marketplace and restructuring of the delivery system advance these principles for all children. Children's health care encompasses health promotion and disease prevention strategies that are necessarily broad and increasingly specify multisector approaches that integrate medical, public health, educational, and social services. Consequently, consolidating personal medical care services and other services heretofore delivered by the community health sector into privately managed, vertically integrated delivery systems may not produce the scope and horizontal integration of health and related services needed to rationalize the delivery system for many children. Managed care arrangements may effectively organize primary and specialty medical services for relatively healthy populations. However, the increasingly prevalent new morbidities and the complex socioeconomic and environmental conditions faced by many families often require intense, sustained, and coordinated health services that neither the current system nor the emerging managed care arrangements are structured to provide.[16]

Child Health Service Sectors

The U.S. child health system has been characterized as a patchwork of disconnected programs, each with distinct eligibility, administrative, and funding criteria.[17] The three distinct yet interdependent sectors that constitute child health services have unique histories, mandates, organizational characteristics and constraints, and funding streams.[18] They are the personal medical and preventive services sector; the population-based, community health services sector; and the health-related support services sector.

Personal Medical and Preventive Services. Personal medical and preventive health services for children include primary and specialty medical services, which are generally delivered in private and public medical offices, hospitals, and laboratories. Restructuring the organization of the personal health service care sector, where the majority of health care dollars are spent, is the major focus of current health system change. Personal medical services are principally funded through private health insurance, by the federal Medicaid program, and by out-of-pocket payments from families.[19]

Population-Based Community Health Services. The second sector of child health services includes population-based health promotion and disease prevention services, such as immunization delivery and monitoring programs, lead screening and abatement programs, and child abuse prevention. Other community health services are special child abuse treatment programs and rehabilitative services for children with complex congenital conditions or other chronic and debilitating diseases. Community-based programs provide assurance and coordination functions for children's health services, such as case management and referral programs for children with chronic diseases, and early intervention and monitoring programs for infants at risk for developmental disability. Funding for this sector comes from federal programs such as Medicaid's Early Periodic Screening, Diagnosis, and Treatment program (EPSDT), Title V (Maternal and Child Health) of the Social Security Act, and many other categorical programs.[20]

Health-Related Support Services. The third sector of the child health system includes health-related support services, such as nutrition education, early intervention, rehabilitation, and family support programs. Among the services in this sector are parent education and skill building in families with infants at risk for developmental delay due to physiological (such as low birthweight) or social (such as very low income) problems, or special education and psychotherapy for children with HIV. Funding for these services comes from diverse agencies, among them the U.S. Department of Agriculture (funding the Supplemental Food Program for Women, Infants, and Children, or WIC) and the Department of Education (funding the Individuals with Disabilities Education Act, or IDEA).

Fragmented Delivery System

These three child health sectors have evolved separately,[21] and the patchwork of programs that make up each sector poses real challenges to forging a continuum of integrated services. Incremental federal and state funding for children's health programs has produced this array of categorical, condition-specific, means-tested programs that are not well integrated within or between the child health service sectors. Many of these programs were developed to fill gaps or to address an emerging need (child abuse, HIV, mental health problems, lead toxicity), yet there is often little coordination within the federal, state, or local governing authorities, nor any attempts to link with private sector efforts. Program administrative mandates and categorical or block grant criteria often determine the number of children who can be served.

Some states have moved to establish omnibus coordinating agencies or administrative councils for children and family services. The Maternal and Child

Health Bureau is the single federal agency charged with improving the health status and organization of service systems for children at the federal level. Some have argued that this lone federal agency has neither the authority nor sufficient funding to accomplish its mission.[22]

Integrating Services

Achieving better health outcomes for the growing number of children afflicted with multiple and complex problems requires coordinated health and health-related services that may include primary and specialty medical care, case management, early intervention, and special education.[23] Recent efforts to rationalize the organization and allocation of child health services are exemplified by the infant and toddler portion of the IDEA legislation. The 1986 amendments to this legislation mandate interagency collaboration and regional service integration as part of a state planning process for early childhood intervention services. In many states, this has resulted in organized comprehensive and coordinated assessment and treatment services for infants and young children at risk for development disabilities owing to a variety of adverse perinatal outcomes or environmental factors.

Other examples of integrated delivery models developed for children at risk demonstrate efficiency in providing coordinated, multisectoral services for children. The Child and Adolescent Service System Program (CASSP) is the National Institute of Mental Health initiative to increase states' capacity to create coordinated systems of care in mental health for children and youth.[24] An example of such a mental health service integration model, developed in Ventura County, California, has involved the collaboration of health, juvenile justice, mental health, and education agencies for the purpose of coordinating service delivery to children and reducing out-of-home placement for children with severe mental health conditions. Evaluations of the Ventura Model demonstrate improved mental health outcomes in children and lower frequency of out-of-home placement.[25]

Innovative models, designed to facilitate service coordination by decategorizing funding streams and creating flexible funding pools, include a series of ongoing demonstration projects that have taken place in communities in the United States over the past decade.[26] These projects illustrate some of the strategies used to integrate services and increase children's access to appropriate services, by rationalizing provision of public funds.

Part of the difficulty in integrating health services comes from the sheer volume of categorical programs, as well as the scope of eligibility and financial constraints that inhibit greater coordination.[27] Table 11.1 illustrates part of this challenge. A comprehensive approach to providing preventive, diagnostic,

TABLE 11.1. PUBLIC PROGRAMS IN CHILD HEALTH SERVICE AND HEALTH NEED DOMAINS.

| Health Service | Health Need | | | | |
	Physical	Emotional	Cognitive	Family	Social
Prevention	Title XIX, Title XXI, Title V, Title X, WIC, MCH Block Grant	Title X, PL 99-457	Title XIX, Title X, PL 99-457, Head Start	Title X, Head Start, AFDC, PL 99-457	Title IV, HUD, AFDC
Early identification	Title XIX, Title XXI, Title V, Title X, WIC, MCH Block Grant	Title XIX, PL 99-457	Title XIX, PL 99-457	Title XX, Title IV	Title IV
Diagnosis	Title XIX, Title XXI, Title V, PL 99-457	Title XIX, PL 99-457	Title XIX, PL 99-457	Title XX, Title IV, PL 99-457	Title IV
Treatment	Title XIX, Title XXI, Title V, PL 99-457	Title XIX, PL 99-457	Title XIX, PL 99-457	Title XX, PL 99-457	Title IV
Rehabilitation	Title XIX, Title XXI, Title V, PL 99-457	Title XIX, PL 99-457	Title XIX, PL 99-457		Title IV

Source: Halfon, N., and Berkowitz, G. "Health Care Entitlements for Children: Providing Health Services As If Children Really Mattered." In M. A. Jensen and S. G. Goffin (eds.), *Visions of Entitlement: The Care and Education of America's Children.* Albany, N.Y.: SUNY Press, 1993.

treatment, and rehabilitative services across the physical, emotional, cognitive, and social domains would require integration of many programs and funding sources.

Financing Children's Health Care

Intimately linked to structure and organization of health services is how these services are financed. A range of funding streams currently fund parts of the full continuum of services that children need. However, health insurance remains a principal determinant of children's access to medical care. Financial barriers to medical care result primarily from lack of insurance for primary care services (such as well-child care and immunizations) or specialty child health services (such as mental health services and rehabilitative therapy).

Uninsured Children

Public child health insurance eligibility expansion has occurred as studies continue to document significant differential access to health care for uninsured children. Children without health insurance are less likely to have routine doctor visits or receive care for injuries, and more likely to delay seeking care.[28] In the 1997 National Health Interview Survey (NHIS), parents of uninsured children reported a higher rate of unmet medical, dental, medication, and vision needs than did parents of privately insured children.[29] Delay in care for common childhood conditions that have potentially disabling effects (such as ear infection leading to hearing loss) has been attributed to families' lack of health coverage for the child.[30] Uninsured preschoolers have a lower immunization coverage rate and lower compliance with well-child visit schedules.[31] Uninsured families are also more likely to rely on the emergency room to be their regular source of care, and to inappropriately use costly emergency room and hospital outpatient departments for the child's primary care needs.[32] Lack of health insurance can also result in families restricting their children's participation in sports and other activities because of concerns about their ability to pay for injury care.[33]

The proportion of uninsured children in the United States has increased over the last twenty years. The proportion of children who are uninsured rose 40 percent between 1977 and 1987.[34] By 1989, 13.3 percent of children were uninsured.[35] The percentage of children covered by employer-based insurance dropped steadily for more than a decade. The decline in private insurance coverage for children resulted from elimination of dependent coverage by some employers and from economic shifts toward service jobs without generous health benefits. By 1992, the percentage of children with employer-based coverage had declined to 56.2 percent (from 60.7 percent in 1987), accounting for nearly three million children losing coverage.[36]

The number of uninsured children would have been even greater if expansions of the Medicaid program had not partially compensated for this erosion in employer-based insurance.[37] Between 1989 and 1993, the number of children covered by Medicaid increased 54 percent, from 13.6 percent of U.S. children in 1989 (8.9 million children) to 19.9 percent in 1993 (13.7 million).[38] Although Medicaid extends coverage to children in the lowest-income families, two-thirds of uninsured children live in families with income above the poverty level.[39] In 1992, 21 percent of children with family income of 100–199 percent of the federal poverty level were uninsured,[40] and 74 percent of uninsured children lived in families with one or more working parents.[41] By March 1998, roughly at the time of enactment of the federal State Children's Health Insurance Program (SCHIP), 10.7 million children (representing 15 percent of the U.S. child population) were uninsured.[42] This included a significant number of children who were eligible for but not enrolled in Medicaid.[43]

Specific provisions of the SCHIP legislation addressed some historical limitations of Medicaid.[44] States were required to implement outreach programs and to ensure that children found not to be eligible for SCHIP would be referred to or enrolled in Medicaid if eligible. States also were permitted to extend twelve months of eligibility to a child once Medicaid eligibility was established so that eligibility losses caused by month-to-month income fluctuations could be reduced.

Medicaid Participation. Medicaid participation has been hampered by low reimbursement level and by eligibility rules that cause discontinuities in children's enrollment.[45] Complex Medicaid eligibility criteria and fluctuations in family income result in significant turnover in enrollees each year. It is estimated that 40 percent of Medicaid AFDC enrollees lose Medicaid coverage each year.[46] Duration of enrollment is a critical Medicaid program issue for children. Longitudinal data from 1991 to 1993 showed that only 20 percent of newly Medicaid-eligible children under age sixteen retained coverage after twenty-eight months.[47] Of the children under age sixteen who lost Medicaid coverage, only about 61 percent were insured four months later.

A significant proportion of children who are Medicaid-eligible remain unenrolled. This is particularly true for Latino children.[48] Eligibility expansion has extended coverage, but reasons that eligible children still do not participate include delinking of Medicaid from cash assistance, limited outreach[49] and parent knowledge,[50] and complex rules that are difficult for eligibility workers to administer.[51] In 1993, an estimated 2.3 million uninsured children were Medicaid-eligible.[52] By 1996, this number increased to an estimated 4.3 million.[53]

State Children's Health Insurance Program. Enactment of the State Children's Health Insurance Program in 1997 as Title XXI of the Social Security Act extended health insurance to children who had not been eligible for Medicaid or private, employer-based coverage. SCHIP extended coverage to approximately one-third of the eleven million uninsured children[54] living in families with income between the existing Medicaid eligibility threshold and 200 percent of the federal poverty level. Initially authorized for 1997 through 2001, SCHIP included provisions to prevent children who otherwise could be enrolled in private employer-based insurance from participating in SCHIP.[55]

Private Insurance. Children with employment-based health coverage also are at risk for loss of insurance and disruption of care. Health insurance for children covered under their parents' employment is jeopardized when job loss or job change occurs. As the economy shifts from high-paying, benefit-rich manufacturing jobs to lower-paying, benefit-poor service jobs, dependent coverage is less assured. For example, 25 percent of children from thirteen to eighteen months old in a large health maintenance organization had experienced some disruption of coverage during the previous five-month period.[56] Uninsurance among workers and their families who could receive employer-based insurance but are not enrolled also has been studied.[57]

Even those children and families with health insurance frequently have been underinsured for essential primary medical care, including well-child care, immunizations, and specialty care. In 1992, 50 percent of indemnity insurance health plans covered well-child care and 65 percent of preferred provider organizations (PPOs) covered immunizations.[58] Children with special health care needs caused by a congenital condition, chronic illness, or injury may lack adequate private medical coverage, especially for speech therapy, behavioral therapy, physical therapy, and other essential services.[59] Moreover, despite the demonstrated efficacy of nonmedical social services for health and developmental outcomes, services such as home visitation and health-related consultation are rarely benefits for privately insured children. In contrast, Medicaid generally covers these services.

Cost Sharing. Nearly all health plans apply cost-sharing mechanisms to minimize unnecessary use of medical services and thereby limit expenditures. The RAND Health Insurance Experiment found that placing cost-sharing requirements on families for primary and preventive care services reduced children's use of these discretionary services.[60] Although short-term adverse outcomes from reduced use of medical care were not detected in the RAND study, the sensitivity of children's basic ambulatory medical services to cost sharing was demonstrated.[61] With the expansion of managed care, more preventive services such as immunization and well-child care are routinely covered, and administration fees, deductibles, co-payments, and other cost-sharing mechanisms are less often applied for preventive and primary care visits. In contrast, cost sharing continues to be applied to acute and chronic care services. For many poor, near-poor, and even middle-income families, even nominal cost sharing poses a significant barrier to care.

Nonfinancial Barriers to Care

Children's access to medical care traditionally has been measured by analyzing utilization patterns for specific provider services (such as number of annual physician visits), designated populations (adolescents, children in foster care), children with specific conditions (for instance, those with asthma), or specific services (immunization, prenatal care, and so on).[62] Such analyses have identified many factors that impede use of care and that appear to account for differential utilization rates (such as ethnicity, income, and residence) when controlling for health need (as measured by health status indicators and number and type of conditions).[63] Nonfinancial barriers to care include structural, environmental, and personal barriers such as bureaucratic complexity in the organization of child health services; cultural barriers based on ethnicity or language; and provider distribution or shortage, among others.[64]

Race and Ethnicity. In addition to income, differential access has been consistently documented on the basis of race and ethnicity. Differential access and use associated with race and ethnicity may result from varying modes of utilization, insurance barriers, and the cultural competency of providers. Nonwhite children and adolescents have fewer physician visits and are less likely to have continuity of care.[65] Studies of access to care of Latino children have also indicated a high rate of uninsurance and differential patterns of utilization based on parental immigration status.[66] Problems of care and health outcomes for African American children have been improved when targeted interventions can overcome organizational barriers.[67] A study of African American women receiving prenatal care in an environment that potentially equalizes access to care (a U.S. Army base) detected a lower infant mortality rate and underscores the important role that special barriers have in poor health outcomes for children.[68]

Regular Sources of Care. As Barbara Starfield has demonstrated in numerous reviews of access to care, having a regular source of primary care is particularly important for children.[69] Children with a regular source of care are more likely to receive needed medical services and immunizations, resulting in a higher level of satisfaction reported by the family.[70] Having a regular source of care is principally determined by insurance status, and the insurance effect on access is often mediated by having a regular provider.[71] In several studies, the type and characteristics of the regular care provider have their own independent effect on utilization, irrespective of type of insurance coverage. Therefore, considering the type of a usual source of care is important in analyzing differences in access among children. It is a key indicator of the success of insurance expansions such as SCHIP.[72]

Provider Training. Emerging patterns of morbidity in children, including complex risks, health conditions, and social problems pose new challenges to health care providers and delivery systems.[73] Surveys and anecdotal reports document inadequacies in clinical training for health professionals and their inability to identify, treat, or refer children suffering from complex medical conditions, mental disorders, developmental problems, complex psychosocial problems, and abuse and neglect.[74] In one study, physicians' assessments identified less than 50 percent of emotional problems of the children who were screened.[75] These inadequacies are a function of provider training and knowledge, systemic undervaluing of assessment for new morbidities, and the shortage of community-based treatment resources for these problems.[76]

Distribution of Providers. Geographic access barriers pose problems for both insured and uninsured poor families. Travel time for a family in an underserved urban area or rural location may be substantial[77] and result in reduced use of care.[78] For poor children, a limited supply of local physicians is associated with reduced access to preventive care services[79] and routine emergency room use for nonemergent sick care.[80] Although the overall number of pediatricians has increased over the past two decades, the geographic distribution of pediatricians relative to the child population has not improved significantly.[81] The shortage of local primary care providers for poor children has been further compromised in recent years; the number of office-based physicians delivering primary care services in low-income areas declined by 45.1 percent between 1963 and 1980.[82]

Children who receive care in an office-based setting are more likely to receive continuity of care and coordination of services. One effect of the shortage in office-based primary care providers has been the high, and often inappropriate, rate of emergency department utilization.[83] Persons who identify their regular provider of care as a hospital outpatient department, rather than a medical office, are significantly less likely to see the same provider on a subsequent visit,[84] and young children receive less preventive care, including immunizations, in these settings.[85] In recent years, the outpatient department of a hospital has increasingly replaced the office of a private physician as the site of the regular source of care for poor children.[86]

Improving the Child Health System

The task of integrating personal medical services with complementary community-based health, social, and educational services demands substantial coordination as well as financial incentives. Achieving health system objectives for children requires greater access to health insurance, integration of services, quality measurement, public and community monitoring of performance (including data systems, involvement of communities, and new measures of how well community systems are performing), and tailoring managed care delivery systems to meet the developmental needs of all children and the special needs of vulnerable child populations.[87]

Health Insurance

In the early 1990s, it seemed that national health care reform might provide universal coverage and usher in a more organized system. Instead, state-initiated health insurance expansions for children took center stage. Some states obtained Medicaid demonstration waivers and used this flexibility to convert to managed care systems and to expand coverage for previously uninsured groups.[88] Other states embarked on health insurance expansion for children using state funding (such as Pennsylvania's Child Health Insurance Program, or CHIP), or developed programs that combine public and private revenues (such as Colorado's Child Health Plan). Another form of child health insurance expansion was the Blue Cross and Blue Shield Caring Program for Children.[89] Such privately funded programs primarily covered well-child services and care for acute and chronic illness, but not hospitalization. Thus, program costs were relatively modest.

Enactment of SCHIP in 1997 further strengthened the role of the state in administering unique, state-based health insurance programs for children. State options to determine benefit package, cost sharing, and enrollment mechanisms in SCHIP have contributed to the difference in insurance eligibility and program structure across states.[90] Past experience with children's incomplete participation in Medicaid and their failure to be covered by employer-based insurance when it is available has produced a challenge for SCHIP.[91] Enrollment of eligible children has been a focus of state implementation strategies and will be important for reauthorization of the program. As states experiment with outreach and enrollment procedures, identifying successful methods of enrolling and retaining children in the SCHIP and Medicaid programs is an important objective.[92]

Health System Integration

Expansion of health insurance coverage and system reorganization based on managed care cannot guarantee children's access to a system of health care that is comprehensive and coordinated. Structural and organizational characteristics of the current health system must be addressed to improve allocation and quality of health services for children and families.[93]

The principles of comprehensive, continuous, and coordinated care originally embodied in Medicaid's EPSDT program, and reinforced in 1989 amendments to Title XIX, recognize that access to basic ambulatory medical care does not suffice to meet the needs of children with complex health conditions and environmental risks. For such children, screening, diagnostic, and treatment services must be supplemented with a constellation of supportive services, including outreach, comprehensive case management home visiting, and family counseling services.[94] Several authors have suggested that services should address existing health conditions but should also be sensitive to the functional and developmental capacities of the child as well as to the family's needs and the community environment.[95] This implies a systematic focus on strategically optimizing investment in children's health development.

Programs designed to reduce health risks and promote protective factors have been tested for children at risk of adverse developmental or other outcomes. In an increasingly cost-conscious era, initiatives to broaden and integrate child health services and develop linkage across sectors must demonstrate both effectiveness (improved health outcomes, in an applied setting) and efficiency (cost impact).[96] Home visiting and other early intervention programs targeted to at-risk families have proven cost-effective in improving children's health status, cognitive functioning, and academic performance, while decreasing dependence on public assistance.[97] Until recently, few of these successful demonstration and local community projects have been implemented on a statewide scale. North Carolina's SmartStart, California's Children and Family First Act, and Vermont's Success by Six all report new statewide efforts targeting the health and development of all young children. These are broad, population-based health promotion and disease prevention programs, where the medical sector plays a key role. It is not clear to what degree these new population-based initiatives will become comprehensive and integrated with traditional children's medical services.

The potential of integrated service programs, such as early intervention or school-linked health services, is uncertain in the current managed care marketplace. They are not likely to reduce the short-term costs of a managed care organization by reducing hospitalization or other high-cost medical expenditure. Instead, the savings from these programs may be realized in a lower incidence of special education participation, enhanced family functioning, and lower welfare outlays.[98] Savings are likely to accrue to the education, mental health, juvenile justice, and other business sectors, rather than to the organization that provided the care. It may be more difficult for states to continue to support integrated cross-sector delivery efforts such as early intervention programs, school-based clinics, or many public health safety net programs. Over the past decade, many of these services have been paid for (in the case of early intervention and school-based clinics) or heavily subsidized (in the case of public clinics and hospitals) with Medicaid funds. As Medicaid funds are diverted into commercial managed care contracts, the ability of the state or local community to use these funds for community health programs and health-related support services may be reduced. Continued development of integrated continuums poses a fundamental challenge to states and localities that choose not to earmark some portion of their Medicaid funds, or identify new revenues for this purpose (as California and North Carolina have).

Although direct control over Medicaid funds may decline, the range of mechanisms that states are implementing (combined or separate medical and mental health managed systems, service exclusions, and so on) presents an opportunity to test what types of public-private arrangement prove effective. The infrastructure of the managed care organization may create new opportunities for coordination, if not integration.[99] Greater attention to early childhood development, coupled with the need for Medicaid (and SCHIP) managed care contractors to forge relationships with existing public programs for children, could spur enhanced integration. For example, statewide population-based early childhood health and development promotion programs in California, North Carolina, and Vermont are already being linked with initiatives on the part of local health care providers and managed care organizations. There is a tremendous opportunity to understand which managed care mechanisms serve as barriers or facilitators to quality health care, to identify measures that capture the unique objectives of children's health care, and to use state intervention in Medicaid and SCHIP as a research laboratory.

Measures of Health Care Quality for Children

Government agencies, medical professional organizations, and multidisciplinary expert working groups have all developed normative definitions of comprehensive primary care.[100] For example, standards have been issued by the federal MCHB and the American Academy of Pediatrics for children's medical care, and by the Child Welfare League of America for the health needs of children in foster care.[101] The recent Bright Futures recommendations, funded by the MCHB and the Health Care Financing Administration (HCFA), present a comprehensive set of standards for the content of well-child services.[102] The principles embodied in Bright Futures reaffirm the need for an integrated health care system that is comprehensive, continuous, accessible, coordinated, and accountable. Other research and health care organizations are developing practice guidelines for particular services or medical conditions based on evidence or the consensus of an expert panel.[103] Such guidelines are more readily implemented than the normative standards.

In the private sector, the National Commission for Quality Assurance (NCQA) developed the Health Employer Data Information Set (HEDIS), which compares commercial health plan performance on quality indicators of effectiveness of care, access, and utilization. Many commercial health plans report a subset of HEDIS measures (focusing on maternal and child health) separately for Medicaid enrollees.[104] HEDIS and other quality assurance systems based on administrative data do not capture all domains of quality that are of interest for children's health care. Family satisfaction information collected from patients can supplement utilization and administrative data, particularly for difficult-to-measure constructs such as perceived access. The Consumer Assessment of Health Plans (CAHPS) consumer satisfaction surveys ask parents about their child's health care and have a supplemental survey for parents of children with special health needs.

In 1999, an ambitious national initiative was launched by the Foundation for Accountability (FACCT), the NCQA, and several federal agencies. The Child and Adolescent Health Measurement Initiative (CAHMI) is developing several new quality care measures. Surveys developed by FACCT also ask parents about their child's experience with health care and focus on key areas of child development, primary care services, and care for chronic illness. For example, the FACCT Promoting Healthy Development Survey examines provision of developmentally relevant services to children from birth to three. The Living with Illness survey examines service delivery to children with chronic medical conditions.

There are a number of reasons that developing performance measures and standards of care for children and families is a unique and challenging undertaking.[105] Because children are constantly developing, it is difficult to attribute positive or negative characteristics of their health care to their functioning and future outcomes. The complexity of some constructs that define quality care for children (comprehensive, family-centered, integrated) makes it difficult to create valid quality indicators that can be used for performance comparison. Additionally, the relatively small number and heterogeneity within a group of children with a particular kind of complex medical condition is a methodological challenge in creating standards and performance measures associated with those standards. These are challenges that the pediatric health services research community is attempting to address. In 1997, the Association for Health Services Research (AHSR), with several federal agencies, convened a research agenda setting conference to develop a new, strategic child health services research agenda with a particular focus on quality of care.[106]

Public Accountability and Monitoring

Public accountability for ensuring that all children have access to comprehensive health care has not been part of U.S. child health policy. In the European nations that maintain population-based service delivery models and use public health nurses and other providers to track and monitor infants through the preschool years, compliance with immunization schedules and age-appropriate preventive care visits is substantially higher than in the United States.[107] A combination of universal access to preventive care and integrated health information systems permits such population-based assurance.

Despite recent advances in health information systems, current U.S. data yield little detailed information on quality of care or health outcomes.[108] Data systems currently are not structured or capable of producing child-focused information on encounters with the broader child health system, including the public health, nutrition, and school-based health sectors. Some efforts are under way across the United States to introduce model systems that can be used to ensure delivery of the most basic of medical services for children. An example is the Robert Wood Johnson Foundation's All Kids Count initiative, which supports demonstrations of state and local immunization information and monitoring systems.[109] National surveys such as the National Health Interview Survey (NHIS) and its supplements on children and on individuals with disabilities, and the Medical Expenditure Panel Survey (MEPS), produce much of the national data on children's access to and use of (and costs of) health care.

Data are lacking in some areas, but there still is a role for community performance monitoring.[110] Because children's health services are delivered in multiple sectors, a community rather than a specific public program or commercial managed care organization may have the most to gain or to lose from investing in its children's health. Such a monitoring process would include evaluating which aspects of the system facilitate or hinder access, using information about best practices to make improvements where necessary, and examining improvement by monitoring children's outcomes.

Ideally, community systems should be organized to respond to the determinants of children's health, in terms of availability of services, providers, and programs.[111] Normative standards for children's health care have identified the need for coordination across programs and organizations. To capture the potential contribution to children's health from the sectors responsible for their care, performance should thus be measured at the community level. Consideration of standards of care for children should not neglect administrative and community-level attributes that promote or undermine quality. For example, measures of service and system integration can be applied to evaluate performance within and among the child health service sectors. Defining the critical pathways by which coordination (when successful) takes place constitutes an initial step in developing the measures and the infrastructure for community performance monitoring.[112] Linking the results to specific organizational attributes would then make it possible to improve those system attributes that affect quality. Monitoring these attributes is important for policy and planning purposes.[113] For example, a number of communities are devising population-based report cards on determinants of children's health that, when linked to a monitoring system, can be used to mobilize change.[114] These initiatives may be an initial step toward the population-based accountability that has been lacking for children and families.

Managed Care for Children

Historically, many Medicaid-insured children received medical care in safety-net public health facilities, where provider continuity and comprehensive health care were not always available.[115] Past difficulties in access and fragmentation of the delivery system help to explain the rapid transition in the 1990s from fee-for-service to managed care Medicaid programs. By the late 1990s, forty-one states had converted their Medicaid programs into managed care delivery systems,[116] while many state SCHIP programs also turned to managed care arrangements. Children covered by commercial health insurance also have been affected by these trends. By 1995, approximately six of every ten enrollees in managed care were in for-profit health plans.[117] The effectiveness and improvement of managed care as a delivery system is an important policy question for both publicly and privately insured children.[118]

In early studies, managed care organizations demonstrated marginally higher preventive care utilization for maternal and child health services.[119] In a unique study that randomized families to managed care or to fee-for-service arrangements, managed care plans successfully reduced emergency room use and ambulatory visits for nonsevere conditions but did not appear to reduce medical services for children with acute needs. Thus, the authors concluded that managed care can rationalize care without inappropriate rationing of care.[120] Other studies comparing access and use under fee-for-service or managed care arrangements have found mixed results.[121]

There have been concerns that managed care organizations' lack of experience with comprehensive delivery systems for children, and their tendency to control rather than coordinate services, could jeopardize care for children with chronic illness.[122] Managed care arrangements are largely untested in terms of their ability to cost-effectively manage the care of vulnerable children. Many children with special health needs (such as serious medical conditions) or with special circumstances (foster children, homeless children) have been excluded from previous studies of health outcomes, use, or costs. Even when included in such studies, they often make up such a small proportion of the study sample that evaluation of the impact of managed care on their health outcomes is impossible. In addition, Medicaid beneficiaries (and often commercial insurance enrollees as well) in most states were initially offered a choice between fee-for-service and managed care. Several studies show that children electing not to enroll in managed care are more likely to have certain medical diagnoses or higher health care utilization than children who do enroll.[123] It is thus difficult to compare the experiences of children who elect to enroll and those who do not, particularly without detailed information about their health care needs.

Several studies suggest the kinds of access barriers that children with special health needs might confront within a managed care organization. A survey of pediatricians participating in managed care plans revealed a high rate of denied referrals to specialists for children.[124] Early studies of managed care for children with special health care needs suggested that managed care plans limit mental health and related services, as well as access to specialists.[125] Another survey of administrators from twenty-two managed care plans found that few plans made special efforts to ensure inclusion of pediatric providers in the network.[126]

As managed care expands in the U.S. marketplace, research on the outcomes and effectiveness in such systems is increasingly important.[127] However, it is not only differences between enrolled populations that makes comparison difficult for children. Variation in managed care structures, benefits, and implementation across regions makes it difficult to generalize experience within one region or study to that of other localities. For example, a 1998 survey of state Medicaid programs showed a variety of mixed financing arrangements affecting children's services, including medical and behavioral health contracts, service exclusion, and diagnosis exclusion.[128] In the absence of generalizable findings about managed care impact, certain important focus areas have been identified for Medicaid program oversight of managed care contractors: specificity of pediatric service benefits, requirements for pediatric providers contracting within networks, medical necessity standards tailored for children, quality indicators for children, appropriate payment rates for pediatric services, and promotion of high-quality care.[129]

It is important—but a complex undertaking—to evaluate how contracting arrangements affect care for children. Earlier studies of Medicaid managed care focused on difference between fee-for-service and managed care arrangements rather than on difference within managed care systems.[130] Optimal financing and contracting arrangements within Medicaid managed care are important to identify for children with special health needs and other groups of vulnerable children in particular.[131]

From Social HMOs to HDOs

To overcome the obstacles to comprehensive and coordinated systems of health services for high-risk children and families, new forms of managed health care must be created. This could take the form of social HMOs or health development organizations (HDOs). The social HMO concept augments current vertically integrated medical services with additional health promotion, social services, and enhanced coordination mechanisms to produce appropriate horizontal integration.[132] Demonstration project social HMOs for the frail and elderly population have offered multifaceted risk assessment and an inclusive set of services, resources, case management, and coordination.[133] Evaluation of social HMO experience for the elderly has produced mixed outcomes.[134] Nonetheless the social HMO concept has enormous potential for maximizing the fit between the true health needs of children and an appropriately constructed and integrated delivery system.

An extension of the social HMO concept is what has been termed a health development organization (HDO).[135] The HDO framework creates a mechanism to integrate services not only vertically and horizontally but longitudinally as well, to optimize the health development trajectory of children. HDOs would actively develop the health of the child population by using principles and practices that optimize health development trajectories. These include minimizing the influence of risk factors during a critical developmental period through targeted risk reduction and strategic use of health promotion and other protective factors. This is illustrated in Figure 11.1.

Studies of the commercial managed care sector have examined the proliferation of managed care systems that target particular populations or service needs.[136] This market-based trend toward innovation and diversification could extend to children's services and stimulate new systems of specialty care for children that previously were attempted only within public sector integration initiatives.[137]

Conclusion

Population-based, integrated models of service delivery systems have been developed in European nations and in localized demonstration projects in the United States. Most European countries provide universal health, developmental, and social services to children beginning at conception, including nationally insured health care, maternity leave and support, and child care and development programs.[138] The U.S. health care system continues to produce many important innovations in addressing the special medical and developmental needs of children. Using managed care to rationalize delivery of personal medical services may substantially improve children's access to basic medical care. Nonetheless, many health needs, especially for children with complex medical or socially based health problems, may not be adequately addressed.

FIGURE 11.1. HOW RISK-REDUCTION AND HEALTH-PROMOTION STRATEGIES INFLUENCE HEALTH DEVELOPMENT.

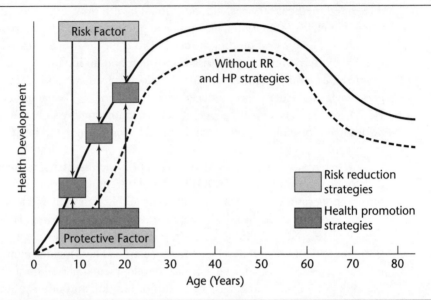

Note: This figure illustrates how risk-reduction strategies can mitigate the influence of risk factors on the developmental trajectory, and how health promotion strategies can simultaneously support and optimize the development trajectory. In the absence of effective risk reduction and health promotion, the developmental trajectory will be suboptimal (dotted curve).

Source: Halfon, N., Inkelas, M., and Hochstein, M. "The Health Development Organization: An Organizational Approach to Achieving Child Health Development." *Milbank Quarterly,* 2000, *78*(3), 447–498.

The evolution of the U.S. health care system into distinct sectors, with fragmented services and categorical funding mechanisms, poses a significant barrier to improved organization of care. Improving the health care delivery system for children means integrating the activities of largely publicly funded community-based health services with privately delivered managed care models. Whether or not the emerging health system more adequately meets the health needs of children and successfully addresses the newer morbidities depends not only on insurance coverage but also upon integrating the disparate sectors of the child health system.

Opportunities exist during this time of great structural change to fashion delivery systems that grant all children access to a continuum of services. However, in the public policy area, insufficient attention has been paid to the unique needs of children and to the design of a system that meets children's needs. The move to managed care may facilitate some of the changes that are necessary to improve services delivered to children, if essential components and safeguards are included. Policy makers, health care providers, and the public at large have to consider how to ensure that children's unique needs are met under the evolving health system if health outcomes are to be improved.

Notes

1. Jameson, E. J., and Wehr, E. "Drafting National Health Care Reform Legislation to Protect the Health Interests of Children." *Stanford Law and Policy Review,* 1994, *5,* 152–176; Halfon, N., Inkelas, M., and Wood, D. "Nonfinancial Barriers to Care for Children and Youth." *Annual Review of Public Health,* 1995, *16,* 447–472; Forrest, C. B., Simpson, L., and Clancy, C. "Child Health Services Research: Challenges and Opportunities." *Journal of the American Medical Association,* 1997, *277,* 1787–1793; Halfon, N., Inkelas, M., and Hochstein, M. "The Health Development Organization: An Organizational Approach to Achieving Child Health Development." *Milbank Quarterly,* 2000, *78,* 447–498.

2. Shonkoff, J. P., and Meisels, S. J. "Early Childhood Intervention: The Evolution of a Concept." In S. J. Meisels and J. P. Shonkoff (eds.), *Intervention Handbook of Early Childhood.* Cambridge, England: Cambridge University Press, 1990.

3. Hertzman, C. "The Lifelong Impact of Childhood Experiences: A Population Perspective." *Proceedings of the American Academy of Arts and Sciences, Daedalus: Health and Wealth,* 1994, *123*(4), 167–180; Sameroff, A. J., and Fiese, B. H. "Transactional Regulation and Early Intervention." In Meisels and Shonkoff (1990); Bronfenbrenner, U. "Ecology of the Family as a Context for Human Development Research Perspectives." *Developmental Psychology,* 1986, *22,* 723–742; Bronfenbrenner, U. *The Ecology of Human Development: Experiments by Nature and Design.* Cambridge, Mass.: Harvard University Press, 1979.

4. Hertzman (1994); Evans, G. "Introduction." In R. G. Evans, M. L. Barer, and T. R. Marmor (eds.), *Why Are Some People Healthy and Others Not? The Determinants of Health of Populations.* Hawthorne, N.Y.: Aldine de Gruyter, 1994; Barker, D. J., and others. "The Relation of Small Head Circumference and Thinness at Birth to Death from Cardiovascular Disease in Adult Life." *British Medical Journal,* 1993, *306,* 422–426; Bakketeig, L. S., and others. "Pre-Pregnancy Risk Factors of Small-for-Gestational-Age Births Among Parous Women in Scandinavia." *Acta Obstetrica Gynecol Scand,* 1993, *72,* 273–279; Werner, E. E. "High Risk Children in Young Adulthood: A Longitudinal Study from Birth to Age 32 Years." *American Journal of Orthopsychiatry,* 1989, *59,* 72–81; Freeman, J. "Prenatal and Perinatal Factors Associated with Brain Disorders." (NIH publication no. 85-1149). Washington, D.C.: U.S. Department of Health and Human Services, 1985.

5. Brooks-Gunn, J., and others. "Early Intervention in Low Birthweight Premature Infants: Results Through Age 5 years from the Infant Health and Development Program." *Journal of the American Medical Association,* 1994, *272,* 1257–1262; Infant Health and Development Program. "Enhancing the Outcomes of Low-Birthweight, Premature Infants: A Multisite Randomized Trial." *Journal of the American Medical Association,* 1990, *263,* 3035–3042.

6. Karoly, L., and others. *Investing in Our Children: What We Know and Don't Know About the Costs and Benefits of Early Childhood Interventions.* Santa Monica, Calif.: RAND, 1998.

7. Brooks-Gunn, J., and others (1994); Zigler, E. F. "Early Childhood Intervention: A Promising Preventative for Juvenile Delinquency." *American Psychologist,* 1992, *47,* 997–1006.

8. Hoeckleman, R. A., and Pless, I. B. "Decline in Mortality Among Young Americans During the 20th Century: Prospects for Reaching National Mortality Reduction Goals for 1990." *Pediatrics,* 1988, *82,* 582–595.

9. Haggerty, R. J., Roghmann, K. J., and Pless, I. B. *Child Health and the Community.* New York: Wiley, 1975; Starfield, B. "Child and Adolescent Health Measures." *Future of Children,* 1992, *2,* 25–39.

10. Halfon, N., and Berkowitz, G. "Health Care Entitlements for Children: Providing Health Services as If Children Really Mattered." In M. A. Jensen and S. G. Goffin (eds.), *Visions of Entitlement: The Care and Education of America's Children.* Albany: SUNY Press, 1993.

11. Fielding, J. E., and Halfon, N. "Where Is the Health in Health Reform?" *Journal of the American Medical Association,* 1994, *272,* 1292–1296.

12. Jameson and Wehr (1994).

13. McGlynn, E., Halfon, N., and Leibowitz, A. "Assessing the Quality of Care for Children: Prospects Under Health Care Reform." *Archives of Pediatric and Adolescent Medicine,* 1995, *149,* 359–368.

14. Newacheck, P. W., and Halfon, N. "The Association Between Mothers' and Children's Use of Physician Services." *Medical Care,* 1986, *24,* 30–33.

15. Carnegie Task Force on Meeting the Needs of Young Children. *Starting Points: Meeting the Needs of Our Youngest Children.* New York: Carnegie Corporation of New York, 1994; National Commission on Children. *Beyond Rhetoric: A New American Agenda for Children and Families.* Washington, D.C.: U.S. Government Printing Office, 1994.

16. Halfon, Inkelas, and Hochstein (2000).

17. Select Panel for the Promotion of Child Health. *Better Health for Our Children: A National Strategy.* Washington, D.C.: U.S. Department of Health and Human Services, 1981; Harvey, B. "Why We Need a National Child Health Policy." *Pediatrics,* 1991, *87,* 1–6; Schlesinger, M., and Eisenberg, L. "Little People in a Big Policy World: Lasting Questions and New Directions in Health Policy for Children." In M. Schlesinger and L. Eisenberg (eds.), *Children in a Changing Health System: Assessments and Proposals for Reform.* Baltimore: Johns Hopkins University Press, 1990.

18. Halfon, Inkelas, and Wood (1995).

19. Lewit, E., and Monheit, A. "Expenditures on Health Care for Children and Pregnant Women." *Future of Children,* 1992, *2,* 95–114; McCormick, M. C., and others. "Annual Report of Access to and Utilization of Health Care for Children and Youth in the United States—1999." *Pediatrics,* 2000, *105,* 219–230.

20. Harvey (1991).

21. Schlesinger and Eisenberg (1990).

22. Grason, H., and Guyer, B. "Rethinking the Organization of Children's Programs: Lessons from the Elderly." *Milbank Quarterly,* 1995, *73,* 565–597.

23. Halfon, Inkelas, and Hochstein (2000).

24. Kahn, A. J., and Kamerman, S. B. *Integrating Services Integration: An Overview of Initiatives, Issues, and Possibilities.* (National Center for Children in Poverty.) New York: Columbia University School of Public Health, 1992.

25. Rosenblatt, A., Attkisson, C. C., and Fernandez, A. J. "Integrating Systems of Care in California for Youth with Severe Emotional Disturbance. II: Initial Group Home Expenditure and Utilization Findings from the California AB377 Evaluation Project." *Journal of Child and Family Studies,* 1992, *1,* 263–286.

26. Newacheck, P., Hughes, D., Halfon, N., and Brindis, C. "Social HMOs and Other Capitated Arrangements for Children with Special Health Care Needs." *Maternal and Child Health Journal,* 1997, *1,* 111–118.

27. Halfon and Berkowitz (1993).

28. Stoddard, J., St. Peter, R., and Newacheck, P. W. "Health Insurance Status and Ambulatory Care for Children." *New England Journal of Medicine,* 1994, *330,* 1421–1425.

29. Newacheck, P. W., and others. "The Unmet Needs of America's Children." *Pediatrics,* 2000, *105,* 989–997.

30. Stoddard, St. Peter, and Newacheck (1994).

31. Wood, D. L., and others. "Access to Medical Care for Children and Adolescents in the United States." *Pediatrics,* 1990, *86,* 666–673; Short, P. F., and Lefkowitz, D. C. "Encouraging Preventive Services for Low-Income Children: The Effect of Expanding Medicaid." *Medical Care,* 1992, *30,* 766–780.

32. Wood and others (1990); Newacheck, P. W., Hughes, D., and Stoddard, J. "Children's Access to Primary Care: Differences by Race, Income, and Insurance Status." *Pediatrics,* 1997, *97,* 26–32.

33. Lave, J. R., and others. "Impact of a Children's Health Insurance Program on Newly Enrolled Children." *Journal of the American Medical Association,* 1998, *279,* 1820–1825.

34. Employee Benefit Research Institute. "Sources of Health Insurance and Characteristics of the Uninsured: Analysis of the March 1992 Current Population Survey." (Report no. 133.) Washington, D.C.: Employee Benefit Research Institute, 1993.

35. U.S. General Accounting Office. *Medicaid: States Turn to Managed Care to Improve Access and Control Costs.* GAO/HRD-93-46. Washington, D.C.: U.S. Government Printing Office, 1993.

36. Newacheck, P. W., Hughes, D. C., and Cisternas, M. "Children and Health Insurance: An Overview of Recent Trends." *Health Affairs,* 1994, *14,* 244–254.

37. Newacheck, Hughes, and Cisternas (1994); Teitelbaum, M. *The Health Insurance Crisis for America's Children.* Washington, D.C.: Children's Defense Fund, 1994.

38. U.S. General Accounting Office (1993).

39. Teitelbaum (1994).

40. Newacheck, P. W., Hughes, D. C., Brindis, C., and Halfon, N. "Decategorizing Health Services: Interim Findings from the Robert Wood Johnson Foundation's Child Health Initiative." *Health Affairs,* 1995, *14,* 232–242.

41. Teitelbaum (1994).

42. Moyer, G. *Chartbook on Children's Insurance Status: Tabulations of the March 1998 Current Population Survey.* Washington, D.C.: Office of Health Policy, Office of the Assistant Secretary for Planning and Evaluation, 1998.

43. Weinick, R. M., Weigers, M. E., and Cohen, J. W. "Children's Health Insurance, Access to Care, and Health Status: New Findings." *Health Affairs,* 1998, *17,* 127–136.

44. Sardell, A., and Johnson, K. "The Politics of EPSDT Policy in the 1990s: Policy Entrepreneurs, Political Streams, and Children's Health Benefits." *Milbank Quarterly,* 1998, *76,* 175–205.

45. Perloff, J., Kletke, P., and Neckerman, K. "Recent Trends in Pediatrician Participation in Medicaid." *Medical Care,* 1986, *24,* 749–760; Davidson, S., and others. "Full and Limited Medicaid Participation Among Pediatricians." *Pediatrics,* 1983, *72,* 552–559.

46. U.S. General Accounting Office (1993).

47. Carrasquillo, O., Himmelstein, D. U., Woolhandler, S., and Bor, D. H. "Can Medicaid Managed Care Provide Continuity of Care to New Medicaid Enrollees? An Analysis of

Tenure on Medicaid." *American Journal of Public Health,* 1998, *88,* 464–466.

48. Halfon, N., and others. "Medicaid Enrollment and Health Services Access by Latino Children in Inner-City Los Angeles." *Journal of the American Medical Association,* 1997, *277,* 636–641; Flores, G., Abreu, M., Olivar, M. A., and Kastner, B. "Access Barriers to Health Care for Latino Children." *Archives of Pediatric and Adolescent Medicine,* 1998, *152,* 1119–1125.

49. Gavin, N., and others. "The Use of EPSDT and Other Health Care Services by Children Enrolled in Medicaid: The Impact of OBRA '89." *Milbank Quarterly,* 1998, *76,* 207.

50. Carrasquillo, Himmelstein, Woolhandler, and Bor (1998); Avruch, S., Machlin, S., Bonin, P., and Ullman, F. "The Demographic Characteristics of Medicaid Eligible Children." *American Journal of Public Health,* 1998, *88,* 445–447.

51. Ellwood, M. "The Medicaid Eligibility Maze: Coverage Expands, But Enrollment Problems Persist." (Occasional paper no. 30.) Urban Institute, 1999. [http://newfederalism.urban.org/ pdf/ occa30.pdf.]

52. Avruch, Machlin, Bonin, and Ullman (1998).

53. Weinick, Weigers, and Cohen (1998).

54. Weinick, Weigers, and Cohen (1998); Thorpe, K. E., and Florence, C. S. "Covering Uninsured Children and Their Parents: Estimated Costs and Number of Newly Insured." *Medical Care, Research and Review,* 1999, *56,* 197–214.

55. Rosenbaum, S., and others. "The Children's Hour: The State Children's Health Insurance Program." *Health Affairs,* 1998, *17,* 75–89.

56. Lieu, T. A., and others. "Risk Factors for Delayed Immunization Among Children in an HMO." *American Journal of Public Health,* 1994, *84,* 1621–1625.

57. Cooper, P. F., and Schone, B. S. "More Offers, Fewer Takers for Employment-Based Health Insurance: 1987 and 1996." *Health Affairs,* 1997, *16,* 142–149.

58. U.S. Department of Labor. "Employee Benefits in Medium and Large Establishments." Bulletin 2422. Washington, D.C.: Bureau of Labor Statistics, 1993.

59. Fox, H. B., and Newacheck, P. W. "Private Health Insurance Coverage of Chronically Ill Children." *Pediatrics,* 1990, *85,* 50–57.

60. Valdez, R. The Effects of Cost Sharing on the Health of Children. (RAND publication no. R-3720-HHS.) Santa Monica, Calif.: RAND, 1986.

61. Valdez, R., and others. "Prepaid Group Practice Effects on the Utilization of Medical Services and Health Outcomes for Children: Results from a Controlled Trial." *Pediatrics,* 1989, *83,* 168–180.

62. Halfon, Inkelas, and Wood (1995).

63. Newacheck, P. W. "Characteristics of Children with High and Low Usage of Physician Services." *Medical Care,* 1992, *30,* 30–42; Wood, D. L., Corey, C., Freeman, H. E., and Shapiro, M. F. "Are Poor Families Satisfied with the Medical Care Their Children Receive?" *Pediatrics,* 1992, *90,* 66–70; Newacheck and Halfon (1986); Guendelman, S., and Schwalbe, J. "Medical Care Utilization by Hispanic Children: How Does It Differ from Black and White Peers?" *Medical Care,* 1986, *24,* 925–940; Wolfe, B. L. "Children's Utilization of Medical Care." *Medical Care,* 1980, *18,* 1196–1207; Dutton, D. B. "Explaining the Low Use of Health Services by the Poor: Costs, Attitudes, or Delivery Systems?" *American Sociological Review,* 1978, *43,* 348–368; Aday, L. A., and Andersen, R. M. "A Framework for the Study of Access to Medical Care." *Health Services Research,* 1974, *9,* 208–220.

64. Halfon, Inkelas, and Wood (1995); Newacheck (1992); Wood, Corey, Freeman, and Shapiro (1992); Dutton (1978).

65. Wood, Corey, Freeman, and Shapiro (1992); Riley, A. W., and others. "Determinants of Health Care Use: An Investigation of Psychosocial Factors." *Medical Care*, 1993, *31*, 767–783; Lieu, T. A., Newacheck, P. W., and McManus, M. A. "Race, Ethnicity, and Access to Ambulatory Care Among U.S. Adolescents." *American Journal of Public Health*, 1994, *83*, 960–965.

66. Halfon and others (1997); Flores, Abreu, Olivar, and Kastner (1998); Holl, J. L., and others. "Profile of Uninsured Children in the United States." *Archives of Pediatric and Adolescent Medicine*, 1995, *149*, 398–406.

67. Orr, S. T., Charney, E., and Straus, J. "Use of Health Services by Black Children According to Payment Mechanism." *Medical Care*, 1988, *26*, 939–947.

68. Rawlings, J. S., and Weir, M. R. "Race- and Rank-Specific Mortality in a U.S. Military Population." *American Journal of Diseases in Children*, 1992, *146*, 313–316; Margolis, P. A., and others. "The Rest of the Access-to-Care Puzzle." *Archives of Pediatric and Adolescent Medicine*, 1995, *149*, 541–545.

69. Starfield, B., and others. "Consumer Experiences and Provider Perceptions of the Quality of Primary Care: Implications for Managed Care." *Journal of Family Practice*, 1998, *46*, 216–226; Starfield, B. "Evaluating the State of Children's Health Insurance Program: Critical Considerations." *Annual Review of Public Health*, 2000, *21*, 569–585.

70. Halfon, Inkelas, and Wood (1995).

71. Kogan, M. D., and others. "The Effect of Gaps in Health Insurance on Continuity of a Regular Source of Care Among Preschool-Aged Children in the United States." *Journal of the American Medical Association*, 1995, *274*, 1429–1435; Halfon and others (1997); Rosenbach, M., Irvin, C., and Coulam, R. "Access for Low-Income Children: Is Health Insurance Enough?" *Pediatrics*, 1999, *103*, 1167–1174.

72. Starfield (2000).

73. Starfield, B., and Newacheck, P. W. "Children's Health Status, Health Risks, and Use of Health Services." In M. J. Schlesinger and L. Eisenberg (eds.), *Children in a Changing Health System*. Baltimore: Johns Hopkins University Press, 1990; Bearinger, L. H., Wildey, L., Gephart, J., and Blum, R. W. "Nursing Competence in Adolescent Health: Anticipating the Future Needs of Youth." *Journal of Professional Nursing*, 1992, *8*, 80–86; Blum, R. W., and Bearinger, L. H. "Knowledge and Attitudes of Health Professionals Toward Adolescent Health Care." *Journal of Adolescent Health Care*, 1990, *11*, 289–294.

74. Friedman, L. S., Johnson, B., and Brett, A. S. "Evaluation of Substance-Abusing Adolescents by Primary Care Physicians." *Journal of Adolescent Health Care*, 1990, *11*, 227–230; Singer, M. I., Petchers, M. K., and Anglin, J. M. "Detection of Adolescent Substance Abuse in a Pediatric Outpatient Department: A Double-Blind Study." *Journal of Pediatrics*, 1987, *111*, 938–941; Goldberg, I. D., Roghmann, K. J., McInerny, T. K., and Burke, J. D. "Mental Health Problems Among Children Seen in Pediatric Practice: Prevalence and Management." *Pediatrics*, 1984, *73*, 278–293.

75. Costello, E. J. "Primary Care Pediatrics, and Child Psychopathology: A Review of Diagnostic, Treatment, and Referral Practices." *Pediatrics*, 1986, *78*, 1044–1051.

76. Office of Technology Assessment. *Adolescent Health*. Vol. III: *Cross-Cutting Issues in the Delivery of Health and Health-Related Services*. OTA-H-469. Washington, D.C.: U.S. Government Printing Office, 1991; Singer, Petchers, and Anglin (1987); Kamerow, D., Pincus, H., and MacDonald, D. "Alcohol Abuse, Other Drug Abuse, and Mental Disorders in Medical Practice." *Journal of the American Medical Association*, 1986, *255*, 2054–2057.

77. Hughes, D., and Rosenbaum, S. "An Overview of Maternal and Child Health Services in Rural America." *Journal of Rural Health*, 1989, *5*, 299–319.

78. Dutton, D. "Children's Health Care 1981: The Myth of Equal Access." In *Better Health for Our Children.* Vol. 4: *Select Panel for the Promotion of Child Health.* DHHS publication no. (PHS) 79-55071. Washington, D.C.: Department of Health and Human Services, 1981.

79. Short and Lefkowitz (1992).

80. Halfon, N., Newacheck, P. W., Wood, D., and St. Peter, R. "Routine Emergency Room Use for Sick Care by U.S. Children." *Pediatrics,* 1995, *98,* 28–34.

81. Chang, R. K., and Halfon, N. "Geographic Distribution of Pediatricians in the United States: An Analysis of the Fifty States and Washington DC." *Pediatrics,* 1997, *100,* 172–179.

82. Kindig, D., and others. "Trends in Physician Availability in 10 Urban Areas from 1963 to 1980." *Inquiry,* 1987, *24,* 136–146.

83. Orr, S. T., Charney, E., Straus, J., and Bloom, B. "Emergency Room Use by Low Income Children with a Regular Source of Health Care." *Medical Care,* 1991, *29,* 283–286; Kasper, J. D. "The Importance of Type of Usual Source of Care for Children's Physician Access and Expenditures." *Medical Care,* 1987, *25,* 386–398; and Halfon, Newacheck, Wood, and St. Peter (1995).

84. Butler, J. A., Winter, W. D., Singer, J. D., and Wenger, M. "Medical Care Use and Expenditures Among Children and Youth in the United States: An Analysis of a National Probability Sample." *Pediatrics,* 1985, *76,* 495–507.

85. Kasper (1987).

86.   Schlesinger, M. "On the Limits of Expanding Health Care Reform: Chronic Care in Prepaid Settings." *Milbank Quarterly,* 1990, *64,* 189–215.

87. Halfon, N., and Hochstein, M. "Developing a System of Care for All: How the Needs of Vulnerable Children Inform the Debate." In R. K. Stein (ed.), *Health Care for Children: What's Right, What's Wrong, What's Next?* New York: United Hospital Fund of New York, 1997.

88. Rosenbaum, S., and Darnell, J. *Medicaid Section 1115 Demonstration Waivers: Approved and Proposed Activities as of November 1994.* Washington, D.C.: Center for Health Policy Research, George Washington University, 1994.

89. Perry, D. "Children's Health Insurance: Beyond Medicaid Coverage." *Health Policy and Child Health,* 1995, *2*(Supplement), 1–4.

90. Newacheck, P. W., Halfon, N., and Inkelas, M. "Monitoring Expanded Health Insurance for Children: Challenges and Opportunities." *Pediatrics,* 2000, *105,* 1004–1007.

91. Cooper and Schone (1997).

92. Halfon, N., Inkelas, M., DuPlessis, H., and Newacheck, P. W. "Challenges in Securing Access to Care for Children." *Health Affairs,* 1999, *18,* 48–63.

93. Halfon, Inkelas, and Hochstein (2000).

94. Halfon and Hochstein (1997); Barnett, W. S., and Escobar, C. M. "Economic Costs and Benefits of Early Intervention." In S. J. Meisels and J. P. Shonkoff (eds.), *Handbook of Early Childhood Intervention.* New York: Cambridge University Press, 1992; Olds, D. "Home Visitation for Pregnant Women and Parents of Young Children." *American Journal of the Diseases of Children,* 1992, *146,* 704–708.

95. Halfon and Hochstein (1997); Starfield (1992); Starfield and Newacheck (1990).

96. Wagner, J. L., Herdman, R. C., and Alberts, D. W. "Well-Child Care: How Much Is Enough?" *Health Affairs,* 1989, *8,* 147–157.

97. Olds, D., and others. "Effect of Prenatal and Infancy Nurse Home Visitation on Government Spending." *Medical Care,* 1993, *31,* 155–174; Olds, D., and others. "Long-Term Effects of Home Visitation on Maternal Life Course, Child Abuse and Neglect, and Children's Arrests: Fifteen Year Follow-up of a Randomized Trial." *Journal of the American*

Medical Association, 1997, *278,* 637–643; Barnett and Escobar (1992); Berrueta-Clement, J. R., and others. *Changed Lives: The Effects of the Perry Preschool Program on Youths Through Age 19.* Ypsilanti, Mich.: High/Scope, 1984; and Karoly and others (1998).

98. Karoly and others (1998).

99. Halfon, Inkelas, and Hochstein (2000).

100. Starfield (1992).

101. Child Welfare League of America. *Standards for Health Care Services for Children in Out-of-Home Care.* Washington, D.C.: Child Welfare League of America, 1988.

102. Green, M. (ed.). *Bright Futures: National Guidelines for Health Supervision of Infants, Children, and Adolescents.* Arlington, Va.: National Center for Education in Maternal and Child Health, 1994.

103. Physician Payment Review Commission. *Annual Report to Congress—1995.* Washington, D.C.: Physician Payment Review Commission, 1995.

104. Physician Payment Review Commission (1995).

105. McGlynn, E. A., and Halfon, N. "Overview of Issues in Improving Quality of Care for Children." *Health Services Research,* 1998, *33,* 977–1000; McGlynn, Halfon, and Leibowitz (1995); Institute of Medicine. *Protecting and Improving Quality of Care for Children Under Health Care Reform: Workshop Highlights.* Washington, D.C.: Institute of Medicine, 1994.

106. Halfon, N., Schuster, M. A., Valentine, W., and McGlynn, E. "Improving Quality of Healthcare for Children: Implementing the Results of the AHSR Research Agenda Conference." *Health Services Research,* 1998, *33,* 955–976.

107. U.S. General Accounting Office. *Preventive Care for Children in Selected Countries.* GAO/HRD-93-62. Washington, D.C.: U.S. Government Printing Office, 1993.

108. McGlynn and Halfon (1998).

109. Wood, D., Saarlas, K. N., Inkelas, M., and Matyas, B. "Immunization Registries in the United States: Implications for the Practice of Public Health in a Changing Health Care System." *Annual Review of Public Health,* 1999, *20,* 231–255.

110. Institute of Medicine (1994).

111. DuPlessis, H. M., Inkelas, M., and Halfon, N. "Assessing the Performance of Community Systems for Children." *Health Services Research,* 1998, *33,* 1111–1142.

112. DuPlessis, Inkelas, and Halfon (1998). Halfon, N., and others. *California Health Report.* (RAND publication DRU-1592-TCWF.) Santa Monica, Calif.: RAND, 2000.

113. Grason, H., and Guyer, B. *MCH Quality Systems Functions Framework.* Baltimore, Md.: Johns Hopkins School of Hygiene and Public Health, 1995.

114. Newacheck, Hughes, Brindis, and Halfon (1995).

115. Dutton (1981); Lion, J., and Altman, S. "Case-Mix Differences Between Hospital Outpatient Departments and Private Practice." *Health Care Financing Review,* 1982, *4,* 89–98; Fleming, N. S., and Jones, H. C. "Practice and Billing Patterns by Site of Care in a Medicaid Program." *Journal of Ambulatory Care Management,* 1985, *8,* 70–80; Halfon, N., and Newacheck, P. W. "Childhood Asthma and Poverty: Differential Impacts and Utilization of Health Services." *Pediatrics,* 1993, *91,* 56–61; St. Peter, R., Newacheck, P. W., and Halfon, N. "Access to Care for Poor Children: Separate and Unequal?" *Journal of the American Medical Association,* 1992, *267,* 2760–2764.

116. Holahan, J., Rangarajan, S., and Schirmer, M. "Medicaid Managed Care Payment Rates in 1998." *Health Affairs,* 1999, *18,* 217–227.

117. Simpson, L., and Fraser, I. "Children and Managed Care: What Research Can, Can't, and Should Tell Us About Impact." *Medical Care,* Research and Review, 1999,

56 (Supplement 2), 13–36; Claxton, G., Feder, J., Shactman, D., and Altman, S. "Public Policy Issues in Nonprofit Conversions: An Overview." *Health Affairs,* 1997, *16,* 9–28.

118. Hughes, D. C., and Luft, H. S. "Managed Care and Children: An Overview." *Future of Children,* 1998, *8,* 25–38; Szilagyi, P. G. "Managed Care for Children: Effect on Access to Care and Utilization of Health Services." *Future of Children,* 1998, *8,* 39–59.

119. Freund, D., and others. "Evaluation of the Medicaid Competition Demonstrations." *Health Care Financing Review,* 1989, *11,* 81–97.

120. Mauldon, J., and others. "Rationing or Rationalizing Children's Medical Care: Comparison of a Medicaid HMO with Fee-for-Service Care." *American Journal of Public Health,* 1994, *84,* 899–904.

121. Szilagyi, P. G., and Schor, E. L. "The Health of Children." *Health Services Research,* 1998, *33,* 1001–1039.

122. Horwitz, S. M., and Stein, R.E.K. "Health Maintenance Organizations vs. Indemnity Insurance for Children with Chronic Illness: Trading Gaps in Coverage." *American Journal of Diseases of Children,* 1990, *144,* 581–586.

123. Scholle, S. H., and others. "Changes in Medicaid Managed Care Enrollment Among Children." *Health Affairs,* 1997, *16,* 164–170; West, D. W., Stuart, M. E., Duggan, A. K., and DeAngelis, C. D. "Evidence for Selective Health Maintenance Organization Enrollment Among Children and Adolescents Covered by Medicaid." *Archives of Pediatric and Adolescent Medicine,* 1996, *150,* 503–507.

124. Cartland, J.D.C., and Yudkowsky, B. K. "Barriers to Pediatric Referral in Managed Care Systems." *Pediatrics,* 1992, *89,* 183–192.

125. Fox, H. B., Wicks, L. B., and Newacheck, P. W. "Health Maintenance Organizations and Children with Special Health Needs: A Suitable Match?" *American Journal of Diseases in Children,* 1993, *147,* 546–552.

126. Fox, H. B., and McManus, M. A. *Strategies to Enhance Preventive and Primary Care Services for High-Risk Children in Health Maintenance Organizations.* Washington, D.C.: Child and Adolescent Health Policy Center, 1995.

127. McGlynn and Halfon (1998).

128. Holahan, Rangarajan, and Schirmer (1999).

129. Fox, H. B., and McManus, M. A. "Improving State Medicaid Contracts and Plan Practices for Children with Special Health Needs." *Future of Children,* 1998, *8,* 105–118.

130. Szilagyi (1998).

131. Ireys, H. "Children with Special Health Care Needs: Evaluating Their Needs and Relevant Service Structures." (Background paper for Institute of Medicine.) Baltimore, Md.: Johns Hopkins University, 1994; Simpson and Fraser (1999).

132. Halfon and Berkowitz (1993).

133. Newacheck, Hughes, Halfon, and Brindis (1997).

134. Leutz, W. N., Greenlick, M. R., and Capitman, J. A. "Integrating Acute and Long-Term Care." *Health Affairs,* 1994, *13,* 58–74.

135. Halfon, Inkelas, and Hochstein (2000).

136. Robinson, J. C. "The Future of Managed Care Organization." *Health Affairs,* 1999, *18,* 7–24.

137. Halfon, Inkelas, and Hochstein (2000).

138. Williams, B. C., and Miller, C. A. "Preventive Health Care for Children: Findings from a 10-Country Study and Directions for United States Policy." *Pediatrics,* 1992, *89*(Supplement), 983–998; Kahn and Kamerman (1992).

CHAPTER TWELVE

MENTAL HEALTH SERVICES AND POLICY ISSUES

Susan L. Ettner

Mental disorders are both common and costly to society. In any given year, about 21 percent of the adult U.S. population suffers from a mental disorder, with about 3 percent suffering from chronic or recurrent and severely impairing disorders.[1] Comparable figures for children and adolescents are 21 percent and 5 percent.[2] Although mental illnesses are not associated with a high mortality rate, they often have their onset in early adulthood, affecting what would normally be the most productive working years. Thus, for example, the Global Burden of Disease Study found that mental illnesses accounted for 15.4 percent of all disability-adjusted life-years, ranking second only to cardiovascular conditions.[3]

In addition to the direct costs of treatment for mental disorders other than dementia, estimated to be about $69 billion, or 7.3 percent of total care costs in 1996,[4] mental illness has been shown to reduce employment rates and work productivity[5] and increase absenteeism.[6] Furthermore, mental illness is often accompanied by drug and alcohol abuse, adding another $13 billion to direct treatment costs.[7] Fifteen percent of adults with mental illness over the course of a year have co-morbid substance disorders[8]; this figure reaches 50 percent for adults with severe mental illness.[9] Other social costs associated with mental illness and substance disorders include violence,[10] homelessness,[11] child abuse,[12] motor vehicle accidents,[13] teenage pregnancy,[14] and marital instability.[15]

Pharmacological advances in treating mental illness began in the 1950s and have continued, improving our ability to care for these disorders in an effective as well as cost-effective manner.[16] Yet despite the large costs that untreated mental illness imposes on society and the great advances in treatment that have been made, the use of mental health services is poorly matched to need. Although 15 percent of adult Americans obtain mental health services each year, only slightly more than half of them have a diagnosable mental or substance disorder, representing less than one-third of all adults suffering from such disorders.[17] In contrast, 4.5 percent of adults without a diagnosable disorder receive mental health care.[18] Similarly, although 21 percent of children receive mental health services in any given year, more than half of children with diagnosable disorders do not receive any treatment.[19] Some of the barriers to mental health care that have been identified are stigma, geographic inaccessibility of providers, financial constraints because of inadequate insurance coverage, and the failure of health care providers to identify the mental health needs of their patients.[20]

In addition to the substantial access barriers facing the patients in greatest need of treatment, substandard quality of care and inappropriate treatment have been long-standing concerns in the mental health sector, dating from the inhumane treatment of the mentally ill in the "lunatic asylums" of the 1700s and 1800s[21] and continuing into the present, with revelations regarding excessive use of restraints and seclusion within certain psychiatric institutions.[22] These access and quality issues suggest the need for a fundamental rethinking of our current mental health policy, defined by Murphy and Dorwart as "a set of governmental systems and regulations that shape the way mental health services are financed and delivered in the United States."[23]

This chapter describes policy issues specific to the mental health services system in the United States. First comes an overview of the nature and treatment of mental illness and the financing and delivery of mental health services. The chapter then summarizes some of the ways in which mental health care differs from health care in general, suggesting the need for separate consideration of mental health services in the policy debate. Some of the concerns for special populations are then described. The chapter concludes with an in-depth discussion of a few of the important issues facing mental health policy makers.

Overview of Mental Illness and the Mental Health Services System

Who are the "mentally ill"? The Surgeon General's Report on Mental Health[24] defines mental disorders as "conditions characterized by alterations in thinking, mood or behavior associated with distress and/or impaired functioning." This definition encompasses a variety of disorders, such as anxiety disorders (which are experienced by about 16.4 percent of adults each year), mood disorders (such as depression and bipolar disorders, also known as manic depression, experienced by about 7.1 percent of adults), schizophrenia (at about 1.3 percent), and numerous other conditions (including dementia).[25] Common manifestations of mental disorder include anxiety, which is characterized by feelings of fear and dread; psychosis, including hallucinations and delusions; mood disturbances, such as prolonged periods of extreme sadness or euphoria; and cognitive impairment, or the inability to organize, process, and recall information.[26]

Distinctions are drawn among mental health problems below the threshold for a standard diagnosis, all diagnosable mental illnesses, serious mental illness (SMI), and severe and persistent mental illness (SPMI). Standard diagnoses are based on criteria outlined in the *Diagnostic and Statistical Manual of Mental Disorders* (DSM), published by the American Psychiatric Association. Serious mental illnesses are those interfering with social functioning; severe and persistent mental illnesses are chronic in addition to being associated with serious functional impairment. Examples of SPMI are schizophrenia, bipolar disorder, certain types of major depression, panic disorder and obsessive-compulsive disorder.[27] Among children, conditions associated with severe functional impairment are instead referred to as serious emotional disturbance (SED). About 5 percent of adults have SMI and 2.6 percent have SPMI;[28] about 9 percent of children aged nine to seventeen have SED.[29] Although even subthreshold mental health problems can cause impairment, persons with persistent and serious mental disorders face major challenges in attempting to live normal lives and are frequently the focus of mental health policy initiatives.

How and where are persons with mental illness treated? Regier and others[30] coined the term "the de facto mental health system" to describe the fragmentation of mental health services delivery in the United States into four sectors: the mental health specialty sector, the general medical sector, the human services sector, and the voluntary support network sector. In addition to psychiatrists, mental health specialists include psychologists, psychiatric nurses, and psychiatric social workers. Among the generalists are primary care physicians, nurse practitioners, and physician's assistants. In the human services sector are social welfare programs and services provided within correctional institutions, schools, and religious institutions. The voluntary support network sector includes self-help groups and other consumer organizations.

Respectively, 5.9 percent, 6.4 percent, 3.0 percent, and 4.1 percent of adult Americans obtain mental health services each year from each of these four sectors; overall, 14.7 percent received services in any of these sectors.[31] Among children and adolescents, 21 percent use mental health services each year, with 8 percent receiving mental health specialty care, 1 percent using services provided by generalists, 11 percent receiving school-based services, and 1 percent obtaining care from other human services programs and the voluntary support network.[32] It should be noted that in addition to the mental health services provided by each of these sectors, informal caregivers play an important role in the care of the mentally ill,[33] despite the fact that persons with severe and persistent mental disorders are less likely to be married[34] and tend to have fewer close ties to friends and relatives[35] and so are less able to turn to family members for support.[36]

Diagnosis and treatment of mental illness takes place in a variety of settings: psychiatric and general hospitals, community mental health clinics, residential treatment centers, psychiatrist and primary care provider offices, and so on. Since the 1960s and 1970s, there has been a shift away from inpatient care toward community-based care, with the "deinstitutionalization" of many long-term psychiatric inpatients.[37] The number of inpatient days attributable primarily to psychiatric disorders declined by about 11.3 million between 1988 and 1994.[38] The recent rise in managed care has further encouraged the shift in care from costly inpatient settings to less intensive outpatient settings.

Although psychiatric hospitalization is becoming an infrequent event even among seriously ill patients, the high cost associated with inpatient episodes ensures that it still accounts for a large proportion of total mental health spending, about one-third of the $69 billion spent in 1996. Inpatient episodes include those occurring in psychiatric hospitals (17 percent of total mental health spending), dedicated psychiatric units within general hospitals (10 percent), and scatter beds or cluster beds within general hospitals (6 percent).[39] Residential treatment centers for children accounted for another 4 percent of total spending, and nursing home and home health agencies 7 percent.[40] The remainder was spent on outpatient mental health clinics (18 percent), psychiatrists (10 percent), psychologists and social workers (14 percent), generalist physicians (5 percent) and psychotropic drugs prescribed in outpatient settings (9 percent).[41]

Because of our poor understanding of the etiology of mental disorders, interventions to prevent mental illness are less well-developed than in other areas of medicine. Those prevention programs that exist in mental health have traditionally focused on children. Thus mental health services for adults consist primarily of treatment of existing disorders, including both active treatment and custodial care. Active treatment of mental illness falls primarily into two categories: psychosocial intervention, employing various forms of psychotherapy, and pharmacotherapy (use of psychotropic drugs). Procedures such as electroconvulsive therapy (ECT) are also used. In addition, persons with SPMI often require a range of other types of supportive services, including income support, assisted housing, family intervention, and vocational rehabilitation.

Given the fragmentation of the delivery system and the diverse needs of persons with severe and chronic mental disorders, case management services are often necessary to ensure that these patients receive the full range of services required for them to lead a relatively normal life. Mental health case managers were originally assigned to assist patients affected by the deinstitutionalization of the 1960s,[42] when long-term inpatients were discharged to what was more the hope than the reality of comprehensive, integrated community care. More recently, private sector case management of mental health services has become popular, although primarily as a means of containing costs. One of the most touted models of care in the public sector has been the Program of Assertive Community Treatment (PACT), which offers individualized case management with a multidisciplinary team approach.[43] PACT is considered to offer integrated, cost-effective care for persons with severe mental illness[44]; it is potentially a model for programs developed by managed care organizations.[45]

Who pays for mental health services? As with the delivery system, the financing of mental health services is fragmented, including private, state, and federal funding streams from multiple sectors (health, social welfare, housing, criminal justice, education).[46] States had the sole responsibility for financing and delivering mental health services until World War II, when the National Mental Health Act introduced the role of the federal government in funding research, training, and development of new mental health programs.[47] The federal government role in financing mental health services increased as a result of the Community Mental Health Center (CMHC) Act of 1965,[48] which paved the way for deinstitutionalization, shifting costs from primarily state-funded public psychiatric hospitals to primarily federally funded outpatient mental health clinics, and devolving responsibility for organizing mental health care from state to local government.[49]

The slow expansion of mental health benefits under Medicaid and Medicare over time has also increased the role of the federal government in financing services, at the same time that private health plans have taken on a larger role with the evolution of the employer-based insurance system. Currently, about 52.6 percent of mental health expenditures are publicly financed, with the remaining 47.4 percent paid by private parties, including private insurance (26.9 percent), out-of-pocket expenditures (17.4 percent) and other private funds (3.2 percent).[50] Medicaid is the most important source of public funds, accounting for 18.9 percent of all mental health expenditures, followed closely by direct state and local funding (17.3 percent), Medicare (14.4 percent) and other federal funding (2.0 percent).[51]

Health Care Policy: Is Mental Health Different?

Although many of the policy questions around delivering and financing mental health services mirror those for medical care, mental health is characterized by certain features that set it apart from medical care and have implications for attempting to subsume mental health into broader health care policies. This section summarizes what is different about mental health care.

Stigma

Historically, a disorder with no known etiology was treated as a mental health problem and stigmatized.[52] Despite the public's increasing understanding of the nature of mental illness, fear, avoidance, and discrimination are still commonplace reactions to persons with mental illness.[53] Stigma poses a substantial psychological barrier to seeking care for mental health problems,[54] particularly in the specialty sector.[55] For this reason, the Surgeon General has identified overcoming stigma as one of the most important steps to improving mental health treatment in the United States.[56] In contrast, stigma does not generally pose a barrier to access for treating a medical condition. With the development of more effective psychotropic medications having fewer side effects,[57] psychiatry is becoming increasingly medicalized over time. The shift toward a medical model for treatment of psychiatric disorders may eventually lessen stigma, though at the possible cost of reducing support for psychosocial interventions.

High Rate of Treatment in the General Medical Sector

Patients with psychiatric disorders often seek care for their condition in the primary care sector instead of the mental health specialty sector. Data from the two largest epidemiological studies of the prevalence and treatment of psychiatric disorders in the United States, the Epidemiological Catchment Area (ECA) study and the National Comorbidity Survey (NCS), showed that only slightly more than one-quarter of adults with a diagnosable mental or addictive disorder in a given year receive any treatment; of those receiving services, only about half are treated in the specialty sector. Use of mental health specialty services is even lower for children and the elderly. Even among the most impaired children—those with SED—only 40 percent of those receiving any treatment obtained specialty mental health services.[58] Among elderly Medicare beneficiaries receiving physician services for a psychiatric condition, only 29 percent saw a specialist at least once.[59]

The degree to which primary care providers and other generalists can effectively substitute for mental health specialists in the treatment of psychiatric disorders is controversial.[60] Mental health treatment provided by generalists tends to focus on psychotropic drug prescriptions, with about two-thirds of such drugs prescribed by primary care providers and medical specialists other than psychiatrists.[61] Episodes of mental health treatment in the general medical sector tend to be shorter and less costly than episodes involving mental health specialty care.[62]

However, evidence on the relative quality of psychiatric care provided in the two sectors is limited, with somewhat mixed evidence suggesting that mental health specialists may provide more appropriate care.[63]

The issue of whether generalists are being substituted for specialists, and the implications of such substitution, arise in other areas of medicine as well. However, mental health services may be particularly prone to delivery through the general medical sector, because of three factors. The first is the stigma associated with visiting a mental health specialty provider such as a psychiatrist. The second is that insurance benefits are structured in such a way as to favor providing mental health services as part of a primary care visit.[64] The third is the geographic maldistribution[65] and inadequate supply of mental health specialists in many parts of the United States.[66] Distance and provider supply have been shown to influence mental health services utilization and the choice between specialist and generalist care.[67]

Role of State and Local Governments in Financing and Delivery

The public sector has always played a larger role in financing and delivering mental health services than for medical care. For example, federal and state funding accounted for 56.3 percent of all mental health and substance abuse spending in 1996, but only 47.5 percent of all health care spending.[68] Public financing of mental health services has been argued in part as a response to the external costs imposed on society by mental illness and addictive disorders, including unemployment, crime, violence, and homelessness.[69] The availability of publicly funded services may, however, amount to a disincentive for employers to offer behavioral health care benefits to workers.[70]

The difference between sources of financing for mental health versus medical care is particularly noticeable for direct state and local funding, at 19.4 percent of all behavioral health versus 7.2 percent of general health expenditures.[71] Although the federal government has been playing an increasing role over time in financing behavioral health care, state and local government are still the most important public payers when looking at combined mental health and substance abuse expenditures, accounting for 18.7 percent of expenditures.[72]

The high proportion of mental health and substance abuse funding that comes directly from states is largely attributable to the historical role played by public psychiatric hospitals, which have been operating since the middle of the nineteenth century; at their peak in 1955 they had a resident census of 558,922.[73] Although closing or downsizing state mental hospitals has become commonplace, they continue to constitute the largest single expenditure for a mental health care specialty organization in the United States.[74] Only about 26 percent of nonfederal general hospitals in the United States are run by state and local governments,[75] but about 36 percent of psychiatric hospitals are public.[76] The shift from inpatient to outpatient care under deinstitutionalization has reduced the importance of state hospitals, but the state plays an ongoing role in organizing care for the mentally ill. For example, the replacement of the CMHC program with state block grants in the 1980s reduced federal control over delivery of services and allowed states to tailor programs to meet the needs of their particular patient populations.[77]

Private Insurance Coverage

Private insurance coverage for mental health and substance abuse treatment tends to be much less generous than for medical care. A recent study showed that 9 percent of small firms and 1 percent of large firms did not offer any mental health or substance abuse benefits to employees in the health plan with the greatest enrollment.[78] Employers routinely impose higher cost-sharing requirements and lower maximum lifetime dollar limits for mental health services than for medical care. Other restrictions are also commonly imposed on behavioral health care that do not apply to medical care, such as limiting the number of outpatient visits (typically twenty) or inpatient days (usually thirty). Although the Health Maintenance Organization Act of 1973 requires that HMOs pay for mental health and substance abuse services in order to be certified, only minimal coverage is required.[79]

One implication of differential coverage of medical and mental health care is that an employee who develops breast cancer can get most of her treatment reimbursed, while a comparable employee with onset of bipolar disorder (another chronic, costly, and partially heritable disorder) cannot. The cost-offset criterion often used by managed care organizations (MCOs) for broadening mental health services coverage is further evidence of inequity in insurance coverage; requiring that expansion in psychiatric treatment must achieve cost-neutrality through commensurate reduction in medical costs is a much stricter standard than the cost-effectiveness typically required of medical services. This differential coverage may be due in part simply to stigma or discrimination, but there are economic explanations for the phenomenon as well, including the safety-net coverage provided by the public sector, "moral hazard," and adverse selection.[80]

The demand response to enhanced insurance coverage, known as moral hazard, has been shown to be substantially larger for mental health services than medical care under fee-for-service systems.[81] The RAND Health Insurance Experiment, a randomized study of the effect of insurance on health care costs, found that use of mental health care increased by about twice as much as use of medical care in response to reduced cost-sharing requirements.[82] Mental health service utilization is more responsive to subsidies, which may reflect greater uncertainty about the value of these services. It may also reflect the desirability of certain types of behavioral health care among populations with less acute need for such services. As one example, most people will not choose to undergo cardiac surgery in the absence of clear-cut indications for such treatment, even if it is fully covered by their insurance. In contrast, free psychotherapy might well prove highly attractive to many well-educated, psychologically minded individuals with no diagnosable psychiatric disorder. Anecdotal evidence about the popularity of Prozac and other selective serotonin reuptake inhibitors (SSRIs) among persons without a standard diagnosis of a depressive disorder suggests that in the absence of direct controls (utilization review, or "gatekeeping"), more generous coverage of behavioral health care could lead to increased utilization among a wider population than was originally intended.

In terms of the moral hazard problem, mental health care is similar to long-term care, where calls for enhanced insurance coverage of services such as home health care have led to predictions of a "woodwork effect," that is, service utilization that would not have occurred in the absence of insurance coverage. The woodwork effect in mental health suggests that relatively healthy people might engage in extended psychotherapy or take Prozac to lose weight if insurers offer better coverage for these services. Thus concerns about skyrocketing costs in response to insurance subsidies may in part explain the current inequitable situation in which insurance coverage of behavioral health is much poorer than for medical care. As with the long-term care proposals, which typically set explicit functional criteria to determine which patients are eligible for benefits, mental health coverage can more easily be expanded in conjunction with care management processes that limit benefits to patients for whom medical necessity can be documented.

In addition to moral hazard, insurers may be reluctant to offer generous mental health and substance abuse benefits because of the potential for adverse selection. Individuals suffering from mental illness have been shown to have higher medical as well as behavioral health care costs,[83] and the chronic nature of mental disorders suggests that there is greater potential for a patient to self-select into the insurance plans offering the best behavioral health care benefits. In contrast, patients and insurers cannot predict very well which patients will experience acute medical conditions during the next year, eliminating the potential both for those patients to self-select into generous insurance plans and for insurers to avoid enrolling them. Plans seeking to avoid enrolling a disproportionate number of patients with behavioral health care needs often engage in a "rush to the bottom," resulting in minimal coverage of these services.

One proposed remedy is to mandate benefits, which would allow insurers to offer coverage without fear of attracting all of the costly patients. It should be noted, however, that mandated benefits cannot prevent all forms of "cream-skimming" and "dumping." For example, MCOs may try to discourage patients with mental illness from enrolling by purposely trying not to develop a reputation for providing high-quality behavioral health care, by engaging in strict utilization review that effectively limits covered benefits, or by limiting provider networks so that a long waiting period for a mental health specialty visit effectively rations care.

Medicare and Medicaid Coverage

Differential coverage of mental health and medical care can be seen not only with private insurance but with publicly funded programs as well. Medicare and Medicaid insurance are particularly important sources of insurance coverage for those with serious and persistent mental illness, since their capacity for gainful employment is impaired. Thus they are less likely to be covered by employer-based insurance, but they often qualify for disability-related income support and health insurance benefits through either the Supplemental Security Income (SSI) or the Social Security Disability Insurance (SSDI) program. (The programs play a large role in covering those with physical disability as well. However, mental illnesses such as schizophrenia or bipolar disorder have earlier onset than many medical disorders, leading to a high proportion of disability related to mental illness—about 22 percent of disabled Medicare beneficiaries qualify on the basis of psychiatric impairment.[84]) Thus it is important to understand the limitations of public insurance coverage of mental health services relative to medical care.

Although the Omnibus Budget Reconciliation Act of 1989 removed the last of Medicare's payment limits for outpatient mental health care, Medicare continues to impose a 50 percent co-payment rate for outpatient mental health services other than initial diagnostic services and psychotropic drug management, in contrast to the usual 20 percent coinsurance rate for medical care. In addition, in an effort to prevent states from shifting the cost of psychiatric hospital care onto the federal government,[85] Medicare limits lifetime coverage of psychiatric hospital care to 190 days, although no such restrictions are placed on general hospital stays. Furthermore, Medicare's failure to cover outpatient prescription drugs has a disproportionate impact on the out-of-pocket costs for those with mental illness, for whom drug therapy is often a critical component of treatment.

Medicaid offers more comprehensive coverage of outpatient mental health care than Medicare and pays for most prescription drugs. However, its coverage of psychiatric inpatient facilities is less generous. Again, this is probably due to the desire to avoid having federal funds replace direct state and local funding; the federal government prohibits state Medicaid programs from covering care provided to adults from twenty-two to sixty-four years old within "institutions for mental disease," or IMDs (psychiatric hospitals and nursing homes specializing in psychiatric services). Although the elderly are generally covered because Medicaid is the secondary payer after Medicare rather than the primary payer, some states exclude psychiatric hospital care from Medicaid coverage for children as well as for nonelderly adults.

Differential coverage of mental health and medical care, or psychiatric and general hospital stays, puts beneficiaries at risk for high out-of-pocket costs and also distorts incentives. As one example, the IMD exclusion amounts to an incentive for states to treat Medicaid beneficiaries in need of inpatient mental health services in general, rather than psychiatric, hospital settings. It has also been cited as one reason for underdetecting mental health problems within nursing homes, which are fearful of losing Medicaid funding.[86] As another example, on the margin the treatment choices of Medicare beneficiaries with depression may be skewed toward ECT, a service that is covered under Medicare, and away from antidepressants, which are not reimbursed in outpatient settings.

Medicare Reimbursement Methodology for Inpatient Care

Psychiatric hospitals and certain psychiatric specialty units within general hospitals have been exempted from payment under the Prospective Payment System (PPS), Medicare's reimbursement methodology for acute general hospitals, since its introduction in 1983. This exemption results from the high degree of heterogeneity that was found in the cost of inpatient episodes within psychiatric diagnosis-related groups (DRGs) and the relationship of hospital specialty to variability in costs within DRGs.[87] Implementation of PPS for psychiatric facilities was predicted to result in an inequitable situation for psychiatric hospitals, as well as to generate incentives for hospitals to skim the healthiest patients and dump the sickest patients within DRGs. As a result, psychiatric specialty facilities are instead reimbursed under the Tax Equity and Fiscal Responsibility Act (TEFRA) of 1982.

Like PPS, TEFRA reimbursement is based on the notion of a target amount paid for each admission. Unlike PPS, TEFRA target amounts are based in part on the historical cost structure of the facility. Furthermore, providers can apply for an increase in their target amount, for example, if they can document an increase in patient case mix. Facilities with average costs above the target amount bear the extra costs, much like under PPS, but it has been argued that facilities with average costs well below target amounts operate under incentives similar to cost-based reimbursement.[88] In addition to offering fewer incentives for cost containment than PPS, TEFRA rules are considered by some commentators to be inequitable.[89] They also allow permit additional "gaming" on the part of general hospitals. Whether general hospitals apply for PPS exemption for their psychiatric units has been shown to depend on which reimbursement methodology—PPS or TEFRA—would prove to be most lucrative.[90] Those with exempt units may also choose whether to treat each psychiatric patient in the unit or a scatter bed, which may again depend on their expected reimbursement under each system.

Treatment Variability

It has been argued that there is less consensus about the effectiveness of treatment in psychiatry than in other fields of medicine.[91] This uncertainty may stem from the difficulty in evaluating psychosocial interventions that cannot easily be standardized. For example, psychotherapy is generally manualized for research studies, yet the individualized aspects of psychotherapy may be precisely what makes it work. As a result of this uncertainty, treatment variability also seems to be greater in mental health than medical care.[92] This uncertainty about which treatments actually work and variability in using treatments probably contributes to the reluctance of insurers to cover mental health services and the failure of patients to obtain appropriate care.

Information Deficits

Poor consumer information may have even greater implications for quality of care among patients with psychiatric disorders than it does for patients with medical conditions. The classic economic theory of markets is predicated on the assumption that consumers make rational choices based on perfect information. If so, market forces should prevent health care providers from offering suboptimal quality, since patients would avoid these providers, eventually driving them out of the market. Yet health care markets are more often characterized by imperfect information; even well-educated patients often know little about their condition, possible courses of treatment for it, and the quality of care being given.

The assumption of perfect consumer information is particularly difficult to justify when the patients involved have psychiatric disorders. Many people suffer from cognitive and perceptual deficits that hinder their ability to compare the quality of competing health care providers and make rational market choices. Moreover, patients with psychiatric disorders are less likely to be married or to have close family ties, thus lacking support from family members who might act as their advocate in choosing a health care provider. Market failures due to imperfect information are therefore likely to be exacerbated among patients with psychiatric disorders. Furthermore, the patient in greatest need of services—one with a severely disabling disorder such as schizophrenia—is precisely the one most likely to suffer impaired judgment.

Special Populations

Poor access to mental health care is a problem for many Americans, and to a certain extent the reasons for inadequate treatment cut across demographic groups. However, certain issues are of particularly great concern for populations such as the elderly, children, members of minority groups, and residents of rural areas.

Elderly

Rates of mental disorders generally appear to be as high among older adults as younger.[93] The loss of loved ones, which is common at an older age, frequently triggers depression, and the suicide rate is highest among older Americans.[94] Yet despite their equivalent need for services, the elderly are less likely than the nonelderly to be diagnosed and treated for mental illness[95]; when they do obtain care, they are less likely to receive services from the mental health specialty sector.[96] Suboptimal use of services among the elderly is probably due to both provider and patient factors. Providers often do not recognize the signs of mental illness among the elderly, failing to distinguish it from the normal aging process.[97] Cognitive impairment and differences in how the disorders present can make mental illness difficult to diagnose among the elderly. In turn, elderly patients tend to have greater perception of stigma than the nonelderly,[98] and traveling to obtain specialty care poses greater difficulties for the elderly because of their physical frailty. Financial barriers contribute to their lower use of behavioral health care as well, although it is unclear whether these barriers are greater for the elderly than for younger patients, for whom the cost of treatment is also a major concern, particularly given their higher rate of uninsurance.

Finally, the elderly and their caregivers suffer from the added burden of Alzheimer's disease and other dementias, which add another \$18 billion in treatment costs to the \$69 billion associated with other mental disorders. The prevalence rate for dementia rises with age, with approximately 8–15 percent of the elderly suffering from Alzheimer's disease.[99] Dementia and other organic disorders are a frequent cause of psychiatric hospitalization among the elderly, accounting for 64,596 inpatient stays in 1990.[100] Although treatment options for dementia are currently very limited, family members and other community caregivers often experience difficulty managing the behavior of these patients. These difficulties sometimes necessitate hospitalizing agitated patients simply to get them under control, even though their illness cannot be treated as effectively as other mental disorders. As with all mental illness, caregiver burden is a major concern for the family members of patients with dementia.

Children

Roughly 21 percent of children from nine to seventeen have a diagnosable mental disorder each year, with about 5 percent experiencing severe impairment as a result.[101] Suicide is a major concern for this age group, being the third leading cause of death among adolescents, at a rate of about 9.5 per hundred thousand.[102] Although 21 percent of children ages nine to seventeen receive mental health services each year, as with adults a portion of this use is accounted for by children without a diagnosable disorder. Thus 11 percent of children, or roughly half of all children with mental disorders, have a mental disorder that is left untreated. As with the elderly, diagnosis of mental illness is generally more difficult in the case of children and relies heavily on proxy respondents, such as parents and teachers. Among children who receive mental health services, the majority of these services are provided within schools.[103] Only 20 percent of children with SED receive mental health specialty services.[104] Inadequate access to specialty care among children is exacerbated by a shortage of child psychiatrists and other mental health specialists focusing on children.[105] Another problem specific to child mental health services is the lack of studies documenting the safety and efficacy of drugs for this age group, leading to concerns about potentially inappropriate off-label use of psychotropic medication among children.

Minorities

Mental disorders are generally as common among members of racial and ethnic minority groups as for nonminorities,[106] or more common, especially because of their higher rate of risk factors for mental illness (such as low socioeconomic status). High suicide rates are a particular concern among Native Americans.[107] Yet members of minority groups tend to have fewer outpatient visits than nonminorities[108] and less frequent use of mental health specialists.[109] Interestingly, though, African Americans are admitted to inpatient care at a much higher rate than whites.[110]

Reasons for differential treatment pattern are likely to vary across populations. For example, African Americans are thought to experience greater distrust of the system,[111] while Asian Americans may find mental health services to be particularly stigmatizing.[112] Recently immigrated Hispanic Americans and Asian Americans are likely to experience language barriers. Some barriers to accessing care (notably financial) cut across all racial and ethnic groups but are likely to pose greater constraints for members of minority groups, who are less wealthy on average than nonminorities. Finally, few providers of mental health services are members of minority groups themselves,[113] and patients are less likely to drop out of treatment if providers share their language and ethnicity.[114] To address the issue that inadequate cultural competence is a deterrent to receiving appropriate treatment, the Surgeon General has called for mental health services to be tailored to the demographic and cultural characteristics of the patient being treated.[115]

Rural Residents

The distance to a provider tends to be longer in rural areas, suggesting greater time and transportation costs associated with obtaining care. Furthermore, geographic accessibility of mental health specialists is limited in rural areas,[116] leading to heavier reliance on primary care providers than in urban areas.[117] Thus lack of physical proximity to providers of mental health services is a major concern among rural populations. These problems have led to proposed solutions such as "telepsychiatry," but there is not yet sufficient information to evaluate whether these innovations can address access issues on a large scale. The geographic barrier to accessing specialty services is exacerbated by the greater stigma experienced by a rural resident in obtaining mental health care, since those in a rural area have less anonymity.[118]

Current Mental Health Policy Issues

Many of the limitations of the U.S. mental health services delivery system are best addressed through interventions aimed at patients and providers, or they depend primarily on decisions made by private parties, such as insurers and employers. This section focuses instead on some of the actions that can be taken at the federal and state levels to improve mental health care.

Safety-Net Providers

Prior to the 1970s, most inpatient mental health care was provided within mental hospitals directly owned and operated by the states. Between 1970 and 1992, however, all of the net growth in the number of psychiatric hospitals in the United States occurred in the private sector, increasing the proportion of psychiatric hospitals run privately from 33 percent to 64 percent.[119] Over the same time period, the number of general hospitals with psychiatric units grew from 664 to 1,516.[120]

The movement from state psychiatric hospitals into private psychiatric and general hospitals continued into the 1990s, fueled in part by the closing of public facilities in many parts of the country on account of state budget deficits, deteriorating physical facilities, and the perception that direct public provision of services is less efficient than contracting with private parties to provide the services (known as the make-versus-buy debate).

Earlier predictions maintained that the state mental hospital would not survive as an institution. Between 1990 and 1997, the inpatient census in state psychiatric hospitals declined by 37 percent. Yet the reality is that even though state mental hospitals are experiencing reduction in patient population, they are unlikely to disappear altogether, at least in the foreseeable future. Currently 239 state psychiatric hospitals remain open, accounting for about 45 percent of state mental health budgets (National Association of State Mental Health Program Directors data).

Privatization has led to cautions about declining access to care for the sickest and most costly patients. Concern about the financial incentives for private hospitals to skim the relatively healthy patients and dump the sickest ones have been heightened by the concurrent trend toward for-profit psychiatric hospitals, in part because of for-profit conversions and growth in for-profit psychiatric hospital chains. In contrast to the general hospital sector, in which only 13 percent of hospitals are for-profit, 43 percent of psychiatric hospitals are for-profit.[121] Although the evidence on case mix and quality differences between public, private for-profit, and private not-for-profit providers is mixed,[122] the growing dominance of private, for-profit providers in the psychiatric sector has nonetheless been controversial.[123] It would be arguably premature for states to relinquish all direct control over delivering inpatient psychiatric services before ensuring that a safety-net provider exists.

Certainly for the most vulnerable patients, public hospitals continue to play a critical role. State hospitals are among the few willing to admit patients who are violent or disruptive, require long stays, or are uninsured.[124] Thus in the absence of alternative arrangements to guarantee access to private hospitals for these patients, it is important for states to maintain ongoing financial and political support for public psychiatric hospitals, including initiatives to improve the quality and cost-effectiveness of care provided in those institutions.

Managed Behavioral Health Care Under Public Programs

Following the trend in private insurance, public insurance programs are moving into managed care at a rapid rate. Thirty-five percent of elderly Medicare beneficiaries are expected to be in managed care plans by 2007.[125] State Medicaid programs have moved even more rapidly to enrolling beneficiaries in managed care plans. By 1998, the proportion of Medicaid beneficiaries enrolled in MCOs was 54 percent (a dramatic increase from the 14 percent in 1993), and all but three states had some form of Medicaid managed care program (according to the Health Care Financing Administration Website, www.hcfa.gov). In contrast to Medicare, Medicaid managed care programs are generally mandatory and often cover the disabled. Although the initial focus of Medicaid managed care programs was women and children on public assistance, currently twenty-nine states have managed care programs for disabled SSI recipients,[126] a population with a high incidence of mental illness and substance abuse. Currently twenty states also have non-Medicaid managed care programs that include behavioral health care.[127]

The fundamental ability of managed care plans to meet the needs of patients with chronic and costly illness has been questioned. Reservations notwithstanding, under the inexorable pressure of cost containment, continued enrollment of publicly insured patients in managed care plans seems certain. The question for mental health policy makers is therefore how to structure public managed care programs to ensure the best possible access to behavioral health care. In this context, several decisions face the public purchaser seeking to contract with a health plan to cover their beneficiary population.

The first question is whether mental health and substance abuse services should be "carved in" or "carved out." Managed behavioral health care carve-out vendors are essentially MCOs that cover only mental health services (and typically substance abuse services as well). It has been estimated that as much as 40–45 percent of all employer-based mental health care coverage in 1994 may have been part of a carve-out,[128] with a total of more than 162 million people currently enrolled.[129] Carve-out services can be used in conjunction with either fee-for-service or a managed care arrangement for medical care, and many HMOs also have internal behavioral health care carve-outs.

Carve-out vendors are sometimes, but not always, put at risk for service use of the enrollees. In risk-based carve-outs, the vendor receives a capitated payment and is at full or partial risk for the actual costs of the patient population. Almost half of the lives covered by carve-outs are enrolled in risk-based programs.[130] In administrative services only (ASO) contracts, the purchaser pays the carve-out vendor a fee to manage the care of the patient population. The vendor is not at risk for the utilization of the patients per se; however, the amount of the administrative payment can be specified to depend on the vendor's performance, so the vendor receives a reduced fee in the event that behavioral health care costs are not sufficiently contained. In either case, the vendor has a financial incentive to reduce costs. Furthermore, given the volatility of the market for behavioral health care carve-outs, the desire to develop a reputation for effectively managing care is arguably another important incentive for vendors to contain costs.[131] Consistent with these incentives, the literature on the effects of managed behavioral health care carve-outs has reliably shown large reductions in utilization and costs, particularly on the inpatient side.[132]

Currently, Medicare managed care plans are all carve-ins, with a single capitation payment covering both behavioral health and medical care. In contrast, Medicaid programs have made extensive use of carved-out and stand-alone models of managed behavioral health care for their populations, even when coverage of medical care remains fee-for-service. Persuasive arguments can be made for or against carving out behavioral health care. Arguments in favor of carve-outs[133] are that a vendor specializing in behavioral health care is better able to manage quality and costs, because of economies of scale and scope in setting up a specialty network; that having a separate budget may protect funding for mental health and substance abuse services within an MCO; and that carving out behavioral health care prevents adverse selection on the part of patients and skimming and dumping of psychiatric patients by competing insurance plans as long as only a single vendor is used.

The potential disadvantages of carving out behavioral health care are poor integration of medical and behavioral health care; incentives for cost shifting between the medical and behavioral health care vendors; potential stigmatization of the carved-out services; and potentially less control over providers, since both risk-based and ASO carve-out vendors frequently contract with independent network providers who are paid on a fee-for-service basis. Poor coordination between primary care and mental health care providers is a particular concern for the elderly, for whom mental health and medical problems tend to be closely intertwined. The counterargument is that primary care providers tend to avoid diagnosing mental illness in their patients from lack of knowledge, interest, and time. Thus the positive aspect of cost shifting is that patients may be more likely to receive diagnosis under a carve-out system in which they can be referred elsewhere.

If behavioral health care is carved out, the question is raised whether it is best to have a single carve-out vendor or multiple competing vendors. Closely related to this decision is the choice of using risk versus ASO contracts. In the case of risk-based contracting, the choice of a single vendor has clear-cut benefits in terms of avoiding incentives for vendors to compete to enroll healthy, low-cost patients and avoid sick, high-cost ones. However, competition between vendors ought to produce better incentives to contain costs and offer high-quality services. In theory, risk adjustment of capitation payments to competing behavioral health care carve-out vendors can prevent incentives for cream-skimming and dumping; in practice, it has proven difficult to adjust payments sufficiently to avoid these incentives altogether.[134] Thus it is more common for Medicaid programs to contract with only a single carve-out vendor at a time (even when contracting with multiple competing HMOs for medical care), but to engage in a rebidding process every few years, to establish incentives for the carve-out vendor to do a good job.

Another alternative for public purchasers is to contract with competing vendors, but use mixed payment systems, or "soft" capitation contracts, rather than full capitation mechanisms, so that the purchaser retains some of the risk of the patient's costs and vendors have less cause to engage in patient selection. In a mixed payment system, the vendor receives a payment equal to $\alpha + (\beta \times \text{costs})$, where $0 < \beta < 1$ and α is a fixed payment that is independent of actual costs—for example, $\alpha = (1 - \beta) \times$ expected costs. Thus the vendor bears some, but not all, of the risk associated with higher costs. Soft capitation systems are similar, in that the purchaser bears some of the risk. A per capita target amount and "risk corridors" are set for the expenditures of the carve-out vendor; if the vendor's actual costs exceed the target amount, the purchaser pays a portion of the additional costs. The proportion borne by the purchaser can be specified to depend on how far above the target amount costs actually are; typically the purchaser assumes more risk with further expenditure increases. Conversely, if the vendor's costs fall below the target amount, the purchaser retains some but not all of the difference, with the proportion increasing the further the actual costs lie below the target amount.

The idea is that the purchaser does not want the vendor to suffer huge losses if the target amount dramatically underestimates costs but also does not want the vendor to have an incentive to earn windfall profits by reducing expenditures far below the target amount. Thus, from the point of view of the vendor, mixed payment systems and soft capitation contracts limit the extent of both the up and the down sides to capitation payments.

The impact of managed care on costs, quality, and health outcomes has been a strong focus of research interest in the past decade, yet we still know relatively little about the ability of MCOs to provide high-quality care for persons with severe and chronic mental illnesses, or even for those with more routine behavioral health care needs.[135] It has been argued that certain types of managed care settings pose a unique opportunity for improving the care of the chronically ill,[136] but the strong financial incentives of MCOs to avoid sick patients and offer minimal benefits may dominate their structural advantages in caring for these populations. Given (1) the high degree of variability in the costs of patients with behavioral health problems, (2) the degree of risk aversion of most MCOs, and (3) the inadequacy of risk-adjustment methodologies, using some form of risk sharing between the purchaser and the carve-out vendor is advisable, especially if the purchaser contracts with competing vendors.

Performance-based incentives (based on quality indicators and not just cost-containment goals) should also be incorporated into the contract whenever possible. Measuring and risk adjusting outcomes tends to be even more difficult for behavioral health than medical problems; as one example, mortality is a more useful outcome measure for medical conditions such as myocardial infarction than for even severe mental illnesses such as schizophrenia. Little is known about outcomes for the mentally ill under managed care, although one study suggested that persons with schizophrenia improved less under a mental health carve-out than under fee-for-service.[137] However, both private and public efforts to measure quality of care are under way[138] and should be strongly encouraged, since the ability of behavioral health care carve-out vendors to reduce utilization cannot be interpreted in either a positive or negative light without corresponding information on quality and outcomes.

Parity in Health Insurance Benefits

The issue that has been perhaps most at the forefront of mental health policy initiatives in recent years is parity in health insurance benefits. At least three-quarters of employers restrict coverage of behavioral health care to a greater degree than coverage of medical care, although there is some evidence that the disparity is declining over time.[139] The idea behind parity was to eliminate such inequities in coverage. The federally legislated Mental Health Parity Act of 1996 (PL 104-204) mandated that, beginning in January 1998, health plans offering a mental health benefit could not impose a lower annual and lifetime spending limit on mental health benefits than for medical care. Employers with fewer than fifty workers and those that could show that their premiums increased by more than 1 percent as a result of parity were exempt from this provision. Importantly, however, this legislation did not prevent insurance plans from dropping mental health benefits altogether, requiring higher cost sharing for behavioral health care, or imposing limits on the number of covered outpatient visits or inpatient days; only dollar limits were affected.

Because of the weakness of the Mental Health Parity Act, there has been a strong push to enact parity legislation at the state level that would address some of the limitations of the federal legislation. As of December 1998, fourteen states had passed additional parity legislation that was stronger than the federal legislation.[140] However, as with medical care, the Employee Retirement Income Security Act of 1974 (ERISA) exemption for self-funded employer health plans makes it impossible for states to mandate benefits for all persons with employer-based insurance. Furthermore, as of 1994, only twenty-two states required that health plans cover mental health services at all; nine required that insurers make coverage available but did not require that plans include it, and nineteen had no mental health mandates.[141]

Because of the concerns about moral hazard and adverse selection described earlier, health plans have been reluctant to increase coverage of mental health services. However, to the extent that parity legislation sets a lower bound on behavioral health care benefits for all plans, such legislation should reduce the potential for patient selection into more generous plans. Furthermore, although relatively little is known about the price elasticity of demand for mental health services under managed care,[142] the tradeoff between demand-side and supply-side cost containment suggests that patient cost-sharing requirements can be reduced as long as there is a commensurate increase in utilization management by providers. The majority of privately funded behavioral health care is managed. Thus, it has been argued that more comprehensive coverage of mental health services need not add excessively to costs, so long as the moral hazard is constrained by comprehensively managing care.[143] The negative corollary to this point is that in a managed care environment parity in benefits can be achieved on paper, but without translating into actual practice if gatekeeping is stricter for behavioral health care.

Although a convincing argument can be made for implementing parity in insurance benefits, current legislation does not go very far in addressing financial barriers to mental health care. Since individuals with SPMI are less likely to have insurance coverage through their own (or a spouse's) employer, parity legislation primarily assists persons with less-disabling illnesses. Even for patients with private insurance, current parity legislation contains many loopholes that allow employers to continue differentially restricting use of mental health services. Because parity legislation is designed to address disparity between medical and behavioral health care coverage, at most it can only bring mental health benefits up to the inadequate standard currently set by medical care insurance. As Mechanic[144] notes, many of the long-term care and rehabilitative services required by individuals with mental disorders are generally not covered by private health insurance. Furthermore, parity legislation does not address the large proportion of Americans who are uninsured or publicly insured. Parity legislation is therefore at best a partial solution to concerns about financial barriers to behavioral health care. Thus mental health policy makers should prioritize not only stronger federal parity legislation that applies to all health plans and all states but also inclusion of comprehensive mental health and substance abuse benefits in all health policy initiatives seeking to expand insurance coverage to underinsured and uninsured populations.

Conclusion

Health care policy speaks to many of the same issues facing mental health policy, but additional concerns unique to behavioral health must be addressed. Individuals with severe and chronic psychiatric disorders are among the most vulnerable patient populations, having historically been neglected or mistreated. Given the limited ability of many persons with severe and chronic mental illness to advocate forcefully for themselves, mental health policy makers need to take responsibility for ensuring that these patients have adequate access to the services they need to reenter society. Of particular concern for this population are the limitations of public insurance coverage for psychiatric care, the tenuousness of the psychiatric safety-net system, and the fractured system of delivering and financing mental health services that makes it difficult for these patients to obtain the full continuum of services they need.

Access to care is also a concern for individuals with less-severe, acute disorders, many of whom are covered by employer-based insurance. The inadequate and inequitable coverage of behavioral health care under private insurance plans, potential for dumping or denial of needed care on the part of managed care plans, shortages of mental health specialists and certain types of mental health services in many parts of the country, and stigmatization of psychiatric treatment are among the major impediments to ensuring appropriate care for this population.

Two of the important trends in delivering and financing mental health care are the shift from public to private for-profit providers and the increasing dominance of managed behavioral health care. Additional resources need to be devoted to monitoring these trends and documenting their consequences, to ensure that the access and quality of care available to Americans with medical problems extends to those with mental illness as well.

Notes

1. Regier, D., and others. "The De Facto U.S. Mental and Addictive Disorders Service System. Epidemiologic Catchment Area Prospective 1-Year Prevalence Rates of Disorders and Services." *Archives of General Psychiatry*, 1993, *50*, 85–94; Kessler, R., and others. "Lifetime and 12-Month Prevalence of DSM-III-R Psychiatric Disorders in the United States. Results from the National Comorbidity Survey." *Archives of General Psychiatry*, 1994, *51*, 8–19.

2. Shaffer, D., and others. "The NIMH Diagnostic Interview Schedule for Children, Version 2.3: Description, Acceptability, Prevalence Rates, and Performance in the MECA Study." *Journal of the American Academy of Child and Adolescent Psychiatry*, 1996, *35*, 865–877.

3. Murray, C. and Lopez, A. (eds.). *The Global Burden of Disease. A Comprehensive Assessment of Mortality and Disability from Diseases, Injuries, and Risk Factors in 1990 and Projected to 2020.* Cambridge, Mass.: Harvard School of Public Health, 1996.

4. Mark, T., and others. *National Expenditures for Mental Health, Alcohol and Other Drug Abuse Treatment, 1996.* Rockville, Md.: Substance Abuse and Mental Health Services Administration, 1998; Surgeon General. *Mental Health: A Report of the Surgeon General.* Washington, D.C.: U.S. Government Printing Office, 1999.

5. Ettner, S., Frank, R., and Kessler, R. "The Impact of Psychiatric Disorder on Labor Market Outcomes." *Industrial and Labor Relations Review,* 1997, *51*(1), 64–81; Berndt, E., and others. "Workplace Performance Effects from Chronic Depression and Its Treatment." *Journal of Health Economics,* 1998, *17,* 511–535.

6. Kessler, R. and Frank, R. "The Impact of Psychiatric Disorders on Work Loss Days." *Psychological Medicine,* 1997, *27,* 861–873.

7. Mark and others (1998); Surgeon General (1999).

8. Kessler, R., and others. "The Epidemiology of Co-Occurring Addictive and Mental Disorders: Implications for Prevention and Service Utilization." *American Journal of Orthopsychiatry,* 1996, *1996*(66), 17–31.

9. Drake, R., and Osher, F. "Treating Substance Abuse in Patients with Severe Mental Illness." In S. Henggeler and A. Santos (eds.), *Innovative Approaches for Difficult-to-Treat Populations.* Washington, D.C.: American Psychiatric Press, 1997.

10. Steadman, H., and others. "Violence by People Discharged from Acute Psychiatric Inpatient Facilities and by Others in the Same Neighborhoods." *Archives of General Psychiatry,* 1998, *55,* 1–9; Swanson, J. "Mental Disorder, Substance Abuse, and Community Violence: An Epidemiological Approach." In J. Monahan and H. Steadman (eds.), *Violence and Mental Disorder: Developments in Risk Assessment.* Chicago: University of Chicago Press, 1994; Eronen, M., Angermeyer, M., and Schulze, B. "The Psychiatric Epidemiology of Violent Behavior." *Social Psychiatry and Psychiatric Epidemiology,* 1998, *33*(1), 13–23.

11. Gelberg, L. "Homeless Persons." In R. Andersen, T. Rice, and G. Kominski (eds.), *Changing the U.S. Health Care System.* San Francisco: Jossey-Bass, 1996.

12. Kelleher, K., and others. "Alcohol and Drug Disorders Among Physically Abusive and Neglectful Parents in a Community-Based Sample." *American Journal of Public Health,* 1994, *84,* 1586–1590.

13. Rice, D. and others. *The Cost of Alcohol and Drug Abuse and Mental Illness.* Washington, D.C.: U.S. Government Printing Office, 1990.

14. Kessler, R. "The Social Consequence of Psychiatric Disorders." In M. J. Cox and J. Brooks-Gunn (eds.), *Conflict and Closeness: The Formation, Functioning and Stability of Families.* Hillsdale, N. J.: Erlbaum forthcoming.

15. Kessler (forthcoming).

16. Klerman, G. "Trends in Utilization of Mental Health Services: Perspectives for Health Services Research." *Medical Care,* 1985, *23*(3), 584–597; Nemeroff, C. "Psychopharmacology of Affective Disorders in the 21st Century." *Biological Psychiatry,* 1998, *44,* 517–525.

17. Regier and others (1993); Kessler and others (1996).

18. Kessler, R. C., and others. "Differences in the Use of Psychiatric Outpatient Services Between the United States and Ontario." *New England Journal of Medicine,* 1997, *336*(8), 551–557.

19. Burns, B. E., and others. "Children's Mental Health Service Use Across Service Sectors." *Health Affairs,* 1995, *14,* 147–159.

20. Surgeon General (1999).

21. Grob, G. *The Mad Among Us: A History of the Care of America's Mentally Ill.* Cambridge, Mass.: Harvard University Press, 1994.

22. Meier, B. "A Price Too High? Deal to Save Charter Behavioral May Have Harmed It." *New York Times,* Feb. 16, 2000.

23. Murphy, M., and Dorwart, R. "Mental Health Policy." In D. Calkins (ed.), *Health Care Policy.* Cambridge, Mass.: Blackwell Science, 1995.

24. Surgeon General (1999), Chapter 1, p. 5.

25. Surgeon General (1999).

26. Surgeon General (1999).

27. Surgeon General (1999).

28. Kessler, R., and others. "The 12-Month Prevalence and Correlates of Serious Mental Illness." In R. Manderscheid and M. Sonnenschein (eds.), *Mental Health, United States, 1996.* Rockville, Md.: Center for Mental Health Services, 1996.

29. Friedman, R., and others. "Prevalence of Serious Emotional Disturbance in Children and Adolescents." In R. Manderscheid and M. Sonnenschein (eds.), *Mental Health, United States, 1996.* Rockville, Md.: Center for Mental Health Services, 1996.

30. Regier and others (1993).

31. Regier and others (1993); Kessler and others (1996).

32. Surgeon General (1999).

33. Beeler, J., Rosenthal, A., and Cohler, B. "Patterns of Family Caregiving and Support Provided to Older Psychiatric Patients in Long-Term Care." *Psychiatric Services,* 1999, *50*(9), 1222–1224; Lefley, H. "Aging Parents as Caregivers of Mentally Ill Adult Children: An Emerging Social Problem." *Hospital and Community Psychiatry,* 1987, *38*(10), 1063–1070; Horwitz, A. "Siblings as Caregivers for the Seriously Mentally Ill." *Milbank Quarterly,* 1993, *71*(2):323–339.

34. Kessler (forthcoming).

35. Segal, S., Silverman, C., and Baumohl, J. "Seeking Person-Environment Fit in Community Care Placement." *Journal of Social Issues,* 1989, *45*(3), 49–64.

36. Horwitz (1993).

37. Klerman (1985).

38. Mechanic, D. "Emerging Trends in Mental Health Policy and Practice." *Health Affairs,* 1998, *17*(6), 82–98.

39. Mark and others (1998).

40. Mark and others (1998).

41. Mark and others (1998).

42. Vallon, K., and others. "Comprehensive Case Management in the Private Sector for Patients with Mental Illness." *Psychiatric Services,* 1997, *48*(7), 910–914.

43. Stein, T., and Test, M. "Alternative to Mental Hospital Treatment: Conceptual Model, Treatment Program, and Clinical Evaluation." *Archives of General Psychiatry,* 1980, *37,* 392–397; Rochefort, D., and Goering, P. "'More a Link Than a Division': How Canada Has Learned from U.S. Mental Health Policy." *Health Affairs,* 1998, *17*(5), 110–127.

44. Norquist, G. and S. Hyman. "Advances in Understanding and Treating Mental Illness: Implications for Policy." *Health Affairs,* 1999, 18(5):32–47.

45. Mechanic (1998).

46. Surgeon General (1999).

47. Murphy and Dorwart (1995).

48. Murphy and Dorwart (1995).

49. Hogan, M. "Public-Sector Mental Health Care: New Challenges." *Health Affairs,* 1999, *18*(5), 106–111.

50. McKusick, D., and others. "Spending for Mental Health and Substance Abuse Treatment 1996." *Health Affairs,* 1998, *17*(5), 147–157.

51. McKusick and others (1998).

52. Grob, G. *From Asylum to Community: Mental Health Policy in Modern America.* Princeton, N.J.: Princeton University Press, 1991.

53. Surgeon General (1999); Phelan, J. B., and others. "Public Conceptions of Mental Illness in 1950 in 1996: Has Sophistication Increased? Has Stigma Declined?" Paper presented at American Sociological Association meetings, Toronto, Ont., Aug. 1997; Link, B., and others. "Public Conceptions of Mental Illness: The Labels, Causes, Dangerousness and Social Distance." *American Journal of Public Health*, 1999, *89*(9), 1328–1333.

54. Nunnally, J. *Popular Conceptions of Mental Health: Their Development and Change.* New York: Holt, Rinehart and Winston, 1961; Penn, D., and Martin, J. "The Stigma of Severe Mental Illness: Some Potential Solutions for a Recalcitrant Problem." *Psychiatric Quarterly*, 1998, *69*, 235–247.

55. Sussman, L., Robins, L., and Earls, F. "Treatment-Seeking for Depression by Black and White Americans." *Social Science and Medicine*, 1987, *24*, 187–196; Cooper-Patrick, L., and others. "Identification of Patient Attitudes and Preferences Regarding Treatment of Depression." *Journal of General Internal Medicine*, 1997, *12*, 431–438.

56. Surgeon General (1999).

57. Nemeroff (1998).

58. Burns and others (1995).

59. Ettner, S., and Hermann, R. "Provider Specialty Choice Among Medicare Patients Treated for Psychiatric Disorders." *Health Care Financing Administration Review*, 1997, *18*(3), 1–17.

60. Mechanic, D. "Treating Mental Illness: Generalist vs. Specialist." *Health Affairs*, 1990, *9*(4), 61–75.

61. Pincus, H., and others. "Prescribing Trends in Psychotropic Medications: Primary Care, Psychiatry, and Other Medical Specialties." *Journal of the American Medical Association*, 1998, *279*, 526–531.

62. Frank, R., and Kamlet, M. "Economic Aspects of Patterns of Mental Health Care: Cost Variation by Setting." *General Hospital Psychiatry*, 1990, *12*(1), 11–18; Haas-Wilson, D., Cheadle, A., and Scheffler, R. "Demand for Mental Health Services: An Episode of Treatment Approach." *Southern Economic Journal*, 1989, *56*(1), 219–232; Wells, K. B., and others. "Cost-Sharing and the Use of General Medical Physicians for Outpatient Mental Health Care." *Health Services Research*, 1987, *22*(1), 1–17; Horgan, C. "Specialty and General Ambulatory Mental Health Services: Comparison of Utilization and Expenditures." *Archives of General Psychiatry*, 1985, *42*(6), 565–572; Knesper, D., Pagnucco, D., and Wheeler, J. "Similarities and Differences Across Mental Health Services Providers and Practice Settings in the United States." *American Psychologist*, 1985, *40*(12), 1352–1369; Ettner, S., and Hermann, R. "Differences Between the General Medical and Mental Health Specialty Sectors in the Expenditures and Utilization Patterns of Medicare Patients Treated for Psychiatric Disorders." *Health Services Research*, 1999, *34*(3), 737–760.

63. Sherbourne, C. D., and others. "Subthreshold Depression and Depressive Disorder: Clinical Characteristics of General Medical and Mental Health Specialty Outpatients." *American Journal of Psychiatry*, 1994, *151*(12), 1777–1784; Wells, K., and others. "Use of Minor Tranquilizers and Antidepressant Medications by Depressed Outpatients: Results from the Medical Outcomes Study." *American Journal of Psychiatry*, 1994, *151*(5), 694–700; Sturm, R., and Wells, K. B. "How Can Care for Depression Become More Cost-Effective?" *Journal of the American Medical Association*, 1995, *273*(1), 51–58; Katz, S., and others. "Medication Management of Depression in the United States and Ontario." *Journal of General Internal Medicine*, 1998, *13*(1), 77–85.

64. Mechanic (1998).

65. Knesper, D. J., Wheeler, J.R.C., and Pagnucco, D. L. "Mental Health Services Providers' Distribution Across Counties in the United States." *American Psychologist*, 1984, *39*(12), 1424–1434.

66. Peterson, B., and others. "Mental Health Practitioners and Trainees." In R. Manderscheid and M. Henderson (eds.), *Mental Health, United States, 1998*. Rockville, Md.: Center for Mental Health Services, 1998.

67. Ettner and Hermann (1997); Horgan (1985); Shannon, G., Bashshur, R., and Lovett, J. "Distance and the Use of Mental Health Services." *Milbank Quarterly*, 1986, *64*(2), 302–330; Horgan, C., and Salkever, D. "The Demand for Outpatient Mental Health Care from Nonspecialty Providers." In R. Scheffler and L. Rossiter (eds.), *Advances in Health Economics and Health Services Research*. Greenwich, Conn.: JAI Press, 1987.

68. McKusick (1998).

69. Frank, R., and McGuire, T. "Economics and Mental Health." (Working paper 7052.) Cambridge, Mass.: National Bureau of Economic Research, 1999.

70. Frank, R., Koyanagi, C., and McGuire, T. "The Politics and Economics of Mental Health 'Parity' Laws." *Health Affairs*, 1997, *16*(4), 108–119.

71. McKusick (1998).

72. McKusick (1998).

73. Murphy and Dorwart (1995); Kiesler, C., and Sibulkin, A. *Mental Hospitalization: Myths and Facts About a National Crisis*. Thousand Oaks, Calif.: Sage, 1987.

74. Frank and McGuire (1999).

75. American Hospital Association. *Hospital Statistics*. Chicago: American Hospital Association, 1996.

76. Manderscheid, R., and Sonnenschein, M. (eds.). *Mental Health, United States, 1996*. (Department of Health and Human Services, Center for Mental Health Services, publication no. [SMA] 96-3098.) Washington, D.C.: Superintendent of Documents, U.S. Government Printing Office, 1996.

77. Hogan (1999).

78. Buck, J., and others. "Behavioral Health Benefits in Employer-Sponsored Health Plans, 1997." *Health Affairs*, 1999, *18*(2), 67–78.

79. Murphy and Dorwart (1995).

80. Frank, Koyanagi, and McGuire (1997).

81. Frank and McGuire (1999).

82. Newhouse, J. *Free for All? Lessons from the RAND Health Insurance Experiment*. Cambridge, England: Harvard University Press, 1993.

83. Frank and McGuire (1999); Croghan, T., Obenchain, R., and Crown, W. "What Does Treatment of Depression Really Cost?" *Health Affairs*, 1998, *17*(4), 198–208.

84. Lave, J., and Goldman, H. "Medicare Financing for Mental Health Care." *Health Affairs*, Spring 1990, 19–30.

85. Sherman, J. "Medicare's Mental Health Benefits: Coverage, Use and Expenditures." *Journal of Aging and Health*, 1996, *8*(1), 54–71.

86. Taube, C., Goldman, H., and Salkever, D. "Medicaid Coverage for Mental Illness: Balancing Access and Costs." *Health Affairs*, 1990, *9*, 5–18.

87. Frank and McGuire (1999); Sherman (1996).

88. Cromwell, J., and others. "A Modified TEFRA System for Psychiatric Facilities." In R. Frank and W. Manning (eds.), *Economics and Mental Health*. Baltimore: Johns Hopkins University Press, 1992.

89. Cromwell, J., and others. "Medicare Payment to Psychiatric Facilities: Unfair and Inefficient?" *Health Affairs*, Summer 1991, 124–134.

90. Lave, J., and others. "The Decision to Seek an Exemption from PPS." *Journal of Health Economics*, 1988, *7*, 163–171.

91. Tischler, G. "Utilization Management of Mental Health Services by Private Third Parties." *American Journal of Psychiatry*, 1990, *147*(8), 967–973.

92. Hermann, R. C., and others. "Variation in ECT Use in the United States." *American Journal of Psychiatry*, 1995, *152*(6), 869–875; Phelps, C. "Information Diffusion and Best Practice Adoption." In J. Newhouse and A. Culyer (eds.), *Handbook of Health Economics, vol. 1A*. Amsterdam, Neth.: North Holland Press, 2000.

93. Surgeon General (1999).

94. Hoyert, D., Kochanek, K., and Murphy, S. *Deaths: Final Data for 1997*. Hyattsville, Md.: National Center for Health Statistics, 1999.

95. German, P. S., Shapiro, S., and Skinner, E. A. "Mental Health of the Elderly: Use of Health and Mental Health Services." *Journal of American Geriatric Society*, 1985, *33*(4), 246–252; NIH Consensus Conference. "Diagnosis and Treatment of Depression in Late Life." *Journal of the American Medical Association*, 1992, *268*(8), 1018–1024; Leaf, P. J., and others. "Contact with Health Professionals for the Treatment of Psychiatric and Emotional Problems." *Medical Care*, 1985, *23*(12), 1322–1337.

96. Horgan (1985); Leaf, P. J., and others. "Factors Affecting the Utilization of Specialty and General Medical Mental Health Services." *Medical Care*, 1988, *26*(1), 9–26.

97. NIH Consensus Conference (1992); Unutzer, J., and others. "Depressive Symptoms and the Cost of Health Services in HMO Patients Aged 65 Years and Older." *Journal of the American Medical Association*, 1997, *277*(20), 1618–1623.

98. NIH Consensus Conference (1992); Butler, R., and Lewis, M. *Aging and Mental Health*. St. Louis: Mosby, 1982.

99. Ritchie, K., and Kildea, D. "Is Senile Dementia 'Age-Related' or 'Aging-Related'? Evidence from Meta-Analysis of Dementia Prevalence in the Oldest Old." *Lancet*, 1995, *346*, 931–934.

100. Ettner, S., and Hermann, R. "Inpatient Psychiatric Treatment of Elderly Medicare Beneficiaries, 1990–1991." *Psychiatric Services*, 1998, *49*(9), 1173–1179.

101. Schaffer (1996).

102. Hoyert, Kochanek, and Murphy (1999); Centers for Disease Control. "Suicide Deaths and Rates Per 100,000." [http://www.cdc.gov/ncipc/data/us9794/suic.htm] 1999.

103. Hoagwood, K., and Erwin, H. "Effectiveness of School-Based Mental Health Services for Children: A 10-Year Research Review." *Journal of Child and Family Studies*, 1997, *6*, 435–454.

104. Burns and others (1995).

105. Thomas, C., and Holzer, C. "National Distribution of Child and Adolescent Psychiatrists." *Journal of the American Academy of Child and Adolescent Psychiatry*, 1999, *38*, 9–15.

106. Regier, D., and others. "One-Month Prevalence of Mental Disorders in the United States and Sociodemographic Characteristics: The Epidemiological Catchment Area Study." *Acta Psychiatrica Scandinavica*, 1993, *88*, 35–47.

107. Wallace, J., and others. *Homicide and Suicide Among Native Americans, 1979–1992*. (Violence Surveillance Series, no. 2.) Atlanta: National Center for Injury Prevention and Control, Centers for Disease Control and Prevention, 1996.

108. Neighbors, H., and others. "Ethnic Minority Health Service Delivery: A Review of the Literature." *Research in Community and Mental Health*, 1992, *7*, 55–71; Takeuchi, D., and Uehara, E. "Ethnic Minority Mental Health Services: Current Research and Future Conceptual Directions." In B. Levin and J. Petrila (eds.), *Mental Health Services: A Public Health Perspective*. New York: Oxford University Press, 1996.

109. Sussman, Robins, and Earls (1987); Gallo, J., and others. "Filters on the Pathway to Mental Health Care. II: Sociodemographic Factors." *Psychological Medicine*, 1995, *25*, 1149–1160;

Vega, W., and others. "Lifetime Prevalence of DSM-III-R Psychiatric Disorders Among Urban and Rural Mexican-Americans in California." *Archives of General Psychiatry,* 1998, *55,* 771–778; Zhang, A., Snowden, L., and Sue, S. "Differences Between Asian and White Americans' Help-Seeking Patterns in the Los Angeles Area." *Journal of Community Psychology,* 1998, *26,* 317–326.

110. Snowden, L., and Cheung, F. "Use of Inpatient Mental Health Services by Members of Ethnic Minority Groups." *American Psychologist,* 1990, *45,* 347–355.

111. Sussman, Robins, and Earls (1987); Lin, K., and others. "Sociocultural Determinants of the Help-Seeking Behavior of Patients with Mental Illness." *Journal of Nervous and Mental Disease,* 1982, *170,* 78–85.

112. Uba, L. *Asian-Americans: Personality Patterns, Identity and Mental Health.* New York: Guilford Press, 1994.

113. Peterson and others (1998).

114. Takeuchi, D., Uehara, E., and Maramba, G. "Cultural Diversity and Mental Health Treatment." In A. Horwitz and T. Scheid (eds.), *The Sociology of Mental Health.* New York: Oxford University Press, 1999.

115. Surgeon General (1999).

116. Peterson and others (1998).

117. Lambert, D., and Agger, M. "Access of Rural AFDC Medicaid Beneficiaries to Mental Health Services." *Health Care Financing Review,* 1995, *17*(1), 133–145.

118. Hoyt, D., and others. "Psychological Distress and Help Seeking in Rural America." *American Journal of Community Psychology,* 1997, *25,* 449—470.

119. Manderscheid and Sonnenschein (1996).

120. Mechanic (1998).

121. Levenson, A. I. "The Growth of Investor-Owned Psychiatric Hospitals." *American Journal of Psychiatry,* 1982, *139*(7), 902–907; Ettner, S. L., and Hermann, R. C. "The Role of Profit Status under Imperfect Information: Evidence from the Treatment Patterns of Elderly Medicare Beneficiaries Hospitalized for Psychiatric Diagnoses." *Journal of Health Economics,* 2001, *20*(1), 23–49.

122. Dorwart, R., and others. "A National Study of Psychiatric Hospital Care." *American Journal of Psychiatry,* 1991, *148*(2), 204–210; Schlesinger, M., and Dorwart, R. A. "Ownership and Mental-Health Services: A Reappraisal of the Shift Towards Privately Owned Facilities." *New England Journal of Medicine,* 1984, *311,* 959–965; Mark, T. L. "Psychiatric Hospital Ownership and Performance: Do Nonprofit Organizations Offer Advantages in Markets Characterized by Asymmetric Information?" *Journal of Human Resources,* 1996, *31*(3), 631–650.

123. Levenson (1982); Dorwart and others (1991); Schlesinger and Dorwart (1984); Eisenberg, L. "The Case Against For-Profit Hospitals." *Hospital and Community-Based Psychiatry,* 1984, *35*(10), 1009–1013; Dorwart, R. A., and Epstein, S. S. "Issues in Psychiatric Hospital Care." *Current Opinion in Psychiatry,* 1991, *4,* 789–793; Dorwart, R. A., and Schlesinger, M. "Privatization of Psychiatric Services." *American Journal of Psychiatry,* 1988, *145*(5), 543–553; Levenson, A. I. "Issues Surrounding the Ownership of Private Psychiatric Hospitals by Investor-Owned Hospital Chains." *Hospital and Community Psychiatry,* 1983, *34*(12), 1127–1131; Levenson, A. "The For-Profit System." In S. S. Sharfstein and A. Biegel (eds.), *The New Economics and Psychiatric Care.* Washington, D.C.: American Psychiatric Press, 1985.

124. Fisher, W., and others. "Case Mix in the 'Downsizing' State Hospital." *Psychiatric Services,* 1996, *47,* 255–262.

125. Komisar, H., Reuter, J., and Feder, J. *Medicare Chart Book*. Menlo Park, Calif.: Kaiser Family Foundation, 1997.

126. Substance Abuse and Mental Health Services Administration. "Managed Care Tracking System." [http://www.samhsa.gov/mc/stateprfls] Mar. 15, 2000.

127. Substance Abuse and Mental Health Services Administration (2000).

128. Jensen, G., and others. "Mental Health Insurance in the 1990s: Are Employers Offering Less to More?" *Health Affairs*, 1998, *17*(3), 201–208.

129. Sturm, R. "Tracking Changes in Behavioral Health Services: How Have Carve-Outs Changed Care?" *Journal of Behavioral Health Services and Research*, 1999, *26*(4), 360–371.

130. Oss, M., Drissel, A., and Clary, J. *Managed Behavioral Health Market Share in the United States, 1997–1998*. Gettysburg, Pa.: Open Minds, 1997.

131. Goldman, W., McCulloch, J., and Sturm, R. "Cost and Use of Mental Health Services Before and After Managed Care." *Health Affairs*, 1998, *17*(2), 40–52.

132. For reviews, see Mechanic, D., and McAlpine, D. "Mission Unfulfilled: Potholes on the Road to Mental Health Parity." *Health Affairs*, 1999, *18*(5), 7–21; and Sturm (1999).

133. Frank, R., McGuire, T., and Newhouse, R. "Risk Contracts in Managed Mental Health Care." *Health Affairs*, Fall 1995, 50–64.

134. Ettner, S., and others. "Risk Adjustment of Mental Health and Substance Abuse Payments." *Inquiry*, 1998, *35*(2), 223–239.

135. Mechanic and McAlpine (1999); Pincus, H., Zarin, D., and West, J. "Peering into the 'Black Box': Measuring Outcomes of Managed Care." *Archives of General Psychiatry*, 1996, *53*, 870–877; Lurie, N. "Studying Access to Care in Managed Care Environments." *Health Services Research*, 1997, *32*(5), 691–701.

136. Wagner, E. "Managed Care and Chronic Illness: Health Services Research Needs." *Health Services Research*, 1997, *32*(5), 702–714.

137. Manning, W., and others. "Outcomes for Medicaid Beneficiaries with Schizophrenia Under a Prepaid Mental Health Carve-Out." *Journal of Behavioral Health Services and Research*, 1999, *26*(4), 442–450.

138. Mechanic (1998); Mechanic and McAlpine (1999).

139. Buck and others (1999); Jensen and others (1998).

140. Buck and others (1999).

141. Jensen and others (1998).

142. Frank and McGuire (1999).

143. Goldman, McCulloch, and Sturm (1998).

144. Mechanic (1998).

CHAPTER THIRTEEN

WOMEN'S HEALTH

Key Issues in Access to Insurance Coverage and to Services Among Nonelderly Women

Roberta Wyn and Beatriz M. Solís

Analysis of the current health care system and debates on alternative solutions to increasing coverage, improving access, and controlling costs have often proceeded without regard to the specific implications of the effects on women. Although women and men share the same need for affordable, accessible, and quality care, there are specific health concerns and patterns of use unique to women that are often overlooked. Many health conditions are particular to women, occur with greater frequency among women, or have different consequences for women than for men. These differences affect the amount and kind of health care services needed.

Women have a large stake in how health care services are financed and delivered. They are the coordinators of care for their families and have higher use rates than men.[1] Furthermore, women's less advantaged and less stable economic status places them at particular financial risk for the costs of medical care.

This chapter examines some of the key policy factors related to financing and delivering services for women under sixty-five years of age. First, we examine the adequacy of women's access to health insurance coverage and the ability of that coverage to protect against the costs of health services. This includes current coverage patterns, analysis of the advantages and disadvantages of the current insuring system for women, and the economic importance of coverage. Second, we examine how health insurance coverage affects women's access to care. Lastly, we look beyond financial barriers to other aspects of the health care system that influence access. The population is limited to the nonelderly because much of the chapter focuses on health insurance coverage. Although women over sixty-five also face health insurance access problems, most older women have insurance coverage through Medicare; therefore, their insurance coverage issues differ. (Chapter Nine, on long-term care and the elderly, discusses related issues regarding older women.)

Women's Access to Insurance Coverage

The mechanisms for obtaining health insurance coverage are embedded in complex social and economic situations that differ between women and men and among subgroups of women. The current health insurance structure in the United States is a voluntary system that relies primarily on health insurance obtained from one's own employment or the employment of a spouse or parent, augmented by individually purchased private insurance, and public systems for eligible low-income individuals and families (Medicaid) and for the elderly (Medicare). This patchwork of coverage options leaves many women dependent on coverage through a spouse, reliant on a changing public system, or uninsured. Even though women have a lower rate of being uninsured than men (Table 13.1), they often must rely on complicated arrangements to obtain coverage.

The main source of coverage for both women and men is through employment, obtained either through one's own employment or that of a spouse or

TABLE 13.1. HEALTH INSURANCE COVERAGE BY GENDER, AGES 18–64, UNITED STATES, 1998.

	Percentage Covered	
Health Insurance Coverage	Women	Men
Employment-based coverage, primary	40	55
Employment-based coverage, dependent	28	14
Privately purchased	5	5
Medicaid	7	3
Other coverage*	2	2
Uninsured	18	21
Total	100	100

Note: *Medicare, CHAMPUS, Indian Health Services.

Source: Authors' analysis of the March 1999 Current Population Survey.

parent. Pairing coverage with employment connects two distributive systems: work and insurance. Thus, the factors that determine the distribution of jobs in this society also determine access to employment-based health insurance coverage.[2] This places women at a disadvantage as they have less attachment to the labor market than do men. Even though the proportion of women who work full-time for the full year has increased since the 1980s, fewer than half of working women in 1989 had this labor market status.[3] The remainder were either part-time or seasonally employed, or a combination of the two—work status conditions less likely to involve coverage.[4] Although nearly equal proportions of nonelderly women and men have employment-based coverage (68 percent for women and 69 percent for men; Table 13.1), women are more likely than men to be covered as a dependent (that is, covered through a spouse or parent), and less likely to have coverage directly through their own employer.

Another distinction between men and women is women's greater reliance on Medicaid. Women are twice as likely as men to receive this benefit (Table 13.1) because of income and eligibility requirements that women are more likely to meet. Despite women's greater access to Medicaid than men, this program fails to reach many poor women; in 1997, nearly four out of ten poor women (family income below 100 percent of the poverty level) were uninsured.[5]

Among women, patterns of coverage vary considerably by racial and ethnic background (Table 13.2). Ethnic minority women are less likely than white women to have employment-based coverage. Medicaid coverage, in part, compensates for these lower employment-based coverage rates; black women and Latinas have higher rates of Medicaid coverage than white women.

Yet even with Medicaid serving as a safety net, gaps in coverage persist. Black, Asian American and Pacific Islander (AAPI), and Latina women all have higher uninsured rates than white women. Nearly four out of ten Latinas and one out of four black and AAPI women are uninsured.

Low-income women have high uninsured rates. Four out of ten (39 percent) poor women (family income below poverty) and one-third (32 percent) of near-poor women (family income 100–199 percent of poverty) are uninsured, compared to 12 percent of women with family income at or over 200 percent of poverty.[6]

Issues with Women's Current Coverage Options

Changes in both private sector and public health coverage may affect access to health care for women. In the absence of effective cost controls, it is likely that employment-based coverage as a dependent (also referred to as family coverage) will be ever more difficult to obtain, as employers attempt to reduce health insurance costs. Employers with a high proportion of workers with family coverage

TABLE 13.2. HEALTH INSURANCE COVERAGE BY ETHNICITY, WOMEN AGES 18–64, UNITED STATES, 1998.

Health Insurance Coverage	*Percentage Covered*			
	Latina	Black	White	Asian American and Pacific Islander
Employment-based coverage, primary	25	41	42	38
Employment-based coverage, dependent	20	15	33	26
Privately purchased	3	3	5	5
Medicaid	11	15	4	5
Other coverage*	2	3	2	3
Uninsured	39	23	14	23
Total	100	100	100	100

Notes: * Medicare, CHAMPUS, Indian Health Services.

Source: Authors' analysis of the March 1999 Current Population Survey.

face higher health care costs. Between 1989 and 1996, the premiums for family coverage increased faster than for employee-only coverage, leading some employers to question their role and responsibility to finance health insurance for an employee's family.[7] This concern over rising health insurance costs has led some employers to increasingly restrict access to dependent coverage by increasing employee contributions to dependent coverage, paying incentives to those who chose employee-only coverage, or switching to managed care plans.

Medicaid coverage is also vulnerable to economic constraints to restrict spending and growth. A major change that has occurred in Medicaid is the shift from fee-for-service to managed care delivery system. In 1997, 15.3 million Medicaid beneficiaries were enrolled in managed care, an increase from 2.7 million in 1991.[8] The populations enrolled in these managed care plans are primarily adults in families (the majority of whom are women) and children, who account for nearly three-fourths of Medicaid beneficiaries, although they generated only 27 percent of total program spending in 1996.[9] The elderly and disabled account for the majority of Medicaid spending (64 percent) because of their more intensive use of acute and long-term care services.

Many features of managed care, such as its focus on coordinated care and emphasis on primary care, have the potential to improve access for the Medicaid population. Yet studies comparing Medicaid fee-for-service and Medicaid managed care are mixed, with some measures showing improvements for women enrolled in managed care, and others showing little difference.[10]

Medicaid managed care is being implemented primarily to save costs; thus concern over access and quality has been raised. The incentives in managed care, with the fixed payment reimbursement, could lead to underservice. Furthermore, the limited experience of many managed care plans in working with a low-income population may create barriers to care or insufficient understanding of the range of services a low-income population may need. The Medicaid population is a fluid population with considerable turnover in eligibility. This could limit development of stable relationships with managed care providers and diminish the incentives to provide preventive care. Nonetheless, managed care does have the potential to improve access to care, and in particular to primary and preventive care.

Another major change that affected Medicaid was passage of the Personal Responsibility and Work Opportunity Reconciliation Act of 1996 (PRWORA), known as welfare reform. This legislation replaced Aid to Families with Dependent Children (AFDC) with Temporary Assistance to Needy Families (TANF), a time-limited assistance program. This legislation also severed the automatic link between welfare and Medicaid.[11] Medicaid eligibility standards are tied to state AFDC levels of July 1996, and legislation allows continuance of Medicaid coverage under certain circumstances once a woman becomes employed.

Additionally, under welfare reform, changes were made in the Medicaid eligibility of immigrants, which has restricted access to benefits for certain groups of immigrants and caused a decline in applying for benefits on account of concern over eligibility and immigration status.[12]

After steady enrollment growth during the early 1990s, Medicaid enrollment started to decline in 1995. For adults, enrollment growth fell by 5.5 percent between 1995 and 1997.[13] The findings from a national study of former welfare recipients do not bode well for access to coverage for poor women after welfare reform. After six months off welfare, 34 percent of welfare leavers were uninsured, increasing to 49 percent after one year,[14] even though provisions of the law do allow continued Medicaid eligibility under certain conditions.

Economic Importance of Coverage: Women and Economic Disadvantage

Financing health care and distributing health care costs are particularly important for women. Nonelderly women are more likely than men to use physician services. Women's use of obstetrical/gynecological care explains this difference partially, but not totally.[15] A large gap in use rate between men and women is seen during the reproductive years. Per capita expenditures for women fifteen to forty-four years old are \$2,123 compared with \$1,272 for men, a differential attributable, in part, to the expenses associated with reproductive services for women.[16]

Cost As a Barrier

Financial barriers are often cited by women as a reason for not receiving care. Among women who did not receive clinical preventive services during a one-year period, the most frequently cited barrier was the cost of care, reported by four out of ten nonelderly women and about two out of ten elderly women.[17] Low-income women and those who are uninsured have the lowest clinical preventive use rates and access to care.[18]

Having insurance coverage does not guarantee that medical or preventive services are affordable. Lack of coverage for specific health services and out-of-pocket expenses even when insured (to meet deductibles, co-payments, or coinsurance obligations), increase the financial risk for insured women. Studies have shown that use of services is highest when there is no cost sharing and that cost sharing reduces the amount of effective and less effective medical care alike.[19] Furthermore, coinsurance appears to have a greater effect on low-income persons, reducing their use of effective services relative to the use rate for higher-income people. Not all effects of cost sharing are viewed as detrimental, however. Cost sharing reduces the demand for services and therefore health care expenditures, and cost-sharing obligations can also reduce the use of health care services of little or no value.[20] However, cost sharing does impose a disproportionate burden on low-income persons and can inhibit use of important medical and preventive services.

Women age fifteen to forty-four spend a larger proportion of their income on out-of-pocket medical costs than men of the same age range, in part because of the coverage gaps for preventive and reproductive services.[21]

Health Insurance Coverage and Women's Access to Services

Several studies have documented the relationship between insurance coverage and access to care, building upon the conceptual framework developed by Andersen and colleagues[22] that measures such access indicators as utilization of physician and hospital visits, delayed care, and receipt of preventive care.

Uninsured women are much less likely than those with health insurance coverage to have had a doctor visit in the past year or a regular place where they receive care.[23] Continuity of coverage is also important; lack of continuous health insurance coverage is associated with access problems.[24]

A more specific measure of access than physician and hospital visits is use of clinical preventive services. There is considerable agreement about the efficacy of these services and, in most cases, the frequency at which services should be received. This consensus is an independent criterion of use that can be applied across subgroups of women.

Women who lack health insurance coverage are less likely than those with coverage to receive such screenings as blood pressure test, glaucoma testing, clinical breast examination, mammography, and the Pap test.[25] Many uninsured women also have low income, a factor associated with elevated risk for many of the conditions that these screenings are intended to discover. Thus, the burden of paying for preventive services often falls on those women who are least able to afford such costs. Lack of insurance coverage may well force women and medical providers to prioritize urgent health care problems, compromising access to preventive screenings. This creates an ineffective health care system, one in which advances in prevention and early diagnosis are not fully and adequately used. Diagnosis of disease at an early stage is particularly important for cervical and breast cancer; both morbidity and mortality are reduced if these cancers are detected early.

A further indicator of access for women is use of prenatal services. Studies have documented that uninsured women do not receive adequate prenatal services, as measured by the point during pregnancy when care was initiated and the number of physician visits throughout the pregnancy.[26] During the late 1980s, several legislative options and mandates were enacted to expand Medicaid eligibility for low-income pregnant women and their infants. These expansions required states to cover all pregnant women, as well as children below age six, living in families with income up to 133 percent of the federal poverty level.[27] According to the National Governors' Association Center for Best Practices, as of 1999 thirty-seven states have expanded eligibility for pregnant women beyond the federal mandates.[28] The average Medicaid eligibility level for pregnant women went from 174 percent of poverty in 1997 to 180 percent in 1999.

Health Outcomes

Lack of health insurance coverage not only reduces access to health care but appears to affect health outcomes. Women without health insurance coverage have a more advanced stage of breast cancer at diagnosis and, among those with local and regional disease, poorer survival than women with private coverage.[29] Lack of coverage also affects birth outcomes among women[30] and increases the risk of in-hospital mortality (for both women and men).[31] As access measures increasingly include health status as an outcome, rather than focusing mainly on health care use, more will be known about the connection between access and health status.

Beyond Health Insurance and Cost: Factors Affecting Use

There are several other access barriers that women report in addition to the cost of services. Studies indicate the importance of having a regular connection to the health care system. Having a usual source of care is associated with women's increased use of clinical preventive services and general medical checkups, even among insured women.[32]

Access to a regular provider of care is also an important component of women's health. Women's health care has been characterized as fragmented; many women typically see more than one provider for primary care needs in part because women's health is often split into reproductive needs and all other needs.[33] Because of this fragmentation, women may not receive needed services or may receive repeated services.

Studies have shown that the type of provider seen influences receipt of certain services for women. Women who see an obstetrician/gynecologist are more likely to be screened for breast and cervical cancer than are those whose primary physician is an internist or family practitioner.[34] Physician specialty also affects access to health promotion advice. Internists and family practitioners are more likely to counsel their patients in such areas as exercise, nutrition and diet, and mental health issues, whereas obstetricians/gynecologists are more likely to ask about sexual practices and sexually transmitted diseases.[35]

Practice and referral patterns of physicians are important determinants of using clinical preventive services for women; nearly three-quarters of women who have mammograms reported physician recommendation as the reason for the screening.[36] To facilitate access to women's reproductive health care, legislation has been passed in approximately 60 percent of states that allow women enrolled in managed care plans some level of direct access to an obstetrician/gynecologist without first obtaining a referral from a primary care physician.[37]

Enhancing the accessibility of services for women is also crucial. Factors such as geographic location of services, availability of child care, and cultural sensitivity of services all influence access to the health care system.[38] Time constraints also impede women's access to care. Multiple roles and responsibilities (paid employment, care of children and parents, household work) all compete for women's time. Women often make tradeoffs to allocate the time and resources available.

In one study, more than one-quarter of women who did not receive a recommended clinical preventive service reported time constraints as a factor.[39]

Policy Implications and Future Research

The current insurance system leaves many women uninsured; low-income women and women of color are especially at risk of not having insurance coverage. Women without insurance coverage are at serious risk of delaying or not receiving needed care and of not being screened for early detection of disease. Costs remain a barrier even for insured women, suggesting that any coverage that imposes large deductibles and coinsurance obligations would hinder use of necessary services, especially for economically disadvantaged women. Lack of coverage for specific services also reduces the use of necessary care, such as preventive screenings. Limited coverage of important services, such as reproductive care, restricts the choices that women have available to them. These problems with benefit coverage emphasize the importance of comprehensive coverage.

Particular consideration of low-income women is required in formulating new health policy regarding financing of services. They have the lowest rates of screening for certain clinical preventive services and the poorest health status, and they are the most vulnerable to the effects of costs.

However, unintended effects of welfare reform legislation may make health insurance coverage even harder for low-income women to obtain. Medicaid enrollment is declining after a decade of growth, attributable in large measure to welfare reform legislation.[40] Among former welfare recipients, one-third (34 percent) are uninsured in the first six months of leaving welfare; after twelve or more months, about one-half are uninsured.[41]

In addition to financial access to health services, the organization of health care needs to facilitate access to a regular source and provider of care to increase the continuity of care women receive. Appropriate incentives need to be in place in the health care system to encourage physician promotion of primary and preventive care. Women may benefit from having a women's health specialist as a primary care provider,[42] an area that requires additional consideration and research. The trend toward defining gynecologists as primary care providers would increase access to certain types of preventive screenings for women, but it is not clear what effect this designation will have on women's overall access to nonreproductive-related primary care services.

We need further research on special measures needed to reach women who historically have been underserved by the health care system, such as ethnic minority women, low-income women, and those with less formal education. These population groups often experience the worst health status and are typically less likely to have access to primary care and preventive care services; once in the system, they may also experience disparity in medical treatment.

In addition to the financial and structural barriers that women face, many women experience competing social roles and responsibilities that interfere with their own needs for appropriate health care. Many women report time constraints as a deterrent to use of services. Some of these barriers can be addressed by the health care system; extending hours, bringing services into the community where women live and work, and providing child care access could remove some of these barriers.

Facilitating access to the health care system is only part of the process of improving the health of women. Additional research is needed on the coordination and process of care once a woman has been screened and identified as needing further diagnostic work and treatment. We must continue to investigate disparity in access to services, treatment approaches, and clinical outcomes between women and men, and among subgroups of women, to understand and eliminate the causes of any inequity in the health care system.[43]

Notes

1. Sandman, D. R., Simantov, E., and An, C. *Out of Touch: American Men and the Health Care System.* New York: Commonwealth Fund, 2000.
2. Jecker, N. S. "Can an Employer-Based Health Insurance System Be Just?" *Journal of Health Politics, Policy, and Law,* 1993, *18*(3), 657–673.
3. Population Reference Bureau. *What the 1990 Census Tells Us About Women: A State Factbook.* Washington, D.C.: Population Reference Bureau, 1993.
4. Schauffler, H. H., and Brown, E. R. *The State of Health Insurance in California, 1998.* Berkeley: Health Insurance Policy Program, University of California, Berkeley, and UCLA Center for Health Policy, 1999; U.S. Department of Census. *Current Population Reports: Health Insurance Coverage.* Washington, D.C.: U.S. Department of Commerce, 1999.
5. Kaiser Commission on Medicaid and the Uninsured. *A Profile of the Low-Income Uninsured.* Washington D.C.: Kaiser Commission on Medicaid and the Uninsured, 1999.
6. Based on authors' analyses of the March 1999 Current Population Survey.
7. U.S. General Accounting Office. "Employer-Based Health Insurance: Costs Increase and Family Coverage Decreases." (Report to the Ranking Minority Member, Subcommittee on Children and Families, Committee on Labor and Human Resources, US Senate. GAO/HEHS-97-35.) Washington, D.C.: U.S. General Accounting Office, Feb. 1997.
8. Kaiser Commission on Medicaid and the Uninsured. *Medicaid Facts. Medicaid and Managed Care.* Washington, D.C.: Henry J. Kaiser Family Foundation, 1998.
9. Kaiser Commission on Medicaid and the Uninsured (1998).
10. Rowland, D., Rosenbaum, S., Simon, L., and Chait, E. *Medicaid Managed Care: Lessons from the Literature.* Washington, D.C.: Henry J. Kaiser Family Foundation, 1995; Salganicoff,

A., Wyn, R. and Solís, B. "Medicaid Managed Care and Low-Income Women: Implications for Access and Satisfaction." *Women's Health Issues,* 1998, *8,* 339–349.

11. Ellwood, M. "The Medicaid Eligibility Maze: Coverage Expands, But Enrollment Problems Persist. Findings from a Five State Study." Washington, D.C.: Henry J. Kaiser Family Foundation, 1999.

12. Zimmerman, W., and Tumlin, K. *Patchwork Policies: State Assistance for Immigrants Under Welfare Reform.* (Occasional paper no. 24.) Washington, D.C.: Urban Institute, 1999.

13. Kaiser Commission on Medicaid and the Uninsured. *Medicaid Facts. Medicaid Enrollment and Spending Trends.* Washington, D.C.: Henry J. Kaiser Family Foundation, 1999.

14. Garrett, B., and Holahan, J. *Welfare Leavers, Medicaid Coverage, and Private Health Insurance.* (New Federalism, Series B, No. B-13.) Washington, D.C.: Urban Institute, Mar. 2000.

15. Sandman, D., Simantov, E., and An, C. *Out of Touch: American Men and the Health Care System.* New York: Commonwealth Fund, 2000.

16. Women's Research and Education Institute. *Women's Health Insurance Costs and Experiences.* Washington, D.C.: Women's Research and Education Institute, 1994.

17. Wyn, R., Brown, E. R., and Yu, H. "Women's Use of Preventive Health Services." In M. Falik and K. Scott Collins (eds.), *Women's Health: The Commonwealth Fund Survey.* Baltimore, Md.: Johns Hopkins University Press, 1996.

18. Collins, K. S., and others. *Health Concerns Across a Woman's Lifespan: The Commonwealth Fund 1998 Survey of Women's Health.* New York: Commonwealth Fund, 1999.

19. Lohr, K., and others. "Effect of Cost-Sharing on Use of Medically Effective and Less Effective Care." *Medical Care, 24*(9, Supplement), 1986, S31–S38.

20. Rice, T., and Morrison, K. "Patient Cost Sharing for Medical Services: A Review of the Literature and Implications for Health Care Reform." *Medical Care Review,* 1994, *51*(3), 235–287.

21. Women's Research and Education Institute. *Women's Health Insurance Costs and Experience.* Washington, D.C.: Women's Research and Education Institute, 1994, pp. 6–10.

22. Andersen, R. M., and Davidson, P. "Measuring Access and Trends." In R. M. Andersen, T. H. Rice, and G. F. Kominski (eds.), *Changing the U.S. Health Care System.* San Francisco: Jossey-Bass, 1996.

23. Collins and others (1999).

24. Commonwealth Fund. *Health Insurance Coverage and Access to Care for Working-Age Women.* New York: Commonwealth Fund, 1999.

25. Collins and others (1999); Hoffman, C. *Uninsured in America: A Chart Book.* Washington, D.C.: Henry J. Kaiser Family Foundation, 1998.

26. U.S. General Accounting Office. "Prenatal Care: Medicaid Recipients and Uninsured Women Obtain Insufficient Care." (Publication no. GAO/HRD-87-137.) Washington, D.C.: U.S. General Accounting Office, 1987.

27. Rowland, D., and Salganicoff, A. *The Key to the Door: Medicaid's Role in Improving Health Care for Women and Children.* Washington, D.C.: Henry J. Kaiser Family Foundation, 1999.

28. National Governors' Association. "Center for Best Practices, Issue Brief. Income Eligibility for Pregnant Women and Children." Washington, D.C.: National Governors' Association, 2000.

29. Ayanian, J., Kohler, B. A., Abe, T., and Epstein, A. M. "The Relation Between Health Insurance Coverage and Clinical Outcomes Among Women with Breast Cancer." *New England Journal of Medicine,* 1993, *329*(5), 326–331.

30. Braverman, P., and others. "Adverse Outcomes and Lack of Health Insurance Among Newborns in an Eight-County Area of California, 1982–1986." *New England Journal of Medicine,* 1989, *321*(8), 508–513.

31. Hadley, J., Steinberg, E. P., and Feder, J. "Comparison of Uninsured and Privately Insured Hospital Patients: Condition on Admissions, Resource Use, and Outcome." *Journal of the American Medical Association,* 1991, *265*(3), 374–379.

32. Brown, E. R., and others. "Women's Health-Related Behaviors and Use of Preventive Services." (Report to the Commonwealth Fund.) New York: Commonwealth Fund, Commission on Women's Health, 1995.

33. Clancy, C. M., and Massion, C. T. "American Women's Health Care: A Patchwork Quilt with Gaps." *Journal of the American Medical Association,* 1992, *268*(14), 1918–1920.

34. Lurie, N., and others. "Preventive Care for Women. Does the Sex of the Physician Matter?" *New England Journal of Medicine,* 1993, *329*(7), 478–482.

35. American College of Obstetricians and Gynecologists. "Issues in Women's Health." (ACOG News Release.) Oct. 29, 1993.

36. Romans, M. C., and others. "Utilization of Screening Mammography 1990." *Women's Health Issues,* 1991, *1*(2), 68–73.

37. Families USA Foundation. *Hit and Miss: State Managed Care Laws.* Washington, D.C.: Families USA Foundation, July 1998; Henry J. Kaiser Foundation. "An Issue Brief. State Policies on Access to Gynecological Care and Contraception." Washington, D.C.: Henry J. Kaiser Foundation, 1999.

38. Woloshin, S., and others. "Language Barriers in Medicine in the United States." *Journal of the American Medical Association,* 1995, *273*(9), 724–728; Solis, J. M., Marks, G., Garcia, M., and Shelton, D. "Acculturation, Access to Care, and Use of Preventive Services by Hispanics: Findings from HHANES 1982–84." *American Journal of Public Health,* 1990, *80,* 11–19.

39. Wyn, Brown, and Yu (1996).

40. Kaiser Commission on Medicaid and the Uninsured. *Medicaid Facts, Medicaid Enrollment and Spending Trends.* Washington, D.C.: Henry J. Kaiser Family Foundation, 1999.

41. Garrett and Holahan (2000).

42. Clancy and Massion (1992); Johnson, K., and Hoffman, E. "Women's Health: Designing and Implementing an Interdisciplinary Specialty." *Women's Health Issues,* 1993, *3*(2), 115–119.

43. Council on Ethical and Judicial Affairs, American Medical Association. "Gender Disparities in Clinical Decision Making." *Journal of the American Medical Association,* 1991, *266*(4), 559–562; Council on Ethical and Judicial Affairs, American Medical Association. "Black-White Disparities in Health Care." *Journal of the American Medical Association,* 1990, *263*(7), 2344–2346.

CHAPTER FOURTEEN

HOMELESS PERSONS

Lillian Gelberg and Lisa Arangua

Homelessness has reached crisis proportions in the United States today. It is estimated that 3.5 million people are currently without a home.[1] However, the crisis is much worse than this; nationally, 14 percent of the U.S. population (26 million people) have been homeless at some time in their lives and 5 percent (8.5 million people) have been homeless within the past five years.[2] Los Angeles is known as the homeless capital, although some would argue that New York holds this infamous distinction. Seventy-one percent of homeless persons live in central cities, while 21 percent live in suburban areas and 9 percent live in rural areas.[3]

History of Homelessness

A discussion of how the United States has dealt with the homeless is relevant because homeless policies have come full circle. The picture of the homeless population of the United States has changed over the years.[4] Homelessness was first encountered in colonial North America as a result of rapid economic changes, fluctuations in immigration and seasonal and wage labor, and sickness and disease. An increasing number of families sank to the level of destitution. There was no in-kind or cash aid for the destitute. As a result, the colonies became deluged with people who had marginal means to survive.[5]

In American history, there have been two responses to homelessness (patterned after English poor law principles): outdoor relief (basic assistance given outside a public institution) and institutionalized relief (public poorhouses, also known as indoor relief or shelter relief). By this early period of American history, a clear distinction was already being made about the deserving and undeserving poor—a principle that still endures today. The undeserving poor, referred to in colonial times as paupers, were considered idle and able-bodied, and their inability to support themselves or their families was considered an individual and moral failure. Policies for the undeserving poor never focused on systemic failure as a cause of poverty but instead placed blame on the moral degeneracy of the individual. As Cotton Mather put it, "For those who indulge themselves in idleness, the express command of God unto us is, that we should let them starve.[6]

Throughout most of the nineteenth century, the major policy response to the homeless was outdoor relief. As with our current entitlement programs for the poor, critics believed that outdoor relief served to sustain homelessness. According to Alexis de Tocqueville, the outdoor relief system bred the very condition it sought to remedy: "man had a natural passion for idleness," and by providing the means of subsistence outdoor relief freed the homeless from an obligation to work.[7] Critics of poor relief policies also sought the more punitive approach of reduction in aid as a means of encouraging work. The Royal Poor Law Commission Report of 1834 stated that "while relief should not be denied the poor, life should be so miserable for them that they would rather work than accept public aid."[8] Current block grant and entitlement policies for the poor (that is, welfare, shelter relief) continue to allude to these same principles.[9]

However, reformers' views of relief recipients were contrary to those who actually received relief.[10] Very few of those receiving relief could work. The majority were in fact single mothers, children, the aged, and the sick. Nevertheless, reformers felt that the very existence of outdoor relief would deter the able-bodied from self-sufficiency; hence relief was a threat to the work ethic.[11]

During the middle and late nineteenth century, theories regarding the destitute took a less draconian posture. There was less emphasis on differentiating between the deserving and undeserving poor. The idle, able-bodied person was considered a victim of external forces beyond his control, such as poor educational or religious upbringing.[12] From this theory emerged the institutionalization of the homeless. The main objective behind institutionalization was that the external forces that caused the homeless condition were mutable and could be reversed.

But institutionalization was later perceived as a more expensive and less effective form of relief. Mothers and children were mixed together with substance abusers and the mentally ill. The rehabilitation rate was low and mortality was high.[13]

As the twentieth century opened, theories about the deserving and un-deserving poor reemerged. Homelessness was once again blamed on individual degeneracy rather than on economic conditions. The ineffectiveness of major policies for the homeless triggered a public campaign that fully dissolved these programs. The lack of safety-net programs resulted in parents' giving up their children to the child welfare system in order to find work. Middle-aged, unemployed men began to flood the streets.

It was during this time that we began to see the emergence of the "skid row" population, which actually developed as a result of industry's need for a mobile, semiskilled labor class. The term derived from the skid roads, or skidways, used by Seattle's lumberjacks employed as seasonal labor to slide logs to the mills. These skid roads (later, skid rows), with their flophouses, taverns, brothels, labor agencies, inexpensive eating places, and location near transportation stations, served as centers for unattached seasonal laborers. They were populated by middle-aged white men, predominately Northern European immigrants, employed in seasonal and temporary work.[14] During the twentieth century, the skid row populations grew during depression and at the end of a war in proportion to increasing unemployment. The Great Depression, with 25 percent unemployment, brought a large cross-section of the general population to skid row in search of work and housing.[15]

With the economic boom years after World War II, and welfare reform, skid rows decreased in size. With less need for an unskilled labor pool, skid row became a haven for mainly white, middle-aged, alcoholic men.[16] However, they did not disappear. In the 1950s, with the civil rights movement, development of psychotropic drugs, loss of funding for state mental institutions, and inadequate funding of community-based mental health services, we began to see an increasing number of alcoholic and mentally ill men and women living on the streets.[17]

In the 1970s, 1980s, and 1990s, homeless trends of the past became prelude to current trends. The effect of reducing welfare benefits relative to inflation was to increase the number of homeless families. Urban development, loss of low-income housing, and high unemployment resulted in more homeless persons who were members of minority groups. Politically expedient policies—such as street sweeps of the homeless and reduction in public aid to the homeless—dominate the public discourse. Not since the Great Depression have we seen so many homeless persons and such a broad cross-section of society represented in their ranks.[18]

As in the past, most homeless are burdened with unattended mental and physical health problems, which hinders their ability to work. Because of the prevalence of infectious disease, they have the potential to spread tuberculosis and the like to other homeless persons and the general population. Planning for appropriate and effective health services for the homeless requires attention to the unique characteristics of this population—both as individuals and as patients—in terms of health status, barriers to obtaining and adhering to prescribed medical care, and integration of housing and health services.

Who Are the Homeless?

Although in recent generations the homeless population primarily consisted of middle-aged, alcoholic white men, the distant past has become prologue to the current demographic profile of the homeless population, which consists of men, women, and children. About two-thirds of the currently homeless are single men (67 percent) and 20 percent are single women.[19] About 34 percent of homeless women and 8 percent of homeless men are currently married.[20] Fifteen percent of homeless persons are parents with children.[21] Sixty percent of homeless women and 41 percent of homeless men have at least one minor child, but of these only 39 percent of women and 3 percent of men currently live with those children.[22] Homeless persons are young; a majority of the currently homeless are between the ages of twenty-five and forty-four, most children (62 percent) are under the age of eight, only 1 percent are unaccompanied youths or teen parents under the age of eighteen, and only 2 percent of the homeless are older than sixty-five.[23] About 23 percent of homeless persons are veterans.[24]

The economic picture of homeless persons is dismal, as would be expected, and suggests that they are severely lacking in the educational and financial resources necessary to access health care. Thirty-nine percent have not graduated from high school, 34 percent have a high school diploma or GED, and 28 percent have some post–high school education.[25] Further, in 1996, the mean monthly income for a homeless family was $475 (46 percent of the federal poverty line for a family of three). All other homeless persons reported a mean monthly income of $348, or 51 percent of the federal poverty level for one person.[26] Despite these figures, only 28 percent receive income maintenance.[27] Fifty-five percent do not have medical insurance, compared to 32 percent of formerly homeless persons and 17 percent in the general population.[28]

From a public policy standpoint, it is important to distinguish between the incidence and course of homelessness.[29] Half of the homeless population may be considered to be newly homeless (homeless one year or less) and one-fifth are long-term homeless (homeless for more than two years).[30] The distinction between homeless and nonhomeless impoverished is not a clear one, since people cycle in and out of homelessness during their lifetimes.[31] However, most preventive policies have focused on the conditions of the long-term homeless (mental illness, substance abuse, and criminal activity), a population which is overrepresented in enumeration samples of homeless persons. The consequences of focusing on the long-term homeless are seen not only in punitive policies that attribute social problems to individual shortcomings (as the history of homeless policies attests) but also in policies having limited impact on the incidence of homelessness. This distinction between long-term and short-term homelessness redirects policy to focus on variation in the homeless population—why people become homeless, why they cycle in and out of homelessness and why some remain homeless for a long period of time—rather than focusing on providing housing as a first step.[32]

The shortage of adequate low-income housing is the major precipitating factor for homelessness. Unemployment, personal or family life crisis, increase in rent out of proportion to inflation, and reduction in public benefits can also directly result in the loss of a home. Early findings on the impact of recent federal welfare reform policy have shown that reduction or elimination of public assistance benefits resulted in homelessness.[33] Illness, on the other hand, tends to result in loss of a home more indirectly, by way of these more direct precipitating factors. Other indirect precipitants of homelessness are deinstitutionalization from a public mental hospital, substance abuse, and overcrowding of prisons and jails from which prisoners who are not self-sufficient are often released.[34]

Health Status

The health impact of lack of housing is a pervasive issue among homeless persons (lack of housing affects the health of all homeless persons), whether newly homeless, long-term homeless, formerly homeless, or episodically homelessness. Even a relatively short bout of homelessness exposes an individual to severe deprivation (hunger, lack of adequate hygiene) and victimization (physical assault, robbery, rape).[35] The homeless—adults and children—have a very high prevalence of untreated acute and chronic medical, mental health, and substance abuse problems. They are exposed to illness thanks to overcrowding in shelters and exposure to heat and cold.[36] Further, those homeless persons who have a substance abuse or mental health problem, or a physical disability, are at increased risk of not exiting a shelter environment.[37]

A dearth of prospective research makes it difficult to identify whether certain health conditions precede, cause, or result from the homeless experience. However, research has found that unstable housing—such as extreme overcrowding, substandard housing (lack of heat, dilapidated living conditions) or loss of housing altogether contributes significantly to poor health outcomes, and that stable housing plays a critical role in improving these health conditions.[38]

The significant impact of housing on health produces a striking difference in health outcomes between the homeless and their housed counterparts. Significant difference in health outcomes emerges when we compare the homeless to their poor, but stably housed, peers. Homeless mothers were more likely than poor but stably housed mothers to experience spousal abuse, child abuse, drug use, and mental health problems.[39] In contrast, when we compare homeless mothers to their marginally housed peers, quite a different picture emerges. There is no significant difference in the mental and physical health of homeless mothers and their poor but marginally housed peers.[40] This relationship between housing and health is important and suggests why we must view the entire ecology of homelessness, including the impact of lack of housing on well-being, rather than focus narrowly on the health and mental health problems of the homeless.

Physical Illness

Homeless persons are subject to the same risk factors for physical illness as the general population, but they may be exposed to an excessive level of such risk. They also experience risk factors unique to homelessness: excessive use of alcohol, illegal drugs, and cigarettes; sleeping in an upright position (resulting in venous stasis and its consequences); extensive walking in poorly fitting shoes; and inadequate nutrition.[41]

Further, homelessness itself is physically dangerous, as homeless persons are at risk for assault and victimization, as well as exposure to the elements. Homeless people are at great risk of being victimized because they lack personal security, whether they live in a shelter or outdoors. They are exposed to illness owing to overcrowding in shelters and exposure to heat and cold.[42]

Consequently, the homeless have much higher incidence of physical illness than the general population. About 37 percent of homeless persons report having poor health, compared to 10 percent in the general population.[43] Homeless persons who are older, women, those with less education, and those who indicate a physical or mental health condition are more likely to report their health status as fair or poor. If one controls for these contributors to poor health status, length of time being homeless is significantly associated with the homeless perceiving themselves to have fair health status.[44] Studies have found that one-third to one-half of homeless adults have at least one chronic condition.[45] Thus, illness appears to be taking its toll, preventing some of the homeless from escaping their predicament. For example, one-quarter of homeless adults report that their poor health prevented them from working or going to school.[46]

Even more seriously, the age-adjusted mortality rate is three to four times higher in the homeless population (New York City shelters) than in the general population.[47] Among homeless men, prior use of injection drugs, incarceration, and chronic homelessness increased the likelihood of death.[48]

Risk factors for death among homeless patients in another study in Boston in forty sites offering health care for the homeless include AIDS, renal disease, symptomatic HIV, history of cold-related injury, liver disease, arrhythmia, substance abuse, and chronic homelessness.[49] Homeless children experience a higher number of acute illness symptoms (fever, ear infection, diarrhea, asthma, and so on), and their mothers are more likely to report that their children are in fair or poor health than their housed counterparts.[50]

The most common group of self-reported physical illnesses among homeless adults is arthritis, rheumatism, and joint problems. The next most common self-reported medical conditions are chest infection, cold, cough or bronchitis, high blood pressure and problems walking, lost limb, or other handicaps.[51] From objective clinic reports, the most common physical illnesses among homeless adults are infectious disease; dental problems; vision problems; skin and ear problems; gastrointestinal disease; female genitourinary problems; and inadequate nutrition, immunization, and cancer screening.[52] Inadequate immunization, although not a physical illness, reflects the lack of preventive health care in this population.[53]

Communicable Disease

The data suggest that prevention, diagnosis, and treatment of infectious disease among the homeless population needs to be addressed by health care, housing, and social service providers. Contagious diseases, such as tuberculosis[54] and HIV infection,[55] are more common among the homeless than the general population.

Increased risk of tuberculosis in this population is well documented.[56] The prevalence of tuberculosis infection among homeless adults ranges from 32 percent in San Francisco[57] and Los Angeles[58] to 43 percent in New York.[59] The rate is three to six times greater than the 5–10 percent prevalence of TB infection among the general population.[60] The rate of active tuberculosis among men in a New York shelter clinic is 6 percent.[61] The rate of positive tuberculosis skin test has been found to be related to duration of homelessness,[62] living in a crowded shelter or single-room occupancy hotel,[63] injection drug use,[64] and increasing age.[65] The homeless can spread communicable diseases such as tuberculosis to others. Homeless persons may also be more infectious than other persons with TB[66]; a homeless person with undiagnosed pulmonary tuberculosis who frequented a neighborhood bar infected 42 percent of the regular customers of that bar.[67] Tuberculosis may be more difficult to treat among the homeless because of the difficulty of screening, following, and maintaining TB treatment for this population, and because many have multidrug-resistant organisms.[68]

The prevalence of HIV infection among the homeless is higher than in the housed population. Studies reveal an HIV infection rate of 9 percent among San Francisco's homeless adults.[69] Among 649 women in the same study, HIV seroprevalence was 6.3 percent.[70] Risk factors for HIV infection included being black, injection drug use, and chronic homelessness.[71] The rate of HIV infection nationally is estimated to be between 0.3 percent and 0.4 percent.[72] Regarding the rate of HIV in clinic populations, in a treatment sample of homeless clients of a primary care clinic in Denver the overall seroprevalence of HIV was 0.9 percent (1.3 percent for men and 0.1 percent for women).[73] In a treatment sample of 17,292 homeless adult clients of the Boston Health Care for the Homeless Program, AIDS was the leading cause of death among persons age twenty-five to forty-four.

Moreover, studies have found an association between HIV infection and serious mental illness among homeless persons. In a New York shelter, HIV prevalence among homeless psychiatric patients was 19 percent.[74] Two important risk factors for HIV infection among persons with serious mental illness are depression leading to risky intravenous drug use practices, and risky sex conduct.[75]

The homeless population has also experienced outbreaks of several other infectious diseases, often as a result of overcrowding, poor sanitation, and exposure to others who are likewise at risk of disease. Outbreaks have been reported of meningococcal disease,[76] pneumococcal pneumonia,[77] diphtheria,[78] hepatitis B,[79] hepatitis C,[80] and bartonella quintana.[81]

Women's Health

Homeless women are severely in need of women's health services,[82] yet pregnancy and recent childbirth are risk factors for becoming homeless.[83] Among homeless women interviewed in Los Angeles, 41 percent had used no contraceptive method of any kind during the past year, although the average reported frequency of vaginal intercourse during that time was once per week.[84] Less than 10 percent use condoms regularly, despite a lifestyle that places them at great risk for AIDS and other sexually transmitted diseases.[85] Sixty percent of homeless family planning clinic users had a history of a sexually transmitted disease, and 28 percent had a history of pelvic inflammatory disease.[86] About half of homeless women age forty or older did not receive a clinical breast exam in the past year, and 53 percent of homeless women who are forty or older did not receive a mammogram in the past year.[87] In addition, 46 percent of homeless women did not receive a Pap smear in the past year,[88] compared to less than 23 percent of women in the general population.[89] This is alarming, given that 23 percent of homeless family planning clinic users had an abnormal Pap smear.[90]

Regarding homeless women's obstetrical history, 76 percent of homeless women have at least one natural child.[91] Homeless women are more likely to be pregnant (11 percent of homeless adults, 24 percent of sixteen-to-nineteen-year-old homeless youths) than their poor but housed peers (5 percent).[92] In addition, they are more likely to receive inadequate prenatal care than poor but housed women (56 percent versus 15 percent).[93] It follows that homeless women are more likely than impoverished but housed women to have poor birth outcomes (16 percent versus 7 percent low-birthweight newborns).[94] In New York City, infant mortality was highest among the homeless (24.9 per thousand live births) as compared to poor housed women (16.6 per thousand live births), and nonpoor housed women (12.0 per thousand live births).[95] In Los Angeles, homeless women had a higher rate of premature births (18.5 percent versus 11 percent of the general population).[96] However, the rate of infant mortality for homeless women was the same as that for housed women.[97]

Violence

Violent and abusive behaviors continue to be a major cause of physical and emotional injury in the United States, but homeless persons suffer disproportionately from its far-reaching consequences. More than half of homeless persons report having been criminally victimized while homeless (36.6 percent of the general population have been victimized in the past year).[98] Homeless men experience a slightly higher rate of recent physical victimization than homeless women (20 percent versus 18 percent respectively); however, homeless women experience a higher rate of recent sexual violence (9 percent versus 1 percent respectively).[99] In a recent study, 13 percent of homeless women report being sexually assaulted or raped in the past year alone,[100] compared to 2.7 percent of women in the general population.[101]

Serious mental illness is a significant predictor of victimization for both homeless men and women. Forty-four percent of homeless persons with serious mental illness have been criminally victimized within the past two months alone.[102] Among seriously mentally ill homeless persons, recent victimization is a predictor of future victimization as well as increased length of time homeless.[103] Moreover, the co-morbidity of serious mental illness and substance abuse also predicts victimization among homeless persons. The more severe a homeless person's mental health and substance abuse disorders, the more likely he or she is to have been victimized.[104]

Victimization prior to age eighteen is also widespread among homeless persons. Twenty-two percent of the homeless report physical abuse as a child or youth, and 13 percent report sexual abuse.[105] Child physical and sexual abuse history is also found to be a strong precursor to adult homelessness.[106]

Homeless persons with mental illness are more likely to have experienced sexual or physical abuse as a child. Mental illness and substance abuse in homeless women were associated with history of both physical and sexual abuse; however, in homeless men, only mental illness was associated with physical abuse history.[107] Moreover, there is overlapping evidence that the prevalence of childhood abuse in homeless women with serious mental illness is substantially higher than among homeless women in general, and the intensity of exposure to that violence contributes to the severity of their psychiatric symptoms.[108]

Adolescents

Homeless youths in the United States are a unique subpopulation of homeless persons. The current estimates of homeless youths range from one hundred thousand to five hundred thousand.[109] Eight percent of adolescents in a nationally representative sample of young people reported that they were homeless at least one night in the past twelve months.[110] Homeless youths in the United States are defined as individuals under nineteen years of age who meet at least one of these criteria: (1) they have run away from home or their alternative care placement and remained away for a long period of time with little or no connection to family or caretakers; (2) they have been forced out of their home or foster care placement, have been abandoned by their parents, or have left home for the streets with their parents' knowledge and consent; or (3) they have no stable place of residence; lack adult supervision, guidance and care; and have little likelihood of reunification with parents.[111]

Youths become homeless largely as a result of persistent family dysfunction, specifically parental neglect, physical or sexual abuse, family substance abuse, and family violence.[112] Given their family problems, it is not surprising that homeless youths suffer from a high rate of developmental health problems: poor coping skills, suicidal tendencies, substance abuse, depression, and other mental health problems resulting in a high frequency of psychiatric hospitalization.[113] Moreover, 28 percent of street youth and 10 percent of shelter youth have participated in survival sex (sold sex for food, clothing, or shelter), and research has found that family abuse, including physical abuse, is a strong correlate of survival sex among these young people.[114]

Homeless youth also suffer from victimization and health problems that largely extend from their homeless condition. They experience an extremely high rate of psychological maladjustment and victimization while homeless.[115] Assault and robbery were especially frequent, having been reported as experienced in one-fourth to one-half of homeless youths, and having been raped in the past three months was reported by one in ten of these youths.[116] The traumatic

experience of living on the streets seems to supercede that of the family characteristics that may have led to their homelessness, although this finding deserves
further research.[117]

Homeless youth also experience physical health conditions that exceed the
incidence among youth in the general population. These include hepatitis,[118]
HIV[119] (with seroprevalence of 5 percent among homeless youth in a New York
City shelter clinic[120]), respiratory problems (asthma and pneumonia, scabies
and trauma), and pregnancy.[121]

Dental Health

One of the more overt identifiers of poverty in the United States is poor dental
health. It is one of the major health problems reported by homeless individuals.[122]
However, few statistics exist on the prevalence of dental problems specifically
among homeless persons. Ninety-one percent of homeless persons who have
contact with a shelter-based dental program are found to have untreated caries.[123]
Moreover, homeless persons living in the community are one-third as likely as
domiciled adults to have obtained dental care in the past year; consequently
they are twice as likely to have gross dental decay (57 percent versus 23 percent).[124]
Given this high rate of dental disease, dental care should be an integral part of
any health care services package developed for the homeless population.

Mental Illness and Substance Abuse

The media has made the public aware of the high prevalence of mental illness
and substance abuse among the homeless and their desperate need for effective
mental health and substance abuse treatment. Moreover, alcohol, drug abuse,
and mental health problems among the homeless dominate the research on homeless inquiry. Regarding lifetime incidence, more than three-quarters (86 percent)
of homeless persons have experienced at least one alcohol, drug, or mental
health problem in their lifetime, with 57 percent having mental health problems,
62 percent having alcohol problems, and 58 percent having drug problems. The
rates of recent psychiatric problems are also very high: two-thirds (66 percent) of
homeless persons have experienced at least one alcohol, drug, or mental health
problem during the past month. Thirty-nine percent had mental health problems
in the past month, 38 percent had alcohol problems, and 26 percent had drug
problems.[125]

Regarding diagnostic data, one-third of homeless adults suffer from current
serious mental illness, including schizophrenic, affective, personality or character,
and cognitive disorders.[126] Further, one third have substance abuse disorder.[127]

About 17 percent have dual diagnoses of chronic mental illness and chronic substance use.[128] The latter individuals pose a challenge to developing services that successfully address both aspects of their illness.[129] In addition to intrinsic illness processes, environmental stresses and homeless appearance must be considered in order to avoid inaccurate diagnosis of mental illness among homeless individuals. These individuals may experience chronic isolation, geographic mobility, disturbed sleep, and fear of victimization, and they may show disheveled appearance and signs of lack of self-care.[130]

A similarly high prevalence of mental problems has been found among homeless children and mothers. It has been reported that 47 percent of homeless children age five or younger are developmentally delayed, and 31 percent of those older than five are clinically depressed.[131] Homeless and low-income children experience significant adversity in their lives, but homeless preschool children face more stress.[132] Moreover, homeless children are further behind academically than their housed counterparts.[133] Mothers' emotional status (in addition to various stressors) strongly predicts children's negative emotional outcomes.[134] More than two-thirds (73 percent) of homeless mothers have a lifetime diagnosis of one or more mental health disorders (mood, anxiety, or substance use disorder). For homeless mothers, posttraumatic stress disorder, substance abuse disorders, and major depression are disproportionately represented, with the lifetime rate of posttraumatic stress disorder three times greater than in the general female population.[135]

Access to Health Care

It is important to recognize that the majority of homeless persons (75 percent) have used health services in the past year,[136] which may represent good access to care—but it may also underscore the poor health status of homeless persons. However, 24 percent of homeless persons report they needed to see a doctor in the last year but were not able to.[137] Moreover, a look at homeless persons' sources of health care use suggests inappropriate health care delivery. For example, more than one-half (57 percent) lack a regular source of care (which has been acknowledged as an important indicator of access to medical care), compared to 24 percent of the poverty population in the United States and 19 percent of the general population.[138]

The majority of homeless persons seek care at places that do not provide continuous quality care. Of those homeless persons who sought care in the past year, 32 percent report receiving medical care at a hospital emergency room, 27 percent at a hospital outpatient clinic, 21 percent receive care at a community health clinic, 20 percent at a hospital as an inpatient, and 19 percent report receiving care at a private doctor's office.[139] The high rates of emergency room use and hospitalization in this young population represent the substitution of inpatient and emergency room care for outpatient ambulatory care services. Homeless persons' limited access to ambulatory care is due to individual factors (competing needs, substance dependence, mental illness) as well as system factors (availability, cost, convenience, appropriateness of care).

Use of Physical Health Services

Homeless adults are more likely than the general population to report having had a medical hospitalization during the preceding year.[140] For example, a Hawaiian study found that homeless persons' age and sex-adjusted acute care hospitalization rate was 542 per thousand person-years, as compared with the general population rate of 96 per thousand person-years. In this study, homeless adults were admitted to acute care hospitals for 4,766 days compared with a predicted 640 days, resulting in costs of $2.8 million per year for excess hospitalization.[141] Further, when hospitalized, homeless adults are most likely to be admitted to general county hospitals.[142] A study in New York found that homeless adult patients' hospital length of stay exceeded the mean general admission by 36 percent.

About three-quarters of hospitalized homeless adults were hospitalized for conditions for which hospitalization is often preventable (substance abuse, mental illness, trauma, respiratory disorders, skin disorders, and infectious diseases other than AIDS).[143] Another study found that following hospital discharge, 40 percent of homeless adults were readmitted to the hospital within fourteen months, usually with the same diagnosis as on the initial hospitalization. These high hospitalization and readmission rates resulted in costs at a major urban hospital of more than $1.8 million during the three-month study.[144] The finding that most of the homeless inpatients were admitted for problems that could have been treated less expensively in an outpatient setting suggests difficulty in sustaining treatment intensity for homeless persons outside of the hospital. These data imply an ineffective local service delivery system for the homeless population.

Despite higher rates of medical hospitalization and disease, homeless adults are in fact less likely to use medical ambulatory services than the general population. Homeless adults have a lower number of ambulatory physician contacts in the past year (2.9) than the poverty group (6.3) and the general population (5.5).[145] This suggests that the homeless may delay seeking medical attention at a time when severe stages of illness could be prevented.

Different design approaches must be applied to the distinct needs of certain subpopulations of the homeless. For instance, we need to design health service programs that facilitate health access and health promotion for homeless adolescents, who are at risk for multiple health problems but of whom only 28 percent used medical care services in the past year.[146] Another distinct subpopulation is homeless children. They are more likely to use ambulatory medical services (two or more emergency department visits during the past year and higher outpatient visit rates for well care and sick care), but they are also more likely to have been hospitalized in the past year than their poor but housed counterparts.[147] These findings highlight not only the poor health status of the homeless but also the need for programs that increase outreach efforts and improve the availability of and access to ongoing primary care services for homeless adolescents and children.

Once homeless persons do get needed medical services, they may find it difficult to comply with treatment. Only 50 percent of homeless patients in New York City who were referred from a satellite clinic to a hospital clinic kept their appointments, and only 25 percent with cardiovascular disease remained in long-term therapy.[148] Further, in a New York City shelter, only six out of fifty homeless individuals requiring isoniazid prophylaxis for tuberculosis were found to be taking their medications; not one completed the full year of treatment,[149] and only four of thirty acutely psychotic homeless patients were taking the psychotropic medications that had been prescribed for them.[150]

Success of interventions and compliance with medical regimens is affected by the social situation of the homeless.[151] Their social conditions, competing needs, and unique lifestyles all combine to make more traditional approaches to health care delivery less effective for homeless patients even when compared to poor domiciled patients.

Use of Mental Health and Substance Abuse Services

As noted above, mental illness and substance abuse is more prevalent among homeless people than in the general population. Consequently, of the hospital admissions for homeless persons, the vast majority (51.5 percent) were for treatment of substance abuse or mental illness, compared to 19.7 percent for other low-income patients.[152] A large proportion (15 percent to 44 percent) of homeless adults report having had a previous psychiatric hospitalization.[153] The age- and sex-adjusted rate of admission of homeless to Hawaiian state psychiatric hospitals was 105 per thousand person-years, compared with the general population rate of 0.8 per thousand person-years.[154]

Despite their high prevalence of current mental illness and prior psychiatric hospitalization, most homeless individuals have not recently used existing outpatient mental health and substance abuse systems for care. Only 18 percent of homeless people in Baltimore's shelters had used outpatient mental health services during the six months preceding a study,[155] and the majority of those with previous mental hospitalization had not made an outpatient mental health visit in the past five years.[156] Although 51 percent of homeless persons with chronic mental illness have used outpatient mental health services at sometime in their lifetimes, compared to 38 percent who used inpatient services, only 14 percent have used these services in the past two months, compared to 5 percent who used inpatient services.[157] Seventy-three percent of homeless clients who report inpatient treatment for mental health problems received this treatment before they became homeless.[158] There is also high prevalence of inadequately treated mental illness within the homeless population: 25 percent of homeless adults considered committing suicide, and 7 percent attempted suicide during a yearlong period.[159] These data suggest that homeless persons who are mentally ill are in need of continuity of mental health services but are not receiving these services within an outpatient setting.

The data on lack of outpatient treatment are even more striking for use of outpatient substance abuse services. Only 26 percent of homeless persons with recent substance abuse problems (within the past six months) have used outpatient services in their lifetime, compared to 43 percent who used inpatient services.[160] Moreover, about half (52 percent) of those with recent substance abuse dependence had ever received treatment from the formal substance abuse treatment delivery system.[161] Recent residential treatment (past two months) for substance abuse problems was far more common than recent outpatient treatment. Only 7 percent of homeless persons with substance abuse problems used outpatient substance abuse services in the past two months, compared to 16 percent who used inpatient services during this time period.[162] The limited-use outpatient treatment, as well as the lack of any treatment use among recent substance abusers, suggests closer examination of system-level characteristics that may interfere with the homeless receiving the services that they need.

Barriers to Health Care

Compounding their increased risk for disease is evidence that homeless people encounter major obstacles to obtaining needed medical and psychiatric services. About one-quarter of homeless persons stated that they needed to see a doctor in the past year but were not able to do so,[163] and more than half did not have a regular source of care.[164] Some homeless persons do seek care for their health problems, but certain segments of the population are less likely to obtain care even if they are sick or have a regular source of care. For instance, homeless adults with little education and without health insurance are less likely to seek care even if they are sick.[165] Persons who are less likely to have a regular source of care are young, are Hispanic, do not have health insurance, are long-term homeless (five or more years since last housed), have subsistence difficulties, or are socially isolated.[166]

Homeless persons with mental health problems are less likely to seek mental health services if they do not receive mental health advice or referrals from service providers outside the mental health system or if they have affective disorders (such as depression).[167] Homeless with substance abuse problems were less likely to seek treatment for these problems if they did not get help accessing these services, spent more time in places that were not meant for sleeping, and lived in service-poor environments.[168] Delay in seeking care or the lack of a regular source of care may result in health care practitioners' having to manage conditions that would have been easier to treat had the individual sought help earlier.

Homeless individuals face numerous problems in obtaining appropriate health care: cost, transportation, competing needs, mental illness, the homeless lifestyle, personal barriers, lack of availability of health services, medical provider bias, insufficient discharge planning from hospitals, and lack of recuperative care.

Cost. First, there are the financial barriers and problems in satisfying eligibility requirements for health insurance. One fifth of homeless adults who had not obtained needed medical care stated that this was due to inability to pay for medical services.[169] Only one-third[170] to nearly one-half[171] of the homeless in the community have any form of health insurance (Medicaid, Medicare, Veterans Affairs, or private insurance), and most have no cash resources at all.[172]

Transportation. Accessible transportation to medical facilities is often unavailable to this population.[173]

Competing Needs. The homeless have competing needs, and it is understandable that they may place greater priority on fulfilling their basic needs for food, shelter, and income than on obtaining needed health services or following through with a prescribed treatment plan.[174] Although we typically think of homeless people as having an inordinate amount of time on their hands, often they must deal with the varied schedules and locations of several service facilities to ensure that all their needs are met.[175] For instance, it is not uncommon for a homeless person to begin the day early in the morning by queuing up at a soup line for breakfast, then walking to the next soup line to join the long queue for lunch, and then walking back to the shelter to wait in line once again in hope of securing a bed for the night.

Even medical care for an active disease may seem less important than other needs, and preventive health care sometimes loses out completely. For example, in a New York City study that reviewed the hospital records of both homeless and poor domiciled children, immunizations were delayed in 70 percent of homeless children in the study, compared to 22 percent of immunization delay for domiciled children.[176] Other studies of mothers' self-report of immunization delay have produced divergent results: several studies found that immunizations were delayed in about 30 percent of homeless children, while one study reported only 5 percent of immunization delay among homeless children.[177] About a half to a third of the homeless persons who said they had not obtained needed medical care stated that this was because their medical problem was not sufficiently serious to warrant their attention.[178]

Mental Illness. Those homeless individuals who experience psychological distress as well as disabling mental illness may be in the greatest need of health services[179] and yet may be the least able to obtain them.[180] This may be[181] attributable to such individual characteristics of mental ill health as paranoia, disorientation, unconventional health beliefs, lack of social support, lack of organizational skills to gain access to needed services,[182] or fear of authority figures and institutions as a result of previous institutionalization.[183] Further, mentally ill homeless adults often require services, largely unavailable today, that are able to handle multifaceted problems including mental illness, substance abuse, physical illness, criminality, and such social service–related problems as housing and employment.[184]

What is needed are nontraditional services that would fulfill basic needs before addressing psychodynamic issues.[185] Comprehensive case management is needed that would address such homeless mentally ill persons' housing, social support, employment, vocational rehabilitation, mental health, and physical health needs.[186] Such services would be best provided by a multidisciplinary team and health service center.

Lifestyle. The social conditions of street life itself may affect compliance with medical care. There is usually a lack of proper sanitation;[187] no stable place to keep medications safe, intact, and refrigerated;[188] and inability to obtain the proper food for a medically indicated diet such as diabetes mellitus or hypertension.[189] Lacking social support, homeless persons often do not have anyone who can transport them to a clinic or care for them if needed after giving birth or experiencing a major illness.[190] Although most homeless persons are long-term residents of their community, many are quite mobile within a city in their search for subsistence resources. This mobility makes continuity of care difficult.[191] Keeping follow-up appointments—necessary for continuous, comprehensive care—is difficult for homeless people because of their competing needs and different time orientation.[192]

Personal Barriers. Homeless people at times present barriers to their own care. Because an exhibition of toughness is necessary to survive on the streets, homeless persons may at times deny that they have health problems in an attempt to maintain a sense of their own endurance. However, while attempting to present a tough façade, they actually may be afraid to venture out of the immediate geographical area to which they have become somewhat acclimated, which presents a barrier to seeking medical services in another area. They may be too embarrassed to have medical professionals see them in a condition of poor personal hygiene. They may fear that their meager financial resources will be taken away to pay for the medical care they receive.

Fear of authority figures and need to control a situation concerning themselves are additional factors that keep homeless people from seeking medical care.[193] Fear of those in a position of authority is prevalent over the spectrum of the homeless population and can result in failure to seek medical care. For example, homeless undocumented immigrants have reason to fear that medical providers will call in immigration and naturalization authorities; runaway teenagers and homeless women with children may fear child protective service workers; and drug abusers or ex-cons may fear the police.[194]

Unavailability of Health Services. There is a lack of facilities that can adequately treat homeless people. The offices of most middle-class physicians will not welcome an unwashed, ungroomed individual.[195] As a result, national health care reform and universal coverage may not solve the access problems of homeless people, as is evident in their barriers to care in Great Britain today.[196] Availability and accessibility of primary care for many homeless persons in Great Britain is quite limited despite the elimination of hospital and medication charges.[197]

Further, health care facilities designed for the poor, or for emergency treatment, are not set up to provide the basic care that the homeless population requires, and they may not be set up to take into consideration the culture of homelessness. Homeless people often cannot keep the scheduled appointments that are required in most primary care operations, thus creating barriers to first contact as well as follow-up care. However, the purpose of an emergency room is to provide urgent or emergent care to people who arrive without prior scheduling. This is often why homeless individuals use emergency rooms as their source of medical care, but emergency rooms cannot provide the continuous comprehensive medical care that the complex problems of the homeless require.[198]

Many primary care settings that were designed for the housed poor are not set up to treat homeless patients. Public health systems for the poor tend to be based on clinics designed for specific, targeted programs such as family planning, prenatal care, tuberculosis testing and treatment, mental health and substance abuse treatment, or immunization, yet the multiple medical and social problems of homeless persons do not neatly fit into such types of services. For instance, underuse of outpatient mental health and substance services by the homeless has much to do with the fragmentation of these services from other health and human service settings, which threaten the availability and accessibility of services for homeless persons. However, the extent of mental health and substance abuse services that are integrated with other service settings is very limited and has been diminishing over time.[199] Thus, many homeless persons end up seeking medical care late in the course of their diseases or for traumatic or life-threatening conditions.

Bias. Homeless people may sense from the medical profession itself a barrier to obtaining needed medical care. Medical providers may consider homeless persons to be undesirable patients because of their poor hygiene or their mental illness, or because of assumptions that they are coming to the hospital for shelter and not for a medical problem.[200] Clinic directors reported that in more than 50 percent of clinics, physician recruitment was hampered by poor working conditions, inadequate salaries, physician bias against working with the homeless, and the lack of respect this work receives from the medical profession.[201] Being treated with lack of respect does not encourage follow-up care or compliance with care.

Health care practitioners, usually middle-class people, may view various aspects of health care quite differently than do their homeless patients. The attitudes of homeless patients in regard to establishing priorities, adhering to schedules, and keeping appointments can differ from those of their providers, setting up the possibility of conflict and failure.[202] Treatment plans are often automatically based on the assumption that the patient has a home. However, most homeless persons lack reliable access to a place where they can recuperate (in bed, if indicated) and properly store medication. Ordinary and uncomplicated postclinic care such as cleansing a wound with soap and hot water may be extremely difficult to implement. Prescribed dietary regimens, which may involve taking medications with meals, are impractical if the patient is without a reliable place to store groceries. Because shelters, soup lines, and garbage cans provide an unreliable source of nutritious food, homeless people have little control over what they eat. Needles and medications with recreational use (for example, valium) are highly valued on the street and can make homeless patients a target for victimization.[203]

Inadequate Discharge Planning. For homeless inpatients there is also a lack of adequate discharge planning. They are discharged directly from the hospital to the streets; even homeless mothers are discharged in that way with their newborn infants soon after childbirth. Readmission of homeless patients to hospitals is not uncommon.[204]

Lack of Recuperative Care. Finally, there is a lack of recuperative services for homeless patients. When they are inappropriately discharged from a hospital, they are often unable to manage the necessary recuperation. Recuperation cannot be adequately managed on the streets or accommodated in a shelter. Few health centers that care for the homeless offer recuperative care services because of the cost as well as restrictive licensing in many cities. Reports by hospital staff show that longer hospital stays among homeless patients are primarily due to lack of housing. The leading cause of long stays cited was placement problems among homeless psychiatric patients. Public hospitals have been under court order since 1991 to place all such patients in supportive housing at the time of discharge. However, because of a shortage of supportive housing in New York City and the continued downsizing of state psychiatric hospitals, this process can be delayed for months. Physicians also reported delaying the discharge of homeless patients who required follow-up care, knowing that these patients' access to ambulatory care and clean environments or their compliance with treatment might be limited.[205]

Research on the Poor

Since the War on Poverty in the 1960s, there has been explosive growth in collecting and analyzing poverty-related data from administrative systems, surveys, and program evaluations. Funding for this research has been primarily by the federal government, followed by local governments and private foundations. These data have been used by elected officials not only to identify important public policy issues but also to monitor the progress of publicly funded poverty programs in meeting their objectives. Increased concern with rigorous methodological standards has encouraged legislators to depend more heavily on research experts for statistics as to the impact of particular legislation than on the testimony from lobbyists. The U.S. Congressional Budget Office and the Office of Management and Budget offer statistics on the cost and benefits of social programs to fuel legislative debate in Washington. Hence, statistics have become the mainstay of legislative debate in the United States, with experts on all sides of an issue offering their estimates of the social impact of a given policy.

History of Research on the Homeless

Despite the lengthy history of homelessness in the United States, homeless inquiry (and therefore long-term national policy on the homeless) did not commence until the 1980s. Most social inquiry on poverty began in the 1960s, but the delay in research on the homeless resulted in part from the political perception that homelessness was an isolated issue affecting a few urban areas.[206] This delay in research also derived from the difficulty in measuring homelessness. Conventional censuses and samples by design (for example, household samples) missed the homeless. Sampling frames for homeless would be subject to more costly data collection methods (such as in-person interviews).[207] The difficulty of measuring and enumerating the homeless restricted estimates of the size and composition of the population to anecdotal accounts. Recognition of homelessness as a major public policy issue was first highlighted on the local level by Baxter in 1981[208] and then on the national level in a fifty-five-city survey of hunger and homelessness published by the U.S. Conference of Mayors in 1982.[209] These studies were soon followed by the first hearings on homelessness in the U.S. Congress since the Great Depression.

By the time homelessness entered the national political agenda, social research methods affecting poverty-related policies began to shift. In the 1960s and 1970s, the federal government sponsored a series of large-scale welfare, job-training, and education experiments. Although much was learned from these experiments, they were costly, took several years to complete, and often produced inconclusive results. Moreover, the 1980s witnessed decreased government support of poverty-related research and programs stemming from strong public sentiment for lower taxes and smaller increases in budget growth at all levels of government—a sentiment that has continued into the 1990s. As a result, few new experiments have been launched by federal agencies. The federal and local governments, as well as most private foundations, instead choose to sponsor short-term assessment studies to support evaluation of relatively small demonstration projects, and to make longitudinal and cross-sectional survey data files available to academics and others for multivariate analyses.

In the mid-1980s, as a result of increased interest in homelessness and decreased government support of poverty programs, the Robert Wood Johnson Foundation (one of the nation's largest philanthropies) in conjunction with the Pew Charitable Trusts (one of the nation's largest general funds) sponsored the Health Care for the Homeless (HCH) demonstration project.[210] This nineteen-site, four-year project focused on comprehensive health care for the homeless. Evaluators for the demonstration projects found that in the first two years of the program, one hundred thousand patients had been seen.[211] Two-thirds of the visits were for acute problems, and one-third for chronic conditions. The homeless were six times as likely to have a neurological disorder, five times more likely to have hepatitis, four times more likely to have respiratory or nutritional disorders, and two to three times more likely to have skin problems or to suffer from trauma.[212]

In response to the results provided by this and other private initiatives, in July 1987 Congress passed the Stewart B. McKinney Act (Public Law 100-77), the first major legislation on homelessness. Title VI of the McKinney Act established a primary health services program, which is structured similar to the RWJ Health Care for the Homeless demonstration programs. The McKinney Act was the government's first attempt at a long-term national policy to respond to the needs of the homeless.

Approaches to Studying the Homeless

One issue that has plagued research on both poverty and homelessness is the need for widely accepted definitions of these conditions. To devise effective programs and policies and to allocate appropriate resources, it is essential to know with some confidence the total number of people affected and the fluctuations of this number over time. A primary obstacle to developing credible data is the absence of broadly accepted definitions of the problem condition.

The U.S. poverty measure is an important indicator of well-being in America and sharply affects public policy and programming for the poor. For the past decade, there has been heated debate that the current measure used to estimate the poverty rate is outdated and does not accurately reflect the nation's poverty population, nor does it adequately serve policy makers or researchers.[213] The measure was originally developed in the early 1960s as an indicator of the number and proportion of people with inadequate income for needed consumption of food and other goods and services. It does not account for many of the key welfare programs designed to alleviate poverty, such as food stamps and the Earned Income Tax Credit. Beginning in 1992, the Panel on Poverty and Family Assistance of the National Academy of Sciences/National Research Council (NRC) conducted a thorough review of the poverty measure and recommended replacing it with a new measure, based on a commonly accepted notion of economic deprivation and accounting for the impact of social welfare programs on the poor.[214] The Census Bureau corroborated with this conjecture in its recent announcement of the 1998 poverty rate when it acknowledged the flawed and antiquated nature of the current measure and stressed the need to update it.[215]

As with standard definitions of the poverty measure, researchers have confronted similar debates over the biasing effects of certain definitions of the homeless. Early studies focused on the literal homeless, defined as those who sleep in shelters provided primarily for homeless persons, or in places—public or private—not intended as dwellings. However, these early studies found one-third of people in housing situations not considered by most standards as conventional housing were sleeping in a shelter or a public place on any given night and had spent at least one night during the previous week in someone else's home or in a hotel.[216] Recently, many homeless researchers[217] have adopted the same definition of *homeless* that garners greater public interest, a definition also used in the McKinney Act of 1987—namely, an individual who lacks a fixed, regular, and adequate nighttime residence that is (1) a supervised publicly or privately operated shelter designed to provide temporary living accommodations (including welfare hotels, congregate shelters, and transitional housing for the mentally ill); (2) a public or private place that provides a temporary residence for individuals intended to be institutionalized; or (3) public or private place not designed for, or ordinarily used as, regular sleeping accommodations for human beings. This definition ultimately includes homeless persons who are more likely to incur greater public cost (that is, service users and the more vulnerable homeless persons—those living on the street), and hence invoke the public interest.

Since research on homelessness did not keep pace with other research on poverty, most methods to estimate the composition and size of the low-income group (derived from common definitions) were also applied to the homeless. The most widely used method for national estimates of poverty has been the simple head-count ratio (the poverty rate or proportion of people who are poor).[218] In 1990, the Census Bureau used the head-count ratio to enumerate the homeless population in the United States. These counts took place in five cities (Chicago, Los Angeles, New Orleans, New York, and Phoenix) that were chosen purposely to represent differing regions and weather conditions and to include the two cities believed to have the largest homeless populations (New York and Los Angeles).

Head-count ratio has been largely criticized by poverty and homeless researchers alike for its failure to gauge the depth and dimensions of the condition being enumerated. Such a ratio gives an accurate portrayal of the currently poor or homeless population and useful information for purposes such as projecting service needs (number of shelter beds needed, number of persons or families in need of affordable housing, potential patient population for safety-net clinics). However, since the head-count ratio reduces individuals easily or accurately into a single type, if relied on for inference as to the population of persons who become poor or homeless these samples can systematically bias estimates. For instance, although the head-count ratios suggest that homelessness is a persistent problem affecting seriously disabled and deviant individuals, studies of formally homeless people suggest that a large number experience homelessness in short spells and are fairly ordinary Americans.[219]

There is a need for information in simple, disaggregated form that examines incident cases of a representative sample of homeless persons to assess persistence of homelessness and associated risk factors. This has recently been done to a large extent in the Housing and Urban Development/Urban Institute report cited throughout this chapter. Another example is that the head-count ratio does not produce statistics on individual or family resources, nor does it yield statistics that exclude all government benefits from income.[220] These measures can assess important public policy issues, such as appropriate policy interventions for different groups of persons and the impact of government benefits on poverty.

As should be made apparent from this discussion, poverty and homelessness have been treated as mutually exclusive—rather than intersecting—conditions. Since its inception, the annual poverty rate has excluded from its sample some high-risk poverty groups, such as the homeless and people in institutions. This exclusion has largely resulted from the standard methodology (household surveys) used to estimate poverty, which fails to capture these groups. Since 1967, the Census Bureau has developed the poverty statistic by comparing the official poverty threshold with an estimate of resources for each family (or individual) in the Current Population Survey for March of each year, which includes about sixty thousand households. In its review of the poverty measure, the National Research Council urged the Census Bureau to use its special operations of the decennial census (which counts people without conventional housing) to more closely approximate the poverty rate, and to make comparisons between housed and unconventionally housed poor persons.[221] However, although the National Research Council did acknowledge the doubtful quality of census estimates on the homeless, it made no recommendations on how to improve these counts, nor did it propose alternative sampling methodologies to improve a survey's ability to count the homeless.[222]

To reconcile the gap in comparison data between the homeless and their housed peers, homeless researchers have conducted a series of studies on these population groups. Even so, the samples have been small and focus on specific subpopulations (say, women with children). These studies have compared indicators of deprivation among housed and homeless poor persons—economic, physical, psychological, and social deprivation. The comparisons have contributed to our knowledge base by directly assessing the differences in well-being among homeless and housed persons as well as focusing public and private sector policies on ameliorating the various dimensions of deprivation among these populations.

Unfortunately, the limited sample size of studies on the homeless and their housed peers precludes reliable results about these groups. To allow reliable comparisons as well as constitute the basis for firm and precise national estimates of poverty, alternative sampling methodologies need to be closely examined so that an annual, supplemental survey of the homeless is included in the poverty series.[223] Recent homeless research itself lends information on effective sampling methodologies that would be useful for a large supplemental probability survey of the homeless.[224] Most studies on the homeless have been based on small convenience samples, but several recent studies have used large community-based probability samples of the homeless.[225] Most of these used a service-setting sampling approach and a multistaged sampling procedure: conventional area sampling methods, with probabilities proportionate to population size; a systematic sample of programs (shelters, meal programs) selected with probability proportional to size; and random sampling of homeless people who use homeless programs on randomly selected days and times (in some cases, enumeration of shelter inhabitants were undertaken).

This sampling method would result in lower-bound estimates (population may be underestimated in rural areas and other locations where there are few or no homeless services). The focus on the service program as the ultimate sampling unit takes into account critical public policy concerns, such as the amount of turnover within the homeless population, variation in the length of a homeless spell, multiple contact with homeless services by a single client, and seasonal variation in homelessness.[226] Other community-based probability studies apply more inclusive sampling frames (say, combining a service-setting sampling approach with a blitz sampling approach—a one-night enumeration).[227] These studies have found that less inclusive sampling frames can substantially affect population estimates, but they do not consistently produce biased estimates of population characteristics.[228]

However, a supplemental survey of the homeless would be costly. The March Current Population Survey, which is used to estimate poverty, uses telephone interviews as its primary survey research method. Any survey on the homeless would require face-to-face interviews, which is an expensive research method. Moreover, the study would incur even greater costs if it included methods used in an inclusive sampling frame, combining a service-setting sampling approach with a blitz sampling approach, which is usually time consuming and expensive.

Still, the benefits of a well-designed annual study of the homeless arguably outweigh the cost. Studies have shown that phone coverage is high in the United States, and point estimates based on telephone surveys are generalizable to the entire population, but coverage is low for poor (especially homeless) persons. This suggests that telephone interviewing of representative samples of poor persons is likely to be seriously affected by coverage bias. Moreover, an annual survey of homeless persons will yield comparison data on perhaps the most vulnerable population of poor persons, and it could also monitor the performance, impact, and unmet service needs of publicly funded (McKinney) programs for homeless persons.

Poverty and homeless researchers alike are currently investigating more cost-effective methods of data collection for policy relevant research. This has resulted from decreased government support of poverty-related research and programs and also the Government Performance and Results Act of 1996, which obligates federal departments to report on the performance of all funded programs in meeting their specified objectives. Researchers have focused their efforts on using administrative data sources as a cost-effective means to monitor performance, document unmet needs, and describe program impact.

Administrative data are data used in ongoing record keeping for social welfare, health, and other public agencies and programs. For many types of analysis and research, administrative data offer advantages that are only accentuated by policy and program changes. These advantages include detail and accuracy of program information, large sample sizes that permit more types of analysis, state-specific data that can reflect state programs, low cost relative to alternative forms of data sources, data on the same individual over a long period, and the ability to obtain many kinds of information through links to other datasets.[229] Administrative data possess some limitations that diminish their application in certain types of research; among the shortcomings are the inability to (1) estimate such things as the rate of program participation; (2) measure all outcomes such as indicators of well-being that would not be tracked in the program-based data; and (3) measure anything if a person is "off the program."[230]

Even so, researchers see the opportunity to offset these limitations through linking data. Administrative data from one program seldom contain enough information for useful evaluation, but by linking administrative data from a number of programs and across time, it is possible to explain an array of explanatory and outcome variables. Further, linking information from state administrative databases with survey data on individuals and households has considerable promise in estimating measures of well-being.[231]

Administrative data are playing an increasingly prominent role in informing research and policy analysis on our nation's poor and disadvantaged. Homeless and poverty researchers are currently examining how to use administrative data to determine (1) average daily census of service users; (2) incidence, or the number of new records of persons or families; and (3) prevalence, or the number of all unduplicated cases of persons or families.[232] In this climate of scarce resources and citizen reluctance to support big government, these researchers have come to understand the potential of administrative data to describe prevalence, incidence, and program impact. These researchers are also strongly encouraging policy makers, program managers, funding agencies, and foundations to join in the effort to strengthen administrative data and to ensure that administrative data play an expanding role in monitoring the well-being of the nation's disadvantaged.

Health Programs for Homeless People

A variety of programs have been developed to address the health care needs of the homeless, but there is no effort to integrate these systems or to ensure permanent funding. Without adequate and permanent funding, their support is in jeopardy every year.[233] Within the federal government, most of the services fall under the umbrella of the 1987 McKinney Act, the first comprehensive federal legislation to address the health, education, and social welfare needs of homeless persons. In this section, we focus on several programs that have addressed the health of homeless persons.

Health Care for the Homeless

Federal efforts to provide medical services to the homeless population are primarily conducted by the HCH program. Community health centers supported by the 1985 Robert Wood Johnson Foundation/Pew Memorial Trust Health Care for the Homeless Program, subsequently covered by the McKinney Act, have addressed many of the access and quality-of-care issues raised in this chapter.[234]

A critical aspect of HCH is outreach. Teams of health care professionals bring a wide range of services to homeless persons in shelters, hotels, soup lines, beaches and parks, train and bus stations, religious facilities, and other places where homeless people are found. This reduces barriers to care such as lack of transportation, lack of information about available facilities, and psychological problems. Outreach teams are typically based in health care centers, to which clinicians can refer homeless patients who need additional medical attention. A walk-in appointment system reduces access barriers at these medical facilities. Medical care, routine laboratory tests, substance abuse counseling, and some medications are provided free of charge to reduce the cost barrier.

HCH programs try to employ staff (physicians, nurses, case mangers, dentists, and so on) who are nonjudgmental and sympathetic to the social problems of homeless people. Physicians and nurse practitioners build trusting relationships with homeless patients. They know that this requires patience. HCH providers try to treat homeless patients with as much respect as affluent patients are customarily given in a private doctor's office. This encourages effective intervention, better compliance, and higher quality and continuity of care. Providers learn to look beyond the presenting problem and are prepared to intervene on many fronts, some of which do not lie within the traditional boundaries of medicine. At the same time, they realize that some homeless patients do not want to address anything other than the problem for which they are seeking care (at least at first).

Medical providers are usually in the primary care disciplines, and therefore capable of treating the common problems faced by homeless people. They can recognize and treat, or refer for treatment, most common primary care problems that are medical, mental, or social in nature, including inadequate vaccination, routine health maintenance and prevention, developmental delay, depression and anxiety, substance abuse, physical and emotional abuse, trauma, skin infestation, peripheral vascular disease, malnutrition and failure to thrive, anemia, dental decay, podiatry problems, and vision impairment.

Providers often work in teams made up of a case manager, nurse, nurse practitioner, social worker, and physician. The case manager coordinates treatment and referral for homeless patients. A referral network of community groups and public agencies are called upon for problems the health center does not have the capability to treat, such as basic needs for shelter, food, and clothing; subspecialty health problems, including serious mental illness and substance abuse; social problems, including lack of income, public benefits, health insurance, and employment, as well as legal problems; emergency care; and hospital care. Transportation vouchers (for public transportation, taxis, or ambulances) are often given out to transport homeless patients to this network of referral facilities. In addition, some facilities offer showers, food, and clothing, as well as health education and preventive care programs. Respite care is provided by a few of these facilities,[235] where the average length of stay is two weeks.[236]

National evaluations of the HCH programs have been conducted.[237] Results reveal that availability and accessibility of services was accomplished to a certain degree—the program treated 23 percent of homeless persons in smaller cities, but only 8 percent of homeless persons in larger cities. The HCH programs were successful at the difficult task of maintaining continuity of care for homeless patients. Half of their clients were seen on more than one occasion. The number of contacts with clients having a chronic medical condition average 4.5, with two-thirds being seen more than once, whereas contacts with the remaining clients averaged 2.3. Compared to patients without targeted conditions (whose average stay in the system was about one month), patients with the targeted chronic medical conditions of tuberculosis, hypertension, peripheral vascular disease, diabetes, or seizure disorder were seen about every two weeks for a period of two to three months. However, these visits may represent provision of more than one type of encounter per patient, so firm conclusions about treatment frequently cannot be drawn from the available data.

There is evidence that the HCH program also provided comprehensive care. Even though 47 percent of patient encounters were for primary care services, 25 percent were for case management and social services, and 28 percent were for substance abuse, mental health, and dental services or referral to a hospital or specialist. A large-scale national evaluation of McKinney-funded HCH programs is nearing completion. No data exist on health status outcomes of the HCH program.

Periodic national evaluations of HCH programs, however, have been limited. The dearth of formal evaluation results from limited resources and variability in population and program characteristics, and also from obstacles in conducting outcome-based cost-benefit analysis. A primary goal of HCH programs is to increase access to outpatient services, and decrease use of costly inpatient services. But measuring access to services may actually result in higher use and greater cost (for lab tests, medication, specialty referral, and hospitalization) as problems that went untreated are assessed. Another goal of HCH programs is to improve health outcomes to decrease long-term costs. Still, HCH projects do not have control over the availability of all necessary resources that have a direct impact on improved health outcomes, such as affordable housing, livable income, or other needed social services. As a result, HCH programs are currently relying on client-based evaluations (a patient satisfaction study that is under way), instead of broad-based evaluations to inform policy.

Mental Health Programs

Title VI of the McKinney Act also has two provisions specific to mental health and substance abuse services for homeless persons, which are overseen by the Center for Mental Health Services of the Substance Abuse and Mental Health Service Administration (PL 100-77, Stewart B. McKinney Homeless Assistance Act, Title VI, Subtitle B). The first is the Mental Health Services for the Homeless Block Grant, which sets aside funds to implement services for homeless persons with mental illness, including outreach services, community mental health services and rehabilitation, referral to inpatient treatment and primary care and substance abuse services, case management services, and supportive services in residential settings. An evaluation of one such program for homeless persons with dual diagnoses of mental illness and substance abuse revealed greater housing stability, a 66 percent decrease in contact with the criminal justice system, a 50 percent decrease in crisis contacts, a 60 percent reduction in hospital admissions, and a 75 percent reduction in use of detoxification services.[238] Projects for assistance in transition from homelessness supplants this program and provides funds for outreach services for homeless persons with mental illness who may also have a substance abuse disorder.

The second provision features two demonstration programs: a mental health demonstration program (called the Demonstration Program for Homeless Adults with Serious Mental Illness) and a substance abuse demonstration program (called the Community Demonstration Grant Projects for Alcohol and Drug Abuse Treatment of Homeless Individuals). These programs are the only demonstration projects in the HCH provisions of the McKinney Act. In 1992, amendments to the McKinney Act consolidated the mental health services demonstration program and the alcohol and drug abuse treatment demonstration program into the Access to Community Care and Effective Services and Supports Program (ACCESS).

ACCESS is an eighteen-site demonstration program in nine states, designed to examine the influence of service system integration on use of services and quality of life for homeless people with severe mental illness as well as those with dual diagnoses of mental illness and substance abuse.[239] At this time, ACCESS provides the only McKinney-funded national evaluation that informs HCH programs of successful service approaches to serving a specific subset of the homeless population: the mentally ill and substance abusers, a population that does not necessarily represent the service needs of the overall homeless population.

Findings from the ACCESS program show significant results for the service delivery structure of the project, service system integration. Fragmentation of service systems has long been recognized as a serious impediment to delivering community-based care for homeless people with severe mental illness and homeless persons in general. The ACCESS program features a broad range of services for the homeless, including mental health care, medical care, and substance abuse treatment. It also offered community survival services such as income support, housing assistance, and social and vocational rehabilitation (services not offered in the HCH programs in general). Service system integration was related to superior housing outcomes; it improved access to housing services three months after program entry, and through the services attainment of independent housing twelve months after program entry. Service system integration was not found to be significantly related to use of services in domains other than housing, but this finding varied among sites.[240]

Studies of the ACCESS program also examined the association between certain personal characteristics and service use. For instance, social supports were positively associated with using medical or surgical outpatient services and substance abuse outpatient treatment. Although a greater level of social support at baseline did not lead to consistent increase in service use over time, it appears that social supports while in the program (intensive case management) were strongly associated with improved access to an array of health and social services.[241] As the first formally evaluated program on a systems integration intervention for the homeless, the ACCESS program produced significant empirical evidence that integrated systems and services can effectively have an impact on outcomes.

There are several other demonstration programs for the homeless mentally ill, not directly supported by McKinney Act funds (ACCESS was the last official McKinney Act funded demonstration project) that could potentially advise service policies for the HCH programs. These programs, although not McKinney-funded, are still supported through funds from the Center for Mental Health Services of the Substance Abuse and Mental Health Service Administration. One such program is the Collaborative Program on Homeless Families: Women with Psychiatric, Substance Use and Co-Occurring Disorders and their Dependent Children, a five-year program that began in FY 1999. The Homeless Families program (for short) will document and examine strategies to provide treatment, housing, support, and family preservation services to homeless mothers with psychiatric or substance abuse disorders who are caring for their children.

The Homeless Prevention Program is a three-year knowledge development program to document and evaluate the effectiveness of homeless prevention approaches in at-risk populations. The interventions are focused on individuals with serious mental illness or substance use disorder, who are formerly homeless or at-risk for homelessness, and who are engaged with the mental health or substance abuse treatment systems. Evaluation results are expected in FY 2000.

The Housing Alternatives program evaluates the effectiveness of housing approaches for persons with serious mental illness—namely, supported housing (independent, scattered-site), linear residential treatment, and modified therapeutic community treatment. Early findings from the program reveal positive outcomes from supported housing programs that combine any assertive community treatment approaches (support teams providing mental health, substance abuse, and support services, and treating the client as a consumer rather than a patient). These programs had high residential tenure rates, and clients had contact with service coordinators if they experienced unhealthy symptoms frequently, reported problems with alcohol or drug use, or used drugs frequently.[242]

Veterans' Programs

Services for homeless veterans are offered through the U.S. Department of Veterans Affairs. The Homeless Chronically Mentally Ill Veterans Program provides outreach, case management services, and psychiatric residential treatment for homeless mentally ill veterans in community-based facilities in forty-five U.S. cities.

The Domiciliary Care for Homeless Veterans Program operates in thirty-one states, addressing the health needs of veterans who have psychiatric illness or alcohol or drug abuse problems. Veterans with such health problems are given room and board in the domiciliary. Services include screening for health problems, medical and psychiatric examinations, treatment and rehabilitation, and postdischarge community support.[243] An evaluation of these programs reveals that one-third of homeless veterans complete residential treatment; of those, one-third are in stable community housing and one-third are employed at the time of discharge.[244]

In the Homeless Chronically Mentally Ill Veterans Program, the number of clinical contacts with program staff and the number of days in residential treatment were associated with improvement in the greatest number of outcomes.[245] In the evaluation of the Domiciliary Care for Homeless Veterans Program, distinct differences in racial outcomes were found. Few differences were found between black and white veterans in terms of program participation, but black veterans showed significant improvement in medical symptomatology, social contacts, and nonviolence, and white veterans showed increased outpatient service use.[246]

Other VA-sponsored health-related programs include a Health Care for the Homeless Veterans Program and the HUD-VA Supported Housing Program. The VA Health Care for the Homeless Veterans Program is an outreach and case management program operating at seventy-one sites across the nation. An evaluation of this program finds that overall satisfaction with residential treatment services was high.[247] Moreover, a higher percentage of dually diagnosed veterans from programs that target dual diagnosis than those from substance abuse programs were discharged to community housing rather than to further institutional treatment.[248] The evaluators suggest that integration of substance abuse and psychiatric treatment may promote faster return to community living for dually diagnosed homeless veterans. The supportive housing program is a joint supported housing program with HUD, making available permanent housing and ongoing treatment services to hard-to-serve homeless mentally ill veterans and those suffering from substance abuse disorders. Rigorous evaluation of this program indicates that the approach significantly reduces the length of homelessness for veterans plagued by serious mental illness and substance abuse disorders.

Other Health Services

The Salvation Army extends a variety of social, rehabilitation, and support services to homeless persons. Their centers include adult rehabilitation programs, food programs, and permanent and transitional housing facilities. Travelers Aid International, a network of social agencies, gives homeless adults and youths short-term counseling, shelter, food, and clothing.[249]

The Better Homes Fund was started by *Better Homes and Gardens* magazine in 1988. The fund offers assistance to homeless families to enable them to escape from homelessness. Local service providers are funded, evaluated, and given training materials to help homeless families attain the social services, support, and skills they need to become housed and remain so.[250]

The Homeless Families Program (HFP), a national demonstration program in nine cities cosponsored by the Robert Wood Johnson Foundation and HUD, awarded its first grants in 1990. This program offered housing combined with appropriately designed health and supportive services for homeless families.[251] HFP found that 85 percent of families were still stably housed eighteen months after entering the program and that access to mental health and substance abuse services improved. However, the system of activities of the HFP projects did not result in broad-based changes: there was no improvement in access to physical health services, case management was in short supply, and the project focused more on families becoming stably housed than becoming self-sufficient. Therefore, the HFP resulted in only 39 percent that were working, preparing for work, or obtaining further education in the program, and only 41 percent of families needing child care services received it at least once throughout the program. The evaluators recommended developing (before program implementation) a clearer theory of how to effect change and better understanding of the nature of the service systems involved.[252]

Homeless Health Care: Future Work

The literature on homeless health care indicates that positive health outcomes for homeless persons are closely linked to stable supportive housing situations that reconnect them to the community. The link between housing and health is based upon the premise that some people need more than just health care in order to have positive health outcomes. At this time, most safety-net health care providers (such as HCH providers) do not have a distinct housing component. Over the last decade, however, demonstration projects for the homeless have shown that service integration (coordinated services but unchanged administrative systems) and systems integration (interagency coordination), when pursued simultaneously, can effectively influence outcomes. Forging advances in an integrated system goes beyond identifying new ways to protect and improve health through this model; it requires moving these innovative approaches to widespread application. This can be achieved by allowing the results from these demonstration projects to bolster political advocacy for health care for the homeless program.

Poor health outcomes for homeless persons are often as much an issue of system-related barriers as patient-related ones. For example, poor adherence to tuberculosis therapy in New York in the 1980s was often blamed on the patients, but adherence improved and case rates declined once the health care system was adapted to meet the needs of the homeless. The directly observed therapy program at the same Harlem hospital reported a 91 percent adherence rate when on-site and home-visit supervised therapy was made available to TB patients. Stein, Lu, and Gelberg's finding—that a longer history of homelessness independent of its relationship with other known risk factors for poor birth outcomes such as lack of prenatal care—appears to be an independent risk factor for poorer birth outcomes.[253] The authors suggest that this finding likely results from inadequate nutrition, neglect of health during homeless times, and chronically stressful and difficult life circumstances. To affect health outcomes, the delivery system must be organized to first stabilize the lives of homeless patients and thus make it possible for them to adhere to their medical needs.

Where possible, stabilization of housing and health problems should be a priority. Not only can supportive housing improve health outcomes for the homeless, but it is also a cost-effective approach. Better access to supportive housing for homeless psychiatric patients could reduce hospital stays by as much as seventy days per admission. Seventy days in a general hospital psychiatric unit, even at a rate of $250 per day for subacute care, costs $17,500, whereas a unit of supportive housing with social services for an entire year costs $12,500 in New York City.[254]

Researchers and policy makers are currently advocating comprehensive systems of care (systems and service integration) to address the needs of homeless individuals. Service integration involves coordinating services, but relationships between service agencies do not fundamentally change. Systems integration requires fundamental change in how agencies share information, resources, and clients.[255] The goals of integration are to improve access to comprehensive services and continuity of care; reduce service duplication, inefficiency, and costs; and establish greater accountability.[256]

Service and system integration is far from a new concept. For the past thirty years, efforts to achieve integration have been variously called community integration, comprehensive services, and continuum of care. In the past, the efforts were not always successful. Among the problems that have weakened efforts at service integration are (1) resistance at all organizational levels, (2) not establishing a communication network between staff of various agencies to garner appreciation of different expertise and to develop a shared commitment to serving the target population, (3) inflexible funding or regulatory relief, (4) no clear sense of what communities offer and what they need to improve, (5) no focus on services and system integration (focus instead on the organizational level and not on service delivery, or no involvement with current or former service recipients in all stages of planning and development), and (6) no staff person dedicated to facilitating long-term systems change or bringing key players to the table and keeping them there.[257]

The recent resurgence of systems integration initiatives included such target populations as the homeless. The myriad needs of the homeless makes integrated systems and service delivery an appropriate response, and it also offers perhaps the best opportunity to assess the extent to which client outcomes are related to integration interventions. There have been several programs on system or service integration for the homeless, but only the ACCESS program has been formally evaluated.[258] It integrated a range of services, including mental health care, medical care, income supports, housing assistance, substance abuse treatment, and social and vocational rehabilitation. Preliminary findings from this study comparing client outcomes found significant access to housing for clients in more integrated sites.[259]

The ACCESS program uses mental health agencies as its principal system of care, but increasing attention is being devoted to models of integration and coordination that use the primary care sector as the principal system of care. A large body of literature shows that the primary care sector is often the only source of care for a significant portion of individuals with substance abuse and psychiatric disorders, making primary care physicians well positioned to identify these problems and intervene.[260] Primary care physicians can identify preclinical substance abuse and psychiatric disorders in the context of patient contact for other problems, and their influence with their patients can facilitate effective intervention.[261]

Screening is the essential first step, and many professional organizations, such as the American Medical Association and the American Society of Addiction Medicine, recommend that physicians routinely screen patients for these disorders.[262] Though primary care clinicians receive some training in providing mental health care, it is not enough to meet the need. Recent research demonstrates that primary care clinicians do a better job detecting, treating, and referring these problems when working in a collaborative relationship with mental health and substance abuse service providers, and this approach is also more cost-effective. Psychiatric illness—primarily depression, somatization, anxiety, and substance abuse—accounts for the majority of disability days per month even when controlling for physical illness.[263] Evidence shows that collaborative relationships between primary care physicians and mental health and substance abuse service providers can decrease health resource use in the U.S. health care system.

But before health providers and policy makers consider the success and need for integrated health services for the homeless, they must first address a far graver concern: the long-term sustainability of health safety-net systems that serve as the bulwark for integrated system initiatives. In the absence of universal, comprehensive coverage, the health care safety net has served as the default system for caring for many of the nation's uninsured and vulnerable populations. Core safety-net providers typically include public hospitals; federal, state, and locally supported community health centers (CHCs); federally qualified health centers (FQHCs) or clinics such as Health Care for the Homeless clinics; and local health departments. Some safety-net programs are targeted specifically to the general homeless population (as with HCH programs) or specific groups within this population, such as children, youths, or veterans. Other safety-net programs are nontargeted, available to the low-income population as a whole or specific low-income groups such as youths or veterans.[264]

In the past, safety-net providers have served two primary groups of underserved patients: Medicaid recipients and the uninsured. The patient population served by safety-net providers affords continuity of health care: the long-term uninsured can remain long-term users of the safety net, and Medicaid recipients can cycle off Medicaid and become uninsured (as frequently occurs), without much interruption in their health care provider.

Moreover, safety-net providers rely heavily on Medicaid revenues and direct federal, state, and local subsidies as their primary funding sources. However, three competing factors impede on the future viability of the health care safety net: (1) the full impact of Medicaid managed care in an ever more competitive health care marketplace (2) the rising number of uninsured individuals, and (3) the erosion and uncertainty of major direct and indirect subsidies that have helped safety-net functions.[265] Safety-net providers have experienced substantial decreases in their Medicaid revenues as a result of the diversion of Medicaid recipients to managed care plans. Medicaid revenues have helped core safety-net providers defray some of the costs of supporting care for uninsured patients. Moreover, private managed care organizations have no legal responsibility or mission to continue to support the care of patients once they become uninsured, which undermines the continuity of care. To exacerbate matters, the Balanced Budget Act of 1997 reduced some of the major direct public subsidies that have helped finance health care for indigent populations. A number of state and local funds are also being cut or frozen.[266] This financial strain on core safety-net providers comes during a period of growth in the uninsured population, where more than 18 percent (forty-four million people) of the total nonelderly population lack health insurance, an increase of 5 percent (eleven million people) over the past decade.

The shift to Medicaid managed care, the cuts in direct and indirect subsidies, and the increase in the uninsured population have had adverse effects on core safety-net providers as well as on the uninsured and other vulnerable populations who rely on them for care. HCH programs—the core safety-net provider for the homeless—have experienced a 35 percent increase in the number of patients who are uninsured.[267] Thirty percent of HCH projects report decreasing revenue from nonfederal grant sources. Third-party (insurance) revenue is also down, thanks to Medicaid managed care and the increasing number of uninsured patients.[268]

Moreover, it has been argued that the complex and interrelated health conditions of the homeless (including nonmedical factors not usually addressed by managed care entities), the preexisting problem of discontinuity of care resulting from transience, the sensitivity of homeless health care providers, and homeless persons' heavy reliance on clinic-based health care makes the managed care model an inappropriate response to the health care needs of the homeless.[269] Despite the shift to Medicaid managed care, the patterns of health care use among the homeless signify continued use of core safety-net programs.

Implementation of innovative policies (that is integrated systems) for the services that both targeted and nontargeted safety-net programs for the homeless provide have been continuously frustrated by inadequate, untimely, or unsystematic evidence on process and outcome measures. It takes many years to assemble information regarding safety-net providers, and important data is often missing or only describes situations in a few communities.[270] Information on program effectiveness is critical to determine appropriate measures of consumer need, services delivered, and outcomes attained. Such information gives policy makers and practitioners important insight into which policies have the greatest impact on homelessness, and which practices serve homeless people most effectively.[271] More important, the fragility of safety-net providers has the potential to become a national crisis. As a result, efforts must be made to improve the ability to monitor and track the changing structure, capacity, and financial stability of these providers.[272]

The need for better information has been strengthened by the Government Performance and Results Act, which requires not only that public programs provide better information on process and outcomes measures but also that agencies identify cross-cutting responsibilities and specify in their strategic plans how they will work together to avoid unnecessary duplication of effort.

The Results Act requires that the primary agency funding the program facilitate the strategic process and outcome plans. Nontargeted safety-net programs do not have a single established entity to track and monitor activity, since various agencies have responsibility for programs and policies that affect one part of the safety-net delivery system. But targeted safety-net programs for the homeless do have an established entity: the Interagency Council on the Homeless.[273] Currently, targeted programs for the homeless have identified cross-cutting responsibilities related to homelessness under the Results Act, but they have not yet described how they will coordinate or consolidate their efforts at the strategic level, nor have they incorporated results-oriented goals or outcome measures.[274] The council has begun to discuss the need to better connect and monitor targeted homeless assistance programs with nontargeted programs that provide health care services.[275] However, a more concerted effort needs to be directed at improving the capacity and ability to monitor targeted and nontargeted safety-net programs for the homeless. Furthermore, to adequately respond to the Results Act, agencies need to consistently incorporate results-oriented goals and outcome measures relative to the homeless in their performance plans.[276]

The potential created by the Results Act promotes better information regarding the impact of targeted and nontargeted health safety-net programs on the homeless, and the cross-cutting component of the act encourages facilitation of an integrated systems approach. However, to forge advances offered by an integrated system approach requires moving beyond policy prescription to policy development and implementation. In its report "The Future of Public Health," the Institute of Medicine advances this point when it stresses the critical need to advocate for public health, build constituencies, and identify resources by generating supportive and collaborative relationships with public and private agencies and constituent groups for effective planning, implementation, and management of public health policies.[277]

Homeless health programs have already established a venue to facilitate coordination of services—the Interagency Council on the Homeless—which has brought agency representatives together to coordinate administration of programs and resources for assisting homeless people. Council staff and the executive directors of two major homeless advocacy groups believe that the council lost much of its influence in 1994, when Congress stopped its funding and turned it into a voluntary working group, but HUD acknowledges that the council is still very involved in coordinating federal efforts and sharing information.[278] The council serves as a vital mechanism for promoting coordination maintained in the Results Act, and it should be supported and used as such. It is critical that those in health practice for the homeless help to formulate policies on an integrated systems approach achieved in the ACCESS program and use the Interagency Council on the Homeless as a venue to advocate their adoption. Failing to fulfill this responsibility ultimately leads to static policy prescription, which gets lost behind the covers of public health journals and reports, rather than active policy development.

Specific Programmatic Needs

The Health Care for the Homeless program has provided accessible, continuous, comprehensive, appropriate, and sensitive care to homeless people. However, these facilities help only 50 percent of homeless persons in their communities.[279] Currently there are 128 HCH grantees nationally, representing three hundred subcontractors. Thus, one basic starting point in addressing the health care needs of homeless people is to increase the amount, and ensure stability, of funding for this excellent program.

Access to dental care is seriously needed by homeless individuals as well as other impoverished groups in our country,[280] yet poor oral health may prevent homeless individuals from obtaining employment and escaping from the streets. Vision care for homeless persons is also lacking. They can get their vision tested by their primary care providers, but such providers often do not make eyeglasses available.[281] Further, great efforts must be made to address the family planning and prenatal needs of homeless women. Without attention to health care for these women, we will be creating a second generation at risk of poverty and homelessness.

Respite care is severely lacking for the homeless, even in the majority of facilities funded by HCH programs. Currently, a shelter or the street is often the site to which a homeless patient is discharged,[282] and these are inappropriate environments for the sick. Since shelters are, for the most part, open only at night, where do ill homeless persons go for rest, nutrition, and simple basic care? Convalescent facilities are needed so that homeless persons, after being provided medical, surgical, or obstetrical care, are not discharged from an outpatient setting or hospital to the streets when their recuperation requires running water, a bed, refrigeration, or proper nutrition.[283] Respite care would ensure that homeless persons receive care that most others with homes and families routinely enjoy.[284] The homeless need a protected environment in shelters or HCH program facilities for respite, convalescence, and treatment. Given their high rate of excessive hospitalization, such respite care would help homeless individuals stay out of hospitals and reduce hospital stays.

The chronically mentally and physically ill or disabled would rapidly fill up respite care facilities. Therefore, long-term public housing is needed for the chronically ill, including housing to treat homeless persons with tuberculosis, severe mental illness, and substance abuse, as well as hospice facilities for those with terminal illnesses such as AIDS. Community-based screening must be performed to ensure early identification of people with such an illness.[285] Burt and Cohen[286] suggest that, "at the very least, the extent of serious health disabilities suggests that housing solutions must include not simply financial assistance or public housing, but also supportive services that can help the disabled deal with the life crises that can destabilize them and ultimately result in a return to the streets." Such services must be able to treat homeless persons with the dual diagnosis of substance abuse and mental illness.[287]

The reform in medical education toward a humanistic primary care model will, it is hoped, have an impact in creating a cadre of medical providers who are trained to care for vulnerable populations such as the homeless. Fifty percent of McKinney-funded HCH clinics report that they have difficulty recruiting physicians. Perhaps medical education reform, in combination with health care reform, will ameliorate some of the major recruitment barriers experienced by these clinics: poor working conditions, inadequate salaries, physician bias against working with homeless patients, and the lack of respect this work now receives from the medical profession.[288] Since most of the care provided to homeless people is in the emergency room rather than a special clinic for the homeless, all medical and surgical trainees in medical school, residency, and fellowship programs must be trained to develop an appreciation for their patients' housing and poverty status. "It is thus essential that those delivering health care to homeless persons carefully consider how their usual procedures and advice will be heard and experienced by those who do not have a home.[289] Appropriate models of care must be developed, taught to clinicians, and replicated in the community.

Single-payer national health care delivery is the best option for homeless people and is endorsed by the National Health Care for the Homeless Council and

National Coalition for the Homeless.[290] A single-payer plan allows homeless persons to have health care regardless of whether or not they are welfare recipients. Such a plan should guarantee the right to choose one's health care provider. This would allow the homeless to obtain medical care regardless of where they move. Further, free choice gives homeless people the opportunity to select care from programs such as HCH, with providers who have experience in managing the intertwined health and social problems of homeless persons, and it allows these programs to be reimbursed for their efforts. It would make funding of such programs permanent, whereas they are now funded year to year. A single-payer plan should also be designed to augment reimbursement to providers for services they give to homeless and other vulnerable populations, to acknowledge the intensive effort required to assess and treat homeless patients' complex and intertwined medical, mental health, and social problems. It is essential that this plan be universal as well as comprehensive and cover mental health, substance abuse, dental care, vision care, medications, case management, ancillary services, and long-term care. Such a plan would offer comprehensive coverage regardless of income or employment status; no cash contributions should be required of the homeless, given their extreme impoverishment.

Homeless Health Care: Needed Research

Jahiel[291] carefully summarizes the serious need for health services research to evaluate the health care provided to the homeless population, in terms of access, cost, organization, and quality (structure, process, and outcomes) of this care. There is no way of knowing how the homeless population will fit into a managed care delivery system. Evaluation of existing programs is very limited, and lacking are cost-effectiveness studies that compare programs. Research on how to improve the physical and social environments of the homeless is essential. Shelters are dangerous; architecture and urban planning research could resolve this problem. Streets are dangerous, too, which requires the joint efforts of social policy experts, social workers, police, and emergency medical services personnel working together to understand how to prevent crime and its attendant psychological distress.

Conclusion

Perhaps of greatest concern is that our nation seems to have come to accept homelessness as just another negative aspect of modern life, similar in this way to violent crime. It is difficult for health policy makers to address the problems of the homeless population when public support for homeless people is weak at best. Perhaps advocates for the homeless have done a disservice, by focusing on homeless persons' medical, mental health, and substance abuse problems and needs rather than on the core issues of lack of low-income housing, and the breakdown of social cohesiveness and community relations in this country. As Gary Blasi suggests:

> Mass homelessness is now seen as an acceptable feature of American life. Institutional forces have been aggravated by conservative political forces, aimed at demonstrating either that homelessness is not much of a problem after all, or that such problems as there are flow from the personal and moral failures of those who are homeless. Advocates for homeless people, as some of them now recognize, bear considerable responsibility for reinforcing some distortions and introducing others. Indeed it is possible (although by no means uncertain) that by redefining extreme poverty in terms of homelessness, by advocating for 'the homeless' rather than for the extremely poor (including those with disabilities), and by paying inadequate attention to questions of race, advocates unwittingly harmed the ultimate cause they believed they were serving: alleviating the human suffering that attends extreme deprivation.[292]

As a nation, we should not limit our treatment of homelessness to addressing only the physical health, mental health, and substance abuse problems of homeless persons. To end homelessness, we must address our nation's attitudes toward and treatment of the poor, as well as its welfare and housing policies. We need to focus our attention not only on ameliorating or managing homelessness, but also on an effort to end mass homelessness.

Notes

1. Burt, M., and others. "Homelessness: Programs and the People They Serve." Washington, D.C.: Interagency Council on Homelessness, 1999.
2. Link, B., and others. "Lifetime and Five-Year Prevalence of Homelessness in the United States." *American Journal of Public Health*, 1994, *84*(12), 1907–1912.
3. Burt and others (1999).
4. Bassuk, E., and Franklin, D. "Homelessness Past and Present: The Case of the United States, 1890–1925." *New England Journal of Public Policy*, 1992, *8*, 67–86.
5. Katz, M. *In the Shadow of the Poorhouse.* New York: Basic Books, 1986.
6. Trattner, W. *From Poor Law to Welfare State.* New York: Free Press, 1989.
7. Trattner (1989).
8. Trattner (1989).
9. Katz, M. *The Undeserving Poor: From the War on Poverty to the War on Welfare.* New York: Pantheon Books, 1990.
10. Katz (1986).

11. Katz (1986).
12. Katz (1986).
13. Katz (1986).
14. Leepson, M. "The Homeless: Growing National Problem." *Editorial Research Reports,* 1982, *11,* 795–812; Vanderkooi, R. "The Main Stem: Skid Row Revisited." In I. Horowitz and C. Nanry (eds.), *Sociological Realities II.* New York: HarperCollins, 1971.
15. Leepson (1982); Hombs, M. E., and Snyder, M. *Homeless in America: A Forced March to Nowhere.* Washington, D.C.: Community for Creative Nonviolence, 1982.
16. Leepson (1982); Lee, B. "The Disappearance of Skid Row: Some Ecological Evidence." *Urban Affairs Quarterly,* 1980, *16*(1), 81–107.
17. Hombs and Snyder (1982).
18. Baxter, E., and Hopper, K. *Private Lives/Public Spaces: Homeless Adults on the Streets of New York.* New York: Institute for Social Welfare Research, 1981; Hopper, K., Baxter, E., Cox, S., and Klein, L. *One Year Later: The Homeless Poor in New York City.* New York: Community Service Society, Institute for Social Welfare Research, 1982.
19. Burt and others (1999).
20. Koegel, P., and Burnam, A. *The Course of Homelessness Study.* Rockville, Md.: National Institute of Mental Health, 1991.
21. Burt and others (1999).
22. Burt and others (1999).
23. Burt and others (1999).
24. Burt and others (1999).
25. Burt and others (1999); Link and others (1994).
26. Burt and others (1999).
27. Burt and others (1999).
28. Burt and others (1999).
29. Phelan, J., and Link, B. "Who Are the Homeless? Reconsidering the Stability and Composition of the Homeless Population." *American Journal of Public Health,* 1999, *89*(9), 1334–1338.
30. Burt and others (1999).
31. Koegel, P. "Through a Different Lens: An Anthropological Perspective on the Homeless Mentally Ill." *Culture, Medicine, and Psychiatry,* 1992, *16,* 1–22.
32. Phelan and Link (1999).
33. Nunez, R., and Cox, C. "A Snapshot of Family Homelessness Across America." *Political Science Quarterly,* 1999, *114*(2), 289–299.
34. Brickner, P. W., and others. *Health Care of Homeless People.* New York: Springer, 1985.
35. Link and others (1994).
36. Fischer, P., and Breakey, W. "Homelessness and Mental Health: An Overview." *International Journal of Mental Health,* 1986, *14,* 6–41.
37. Culhane, D., and Kuhn, R. "Patterns and Determinants of Public Shelter Utilization Among Homeless Adults in New York City and Philadelphia." *Journal of Policy Analysis and Management,* 1998, *17*(1), 23–43.
38. Bauman, K. "Shifting Family Definitions: The Effect of Cohabitation and Other Nonfamily Household Relationships on Measures of Poverty." *Demography,* 1999, *36*(3), 315–325; also includes Smith, S. I., McGuckin, A., and Walker, C. "Health Alliance? The Relevance of Health Professionals to Housing Management." *Public Health,* 1994, *108,* 175–193; Robinson, D. "Health Selection in the Housing System: Access to Council Housing for Homeless People with Health Problems." *Housing Studies,* 1998, *13,* 23–41.

39. Wood, D., Valdez, R. B., Hayashi, T., and Shen, A. "Homeless and Housed Families in Los Angeles: A Study Comparing Demographic, Economic, and Family Function Characteristics." *American Journal of Public Health,* 1990, *80*(9), 1049–1052.

40. Burt and others (1999); Bassuk, E., and others. "The Characteristics and Needs of Sheltered Homeless and Low-Income Housed Mothers." *Journal of the American Medical Association,* 1996, *276*(8), 640–646.

41. Brickner and others (1985).

42. Fischer, P. J., and others. "Mental Health and Social Characteristics of the Homeless: A Survey of Mission Users." *American Journal of Public Health,* 1986, *76*(5), 519–524.

43. Gallagher, T., Andersen, R., Koegel, P., and Gelberg, L. "Determinants of Regular Source of Care Among Homeless Adults in Los Angeles." *Medical Care,* 1997, *35,* 814–830.

44. White, M. C., and others. "Association Between Time Homeless and Perceived Health Status Among the Homeless in San Francisco." *Journal of Community Health,* 1997, *22*(4), 271–282.

45. Burt and others (1999); White and others (1997); Roth, D., and Bean, G. "New Perspectives on Homelessness: Findings from a Statewide Epidemiological Study." *Hospital and Community Psychiatry,* 1986, *37,* 712–719; Bassuk, E., and Rosenberg, L. "Why Does Family Homelessness Occur? A Case-Control Study." *AJPH,* 1988, *78,* 783–788; Morse, G., and Calsyn, R. "Mentally Disturbed Homeless People in St. Louis: Needy, Willing, But Underserved." *International Journal of Mental Health,* 1986, *14,* 74–94.

46. Robertson, M., and Cousineau, M. "Health Status and Access to Health Services Among the Urban Homeless." *American Journal of Public Health,* 1986, *76*(5), 561–563.

47. Barrow, S., Herman, D., Cordova, P., and Struening, E. "Mortality Among Homeless Shelter Residents in New York City." *American Journal of Public Health,* 1999, *89*(4), 529–534; Wright, J. D., and others. *Homelessness and Health.* Washington, D.C.: McGraw-Hill Healthcare Information Center, 1987; Alstrom, C. H., Lindelius, R., and Salum, I. "Morality Among Homeless Men." *British Journal of Addiction,* 1975, *70*(3), 245–252; Hibbs, J., and others. "Mortality in a Cohort of Homeless Adults in Philadelphia." *New England Journal of Medicine,* 1994, *331*(5), 304–309; "Deaths Among Homeless Persons—San Francisco, 1985–1990." *Morbidity and Mortality Weekly Report,* 1991, *40,* 877–880; Hanzlick, R., and Parrish, R. "Death Among the Homeless in Fulton County, Georgia, 1988–1990." *Public Health Reports,* 1993, *108,* 488–491; "Deaths Among Homeless Persons—San Francisco." *Journal of the American Medical Association,* 1992, *267*(4), 484–485.

48. Barrow, Herman, Cordova, and Struening (1999).

49. Hwang, S., and others. "Risk Factors for Death in Homeless Adults in Boston." *Archives of Internal Medicine,* 1998, *158*(13), 1454–1460.

50. Weinreb, L., Goldberg, R., Bassuk, E., and Perloff, J. "Determinants of Health and Service Use Patterns in Homeless and Low-Income Housed Children." *Pediatrics,* 1998, *102,* 554–562.

51. Burt and others (1999).

52. Burt and others (1999); Wenzel, S., Andersen, R., Gifford, D., and Gelberg, L. "Gynecological Symptoms and Conditions and Use of Medical Care Among Homeless Women." *Journal of Health Care for the Poor and Underserved,* forthcoming; Fierman, A., Dreyer, B., Acker, P., and Legano, L. "Status of Immunization and Iron Nutrition in New York City Homeless Children." *Clinical Pediatrics,* 1993, *3,* 151–155; Long, H., and others. "Cancer Screening in Homeless Women: Attitudes and Behaviors." *Journal of Health Care for the Poor and Underserved,* 1998, *9*(3), 276–292.

53. Alperstein, G., Rappaport, C., and Flanigan, J. M. "Health Problems of Homeless Children in New York City." *AJPH,* 1998, *78,* 1232–1233; Wood, D., Valdez, R., Hayashi,

T., and Shen, A. "Health of Homeless Children and Housed, Poor Children." *Pediatrics,* 1990, *86*(6), 858–866; Miller, D., and Lin, E. "Children in Sheltered Homeless Families: Reported Health Status and Use of Health Services." *Pediatrics,* 1988, *81,* 668–673.

54. Brickner and others (1985); Barnes, P., and others. "Patterns of Tuberculosis Transmission in Central Los Angeles." *Journal of the American Medical Association,* 1997, *278*(14), 1159–1163; Zolopa, A., and others. "HIV and Tuberculosis Infection in San Francisco's Homeless Adults." *Journal of the American Medical Association,* 1994, *272*(6), 455–461.

55. Zolopa and others (1994); Torres, R., Mani, S., Altholz, J., and Brickner, P. "Human Immunodeficiency Virus Infection Among Homeless Men in a New York City Shelter." *Archives of Internal Medicine,* 1990, *150*(10), 2030–2036.

56. "Tuberculosis Among Residents of Shelters for the Homeless—Ohio, 1990." *Morbidity and Mortality Weekly Report,* 1991, *40,* 869–877.

57. Torres, Mani, Altholz, and Brickner (1990).

58. Gelberg, L., and others. "Tuberculosis Skin Testing Among Homeless Adults." *Journal of General Internal Medicine,* 1997, *12*(1), 25–33.

59. McAdam, J., and others. "The Spectrum of Tuberculosis in a New York City Men's Shelter Clinic, 1982–1988)." *Chest,* 1990, *97*(4), 798–805.

60. Des Prez, R., and Heim, C. "Mycobacterium Tuberculosis." In G. Mandell, G. Douglas, and J. Bennett (eds.), *Principles and Practices of Infectious Diseases.* New York: Churchill Livingstone, 1990.

61. Kline, S., Hedemark, L., and Davies, S. "Outbreak of Tuberculosis Among Regular Patrons of a Neighborhood Bar." *New England Journal of Medicine,* 1995, *333*(4), 222–227.

62. Torres, Mani, Altholz, and Brickner (1990); Gelberg and others (1997).

63. Barnes and others (1997); Torres, Mani, Altholz, and Brickner (1990); Gelberg (1997); Kline, Hedemark, and Davies (1995).

64. Torres, Mani, Altholz, and Brickner (1990).

65. Gelberg (1997).

66. Asch, S., Leake, B., Knowles, L., and Gelberg, L. "Tuberculosis in Homeless Patients: Potential for Case Finding in Public Emergency Departments." *Annals of Emergency Medicine,* 1998, *32,* 144–147.

67. Kline, Hedemark, and Davies (1995).

68. Brudney, K., and Dobkin, J. "Resurgent Tuberculosis in New York City." *American Review of Respiratory Disease,* 1991, *144,* 745–749.

69. Torres, Mani, Altholz, and Brickner (1990).

70. Robertson, M., and others. "HIV Seroprevalence Among Homeless and Marginally Housed Women in San Francisco." Annual meeting of the American Public Health Association, Chicago, Nov. 1999.

71. Robertson and others (1999).

72. Fauci, A., Bartlett, J., and Goosby, E. "Early Treatment of HIV-1 Infection." *Lancet,* 1998, *352*(9144), 1935 [discussion 1936]; McQuillan, G., and others. "Update on the Seroepidemiology of Human Immunodeficiency Virus in the United States Household Population: NHANES III, 1988–1994." *Journal of Acquired Immune Deficiency Syndrome and Human Retrovirology* 1997, *14*(4), 355–360.

73. Shlay, J., and others. "Human Immunodeficiency Virus Seroprevalence and Risk Assessment of a Homeless Population in Denver." *Sexually Transmitted Diseases,* 1996, *23,* 304–311.

74. Susser, E., Valencia, E., and Conover, S. "Prevalence of HIV Infection Among Psychiatric Patients in a New York City Men's Shelter." *American Journal of Public Health,* 1993, *83*(4), 568–570.

75. Rahav, M., Nuttbrock, L., Rivera, J., and Link, B. "HIV Infection Risks Among Homeless, Mentally Ill, Chemical Misusing Men." *Substance Use and Misuse*, 1998, *33*(6), 1407–1426; Hill, P., Harvey, J., and Praaskag, A. *Pandora's Box: Accountability and Performance Standards in Vocational Education*. Santa Monica, Calif.: RAND, 1993; Susser, E., and others. "Sexual Behavior of Homeless Mentally Ill Men at Risk for HIV." *American Journal of Psychiatry*, 1995, *152*, 583–587.

76. Filice, G., and others. "Group A Meningococcal Disease in Skid Rows: Epidemiology and Implications of Control." *American Journal of Public Health*, 1984, *74*(3), 253–254; Counts, G., and others. "Group A Meningococcal Disease in the U.S. Pacific Northwest: Epidemiology, Clinical Features, and Effect of a Vaccination Control Program." *Reviews of Infectious Diseases*, 1984, *6*(5), 640–648.

77. DeMaria, A., and others. "An Outbreak of Type 1 Pneumococcal Pneumonia in a Men's Shelter." *Journal of the American Medical Association*, 1980, *244*(13), 1446–1449.

78. Heath, C., and Zusman, J. "An Outbreak of Diphtheria Among Skid-Row Men." *New England Journal of Medicine*, 1962, *267*(16), 809–812; Pedersen, A., and others. "Diphtheria on Skid Row, Seattle, Washington, 1972–1975." *Public Health Reports*, 1977, *92*(4), 336–342.

79. Busen, N., and Beech, B. "A Collaborative Model for Community-Based Health Care Screening of Homeless Adolescents." *Journal of Professional Nursing*, 1997, *13*, 316–324; Morey, M., and Friedman, L. "Health Care Needs of Homeless Adolescents." *Current Opinions in Pediatrics*, 1993, *5*(4), 395–399; Wang, E., King, S., Goldberg, E., and Milner, R.R.S. "Hepatitis B and Human Immunodeficiency Virus Infection in Street Youths in Toronto, Canada." *Pediatric Infectious Diseases Journal*, 1991, *10*, 130–133.

80. Vidal-Trecan, G., and others. "Patterns of Sexual and Injecting Risk Behaviours in French Intravenous Drug Users Not Reporting HIV and Hepatitis C Virus Seropositivities." *Addiction*, 1998, *93*, 1657–1668; Zanetta, D., and others. "HIV Infection and Related Risk Behaviors in a Disadvantaged-Youth Institution of Sao Paulo, Brazil." *International Journal of STD and AIDS*, 1999, *10*, 98–104; Hagan, H., and others. "Syringe Exchange and Risk of Infection with Hepatitis B and C Viruses." *American Journal of Epidemiology*, 1999, *143*, 203–213.

81. Jackson, L., and Spach, D. "Emergence of Bartonella Quintana Infection Among Homeless Persons." *Emerging Infectious Diseases*, 1996, *2*(2), 141–143.

82. Institute of Medicine. *Homelessness, Health, and Human Needs*. Washington, D.C.: National Academy Press, 1988.

83. Weitzman, B. C. "Pregnancy and Childbirth: Risk Factors for Homelessness?" *Family Planning Perspectives*, 1989, *21*(4), 175–178.

84. Gelberg, L., and others. "Use of Birth Control Among Homeless Women: Prior Use and Willingness to Use in the Future." (Draft.) UCLA Department of Family Medicine, 1999.

85. Shuler, P. A., Gelberg, L., and Davis, J. E. "Characteristics Associated with the Risk of Unintended Pregnancy Among Urban Homeless Women." *Journal of the American Academy of Nurse Practitioners*, 1995, *7*, 13–22; Brickner, P., and others. *Under the Safety Net: The Health and Social Welfare of the Homeless in the United States*. New York: Norton, 1990.

86. Brickner and others (1990).

87. Long and others (1998).

88. Long and others (1998).

89. Blackman, D., Bennett, E., and Miller, D. "Trends in Self-Reported Use of Mammograms, 1989–1997, and Papanicolaou Tests, 1991–1997—Behavioral Risk Factor Surveillance System." *Morbidity and Mortality Weekly Report*, 1999, *48*(SS06), 1–22.

90. Shuler, P. A. "Homeless Women's Holistic and Family Planning Needs: An Exposition and Test of the Nurse Practitioner Model." University of California, Los Angeles, 1991; Burnam, M. A., and Koegel, P. *The Course of Homelessness Among the Seriously Mental Ill: An NIMH Funded Proposal.* Rockville, Md., 1989.

91. Burt and others (1999).

92. Chavkin, W., Kristal, A., Seabron, C., and Guigli, P. "The Reproductive Experience of Women Living in Hotels for the Homeless in New York City." *New York State Journal of Medicine,* 1987, *86,* 10–13.

93. Paterson, C. M., and Roderick, P. "Obstetric Outcome in Homeless Women." *British Medical Journal,* 1990, *301,* 263–266; Gelberg, L. "Homeless Women's Access to Women's Health Services." Robert Wood Johnson Foundation, Generalist Physician Faculty Scholar's Program, annual meeting, San Diego, Dec. 1997.

94. Alstrom, Lindelius, and Salum (1975); Brickner and others (1990); Paterson and Roderick (1990); Stein, J. A., Lu, M., and Gelberg, L. "Homelessness History and Adverse Birth Outcomes Associations with Prenatal Care, Dysfunctional Behaviors, Medical Risk, and Ethnicity." *Health Psychology,* 2000, *19*(6), 524–534; Nyamathi, A. "Sense of Coherence in Minority Women at Risk for HIV Infection." *Public Health Nursing,* 1993, *10*(3), 151–158; Stein, J. A., Lu, M. C., and Gelberg, L. "Severity of Homelessness and Adverse Birth Outcomes." *Health Psychology,* 2000, *19*(6), 524–534.

95. Paterson and Roderick (1990).

96. Stein, Lu, and Gelberg (2000).

97. Mowbray, C., Johnson, V., Solarz, A., and Combs, C. "Mental Health and Homelessness in Detroit: A Research Study." Detroit: Michigan Department of Mental Health, 1986.

98. Burt and others (1999).

99. Burt and others (1999); Wenzel, S., Koegel, P., and Gelberg, L. "Antecedents of Physical and Sexual Victimization Among Homeless Women: A Comparison to Homeless Men." *American Journal of Community Psychology,* 2000, *11,* 212–230; Wenzel, S., Koegel, P., and Gelberg, L. "Antecedents of Physical and Sexual Victimization Among Homeless Women: A Comparison to Homeless Men." *American Journal of Community Psychology,* 2000, *28*(3), 367–390.

100. Wenzel, S., Leake, B., and Gelberg, L. "Health of Homeless Women With Recent Experience of Rape." *Journal of General Internal Medicine,* 2000, *15*(4), 265–268.

101. Rennison, C. "Criminal Victimization 1998, Changes 1997–98 with Trends 1993–98." Washington, D.C.: U.S. Department of Justice, 1999.

102. Lam, J., and Rosenheck, R. "The Effect of Victimization on Clinical Outcomes of Homeless Persons with Serious Mental Illness." *Psychiatric Services,* 1998, *49*(5), 678–683.

103. Lam and Rosenheck (1998).

104. Wenzel, Koegel, and Gelberg (2000); Lam and Rosenheck (1998).

105. Burt and others (1999).

106. Wenzel, Koegel, and Gelberg (2000); Herman, D., Susser, E., Struening, E., and Link, B. "Adverse Childhood Experiences: Are They Risk Factors for Adult Homelessness?" *American Journal of Public Health,* 1997, *87*(2), 249–255; Bassuk, E., Melnick, S., and Browne, A. "Responding to the Needs of Low-Income and Homeless Women Who Are Survivors of Family Violence." *Journal of the American Medical Women's Association,* 1998, *53,* 57–64.

107. North, C., Smith, E., Pollio, D., and Spitznagel, E. "Are the Mentally Ill Homeless a Distinct Homeless Subgroup?" *Annals of Clinical Psychiatry,* 1996, *8*(3), 117–128.

108. Davies-Netzley, S., Hurlburt, M., and Hough, R. "Childhood Abuse as a Precursor to Homelessness for Homeless Women with Severe Mental Illness." *Violence and Victims,* 1996,

11(2), 129–142.; Goodman, L., Dutton, M., and Harris, M. "The Relationship Between Violence Dimensions and Symptoms Severity Among Homeless, Mentally Ill Women." *Journal of Trauma and Stress,* 1997, *10*(1), 51–70; Browne, A., and Bassuk, S. "Intimate Violence in the Lives of Homeless and Poor Housed Women: Prevalence and Patterns in an Ethnically Diverse Sample." *American Journal of OrthoPsychiatry,* 1997, *67*(2), 261–278; Goodman, L., and Dutton, M. "The Relationship Between Victimization and Cognitive Schemata Among Episodically Homeless, Seriously Mentally Ill Women." *Violence and Victims,* 1996, *11*(2), 159–174.

109. Dietz, P., and Coburn, J. "To Whom Do They Belong? Runaway, Homeless and Other Youth in High-Risk Situations in the 1990s." Washington, D.C.: National Network for Runaway and Youth Services, 1991.

110. Ringwalt, C., Greene, J., Robertson, M., and McPheeters, M. "The Prevalence of Homelessness Among Adolescents in the United States." *American Journal of Public health,* 1998, *88*(9), 1325–1329.

111. Smollar, J. "Homeless Youth in the United States: Description and Developmental Issues." In M. Raffaelli and R. Larson (eds.), *Homeless and Working Youth Around the World: Exploring Developmental Issues.* San Francisco: Jossey-Bass, 1999.

112. MacLean, M., Embry, L., and Cauce, A. "Homeless Adolescents' Paths to Separation from Family: Comparison of Family Characteristics, Psychological Adjustment, and Victimization." *Journal of Community Psychology,* 1999, *27*(2), 179–187.

113. Ensign, J., and Santelli, J. "Health Status and Service Use: Comparison of Adolescents at a School-Based Health Clinic with Homeless Adolescents." *Archives of Pediatrics and Adolescent Medicine,* 1998, *152*(1), 20–24; Unger, J., and others. "Homeless Youths and Young Adults in Los Angeles: Prevalence of Mental Health Problems and the Relationship Between Mental Health and Substance Abuse Disorders." *American Journal of Community Psychology,* 1997, *25*(3), 371–394; Greene, J., Ennett, S., and Ringwalt, C. "Substance Use Among Runaway and Homeless Youth in Three National Samples." *American Journal of Public Health,* 1997, *87*(2), 229–235; Greene, J. and Ringwalt, C. "Youth and Familial Substance Use's Association with Suicide Attempts Among Runaway and Homeless Youth." *Substance Use and Misuse,* 1996, *31*(8), 1041–1058.

114. Greene, J., Ennett, S., and Ringwalt, C. "Prevalence and Correlates of Survival Sex Among Runaway and Homeless Youth." *American Journal of Public Health,* 1999, *89*(9), 1406–1409.

115. Kipke, M., Simon, T., Montgomery, S., Unger, J., and Iversen, E. "Homeless Youth and Their Exposure to and Involvement in Violence While Living on the Streets." *Journal of Adolescent Health,* 1997, *20*(5), 360–367.

116. MacLean, Embry, and Cauce (1999).

117. Whitbeck, L., Hoyt, D., and Yoder, K. "A Risk-Amplification Model of Victimization and Depressive Symptoms Among Runaway and Homeless Adolescents." *American Journal of Community Psychology,* 1999, *27*(2), 273–296.

118. Alderman, E., and others. "Are There Risk Factors for Hepatitis B Infection in Inner-City Adolescents That Justify Prevaccination Screening?" *Journal of Adolescent Youth,* 1998, *22*(5), 389–393; Toy, E., and others. "Hepatitis B Virus Infection Among Street Youths in Montreal." *Canadian Medical Association Journal,* 1999, *161*(6), 693–698.

119. Walters, A. "HIV Prevention in Street Youth." *Journal of Adolescent Health,* 1999, *25*(3), 187–198.

120. Stricof, R., Kennedy, J., Nattell, T., and Weisfuse, I.N.L. "HIV Seroprevalence in a Facility for Runaway and Homeless Adolescents." *American Journal of Public Health,* 1991, *81* (supplement), 50–53.

121. Ensign and Santelli (1998); Greene, J., and Ringwalt, C. "Pregnancy Among Three National Samples of Runaway and Homeless Youth." *Journal of Adolescent Health*, 1998, *23*(6), 370–377.

122. Mowbray, Johnson, Solarz, and Combs (1986).

123. Kaste, L., and Bolden, A. "Dental Caries in Homeless Adults in Boston." *Journal of Public Health, Dentistry*, 1995, *55*(1), 34–36.

124. Gelberg, L., Linn, L. S., and Rosenberg, D. J. "Dental Health of Homeless Adults." *Special Care in Dentistry*, 1988, *8*, 167–172.

125. Burt and others (1999).

126. Fischer and others (1986); Institute of Medicine (1988); Koegel, P., Burnam, A., and Farr, R. "The Prevalence of Specific Psychiatric Disorders Among Homeless Individuals in the Inner City of Los Angeles." *Archives of General Psychiatry*, 1988, *45*, 1085–1092; Bassuk, E., Rubin, L., and Lauriat, A. "Is Homelessness a Mental Health Problem?" *American Journal of Psychiatry*, 1984, *141*, 1546–1550; Sacks, J., Phillips, J., and Cappelletty, G. "Characteristics of the Homeless Mentally Disordered Population in Fresno County." *Community Mental Health Journal*, 1987, *23*, 114–119; Arce, A., Tadlock, M. T., Vergare, M. J., and Shapiro, S. H. "A Psychiatric Profile of Street People Admitted to an Emergency Shelter." *Hospital and Community Psychiatry*, 1983, *34*, 812–817; Smith, E. M., North, C. S., and Spitznagel, E. L. "Alcohol, Drugs and Psychiatric Comorbidity Among Homeless Women: An Epidemiologic Study." *Journal of Clinical Psychiatry*, 1993, *54*, 82–87; Susser, E., Conover, S., and Struening, E. "Problems of Epidemiologic Method in Assessing the Type and Extent of Mental Illness Among Homeless Adults." *Hospital and Community Psychiatry*, 1989, *40*, 261–265.

127. See all the works cited in note 126. See also Koegel, P., and Burnam, M. "Alcoholism Among Homeless Adults in the Inner City of Los Angeles." *Archives of General Psychiatry*, 1988, *45*(11), 1011–1018; and Struening, E., and others. "A Typology Based on Measures of Substance Abuse and Mental Disorder." *Journal of Addiction and Disease*, 1991, *11*, 99–117.

128. Koegel, P., and others. "Utilization of Mental Health and Substance Abuse Services Among Homeless Adults in Los Angeles." *Medical Care*, 1999, *37*(3), 306–317.

129. Wright and others (1987); Koegel, Burnam, and Farr (1988).

130. Chafetz, L., and Goldfinger, S. "Residential Instability in a Psychiatric Emergency Setting." *Psychiatric Quarterly*, 1984, *56*(1), 20–34.

131. Bassuk, E. L., Rubin, L., and Lauriat, A. S. "Characteristics of Sheltered Homeless Families." *American Journal of Public Health*, 1986, *76*, 1097–1101.

132. Bassuk, E., and others. "Determinants of Behavior in Homeless and Low-Income Housed Preschool Children." *Pediatrics*, 1997, *100*(1), 92–100.

133. St. Lawrence, J., and Brasfield, T. "HIV Risk Behavior Among Homeless Adults." *AIDS Education and Prevention*, 1995, *7*(1), 22–31.

134. Bassuk and others (1997); Zima, B. T., Wells, K. B., Benjamin, B., and Duan, N. "Mental Health Problems Among Homeless Mothers." *Archives of General Psychiatry*, 1996, *53*, 332–338.

135. Bassuk, E., Buckner, J., Perloff, J., and Bassuk, S. "Prevalence of Mental Health and Substance Use Disorders Among Homeless and Low-Income Housed Mothers." *American Journal of Psychiatry*, 1998, *155*(11), 1561–1564.

136. Burt and others (1999).

137. Burt and others (1999).

138. Gallagher, Andersen, Koegel, and Gelberg (1997).

139. Burt and others (1999).

140. Fischer and others (1986); Cohen, C., Teresi, J., and Holmes, D. "The Physical Well-Being of Old Homeless Men." *Journal of Gerontology,* 1988, *43,* 121–128; Robertson, M., Ropers, R., and Boyer, R. "The Homeless of Los Angeles County: An Empirical Evaluation." Los Angeles: UCLA School of Public Health, 1985.

141. Martell, J., and others. "Hospitalization in an Urban Homeless Population: The Honolulu Urban Homeless Project." *Annals of Internal Medicine,* 1992, *116,* 299–303.

142. Fischer and others (1986); Robertson and Cousineau (1986).

143. Salit, S., and others. "Hospitalization Costs Associated with Homelessness in New York City." (Special article.) *New England Journal of Medicine,* 1998, *338*(24), 1734–1740.

144. Kelly, J. T., and Goldfinger, S. M. "Homeless Inpatients: Medical, Surgical, and Psychiatric Problems." San Francisco: University of San Francisco, 1985.

145. Gallagher, Andersen, Koegel, and Gelberg (1997).

146. DeRosa, C., and others. "Service Utilization Among Homeless and Runaway Youth in Los Angeles, California: Rates and Reasons." *Journal of Adolescent Health,* 1999, *24*(3), 190–200.

147. Weinreb, Goldberg, Bassuk, and Perloff (1998).

148. Brickner, P. W., and Kaufman, A. "Case Finding of Heart Disease in Homeless Men." *Bulletin of the New York Academy of Medicine,* 1973, *49,* 475–484.

149. McAdam, J., Brickner, P., and Glicksman, R. "Tuberculosis in the SRO/Homeless Population." In P. Brickner and others (eds.), *Health Care for Homeless People.* New York: Springer, 1985.

150. Bassuk, Rubin, and Lauriat (1984).

151. Gallagher, Andersen, Koegel, and Gelberg (1997); Kinchen, K., and Wright, J. "Hypertension Management in Health Care for the Homeless Clinics: Results from a Survey." *American Journal of Public Health,* 1991, *81,* 1163–1165.

152. Salit (1998).

153. Koegel, Burnam, and Farr (1988); Rossi, P. H., Wright, J. D., Fisher, G. A., and Willis, G. "The Urban Homeless: Estimating Composition and Size." *Science,* 1987, *235*(4794), 1336–1341; Segal, S., Baumohl, J., and Johnson, E. "Falling Through the Cracks: Mental Disorder and Social Margin in a Young Vagrant Population." *Social Problems,* 1977, *24*(3), 387–401; Kroll, J., and others. "A Survey of Homeless Adults in Urban Emergency Shelters." *Hospital and Community Psychiatry,* 1986, *37,* 283–286; Gelberg, L., Linn, L., and Leake, B. "Mental Health, Alcohol and Drug Use, and Criminal History Among Homeless Adults." *American Journal of Psychiatry,* 1988, *145,* 191–196; Roth, D., Bean, G., and Hyde, P. "Homelessness and Mental Health Policy: Developing an Appropriate Role for the 1980s." *Community Mental Health Journal,* 1986, *22,* 203–214.

154. Martell and others (1992).

155. Fischer and others (1986).

156. Gelberg, L., and Linn, L. "Social and Physical Health of Homeless Adults Previously Treated for Mental Health Problems." *Hospital and Community Psychiatry,* 1988, *39*(5), 510–516.

157. Koegel and others (1999).

158. Burt and others (1999).

159. Robertson, Ropers, and Boyer (1985).

160. Koegel and others (1999).

161. Koegel and others (1999).

162. Koegel and others (1999).

163. Burt and others (1999).

164. Gallagher, Andersen, Koegel, and Gelberg (1997).

165. Padgett, D., Struening, E., and Andrews, H. "Factors Affecting the Use of Medical, Mental Health, Alcohol, and Drug Treatment Services by Homeless Adults." *Medical Care*, 1990, *28*, 805–821.

166. Gallagher, Andersen, Koegel, and Gelberg (1997).

167. Koegel and others (1999).

168. Koegel and others (1999).

169. Cohen, Teresi, and Holmes (1988).

170. Fischer and others (1986); Gallagher, Andersen, Koegel, and Gelberg (1997).

171. Burt and others (1999).

172. Koegel, P., and Gelberg, L. "Patient-Oriented Approach to Providing Care to Homeless Persons." In D. Wood (ed.), *Delivering Health Care to Homeless Persons: A Guide to the Diagnosis and Management of Medical and Mental Health Conditions*. New York: Springer, 1992.

173. Robertson and Cousineau (1986).

174. Gallagher, Andersen, Koegel, and Gelberg (1997); Sacks, Phillips, and Cappelletty (1987); Gelberg and Linn (1988); Bangsberg, D., Tulsky, J., Hecht, F., and Moss, A. "Protease Inhibitors in the Homeless." *Journal of the American Medical Association*, 1997, *278*(1), 63–65; Gelberg, L., Gallagher, T. C., Andersen, R. M., and Koegel, P. "Competing Priorities as a Barrier to Medical Care Among Homeless Adults in Los Angeles." *American Journal of Public Health*, 1997, *87*(2), 217–220; Ball, F. J., and Havassy, B. E. "A Survey of the Problems and Needs of Homeless Consumers of Acute Psychiatric Services." *Hospital and Community Psychiatry*, 1984, *35*, 917–921.

175. Koegel and Gelberg (1992).

176. Fierman, A. H., and others. "Status of Immunization and Iron Nutrition in New York City Homeless Children." *Clinical Pediatrics*, 1993, *32*(3), 151–155.

177. Miller and Lin (1988); Orenstein, J. B., Boenning, D. A., Engh, E. P., and Zimmerman, S. J. "Emergency Care of Children in Shelters." *Pediatric Emergency Care*, 1992, *8*(6), 313–317; Weinreb, Goldberg, Bassuk, and Perloff (1998).

178. Robertson and Cousineau (1986); Geber, G. "Barriers to Health Care for Street Youth." *Journal of Adolescent Health*, 1997, *21*(5), 287–290.

179. Wright and others (1987); Susser, E., and others. "Injection Drug Use and Risk of HIV Transmission Among Homeless Men with Mental Illness." *American Journal of Psychiatry*, 1996, *153*(6), 794–798; Lam, J., and Rosenheck, R. "Street Outreach for Homeless Persons with Serious Mental Illness: Is It Effective?" *Medical Care*, 1999, *37*(9), 894–907; Crystal, S. "Homeless Men and Homeless Women: The Gender Gap." *Urban and Social Change Review*, 1984, *17*, 2–6.

180. Gelberg and Linn (1988).

181. Gelberg, L., and Linn, L. "Psychological Distress Among Homeless Adults." *Journal of Nervous and Mental Disease*, 1989, *177*(5), 291–295.

182. Lam and Rosenheck (1999); Bachrach, L. "Issues in Identifying and Treating the Homeless Mentally Ill." In H. R. Lamb (ed.), *Leona Bachrach Speaks: Selected Speeches and Lectures by L. Bachrach*. San Francisco: Jossey-Bass, 1987.

183. Roth and Bean (1986).

184. Morse and Calsyn (1986); Gelberg, Linn, and Leake (1988); Gelberg and Linn (1988); Crystal (1984); Rosenheck, R., and others. "Service System Integration, Access to Services, and Housing Outcomes in a Program for Homeless Persons with Severe Mental Illness." *American Journal of Public Health*, 1998, *88*(11), 1610–1615.

185. Morse and Calsyn (1986); Bachrach (1987); Rog, D., Holupka, C., and Brito, M. "The Impact of Housing on Health: Examining Supportive Housing for Individuals with Mental Illness." *Current Issues in Public Health,* 1996, *2,* 153–160.

186. Lam and Rosenheck (1999).

187. Baxter and Hopper (1981).

188. Wright and others (1987); Brickner, P. W., and others. "Medical Aspects of Homelessness." (Unpublished data.) *Department of Community Medicine, St. Vincent's Hospital and Medical Center of New York,* 1984, 1–33.

189. Brickner and others (1984); Wright, J., Rossi, P., and Knight. J. "Health and Homelessness in New York City: Research Report to the Robert Wood Johnson Foundation." Amherst: University of Massachusetts, 1985.

190. Koegel and Gelberg (1992).

191. Koegel and Gelberg (1992); Brickner and others (1984).

192. Koegel and Gelberg (1992).

193. Stark, L. "Barriers to Health Care for Homeless People." In R. Jahiel (ed.), *Homelessness: A Prevention Oriented Approach.* Baltimore: Johns Hopkins University Press, 1992.

194. Jahiel, R. I. *Homelessness: A Prevention-Oriented Approach.* Baltimore: Johns Hopkins University Press, 1992.

195. Stark (1992); Komaromy, M., Lurie, N., and Bindman, A. "California Physicians' Willingness to Treat the Poor." *Western Journal of Medicine,* 1995, *162*(2), 127–132.

196. Reuler, J. "Health Care for the Homeless in a National Health Program." *American Journal of Public Health,* 1989, *79,* 1033–1035.

197. Reuler (1989).

198. Brickner and others (1985).

199. Calloway, M., Topping, S., and Morrissey, J. "Trends in Linkage Behavior Among Providers of Homeless Persons Who Are Seriously and Persistently Mentally Ill." *Association for Health Services Research/Abstract Book,* 1998, *15,* 54–55.

200. Baxter and Hopper (1981).

201. Doblin, B., Gelberg, L., and Freeman, H. "Patient Care and Professional Staffing Patterns in McKinney Act Clinics Providing Primary Care to the Homeless." *Journal of the American Medical Association,* 1992, *267*(5), 698–701.

202. Koegel and Gelberg (1992).

203. Koegel and Gelberg (1992).

204. Stark (1992).

205. Salit and others (1998).

206. Fisher, K., and Collins, J. *Homelessness Healthcare and Welfare Provision.* New York: Routledge, 1993.

207. Rossi, P. *Down and Out in America: The Origins of Homelessness.* Chicago: University of Chicago Press, 1989.

208. Baxter and Hopper (1981).

209. U.S. Conference of Mayors. "A Status Report on Hunger and Homelessness in America's Cities 1982: A 55-City Survey." Washington, D.C.: U.S. Conference of Mayors, 1982.

210. McMurray-Avila, M. *Organizing Health Services for Homeless People.* Nashville, Tenn.: National Health Care for the Homeless Council, 1997.

211. McMurray-Avila (1997).

212. McMurray-Avila (1997).

213. Citro, C., and Michael, R. "Measuring Poverty: A New Approach." Washington, D.C.: National Research Council, 1995.

214. Citro and Michael (1995).

215. Short, K., Iceland, J., and Garner, T. *Experimental Poverty Measures: 1998*. Washington, D.C.: U.S. Bureau of the Census, 1999.

216. Rossi (1989).

217. Burt and others (1999); Jencks, C. *The Homeless*. Cambridge, Mass.: Harvard University Press, 1994; Gelberg, L. "Homelessness and Health." *Journal of the American Board of Family Practice*, 1997, *10*(1), 67–71.

218. Citro and Michael (1995).

219. Phelan and Link (1999).

220. Citro and Michael (1995).

221. Citro and Michael (1995).

222. Citro and Michael (1995).

223. Citro and Michael (1995).

224. Koegel, P., Burnam, A., and Morton, S. "Enumerating Homeless People: Alternative Strategies and Their Consequences." *Evaluation Review*, 1996, *20*(4), 378–403; Dennis, M. "Coverage of a Service-Based Methodology: Findings from the DC*MADS Homelessness Study." Proceedings of *Towards Census 2000: Research Issues for Improving Coverage of the Homeless Population*. Washington, D.C.: Bureau of the Census, Department of Commerce, 1993.

225. Burt and others (1999); Gelberg (1997); Piazza, T., and Cheng, Y. T. "Sample Design for the Study of Alameda County Residents." Berkeley: University of California Survey Research Center, 1992; Koegel, P., and Burnam, M. "The Course of Homelessness Study: Aims and Designs." 119th Annual Meeting of the American Public Health Association, Atlanta, Nov. 1991.

226. Burt and others (1999); Zolopa and others (1994); Gelberg, Gallagher, Andersen, and Koegel (1997); Robertson, M., Zlotnick, C., and Westerfelt, A. "Drug Use Disorders and Treatment Contact Among Homeless Adults in Alameda County, California." *American Journal of Public Health*, 1997, *87*(2), 221–228.

227. Koegel and Burnam (1991).

228. Koegel, Burnam, and Morton (1996).

229. Hotz, V., Goerge, R., Balzekas, J., and Margolin, F. "Administrative Data for Policy-Relevant Research: Assessment of Current Utility and Recommendations for Development." Chicago: Northwestern University/University of Chicago Joint Center for Poverty Research, 1999.

230. Hotz, Goerge, Balzekas, and Margolin (1999).

231. Culhane, D. "Using Administrative Data to Gauge Service Use Dynamics: Methods for Determining Incidence, Prevalence and Census Measures." Washington, D.C.: Homeless Services Data Users Meeting, Dec. 1998.

232. Hotz, Goerge, Balzekas, and Margolin (1999); Culhane (1998).

233. O'Connell, J., Lozier, J., and Gingles, K. "Increased Demand and Decreased Capacity: Challenges to the McKinney Act's Health Care for the Homeless Program." Nashville, Tenn.: National Health Care for the Homeless Council, 1997; U.S. Department of Housing and Urban Development. "Priority: Home! The Federal Plan to Break the Cycle of Homelessness." Washington, D.C.: U.S. Department of Housing and Urban Development, 1994.

234. National Association of Community Health Centers. "Opening Doors to Benefit Programs: A Medicaid Resource Guide for Health Programs Serving the Homeless." Washington, D.C.: National Association of Community Health Centers, 1990.

235. Brickner and others (1985); Jahiel (1992).
236. O'Connell, J., and Lebow, J. "AIDS and the Homeless of Boston." *New England Journal of Public Policy*, 1992, *8*, 541–556.
237. Wright and others (1987); Lewin and ICF. "The Health Needs of the Homeless: A Report of Persons Served by the McKinney Act's Health Care for the Homeless Program." Washington, D.C.: National Association of Community Health Centers (supported by grant from U.S. Department of Health and Human Services), 1989.
238. Mauch, D., and Mulkern, V. "The McKinney Act: New England Responses to Federal Support for State and Local Assistance to Homeless Mentally Ill." *New England Journal of Public Policy*, 1992, *8*, 419–430.
239. National Resource Center on Homelessness and Mental Illness. "National Organizations Concerned with Mental Health, Housing, and Homelessness." Delmar, N.Y.: National Resource Center on Homelessness and Mental Illness, 1995.
240. Rosenheck and others (1998).
241. Lam, J., and Rosenheck, R. "Social Support and Service Use Among Homeless Persons with Serious Mental Illness." *International Journal of Social Psychiatry*, 1999, *45*(1), 13–28.
242. Tsemberis, S. "From Streets to Homes: An Innovative Approach to Supported Housing for Homeless Adults with Psychiatric Disabilities." *Journal of Community Psychology*, 1999, *27*(2), 225–241.
243. National Resource Center on Homelessness and Mental Illness, "National Organizations Concerned with Mental Health, Housing and Homelessness," 1995.
244. Rosenheck, R., Leda, C., and Gallup, P. "Program Design and Clinical Operation of Two National VA Initiatives for Homeless Mentally Ill Veterans." *New England Journal of Public Policy*, Spring/Summer 1992, 315–337.
245. Rosenheck, R., Frisman, L., and Gallup, P. "Effectiveness and Cost Specific Treatment Elements in a Program for Homeless Mentally Ill Veterans." *Psychiatric Services*, 1995, *46*(11), 1131–1139.
246. Leda, C., and Rosenheck, R. "Race in the Treatment of Homeless Mentally Ill Veterans." *Journal of Nervous and Mental Disease*, 1995, *183*(8), 529–537.
247. Kasprow, W., Frisman, L., and Rosenheck, R. "Homeless Veterans' Satisfaction with Residential Treatment." *Psychiatric Services*, 1999, *50*(4), 540–545.
248. Kasprow, Frisman, and Rosenheck (1999).
249. National Resource Center on Homelessness and Mental Illness (1995).
250. Center for Mental Health Services. "Making a Difference: Interim Status Report of the McKinney Demonstration Program for Homeless Adults with Serious Mental Illness." Rockville, Md.: Center for Mental Health Services, 1994.
251. Robert Wood Johnson Foundation. *The Homeless Families Program*. Princeton, N.J.: Robert Wood Johnson Foundation, 1993.
252. Rog, D., and Gutman, M. "The Homeless Families Program: A Summary of Key Findings." Princeton, N.J.: Robert Wood Johnson Foundation, 1999.
253. Stein, Lu, and Gelberg (2000).
254. Salit and others (1998).
255. Dennis, D., Cocozza, J., and Steadman, H. "What Do We Know About Systems Integration and Homelessness?" In L. B. Fosburg and D. L. Dennis (eds.), *Practical Lessons: The 1998 National Symposium on Homelessness Research*. Washington, D.C.: Housing and Urban Development, Department of Health and Human Services, 1999.
256. Randolph, F., and others. "Creating Integrated Service Systems for Homeless Persons with Mental Illness: The ACCESS Program. Access to Community Care and Effective Services and Supports." *Psychiatric Services*, 1997, *48*(3), 369–373.

257. Dennis, Cocozza, and Steadman (1999).
258. Dennis, Cocozza, and Steadman (1999).
259. Rosenheck and others (1998).
260. Fleming, M., and others. "Benefit-Cost Analysis of Brief Physician Advice with Problem Drinkers in Primary Care Setting." *Medical Care,* 2000, *38*(1), 7–18; Fleming, M., and others. "Brief Physician Advice for Problem Alcohol Drinkers: A Randomized Controlled Trial in Community-Based Primary Care Practices." *Journal of the American Medical Association,* 1997, *277*(13), 1039–1045; Friedman, P., Saitz, R., and Samet, J. "Management of Adults Recovering from Alcohol or Other Drug Problems: Relapse Prevention Primary Care." *Journal of the American Medical Association,* 1998, *279*(15), 1227–1231; Kates, N., and others. "Integrating Mental Health Services Within Primary Care: A Canadian Program." *General Hospital Psychiatry,* 1997, *19,* 324–332; Spitzer, R., and others. "Utility of a New Procedure for Diagnosing Mental Disorders in Primary Care: The PRIME-MD 1000 Study." *Journal of the American Medical Association,* 1994, *272*(22), 1749–1756; Wells, K., and others. "Impact of Disseminating Quality Improvement Programs for Depression in Managed Primary Care: A Randomized Controlled Trial." *Journal of the American Medical Association,* 2000, *282*(2), 212–220.
261. Fleming and others (2000); Fleming and others (1997); Wells and others (2000).
262. Institute of Medicine. "Broadening the Base of Treatment for Alcohol Problems: Report of a Study by a Committee of the Institute of Medicine." Washington, D.C.: National Academy Press, 1990; American Society of Addiction Medicine. "Public Policy Statement on Screening for Addiction in Primary Care Setting." *ASAM News,* 1997, *17,* 17–18.
263. Ormel, J., Von Korff, M., and Ustun, B. "Common Mental Disorders and Disability Across Cultures: Results from the WHO Collaborative Study on Psychological Problems in General Health Care." *Journal of the American Medical Association,* 1993, *272,* 1741–1748.
264. Lewin, M., and Alman, S. "American's Health Care Safety Net: Intact But Endangered." Washington, D.C.: National Academy Press, 2000.
265. Lewin and Alman (2000).
266. Holahan, J., Zuckerman, S., Evans, A., and Rangarajan, S. "Medicaid Managed Care in Thirteen States." *Health Affairs,* 1998, *17*(3), 43–63.
267. O'Connell, Lozier, and Gingles (1997).
268. O'Connell, Lozier, and Gingles (1997).
269. HCH Clinician's Network. "Care for the Homeless: Can Managed Care Work for Homeless People? Guidance for State Medicaid Programs." Nashville, Tenn.: National Health Care for the Homeless Council, 1998.
270. Lewin and Alman (2000).
271. Culhane, D., Eldridge, D., Rosenheck, R., and Wilkins, C. "Making Homelessness Programs Accountable to Consumers, Funders, and the Public." In L. B. Fosburg and D. L. Dennis (eds.), *Practical Lessons: The 1998 National Symposium on Homelessness Research.* Washington, D.C.: Housing and Urban Development, Department of Health and Human Services, 1999.
272. Lewin and Alman (2000).
273. Lewin and Alman (2000).
274. U.S. General Accounting Office. "Homelessness: Coordination and Evaluation of Programs Are Essential." Washington, D.C.: U.S. General Accounting Office, 1999.
275. U.S. General Accounting Office (1999).
276. U.S. General Accounting Office (1999).
277. Stoto, M., Abel, C., and Dievler, A. *Healthy Communities: New Partnerships for the Future of Public Health.* Washington, D.C.: National Academy Press, 1996.

278. U.S. General Accounting Office (1999).

279. Doblin, Gelberg, and Freeman (1992).

280. Gelberg, Linn, and Rosenberg (1988).

281. Gelberg, L., Linn, L. S., and Mayer-Oakes, S. A. "Differences in Health Status Between Older and Younger Homeless Adults." *Journal of the American Geriatrics Society,* 1990, *38,* 1220–1229.

282. Stark (1992); Goetcheus, J., and others. "Convalescence: For Those Without a Home: Developing Respite Services in Protected Environments." In P. Brickner (ed.), *Under the Safety Net.* New York: Norton, 1990.

283. Stark (1992).

284. Goetcheus and others (1990).

285. U.S. Department of Housing and Urban Development (1994).

286. Burt, M., and Cohen, B. "America's Homeless: Numbers, Characteristics and Programs that Serve Them." Urban Institute Report 89–3. Washington: Urban Institute, 1989.

287. U.S. Department of Housing and Urban Development (1994).

288. Doblin, Gelberg, and Freeman (1992).

289. Koegel and Gelberg (1992).

290. National Coalition for the Homeless. '*Tis a Gift to Be Simple: Homelessness, Health Care Reform, and the Single Payer Solution.* Nashville, Ky.: National Health Care for the Homeless Council, 1994.

291. Jahiel (1992).

292. Blasi, G. "And We Are Not Seen: Ideological and Political Barriers to Understanding Homelessness." *American Behavioral Scientist,* 1994, *37*(4), 563–586.

PART FIVE

DIRECTIONS FOR CHANGE

CHAPTER FIFTEEN

MANAGED CARE AND THE GROWTH OF COMPETITION

Gerald F. Kominski and Glenn Melnick

A s we enter the twenty-first century, managed care has become an integral part of the U.S. health care system. In the early 1990s, President Clinton presented a plan for national health care reform that was based on a modified version of managed competition first proposed by Alain Enthoven.[1] Through a combination of newly formed health alliances and competitive bidding by health plans, the incentives of the health care market would have been restructured to encourage price competition in the health care market at both the health plan and provider levels.

Although several significant incremental reforms were enacted by Congress during the 1990s, the failure to pass comprehensive national health care reform legislation meant that responsibility for restructuring the health care system fell primarily on the private sector and individual states. This chapter offers a review and synthesis of the empirical literature on the effects of managed care and competition and discusses the implications of current trends, what we have learned to date, and some directions for future research.

Models of Managed Care

Managed care has existed in the United States for more than seventy years. As early as 1932, the Committee on the Costs of Medical Care called for the practice of medicine in the United States to be reorganized into prepaid group practice.[2] This recommendation acknowledged that the incentives of fee-for-service, solo-practitioner medical practice were inefficient compared to a system where physicians coordinated their care and received a fixed payment in advance for their services. Despite these conceptual advantages, the only prominent prepaid group practice for many years was the nonprofit Kaiser Permanente health plan. During the past two decades, managed care has evolved into a broad concept encompassing a variety of managed care organizations (MCOs) or managed care plans (MCPs), some of which barely resemble prepaid group practice.

Health Maintenance Organizations

Health maintenance organizations (HMOs) are the traditional form of managed care. *Group*-model HMOs contract with a single medical group to provide care to plan members, while *staff*-model HMOs employ physicians directly. In group-model HMOs, the medical group contracts exclusively with the HMO. In both these organizational models providers represent a *closed panel*; that is, providers must be staff or medical group members who do not treat patients outside the HMO.

Group- and staff-model HMOs represent a traditional model of managed care that many physicians view as excessively intrusive and many consumers see as too restrictive because of their closed panels. Therefore, alternative models have evolved that allow physicians greater autonomy in how their practices are organized and permit greater choice for plan members. *Network*-model HMOs contract with multiple medical groups, rather than a single group, while HMOs on the *independent practice association (IPA)* model contract with individual physicians in solo practice. Network- and IPA-model HMOs are typically *open panel*; physicians do not contract exclusively with a single HMO and may continue to treat non-HMO patients.

All forms of HMOs employ some form of gatekeeper, a primary care physician who serves as the initial point of contact for receiving care and who must authorize referrals for specialty care. However, in response to competitive pressures during the 1990s, HMOs have begun offering multiple managed care products, including other forms of managed care (described later).[3] For example, some HMOs offer an open-access product that allows self-referral within the network but imposes increased cost sharing on members who choose this option. These hybrid arrangements are likely to continue growing in response to changing perceptions of what best serves the interests of the health plans, providers, and members.

Preferred Provider Organizations

Preferred provider organizations (PPOs) represent a less restrictive form of managed care than the HMO, mainly because they do not require primary care physicians to serve as gatekeepers and thus permit self-referral to specialists. They are generally formed by employers or insurers who contract with physicians and other providers to create a network of participating or preferred providers. These preferred providers generally agree to follow utilization management guidelines and to accept discounted fee-for-service payments as conditions for participating in the PPO. Health plan members are encouraged to use the preferred provider network through reduced cost sharing, although they are generally covered for care provided by nonparticipating physicians.

Point of Service

Point of service (POS) plans are essentially the same as the open-access HMOs we have already described, but they also provide limited coverage for self-referral outside the network. Members may choose the level of managed care they desire at the point of service, with the degree of cost sharing increasing along with freedom of choice. Members in these three-tier plans who use a gatekeeper (HMO tier) have the lowest co-payments, while those self-referring to network providers (PPO tier) have higher co-payments, and those seeking care outside the network (POS tier) have the highest co-payments.

Growth of Managed Care

Without question, managed care has grown substantially since the early 1970s, when Paul Ellwood's advocacy of health maintenance organizations[4] was translated into national policy as the HMO Act of 1973. This legislation gave federal grants and loans to federally qualified HMOs to promote their expansion. More importantly, it required employers with twenty-five or more employees already offering health insurance coverage to offer at least two HMO options, thus promoting the growth of managed care. By the time Harold Luft published his seminal book on HMO performance in 1981, slightly more than seven million U.S. residents were enrolled in HMOs,[5] and almost half of all HMO members were concentrated in California in a single network, the Kaiser Foundation Health Plans.[6] By 1990, enrollment in HMOs increased fivefold to about thirty-five million in almost seven hundred HMOs across the United States. As the 1990s came to an end, HMO enrollment had more than doubled again, to an estimated eighty-one million, or about 25 percent of the U.S. population.[7] Another seventy-five million are currently enrolled in other forms of managed care, including PPOs and POS plans. Among individuals who obtained health insurance through their place of employment, 86 percent were enrolled in some form of managed care as of 1998.[8] Almost 60 percent of individuals with employment-based coverage are enrolled in PPOs or POS plans, indicating a shift away from traditional HMOs.[9]

A number of factors explain the rapid proliferation of managed care during the past two decades. A primary driving force clearly has been employers seeking lower-cost alternatives to indemnity insurance for their employee health benefit plans. At the start of this period of growth, the cost advantages of HMOs were most thoroughly documented by Luft, who found that the long-term cost savings of HMOs were primarily attributable to a lower rate of hospitalization, rather than improved productivity or lower input costs.[10] Thus, although the empirical evidence did not suggest that HMOs would produce substantial savings, they nevertheless gave employers an alternative to the inflationary incentives of indemnity-based, fee-for-service health benefits.

In the early years of managed care, employees faced a complex decision in choosing whether to enroll in an HMO. One major advantage was a reduction in out-of-pocket expenditures associated with most HMOs. Prior to the mid-1980s, however, this financial advantage was offset by having a limited choice of providers and by having to obtain gatekeeper approval before seeking specialty care. These disadvantages of the traditional HMO spurred development of less-restrictive forms of managed care—PPOs and POS plans, discussed earlier. Advocates of managed care cite this ability of the industry to innovate and create new products that vary across markets in response to consumer demand as a major advantage of market-driven reform.

In addition to these cost considerations on the part of employers and employees, managed care also has the potential to improve quality of care, at least in part because of the financial incentives facing providers. In theory, managed care has the potential to improve coordination of care through clinical management of entire episodes of care, develop information systems to assist in care coordination, identify and eliminate wasteful or ineffective practices, and identify and manage care for the costliest conditions (such as those involving chronic illness).

In summary, managed care has grown rapidly during the past two decades, according to some early empirical evidence of cost savings and on the expectation that financial incentives would lead to improved coordination of care and thus better quality. What does the evidence show about how it has actually changed the health care system?

California and the Development of Competitive Markets

An essential element of the development of the managed care market is competition among health plans and the interaction between health plans and consumers. These interrelationships can have important implications for ongoing product innovation and the overall development of the managed care market. To better understand this process, it is instructive to examine the evolution of the managed care market in California and its impact on restructuring the state's health care system.

In June 1982, the California legislature adopted what was to become model legislation for the nation, designed to encourage price competition in the health care sector. The law explicitly permitted formation of health plans that contracted with selected, or "preferred," providers. This legislation allowed the state's Medicaid program, known as MediCal, as well as private insurance companies to contract with a subset of licensed hospitals to which it would channel its enrollees in return for signing participating contracts. The contracts often required price concessions and increased utilization review oversight in order to control both price and use of health services. The law allowed the growth of HMOs and created the conditions necessary for the formation of PPOs.

In the early 1980s, less than 20 percent of the state's insured population was enrolled in managed care plans (most of them being in the Kaiser Permanente HMO). In the years following introduction of the law, the number of plans in California peaked at more than one hundred. Through increased competition and ongoing consolidation as the market matures, the number of plans has been substantially reduced; as of the end of 1999, about fifty-two plans were licensed to operate in the state.[11]

With the passage of California's selective contracting law, health insurance plans had greater flexibility to develop alternative health insurance patterns and to test design features in order to attract subscribers. This increased competition in the health insurance market led to a burst of innovation and a proliferation of choices available to consumers. For example, PPOs grew rapidly by offering a wide choice of providers in their networks. In addition, they combined this feature with lower monthly premiums (compared to prevailing standard fee-for-service indemnity plans) and financial incentives to use network providers, while still affording some financial coverage for out-of-network utilization. The number of people voluntarily selecting these plans that include some reduction in their choice of provider grew dramatically. At the same time, innovations in the HMO market were being tested. The number of HMOs competing with Kaiser and with PPOs grew rapidly.

The new HMOs differed dramatically from Kaiser in ways that made them attractive to both providers and consumers. Physicians could join an HMO either as individuals or as part of an IPA or group practice. Hospitals, likewise, could contract with the plans selectively. Consumers had a wide choice of private providers in these plans, and the monthly premium was generally less than with conventional indemnity plans.

During this same period, employers began changing their fringe benefit contribution rates for health insurance, requiring employees to pay more from their monthly paychecks if they selected plans with higher premiums. The response of consumers to these changes has been remarkable. Voluntary enrollment in managed care plans grew so rapidly that within ten years a majority of the privately insured population had joined some type of managed care plan offering lower monthly premiums in return for some restrictions on choice of provider. This shift from general indemnity health insurance to managed care plans requiring consumers to accept some restrictions on providers and hospitals was largely caused by market forces, but it was also assisted by government action encouraging those forces. The basis for this dramatic restructuring of the health care system is the increased role of price competition in the health care sector among providers and health insurance plans, and more efficient pricing in the health insurance market.

As might be expected, the supply side of the health market also underwent dramatic changes. As the number of people joining managed care health plans grew, health plans had to add capacity to their provider networks to handle the increased volume. Consequently, the percentage of physicians and hospitals contracting with managed care plans has increased substantially. The growth in enrollment in health plans gives the plans greater bargaining power when negotiating with providers for participation in their networks. To counter this growing power on the part of health plans, providers began consolidating to form their own networks. These networks allowed for expanded primary care capacity within local areas as well as wider geographic coverage.

Impact of Managed Care

In the traditional setting, hospitals compete on the basis of services, technology, and amenities to attract physicians and their patients.[12] Physicians' ability to deliver quality care and compete for patients depends in part on the range of services that they can provide. Hospitals partially control the range of available services by deciding what specialized equipment and staff they will invest in. In negotiating with hospitals, physicians can increase their bargaining leverage by credibly threatening to shift their patients to another hospital. Hospitals, in turn, can remove admitting privileges from physicians who do not bring in many patients. Lack of admitting privileges to a highly regarded local hospital could put a physician at a competitive disadvantage.

Price Competition Among Insurers

Introducing selective contracting and managed care risk contracts changes the economic incentives faced by both insurers and providers. The ability to assemble preferred provider networks endows insurers with the potential power to channel patients away from more expensive providers. Insurers, competing with one another for subscribers, have both a financial incentive and the benefit of economies of scale to search the market for an optimal mix of high-quality and low-price providers. Under such conditions, insurance carriers can leverage excess capacity and competitive hospital market conditions to negotiate lower prices with health care providers.

In theory, effective use of the selective contracting mechanism can generate savings for insurers, thereby leading to price advantages over other insurers who pay "too much." Such price advantages could be important in building or maintaining a subscriber base in a competitive insurance market. However, selective contracting plans operate under constraints that in all likelihood prevent them from choosing providers solely by price. If payers use only a price criterion in choosing providers, they may assemble too limited a network, thereby putting themselves at risk of diminishing their subscriber base because of unacceptable quality or access. Thus, payers must assess the relative attractiveness of individual hospitals to consumers before choosing which hospitals to exclude for reasons of high price.

Faced with the pressure to reduce prices or risk being excluded from an insurer's network, providers must also balance tradeoffs in negotiating with selective contracting plans. They must assess their importance to the insurer's network, which determines the likelihood of being excluded should they refuse to grant requested price concessions. Their ability to retain patients should the contract not be offered influences their bargaining position.

Previous research on the early effects of selective contracting in California indicates that restructuring the health care market can lead to increased price competition and lower cost growth. Melnick, Zwanziger, Bamezai, and Pattison found that increasing price sensitivity on the part of buyers has resulted in increased price competition among hospitals, leading them to offer price discounts to secure contracts with managed care plans.[13] Hospitals lowered their costs when faced with competitive pressure on their prices exerted by managed care plans.[14]

Previous published studies showing that competition can lead to smaller increases in hospital costs and prices have been limited in several ways. Because they were done soon after the introduction of price competition, they do not address the question of whether the cost-containment effects can be sustained over a long period of time, or if they are simply a one-time reduction followed by increases at previous rates.

Zwanziger, Melnick, and Bamezai addressed the question of whether price competition in California resulted in a long-term and sustained reduction in hospital expenditures.[15] This analysis was designed to isolate and compare the effects of competition on hospital revenues prior to and following the growth of managed care plans. Hospitals in the most and least competitive market quartiles (as defined by quartile distribution) were identified and their net revenues were calculated for each year from 1980 to 1990, controlling for all other factors. If competition were effective in controlling hospital expenditures, revenues would be lower for hospitals in more competitive markets than for hospitals in less competitive markets after enactment of selective contracting legislation in 1982.

In the period 1980–1982, before the introduction of price competition, hospital expenditures in the most competitive markets (quartile) were 13.75 percent higher than those in the least (quartile) competitive markets. Beginning in the years immediately following the introduction of California's procompetition law, the difference in hospital expenditures between hospitals in the highly competitive markets and least competitive markets began a steady and sustained decline. In 1983–84, hospitals in high-competition markets collected 11.13 percent more revenue than hospitals in the least competitive markets. The difference in net revenue between hospitals in the most competitive and least competitive markets continued to narrow in each subsequent year. Finally, by 1989–90, the difference in net revenues between hospitals in highly competitive markets compared with those in the least competitive markets had reversed its historic relationship. Hospitals in markets with the greatest competitive pressure received 1.62 percent less revenue per year than those facing the least competitive pressure.

Hospital Prices

Despite rapid growth in health plans that feature selective contracting, there is very little empirical evidence in the literature concerning its effects on hospital prices. The desired outcome is lower prices, but some researchers caution that endowing insurers with substantial market power could have a negative impact. For instance, Pauly suggests that in areas where an insurance carrier commands a large share of the health insurance market, it may exploit its position to gain greater discounts.[16] Hospitals in these areas may be so hampered by revenue constraints that serious reductions in quality of care could occur, or financial losses could eventually threaten their viability.

Several studies have addressed these issues both theoretically and empirically.[17] One of the best empirical tests of these issues, to date, was conducted by Staten, Umbeck, and Dunkelberg.[18] They evaluated the effects of hospital market structure and insurer market share on the discount rate that hospitals offered to gain acceptance into the newly formed Blue Cross of Indiana PPO. They compared historical charges with the initial proposed bid for each hospital to calculate the discount rate. These discount rates were regressed on two alternative measures of hospital market structure (sole hospital in the county, or number of hospitals in the county) and two alternative measures of Blue Cross market share (Blue Cross share of the individual hospital's volume, and Blue Cross share of the private market). The ratio of inpatient days per bed for a one-month period was included as a measure of capacity use. The study found that hospitals located in counties with more competitors offered greater discounts and that higher Blue Cross share at either the hospital or the market level did not significantly lower the proposed discounts offered by hospitals.[19]

Melnick, Zwanziger, Bamezai, and Pattison conducted a study of hospital prices that was designed to conduct an improved empirical test of these issues.[20] This study used actual hospital price data from one of the oldest and largest PPOs in the country. The data set contained per diem prices paid by the PPO in 1987, which was nearly five years after its formation. By this time, the PPO and its hospital network had been involved in several rounds of negotiation, allowing provider membership in the PPO to solidify into a more or less stable network and the per diem contract prices to reflect a stable pattern of relative price difference between facilities. In addition, the measure of hospital market structure is empirically derived from patient-origin data.

The results indicated that prices paid to hospitals in the Blue Cross of California PPO network, after controlling for hospital product differences, were strongly influenced by the competitive structure of the hospital market.[21] Hospitals located in less competitive markets were able to secure higher prices. The estimated value of the coefficient for the Herfindahl-Hirschman index (HHI), a measure of market competition, was 0.11–0.13. To illustrate the effect of the HHI on prices, consider a market where a merger leads to three competitors becoming two. Assuming that the competitors have equal market shares, the HHI would change from 0.33 to 0.50, an increase of 50 percent. Such a reduction in the level of competition would lead, on average, to an estimated price increase of approximately 9 percent.

These findings on the relative bargaining position of the hospital and the PPO offer some insight into payer strategies for network design and network pruning. They suggest that consolidating a payer's business in fewer hospitals produces offsetting price effects. The consolidation increases the importance of the PPO to the hospital, enabling the PPO to extract bigger price discounts. At the same time, however, the payer becomes more dependent on those hospitals and must eventually pay them higher rates. Hospital mergers and consolidations in a competitive market also contribute to higher prices, even among nonprofits.[22]

High-occupancy hospitals in markets with little excess capacity receive much higher prices than expected. These results are particularly striking since neither hospital occupancy nor the average occupancy of the other hospitals in the market individually affects prices. Only a relatively small number of hospitals have a high occupancy rate, defined as 75 percent or greater. Still, the results show how important the availability of excess capacity is to the PPO in maintaining a credible threat to move patients elsewhere. If this spare capacity becomes too small, the negotiated price paid by the PPO increases dramatically.

The results illustrate some of the subtleties involved in developing hospital networks. In general, it pays for plans to contract with mid-sized hospitals where they can gain greater leverage with the same patient volume than in larger hospitals, which can absorb a greater number of Blue Cross patient-days without becoming too dependent on a single payer. In addition, these findings suggest that increased consolidation among plans leads to greater hospital cost savings since the importance of a single hospital diminishes, the larger the plan size. Factors other than minimum price are important for the PPO to consider in determining the configuration of its networks.

Kralewski and others identified factors that affect the ability of HMOs to secure hospital discounts.[23] By analyzing hospital-HMO contracts, hospital operating characteristics, and market conditions, they determined that the level of risk sharing, the number of hospitals within a five-mile radius, the proportion of the population enrolled in HMOs, and the number of HMOs operating in the metropolitan statistical area (MSA) were directly related to the ability of HMOs to offer discounts. Further analysis showed that higher cost sharing by enrollees, a larger number of hospitals within a five-mile radius, and more HMOs operating within an MSA results in greater discounts. This suggests that competitive HMO markets do lead to price concessions for hospital services. Hospitals are using discounts as one way to attract HMO business and garner market share.

In addition, Feldman, Kralewski, Shapiro, and Chan found that in competitive health care markets hospitals have to compete with each other for managed care patients by offering discounts for inpatient services.[24] Specifically, staff- and network-model HMOs can extract larger discounts from hospitals compared to an IPA or a group-model HMO because they usually have higher patient enrollment.

HMOs, however, do not always seek the services of hospitals offering the lowest prices. Another study by Feldman and colleagues found that HMOs use different criteria in contracting with hospitals.[25] Low prices, an important element, nonetheless are only one aspect taken into consideration. Of six HMOs reviewed in this study, four network- and group-model HMOs placed price as the most important factor and sought discounts intensely, while two IPA-model HMOs focused more on access and quality rather than seeking the lowest prices. Consequently, these two HMOs contracted with more hospitals within the community.

Health Care Expenditures

Since the time of rapid growth in managed care in the early 1980s, several studies have further confirmed the original findings summarized in Luft's work on HMO performance.[26] The best overall summary of the empirical literature regarding the impact of managed care after 1980 was conducted by Miller and Luft.[27] This literature review supported Luft's earlier findings that HMOs produced significantly lower hospital admission rates compared to indemnity plans. The most significant finding was from the Medical Outcomes Studies, which found admission rates 26–37 percent lower in HMOs.[28]

Discussion of the savings of managed care relative to indemnity insurance is quickly diminishing as a relevant issue in the United States. Given the substantial portion of the population already enrolled in managed care, a more relevant question for the future is, Can competition between health plans control the rate of growth in health care expenditures?[29] As we have discussed, there is empirical evidence that competitive markets have had a lower rate of growth in hospital expenditures. Other evidence supports the conclusion that total health care expenditures grew more slowly in California relative to the rest of the nation in the mid-1990s owing to the increasingly competitive market.[30] However, a number of markets continue to have little competition, and at least 35 percent of employees nationwide are offered only a single health plan by their employers.[31] Therefore, the conditions for managed competition still do not exist in many areas of the United States.[32] Consequently, despite the proliferation of managed care during the 1990s, its potential for containment of national health expenditures has not been fully realized.

Quality of Care

During the 1990s, California was in the forefront in developing a health care market based not only on price competition but also on value-based purchasing.[33] The efforts of several large purchasing groups, notably the California Public Employees Retirement System (CalPERS, representing state, county, and municipal employees), the University of California (UC), the Pacific Business Group on Health (PBGH, representing thirty-three large private and public purchasers), and the Pacific Health Advantage (formerly the Health Insurance Plan of California, representing small employers), were central to transforming the market. PBGH (which includes CalPERS and UC) played a central role in collecting enrollee satisfaction data, requiring that Health Plan Data and Information Set (HEDIS) data made available by participating health plans be audited independently, and conducting several independent surveys assessing health plan performance (including provider satisfaction with health plans).[34] The California Office of Statewide Health Planning and Development (OSHPD), and more recently PBGH, sponsored several major studies to develop risk-adjusted measures of hospital outcomes for individual clinical conditions, such as acute myocardial infarction, that are then published as public report cards.[35]

Although the capacity for meaningful quality reporting is being established in California and other markets across the United States, a fundamental question still remains: Is the overall quality of managed care plans better than that of indemnity plans? Again, Miller and Luft have conducted the most thorough review of the existing literature.[36] They indicate that the evidence regarding HMOs and quality is rather mixed, except with regard to Medicare beneficiaries with chronic conditions who had worse quality in several studies.[37] They conclude that concerns about diminished quality under managed care are not fully warranted, but that quality improvements are also less than anticipated. They cite entrenched patterns of clinical practice, inadequate risk-adjustment methods for capitation rates, and deficient measurement and reporting of quality indicators as continuing barriers to quality improvement.[38]

Future Challenges

Managed care has clearly produced a revolution in the U.S. health care delivery system.[39] The elements of managed competition, outlined by Enthoven more than two decades ago, have slowly evolved in various markets throughout the country, most notably in California. Managed care has become entrenched in the health care market, and the predominant form of health care delivery, albeit in continuously evolving organizational forms. Along with its rapid growth during the 1990s, managed care has also experienced an increasing level of popular dissatisfaction and bad publicity, as newspapers and other media constitute regular outlets for some of the most common complaints against managed care.

This popular discontent is typically referred to as the managed care backlash.[40] The most dramatic examples are individual stories of denied care or benefits. In several extreme cases, denial of treatment has resulted in enormous legal settlements against managed care plans. As managed care has become so pervasive, so have examples of denied treatment—even among health care researchers, as evidenced by several recent accounts in the academic literature documenting the personal experiences of researchers with managed care denials.[41]

Employers are also increasingly dissatisfied with what they view as the unfulfilled promise of managed care. A national coalition of large purchasers who have led the development of value-based purchasing—including PBGH, General Electric, General Motors, and the Buyers Health Care Action Group of Minneapolis—view managed care as entering a period of market gridlock.[42] According to these large purchasers, two important changes are necessary in the current market. First, physicians must take greater responsibility for reorganizing the practice of medicine to improve quality and to achieve greater efficiency, a role the profession has abdicated to managed care.[43] Second, performance and outcomes measures must evolve into a new set of more compelling measures focused on patient safety, and consumers should play a greater role in developing and advocating these new measures. Of course, many current outcome measures, such as the risk-adjusted mortality reports produced in California and elsewhere, are examples of this type of safety-oriented measure. Translating these reports into compelling information that changes consumer and provider behavior continues to be a challenge, however.[44]

National health expenditures and health insurance premiums began to grow more rapidly in 1998,[45] after a period of unprecedented slow growth during the mid-1990s that was viewed by many advocates of managed care as evidence that competition was finally working to contain overall health care costs. If the savings associated with managed care are primarily due to lower hospitalization rates and favorable risk selection, health care costs should begin to increase again as these sources of one-time savings are exhausted. An alternative explanation for the slow growth in health care expenditures during this period is that health plans sustained short-term losses to compete for market share.[46] Kaiser Permanente, for example, incurred losses of more than $500 million in California during this period before seeking premium increases of more than 10 percent in 1999 and 2000. Thus, dissatisfaction with managed care as a cost-containment strategy is likely to increase if health care costs begin accelerating.

Selection bias continues to be an important problem, particularly given the inadequate status of risk-adjustment mechanisms. The promise of managed care and managed competition is difficult to realize fully unless health plans have incentives to enroll all levels of risk. Although adequate risk-adjusted payment systems have been developed for hospital inpatient and outpatient services under the Medicare program, risk-adjusting capitation rates has proven more difficult,[47] primarily because of the difficulty in identifying a priori who in the population is likely to experience high-cost acute events. As with Diagnosis-Related Group, or DRG-based, prospective payment for hospitals, which required more than a decade of methodological development before it was ready for implementation, risk-adjusted capitation may require a large-scale commitment of federal funding over the next few years. After all, if researchers can map the human genome, developing a reasonably reliable predictive model of personal health care expenditures that can be used to risk-adjust capitation rates should be possible.

Conclusion

In summary, there is an emerging empirical literature demonstrating that competition in the hospital sector can lead to lower hospital costs and lower prices for major purchasers. Third-party plans that use selective contracting (PPOs and

HMOs) can leverage competitive market conditions to negotiate lower prices with hospitals. However, the way in which these insurance plans design and manage their hospital networks is important in determining the benefits ultimately derived by the consumers of health care services. The effectiveness of selective contracting as a cost and price control method is highly dependent on the existence of a sufficient level of competition in the market. This suggests that both third-party payers through their contracting activities and government agencies through regulatory oversight must ensure that market conditions remain competitive.

Given the rapid growth of managed care throughout the United States, additional research into the various effects of the significant structural changes brought about by managed care is essential. Along with more analysis on costs, prices, and expenditures, it is necessary to conduct research into the quality and access implications of a competitive system. There has been insufficient research on how managed care plans are able to achieve their cost savings, and whether the savings come from increased efficiency or reduced quality. Further, findings from California indicate that increased price competition leads to reduced access for the uninsured population.[48] These findings underscore the importance of reforming the health insurance system to include everyone.

Notes

1. The elements of managed competition were first described in Enthoven, A. C. "Consumer Choice Health Plan: A National Health Insurance Proposal Based on Regulated Competition in the Private Sector." *New England Journal of Medicine,* 1978, *298,* 709–720; and later refined in Enthoven, A. C., and Kronick, R. "A Consumer-Choice Health Plan for the 1990s." *New England Journal of Medicine,* 1989, *320,* 29–37, 94–101.

2. Committee on the Costs of Medical Care. *Medical Care for the American People: The Final Report.* Chicago: University of Chicago Press, 1932.

3. Gold, M., and Hurley, R. "The Role of Managed Care 'Products' in Managed Care 'Plans.'" *Inquiry,* 1997, *34,* 29–37; and Gabel, J., Whitmore, H., Bergsten, C., and Grimm, L. "Growing Diversification in HMOs, 1988–1994." *Medical Care Research and Review,* 1997, *54,* 101–117.

4. Ellwood, P. and others. "Health Maintenance Strategy." *Medical Care,* 1971, *9,* 291–298.

5. Luft, H. S. *Health Maintenance Organizations: Dimensions of Performance.* New York: Wiley, 1981. See also Luft, H. S. "How Do Health-Maintenance Organizations Achieve Their 'Savings?'" *New England Journal of Medicine,* 1978, *298,* 1336–1343.

6. Gruber, L., Shadle, M., and Polich, C. "From Movement to Industry: The Growth of HMOs." *Health Affairs,* 1988, *7,* 197–208.

7. InterStudy Publications. [http://www.hmodata.com]

8. Levit, K., and others. "Health Spending in 1998: Signals of Change." *Health Affairs,* Jan.–Feb. 2000, *19,* 124–32; and Marquis, M. S., and Long, S. H. "Trends in

Managed Care and Managed Competition 1993–1997." *Health Affairs*, Nov.–Dec. 1999, *18*, 75-88.

9. Levitt, L., and others. *Employer Health Benefits, 1999 Annual Survey.* Menlo Park, Calif.: Henry J. Kaiser Family Foundation, and Chicago: Health Research and Educational Trust, 1999. [http://www.kff.org/content/1999/1538/KFF.pdf]

10. Luft (1981).

11. California Department of Managed Health Care. [http://www.dmhc.ca.gov]

12. Newhouse, J. P. "Toward a Theory of Non-Profit Institutions: An Economic Model of a Hospital." *American Economic Review*, 1970, *60*, 4–74; Pauly, M. V., and Redisch, M. "The Not-for-Profit Hospital as a Physicians' Cooperative." *American Economic Review*, 1973, *63*, 87–99; Harris, J. "The Internal Organization of Hospitals: Some Economic Implications." *Bell Journal of Economics and Management Science*, 1977, *8*, 467–482; and Ellis, R. P., and McGuire, T. G. "Provider Behavior Under Prospective Reimbursement: Cost Sharing and Supply." *Journal of Health Economics*, 1986, *5*, 129–151.

13. Melnick, G. A., Zwanziger, J., Bamezai, A., and Pattison, R. "The Effects of Market Structure and Hospital Bargaining Position on Hospital Prices." *Journal of Health Economics*, 1992, *11*, 217–233.

14. Robinson, J. C. "Decline in Hospital Utilization and Cost Inflation Under Managed Care in California." *Journal of the American Medical Association*, 1996, 276, 1060–1064; Robinson, J. C. "HMO Market Penetration and Hospital Cost Inflation in California." *Journal of the American Medical Association*, 1991, *266*, 2719–2123; and Melnick, G. A., and Zwanziger, J. "Hospital Behavior Under Competition and Cost Containment Policies: The California Experience." *Journal of the American Medical Association*, 1988, *260*, 2669–2675.

15. Zwanziger, J., Melnick, G. A., and Bamezai, A. "Cost and Price Competition in California Hospitals, 1980–1990." *Health Affairs*, 1994, *13*, 1994, 118–126.

16. Pauly, M. V. "Monopsony Power in Health Insurance: Thinking Straight While Standing on Your Head." *Journal of Health Economics*, 1987, *6*, 73–81.

17. Pauly (1987); Pauly, M. V. "Reply: A Response To Market Share/Market Power Revisited." *Journal of Health Economics*, 1988, *7*, 85–87; Pauly, M. V. "Market Power Monopsony, and Health Insurance Markets." *Journal of Health Economics*, 1988, *7*, 111–128; Staten, M., Dunkelberg, W., and Umbeck, J. "Market Share and the Illusion of Power: Can Blue Cross Force Hospitals to Discount?" *Journal of Health Economics*, 1987, *6*, 43–58; and Staten, M., Umbeck, J., and Dunkelberg, W. "Market Share/Market Power Revisited: A New Test for an Old Theory." *Journal of Health Economics*, 1988, *7*, 73–83.

18. Staten, Umbeck, and Dunkelberg (1988).

19. Although the paper by Staten and colleagues (1988) offered the first analysis of hospital prices under PPO arrangements, it has several important limitations. The dependent variable, the discount rate, was calculated using the initial bid proposed by the hospital and not the final price agreed upon between the PPO and the hospital. Thus, their measure is likely to overestimate the final price agreed upon by hospitals in the PPO contract.

20. Melnick, Zwanziger, Bamezai, and Pattison (1992).

21. Melnick, Zwanziger, Bamezai, and Pattison (1992).

22. Keeler, E., Melnick, G. A., and Zwanziger, J. "The Changing Effects of Competition on Non-profit and For-Profit Hospital Pricing Behavior." *Journal of Health Economics*, 1999, *18*, 9–86; and Melnick, G. A., Keeler, E., and Zwanziger, J. "Market Power and Hospital Pricing: Are Nonprofits Different?" *Health Affairs*, May–June 1999, *18*, 167–173.

23. Kralewski, E., and others. "Factors Related to the Provision of Hospital Discounts for HMO Inpatients." *Health Services Research*, 1992, *27*, 133–153.

24. Feldman, R., and others. "Effects of HMOs on the Creation of Competitive Markets for Hospital Services." *Journal of Health Economics*, 1990, *9*, 207–222.

25. Feldman, R., Kralewski, J., Shapiro, J., and Chan, H. C. "Contracts Between Hospitals and Health Maintenance Organizations." *Health Care Management Review*, 1990, *15*, 47–60.

26. Luft (1981).

27. Miller, R. H., and Luft, H. S. "Managed Care Plan Performance Since 1980: A Literature Analysis." *Journal of the American Medical Association*, 1994, *271*, 1512–1519.

28. Greenfield, S., and others. "Variations in Resource Utilization Among Medical Specialties and Systems of Care: Results from the Medical Outcomes Study." *Journal of the American Medical Association*, 1992, *267*, 1624–1630.

29. Enthoven, A. C. "Why Managed Care Has Failed to Contain Health Costs." *Health Affairs*, 1993, *12*, 28–43.

30. Melnick, G. A., and Zwanziger, J. "State Health Care Expenditures Under Competition and Regulation, 1980 through 1991." *American Journal of Public Health*, Oct. 1995, *85*, 1391–1396; Robinson, J. C. "Health Care Purchasing and Market Changes in California." *Health Affairs*, 1995, *14*, 118–130; and Enthoven, A. C., and Singer, S. J. "Managed Competition and California's Health Care Economy." *Health Affairs*, 1996, *15*, 40–57.

31. Levitt and others (1999), Figure 5.2, p. 45. Another recent study estimates that 57 percent of employees have no choice of health plans from their employers, and that employee choice actually declined from 1993 to 1997. See also Marquis and Long (1999).

32. Marquis and Long (1999).

33. Luft, H. S. "Modifying Managed Competition to Address Cost and Quality." *Health Affairs*, 1996, *15*, 24–38.

34. Pacific Business Group on Health. "PBGH's Commitment to Quality Improvement." [http://www.pbgh.org/PBGH_folder/quality.html]

35. See, for example, Kominski, G. F., and Andrews, R. *Report on Health Attack Outcomes in California 1994–1996.* Vol. 1: *User's Guide.* Sacramento: California Office of Statewide Planning and Development, 2001.

36. Miller, R. H., and Luft, H. S. "Does Managed Care Lead to Better or Worse Quality of Care?" *Health Affairs*, Sept.–Oct. 1997, *16*, 7–25.

37. See, for example, Wholey, D. R., Burns, L. R., and Lavizzo-Mourey, R. "Managed Care and the Delivery of Primary Care to the Elderly and the Chronically Ill." *Health Services Research*, 1998, *33*(2), Part II, 322–353.

38. Miller and Luft (1997).

39. Marquis and Long (1999); Bodenheimer, T., and Sullivan, K. "How Large Employers Are Shaping the Health Care Marketplace." *New England Journal of Medicine*, 1998, *338*, 1003–1007, 1084–1087; and Kuttner, R. "The American Health Care System: Employer-Sponsored Health Insurance." *New England Journal of Medicine*, 1999, *340*, 248–252.

40. Blendon, R. J., and others. "Understanding the Managed Care Backlash." *Health Affairs*, July–Aug. 1998, *17*, 80–94; Enthoven, A. C., and Singer, S. J. "The Managed Care Backlash and the Task Force in California." *Health Affairs*, July–Aug. 1998, *17*, 95–110.

41. See, for example, Batavia, A. "Of Wheelchairs and Managed Care." *Health Affairs*, Nov.–Dec. 1999, *18*, 177–182; Singer, S. J. "What's Not to Like About HMOs: A Managed Care Maven Struggles with an HMO Runaround at a Vulnerable Time." *Health Affairs*, July–Aug. 2000, *19*, 206–209.

42. Galvin, R. S. "An Employer's View of the U.S. Health Care Market: As Managed Care Is Maturing into Market Gridlock, Employers and Providers Need a Common Definition of Value." *Health Affairs,* Nov.–Dec. 1999, *18,* 166–170.

43. Gray, B. "Trust and Trustworthy Care in the Managed Care Era." *Health Affairs,* Jan.–Feb. 1997, *16,* 34–49.

44. Epstein, A. M. "Rolling Down the Runway: The Challenges Ahead for Quality Report Cards." *Journal of the American Medical Association,* 1998, *279,* 1691–1696.

45. Levit and others (2000).

46. Sullivan, K. "On the 'Efficiency' of Managed Care Plans." *Health Affairs,* July–Aug. 2000, *19,* 139–148.

47. Newhouse, J. P. "Risk Adjustment: Where Are We Now?" *Inquiry,* 1998, *35,* 122–131; and Dudley, R. A., Rennie, D. J., and Luft, H. S. "Population Choice and Variable Selection in the Estimation and Application of Risk Models." *Inquiry,* 1999, *36,* 200–211.

48. Mann, J., Melnick, G. A., Bemazai, A., and Zwanziger, J. "Uncompensated Care: Hospital Responses to Fiscal Pressures." *Health Affairs,* 1995 *14,* 263–270.

CHAPTER SIXTEEN

MEDICARE REFORM

Jeanne T. Black and Gerald F. Kominski

Medicare was enacted in 1965 as a compromise on the road toward a comprehensive system of national health insurance. Like most great compromises, its original design reflected prevailing concepts about health benefits and health care delivery that have changed substantially in the last thirty-five years. As the second largest social insurance program in the United States after Social Security, Medicare continues to provide tremendous benefit to beneficiaries and their families, who might otherwise individually bear the entire health care costs associated with aging. More than a safety net, Medicare gives seniors and the disabled access to the highest-quality health care. But as the United States enters the twenty-first century, Medicare is facing several significant challenges that threaten the very principles on which the program was originally based.

This chapter begins with a review of the origins of Medicare as an alternative, incremental strategy developed after decades of failed attempts to enact comprehensive national health insurance.[1] We then discuss how Medicare has evolved, including its benefit structure and payment mechanisms, to meet various challenges since its enactment in 1965. Next we review the current challenges facing Medicare, including the demographic threat to its long-term solvency. Finally, we discuss recent proposals to transform Medicare from a defined benefits program to one based on defined contributions, and how such proposals can be expected to affect costs, access, quality, and the scope of benefits.

Origin and Philosophy of Medicare

The United States stands alone among developed nations in not providing universal health coverage to its population. Proposals for national health insurance in the United States were first made before World War I. Following the Great Depression, every decade of the twentieth century saw major proposals put forward that failed to win approval in the U.S. Congress. At the root of this failure are fundamental ideological differences between liberal and conservative policy makers. Historically, liberals have advocated a system of social insurance, while conservatives have favored a welfare approach that extends assistance only to those who cannot fend for themselves in the private market.

The theory of social insurance recognizes that the benefits and costs of capitalism are not equally distributed within society, and that in a democracy government has a role in tempering the impact of a competitive market economy on individuals.[2] Thus, the United States has social insurance programs to cushion the financial impact of occupational injuries, unemployment, and poverty in old age. In general, social insurance programs share three principles:

1. Pooled risk, because serious illness is unpredictable
2. Redistribution of income through the tax system, to achieve affordable coverage for all
3. National administration, to ensure universal access

Although the United States has failed to adopt a system of universal coverage for all residents, it does have a program of social health insurance for its elderly population. The Medicare program, enacted on July 30, 1965, as Title XVIII of the Social Security Act, is the most important piece of health insurance legislation in U.S. history. Its passage raises a fundamental question: Why was Medicare enacted rather than universal health insurance? To answer this question, and to understand how Medicare evolved as well as current proposals for its reform, requires a brief review of the history of national health insurance initiatives in the United States.

The first efforts to promote national health insurance in the United States grew out of the Progressive movement that emerged during the first decade of the twentieth century. Those efforts were based on European models of compulsory social insurance, first enacted into law by Chancellor Otto von Bismarck of Germany in 1883. The leaders of the American Medical Association (AMA), having positive views of the German and British systems, initially were supportive of the progressives' efforts.[3] However, the AMA soon found that local medical societies were vehemently opposed. By 1920, the medical profession solidified its opposition to comprehensive health reform, a position that it maintained throughout the remainder of the twentieth century. Conversely, organized labor, which initially feared that government programs such as compulsory social insurance would lessen workers' need to join labor unions, later became an outspoken advocate of national health insurance.

Calls for health reform to address rising medical costs are not a recent phenomenon. In 1927, eight private foundations established the Committee on the Costs of Medical Care. The committee's final report, published in 1932, called for reorganizing health care delivery into prepaid medical group practice, and for promoting experiments in voluntary health insurance. Voicing its opposition, the *Journal of the American Medical Association* editorialized against "the forces representing the great foundations, public health officialdom, social theory—even socialism and communism" that were threatening the "sound practice of medicine."[4]

Following the Great Depression, President Franklin Delano Roosevelt established the Committee on Economic Security. Its recommendations formed the basis for the package of social legislation known as the New Deal, which included the Social Security Act of 1935. However, the committee's consideration of health insurance brought an immediate storm of criticism from the AMA. As a result, Roosevelt did not publicly support national health insurance, fearing that passage of his entire program—and his reelection—could be jeopardized by its inclusion. At the same time, the AMA, suspicious of future government involvement in health care, began to support the private, voluntary hospital insurance programs begun by Blue Cross and commercial insurance companies, and state Blue Shield programs for surgical and medical expenses.[5]

Despite the failure to enact a national health insurance program as part of the New Deal, support for such a program remained strong in Congress. Every year between 1939 and 1951, a comprehensive health insurance bill sponsored by Senator Robert Wagner (D-N.Y.), Senator James Murray (D-Mont.), and Representative John Dingell, Sr. (D-Mich.), was introduced into Congress. Over this thirteen-year period, the Murray-Wagner-Dingell bills never received enough support to be reported out of committee, and thus these bills never reached a vote on the floor of the House or Senate. In 1948, Harry Truman campaigned for president with national health insurance as part of his Fair Deal platform. Once elected, however, he was unable to overcome the opposition of a coalition of Republicans and Southern Democrats. The AMA mounted a nationwide campaign promoting the horrors of "socialized medicine," and several supporters of national health insurance failed to win reelection in 1950.[6]

By the early 1950s, Truman's advisors in the Federal Security Agency (now the Department of Health and Human Services) were convinced that a new strategy was necessary. They concluded that progress toward national health insurance required a more limited, incremental approach. Popular support for the Social Security program meant that a health insurance program for the elderly stood the greatest chance of approval. Linking a program of Medicare to Social Security had the added benefit of avoiding the stigma associated with a welfare program and portraying Medicare as analogous to private insurance for which the beneficiary has paid.

A program to address the needs of the elderly was also more difficult for the AMA to oppose. In the words of Robert M. Ball, who worked on the initial Medicare proposals and later became a Social Security Commissioner:

> The elderly were an appealing group to cover first in part because they were so ill suited for coverage under voluntary private insurance. They used on average more than twice as many hospital days as younger people but had only about half as much income. Private insurers, who set premiums to cover current costs, had to charge them much more, and the elderly could not afford the charges. Group health insurance, then as today, was mostly for the employed and was just not available to the retired elderly. The result of all this was that somewhat less than half of the elderly had any kind of health insurance, and what they had was almost always inadequate. . . . So the need was not hard to prove, nor was it difficult to prove that voluntary individual insurance was not only not meeting the need, but that it really could not meet the need.[7]

In order to win political support, it also was crucial for Medicare not to be viewed as a threat to the existing health care delivery or financing system. The program was positioned as a solution to the financial difficulties of the elderly that resulted from use of medical services, particularly costly hospitalization, rather than one that would comprehensively address their health needs. As a strategy to temper the AMA's opposition, physician services were not included in the initial Medicare proposals.

Between 1958 and 1963, numerous congressional hearings and intense lobbying took place on the subject of Medicare. Although it was now generally accepted that there was strong public support for a program of health insurance for the elderly, there was vociferous debate between social insurance and welfare advocates regarding the benefits and structure of the program and whether it should be administered by the federal government or by the states. President John F. Kennedy strongly supported providing hospital insurance for the elderly through the Social Security program. However, he was unable to obtain the support of the majority on the House Ways and Means Committee, which had authority for proposed legislation requiring new federal expenditures and whose members included a conservative coalition of Republicans and Southern Democrats opposed to expansion of federal programs. Finally, the landslide Democratic victories in the 1964 elections led President Lyndon Johnson to make hospital insurance for the elderly the first piece of legislation introduced into both houses of Congress as part of his Great Society program.

Competing bills were submitted and considered by the Ways and Means Committee. Under the chairmanship of Representative Wilbur Mills (D-Ark.), a surprising compromise was reached. The Medicare program would provide hospital insurance to all Social Security beneficiaries based on the Blue Cross model and voluntary insurance for physician services based on the health plan for federal employees provided by the Aetna Life Insurance Company. Conservatives had hoped to limit Medicare to state programs serving the very poor elderly. However, in the final bill, benefits for the poor were expanded to cover all ages, to be administered as a joint federal-state program known as Medicaid.

In summary, Medicare emerged out of frustrated efforts to pass national health insurance that began in the early part of the twentieth century. Its proponents conceived it as a social insurance program, and they hoped and expected that it would be a foundation for incremental expansion to other populations and additional benefits. However, the compromises that led to its passage masked these philosophical underpinnings and sowed the seeds for many of the conflicts over Medicare's design and financing that continue into the present.

Evolution of Medicare

In its final form, Medicare included two parts, Hospital Insurance (Part A) and Supplementary Medical Insurance (Part B). The major benefits covered under Part A originally were ninety days of hospital care per episode[8] of care plus sixty lifetime reserve[9] days, one hundred days of post-hospital care per episode in a skilled nursing facility (SNF) if preceded by an inpatient admission, one hundred post-hospital home health visits per year, and one hundred ninety lifetime days of inpatient psychiatric care. Hospice benefits were added later, and home health care was shifted to Part B. Part B covered most physician services, outpatient hospital services, and durable medical equipment. There was no coverage for outpatient prescription drugs, nor any limit on a beneficiary's out-of-pocket expenses. The original Medicare benefits package remains essentially unchanged.

Medicare is financed by a combination of payroll taxes, general revenues, and beneficiary contributions. Part A is a true social insurance program, with eligibility based on payment of payroll taxes that are mandatory for all workers. All beneficiaries eligible for Part A are also eligible for Part B, but participation is voluntary and requires monthly premium payments, which are deducted directly from Social Security checks. These premiums represent approximately 25 percent of Part B costs, with the remainder contributed by federal general revenues. Both Part A and Part B require beneficiary cost sharing. For Part A, this includes a deductible for the first day of hospital care plus coinsurance for hospital care beyond sixty days, and coinsurance for SNF care beyond twenty days as well as for durable medical equipment provided by a home health agency. Part B has an annual deductible and requires 20 percent coinsurance for most services.[10]

Because Part B is voluntary and financed in part by current beneficiary premiums, it intentionally diverges from the social insurance model. The political opponents of social insurance for physician services accepted their inclusion in a separate voluntary insurance plan to preempt future efforts to expand the social insurance component of Part A.

Medicare's framers also knew that political support for the program required that it be modeled on the existing system of health care delivery and financing. As a result, hospital reimbursement was based on existing cost-based agreements with the Blue Cross system, and insurance companies served as payment intermediaries. Similarly, fearing physician refusal to participate in the program, Part B did not establish a fee schedule. Instead, it established payments based on a modified version of the physician's "usual, customary, and reasonable (UCR)" fees charged to privately insured patients; Medicare's version was known as the "customary, prevailing, and reasonable (CPR)" charge. To reassure physicians that the physician-patient relationship would remain intact, Part B allowed physicians to bill patients directly, with the patient to seek payment from the government. In addition, physicians could bill patients for the difference between Medicare's allowed charge for a service and the physician's usual charge, a practice known as balance billing.

Once Medicare had been enacted, transforming it into action was an enormous task. To ensure passage and smooth implementation, Medicare's developers had made accommodations to a wide range of interest groups. One result of these compromises was rapid growth in Medicare expenditures. The cost-based hospital reimbursement system and CPR physician payment system were predictably inflationary, and both hospital charges and physician fees increased sharply in the program's early years. The program's initial emphasis was on removing financial barriers to care, but not on changing the delivery or financing of the health care system. In 1972, Medicare was expanded to cover individuals with end-stage renal disease and disabled people under age sixty-five who had been receiving Social Security disability benefits for two years.

During the 1970s, the rising cost of health care was a growing national concern, and it shaped concerns about the future of Medicare for the next two decades. National health expenditures as a percent of Gross Domestic Product

(GDP) rose from 7.1 percent in 1970 to 8.9 percent in 1980.[11] Medicare's share of national health care costs grew from 10.5 percent to 15.2 percent over the same period.[12] Following the failure of various national health insurance proposals in the 1970s and of legislative and voluntary efforts to control hospital costs, the Medicare program began to adopt a new stance toward provider payment beginning in the mid-1970s. Medicare sponsored several demonstration projects during this period to develop incentive reimbursement programs for hospitals that would encourage greater efficiency and cost containment. Beginning in the 1980s, Medicare received increased Congressional scrutiny because of the growing federal budget deficit. The stage was thus set for Medicare to adopt new policies aimed at restraining costs.

In 1983, the Health Care Financing Administration (the federal agency responsible for Medicare and Medicaid) implemented the Prospective Payment System (PPS) for hospitals. Rather than paying hospitals according to their retrospective costs, PPS paid them a fixed amount relating to the patient's reason for admission, categorized according to a classification system known as Diagnosis-Related Groups (DRGs). PPS had an immediate effect on hospital utilization; length of stay decreased more than 10 percent between 1983 and 1985, and admissions declined as hospitals shifted procedures to the outpatient setting.[13]

Medicare also implemented price controls and global expenditure targets for payment of physician services beginning in 1992. The Medicare Fee Schedule (MFS), based on the Resource-Based Relative Value Scale (RBRVS) developed at Harvard University, had as explicit goals redistribution of payments from surgical to primary care services as well as from urban to rural practitioners. Both the DRG and RBRVS approaches have been adopted by commercial insurance plans as successful cost-containment measures.[14]

Despite successful implementation of hospital and physician price controls, Medicare continued to face challenges in the 1990s, since expenditures continued to grow at a faster rate than revenues. This led to concerns about the long-term solvency of the program, based on projections in the mid-1990s that the program would be in a deficit by the year 2001. To address this impending financing crisis, the Balanced Budget Act (BBA) of 1997 was enacted with strong bipartisan support. The BBA included a number of measures aimed at controlling Medicare spending as well as increased efforts to combat fraud and abuse. These proved even more successful than anticipated. In 1998, the growth rate in Medicare expenditures fell to an unprecedented 1.5 percent,[15] and Medicare costs actually decreased in the six months ending in March 1999.[16] However, by 2000, lawmakers were facing political pressure to return some of these savings from providers seeking higher payments, from health plans seeking higher capitation rates, and from beneficiaries seeking expanded benefits.

Is Medicare Facing a Crisis?

There is no question that the Medicare program faces formidable challenges in the coming decades. As with U.S. health care costs overall, Medicare expenditures have risen steadily as a proportion of GDP. The aging of the baby boom generation is expected to create enormous additional demands. The Medicare benefit package, envisioned initially as just a first step toward comprehensive coverage, has become increasingly inadequate to meet beneficiaries' health needs. The policy question is whether these challenges represent a crisis that requires a radical solution, or whether continued incremental changes will maintain and improve the program as they have in the thirty-five years since its inception. This section discusses the demographic and utilization factors that contribute to rising Medicare costs, forecasts of Medicare insolvency, and the rising financial burden on beneficiaries.

Demographics

The most significant threat to the future of the Medicare program is the aging of the U.S. population. As the baby boom generation (those born between 1946 and 1964) reaches retirement age between 2011 and 2029, this demographic bulge will create an enormous financial burden on Medicare. The number of beneficiaries is estimated to rise from approximately thirty-nine million in 1999 to sixty-nine million in 2025,[17] an increase much greater than that in the number of workers paying into the program. Not only will the proportion of the population age sixty-five and older continue to increase, but the proportion of the oldest old (age eighty-five and older) will be the fastest-growing segment of the elderly.[18]

Demographic changes have political and social implications for the Medicare program in addition to their economic impact.[19] Demographic projections depend on assumptions regarding mortality, fertility, and immigration. Average life expectancy increased throughout the twentieth century as a result of improved standards of living as well as advances in medical care. The key question here is whether historical rates of improvement in mortality will continue, or whether there is a genetically determined limit to the human life span. Whatever the answer to this question, further improvements in average life expectancy will increase the number of years individuals are dependent upon the Medicare program.

Assumptions regarding the number of children born to women of childbearing age affect population growth, the proportion represented by the elderly, and the ratio of tax-paying workers to the number of Medicare beneficiaries. Current forecasts use a fertility rate of slightly below replacement level, consistent with the experience of most European countries. In the long run, however, it is difficult to predict the impact of economic conditions on fertility as well the impact of increased immigration.

In a country with a below-replacement fertility rate, population growth results from both increased longevity and immigration. Most public discussions of the Medicare program do not recognize the impact of immigration, but it is the population factor most subject to policy control. Foreign-born residents represented 9.7 percent of the U.S. population in 1997, and more than 20 percent of the population were either foreign-born or had one or both parents who were.[20] Most immigrants to the United States in the twenty-first century will belong to ethnic groups currently identified as minorities. These groups also tend to have higher fertility rates than the native-born white population; 18 percent of U.S. births in 1995 were to foreign-born women.[21] Therefore, immigration may increase the proportion of younger workers in the population. It will be an increasingly diverse population, however, while Medicare beneficiaries during the next several decades will be predominantly white.

Some policy makers point to the dependency ratio as proof that the Medicare program faces a crisis. The dependency ratio is frequently expressed as the number of contributing workers per beneficiary. Because Medicare Part A is funded through a payroll tax, a decrease in the ratio means an increasing tax burden on workers, unless expenditures per enrollee are reduced. Projections show this ratio decreasing from 3.6 workers per Medicare beneficiary in 2010 to 2.3 in 2030.[22] However, one criticism of the dependency ratio is that is does not take into consideration the other significant group of dependents that workers must also support, namely, children. As the number of children per family has decreased, the total number of dependents per hundred workers actually declined from 90.4 in 1960 to 69.7 in 2000. This number is expected to increase again to 80.2 by 2040, but it is still significantly lower than the 1960 ratio.[23] This broader definition of dependency suggests that although the overall burden on tax-paying workers is less than in the years prior to enactment of Medicare, those sixty-five and over will be demanding a greater share of societal resources during the next few decades. This may create unintended but unavoidable intergenerational conflict in a program that depends on intergenerational transfers.

Because Medicare is a public program for a targeted population group, it is subject to unique political pressures not experienced by universal health care programs. In countries with national health insurance, the risk pool includes the entire population, of which the elderly are a relatively small proportion. Expenditures for individuals under age sixty-five are already counted in the system, so the effect of a growing number of individuals reaching age sixty-five is simply the incremental cost of health care for sixty-five-year-olds versus sixty-four-year-olds.[24] In contrast, the baby boom generation will create a huge budgetary impact in the

United States, because beneficiaries transition from private insurance to public insurance when they become eligible for Medicare. The European countries and Japan have already absorbed the health costs of a population that aged more rapidly than that of the United States. Though there have been signs of strain and incremental reforms in their health systems, these countries continue to provide universal coverage, and cost pressures have not resulted in radical restructuring.[25]

Costs

A generally accepted means of assessing trends in health care expenditures is to examine their relationship to national GDP. Between 1975 and 1995, Medicare expenditures exceeded GDP growth by 3.5 to 4.0 percent per year.[26] Consequently, the Medicare program became an ever larger proportion of the national economy. The trustees of the Part A and Part B trust funds are required by law to make an annual report to Congress that forecasts future expenditures and revenue. The 1998 trustees' report showed Medicare spending growing from 2.7 percent of GDP in 1998 to 5.3 percent in 2025.[27] However, as of 2000, the 2025 estimate had been reduced to 3.95 percent.[28] This change illustrates how sensitive forecasts, particularly long-term ones, are to changes in the underlying economic conditions.

Price, volume, and intensity of service all play a role in medical expenditures. Both the PPS and MFS were mechanisms to limit provider payment and reduce utilization. These approaches to price controls have been effective, but they do not address other underlying determinants of continuing expenditure growth—that is, the diffusion of medical technology and the increasing intensity of services. The growth in health care costs of the elderly has been primarily due to technology driving increasing intensity of services consumed per capita.[29] Analysts differ in their assumptions about how individuals will use services in the future, and the evidence is contradictory. Factors that would increase costs include the fact that the oldest old are far more likely to be institutionalized or to require assistance with activities of daily living.

In addition, utilization rates for procedures such as angioplasty and hip replacement among Medicare beneficiaries have increased dramatically over the past ten years, with some of the largest increases in the population age eighty-five and older. Will the average eighty-five-year-old consume fewer resources because she will be healthier? Or, will she consume the same or more because she will have bypass surgery and a hip replacement in order to continue playing tennis?

Finally, many chronic conditions are not strongly associated with mortality, so that increased longevity will mean more people living with chronic conditions such as dementia.[30] On the other hand, several factors support the notion that per capita use of services may decline as the population ages. For example, a large proportion of Medicare costs is incurred in the last year of a beneficiary's life; thus, increased longevity means that the cost of dying will be spread over a longer period of time. In addition, the cost of dying is lower for the oldest old.[31] The costs for a ninety-three-year-old who dies of pneumonia in a nursing home are less than those for a sixty-eight-year-old who dies in the intensive care unit of complications from open heart surgery. In addition, advances in treatment and improved understanding of risk factors can delay the onset of some chronic conditions.[32]

Efforts to reduce growth in the price and volume of services, through either regulation or competition, were the focus of Medicare reform efforts in the 1980s and 1990s. However, societal choices about the adoption of new technology and who will receive what services are the most difficult issues facing the Medicare program and the U.S. health system in the twenty-first century.

Forecasts of Insolvency

The Medicare Part A Trust Fund has been forecast to become insolvent many times during its history. The frequent declarations of a crisis in Medicare can be explained in part by the nature of economic forecasts. Forecasting requires assumptions about demographics, economic growth, worker productivity, health care costs, and other important variables. Small differences in assumptions compound over time, with the result that analysts' forecasts can vary significantly and change dramatically from year to year. Nevertheless, the Medicare trustees are required by law to project the funds' status seventy-five years into the future. Considering the changes that have occurred since 1925 in medicine, in technology generally, in society, and in the world economy, it is obviously absurd to expect long-term forecasts to be reliable.

Reliable short-term estimates are also difficult to produce. In 1996, the Part A Trust Fund was projected to be bankrupt in 2001.[33] However, the reimbursement changes mandated by the BBA of 1997 were more successful than anticipated in restraining Medicare costs, and by the time of the 1999 trustees' report, bankruptcy of the trust fund had been put off until 2015.[34] As the U.S. economy remained strong, with unemployment levels at historic lows, the 2000 annual report forecast the fund to be solvent until 2025.[35] Despite their inherent instability, these annual forecasts create political pressures and are used to frame the policy debate. Because of the continuing strength of the U.S. economy, the impending crisis in Medicare has subsided temporarily, and pressure for fundamental reform has subsequently been relieved. The next economic downturn may force the insolvency crisis to suddenly reemerge, however.

Benefit Gaps and Rising Out-of-Pocket Expenditures

The Medicare benefit package was modeled after the private health plans of the 1960s, with Part A analogous to Blue Cross hospital coverage and Part B to Blue Shield coverage of physicians' services. The private "Medigap" market developed to offer supplementary insurance, similar to major medical policies sold by many private insurers. Medicare as originally designed was not intended to cover all the medical expenditures of the elderly. Early estimates were that it would pay about 40 percent.[36] In 1994, it was estimated to cover 52 percent.[37] The program has always required beneficiaries to contribute a significant amount toward their covered medical benefits in the form of the part B premium as well as deductibles and coinsurance. However, noncovered services account for the majority of beneficiary out-of-pocket spending. In 1993, the largest component was the cost of long-term care (42 percent), followed by prescription drugs (18 percent).[38]

In 1965, the medical profession, which fought so strenuously against the passage of Medicare, also considered prepaid group practice to be socialized medicine and ostracized physicians who practiced in what are now called group-model HMOs. However, rising health care costs stimulated many changes in the structure of private health plans. As discussed in the previous chapter, by the 1990s HMOs and other forms of managed care had replaced indemnity fee-for-service (FFS) as the predominant type of health plan design. Managed care plans eliminated the distinctions between hospital and physician benefits, which had become unwieldy as health care delivery moved increasingly into ambulatory care. They included benefits for preventive services. Many employers also added prescription drug coverage as an inducement for their employees to switch from costly indemnity plans. Meanwhile, the basic structure of Medicare remained unchanged. What began as a program that mirrored private health insurance in 1965 has become one with a distinctly different benefit structure as we enter the new century.

The traditional Medicare program lacks two important benefits found in most employer-sponsored health plans: prescription drugs and catastrophic coverage. Although prescription drugs are increasingly important in treating the chronic illnesses suffered by the elderly, their cost is rising much more rapidly than that of health care overall. National health spending on prescription drugs rose 15.4 percent from 1997 to 1998. In contrast, total national health expenditures increased 5.6 percent, with increases of only 3.4 percent for hospital care and 5.4 percent for physician services.[39] Although 87 percent of beneficiaries in 1996 had supplemental coverage (through privately purchased Medigap policies, Medicare HMOs, employer-sponsored plans, or Medicaid[40]), more than one-third had no coverage for prescription drugs.[41]

Exacerbating the situation is the fact that the retail pharmacy prices paid by the elderly and others without prescription drug coverage are substantially higher than the prices negotiated by managed care plans. In 1998, the elderly accounted for 34 percent of dispensed prescriptions—and 42 percent of total prescription drug spending.[42] Medicare also has no limitation on beneficiaries' out-of-pocket costs, whereas the typical private insurance plan covers all expenses after the enrollee has incurred a specified amount of coinsurance payment.

Medicare does not cover long-term nursing home care, which is also generally not covered by private employer-sponsored health insurance. Although there is a small private market for long-term care insurance, most nursing home costs are paid by the Medicaid program (for those who are poor or who spend down their assets), or out of pocket. Although the need is great, there are currently no viable reform proposals to include nursing home care as part of the basic Medicare benefit package.

The poverty rate among the elderly has dropped from 28.5 percent in 1966 to 10.5 percent in 1998, equivalent to the rate in the population age eighteen to sixty-four.[43] However, health care costs have risen much faster than the incomes of the elderly. Therefore, out-of-pocket costs represent an increasing proportion of income—the very condition Medicare was enacted to ameliorate. In 1998, average out-of-pocket costs for Medicare beneficiaries represented 18.6 percent of median income, with this proportion projected to rise to 28.6 percent by 2025,[44] not including expenditures for long-term care.

In the 2000 Annual Report of the Public Trustees of the Medicare Trust Funds, Marilyn Moon and Stephen G. Kellison had this to say about the challenges facing Medicare:

> . . . caution is clearly needed in any major restructuring of Medicare. Making changes in increments may be a prudent approach for the future. . . . The approach of the last two decades, seeking improvements in the efficiency and effectiveness of health care delivery, will continue to be an important contributor to Medicare's future. But it is hard to imagine that such efforts alone will allow us to expand coverage from one in every eight Americans to one in every five without additional resources. The challenge facing the future financing of this program is how we as a society share the costs of health care for a much larger aging population.[45]

Reforming Medicare

During the 1990s, the Clinton administration consistently supported use of the private market to achieve cost savings and promote innovation in delivering health services. The Medicare + Choice program was established as part of the BBA of

1997 to expand private sector health plan options for Medicare beneficiaries. Plans participating in Medicare+Choice must cover the basic package of Medicare benefits. They compete within a given market on the basis of supplemental benefits such as prescription drugs, provider networks, and customer service. However, they do not compete on price. Beneficiaries continue to pay the same basic Part B premium, and their total cost sharing cannot be greater than that of traditional Medicare. All plans within a county are paid the same rate per beneficiary, with minimal adjustment for health status. As the name implies, Medicare+Choice has given many beneficiaries the choice between traditional Medicare and a managed care plan similar to that offered by employers in the private sector, while preserving the basic entitlements of the original Medicare program. As of 2000, almost 6.9 million beneficiaries were enrolled in managed care plans.[46]

Since the passage of Medicare in 1965, the political values of the United States have shifted fundamentally. Whereas government was once viewed as a positive force for social change, the prevailing climate holds that government is inefficient and that markets can better meet the desires of individual consumers. This orientation, coupled with cyclic forecasts of trust fund insolvency, has led some policy makers to assert that the Medicare program requires radical restructuring if it is to survive into the new century.

Premium Support Approach

Traditional Medicare is a defined benefits program, in which all beneficiaries are guaranteed a defined set of benefits regardless of ability to pay or health status. As health care costs rise and the beneficiary population increases, this system creates an open-ended financial obligation for the federal government. Policy makers who seek to limit this obligation have proposed replacing the current program with a defined contribution or voucher approach. In its purest form, defined contribution would limit the obligation of the federal government by providing beneficiaries a fixed dollar amount with which they would purchase their own health insurance in the private market. The amount of the government contribution would be adjusted for inflation using a standard economic indicator such as the Consumer Price Index (CPI) or the GDP. Thus, federal Medicare expenditures would be fixed at a targeted level, equal to the government's contribution multiplied by the number of eligible beneficiaries, and beneficiaries would pay any difference between the cost of the plan they chose and the federal contribution. If health care costs continue their historical pattern of rising faster than GDP, the financial risk for these increased costs would be shifted to beneficiaries.

Noting that a strict voucher approach would not be viable either politically or programmatically, economists Henry Aaron and Robert Reischauer proposed a version of the defined contribution approach termed premium support.[47] There are two crucial assumptions underlying this approach: private sector competition is the best means to restrain the rate of cost increases in the Medicare program; and the federal government's financial obligation should be limited in order to impose fiscal discipline on the program and avoid the need for future tax increases to support Medicare.

Under the premium support system, the federal government and beneficiaries would share the risk of rising health care costs. The federal contribution would not be tied to an external economic indicator but would instead be based on bids submitted by private sector health plans seeking to participate in the Medicare program. The traditional Medicare program would be retained, but it would be required to compete with private health plans.

In theory, premium support would offer beneficiaries greater choice, enabling them to select the health plan that best met their needs. Because they would pay the difference between the premium support contribution and the cost of their chosen plan, beneficiaries would have a financial incentive to choose a plan that offered the best value in terms of cost and quality. The beneficiary's required contribution would replace the current Part B premium as well as eliminate the need for Medigap coverage under the traditional program.

The Politics of Premium Support

In addition to creating the Medicare+Choice program and enacting significant cuts in provider reimbursement, the BBA of 1997 also established the National Bipartisan Commission on the Future of Medicare to make recommendations regarding a comprehensive approach to preserve the program, including its long-term financing, covered benefits, and beneficiary contributions.[48] This Medicare Commission was co-chaired by Senator John Breaux (D-La.) and Representative Bill Thomas (R-Calif.). The co-chairs were not interested in incremental reforms; they championed the premium support approach as a means to restructure the entire Medicare program. They cited as a model of premium support the Federal Employees' Health Benefit Program (FEHBP). This program offers a menu of health plan choices to all federal employees based on a competitive contracting process; it served as the original model for managed competition developed by Alain Enthoven.[49]

Under the Breaux-Thomas proposal, as premium support was called, health plans seeking to participate in Medicare in a particular market would submit competitive bids for a standard benefits package. They could also offer a high-option plan with additional benefits, or stop-loss coverage, or both. The competitive bidding process also would apply to the traditional Medicare fee-for-service program. The federal premium contribution would be set at 88 percent of the average bid for the standard benefit plan within each market. A premium subsidy would be provided for individuals up to 135 percent of the federal poverty level.

The Medicare Commission fell one vote short of the number required for formal approval of its recommendation in March 1999, in part because of disagreement regarding the inclusion of prescription drug coverage. At the same time, the sense of fiscal urgency diminished when the Medicare Trustees Annual Report released on March 30, 1999, showed that the projected life of the trust fund had been extended to 2015.[50] Despite the failure of the Medicare Commission to bring a bill to Congress, there remained considerable bipartisan interest in the Commission's concepts. In November 1999, Senators Breaux, Bill Frist (R-Tenn.), Bob Kerrey (D-Neb.), and Chuck Hagel (R-Neb.) introduced a bill based on the Breaux-Thomas proposal, with the addition of a prescription drug option.[51]

Evaluating Premium Support Proposals

There is no reform approach, no system of market incentives or regulatory controls, that will enable the Medicare program to achieve cost savings, preserve access, improve quality, and expand benefits simultaneously. Any reform proponent who claims that a particular approach will do all these things is indulging in wishful thinking and political pandering. The challenge is to weigh carefully the benefits and risks of proposed reforms and to choose those strategies that are most likely to preserve the integrity and basic values of the Medicare program. The premium support approach should be evaluated in terms of the extent to which it is likely to meet goals related to cost, access, quality, and comprehensiveness.

Market Competition and Medicare Expenditures

The premise of the premium support approach is that market competition among private health plans will force them to be more efficient than the traditional Medicare program and thus will restrain growth in Medicare spending. However, the empirical evidence on cost trends does not support this assumption. Between 1969 and 1998, Medicare and private health care expenditures per capita grew at a similar pace overall—an average of 10.0 percent annually for Medicare and 11.2 percent for private insurance.[52] Between 1984 (following implementation of PPS) and 1991, the Medicare growth rate remained *below* the private rate.[53]

The 1990s saw changing patterns of health expenditures that have significant implications for the policy debate regarding Medicare reform. As enrollment in private managed care plans soared in the early 1990s, cost increases among the privately insured dropped significantly below those of Medicare. With increased federal efforts to combat Medicare fraud and abuse and passage of the BBA of 1997, a major reversal took place in 1997, when Medicare growth rates decelerated and dropped below those of private insurance.

These trends continued through the end of the decade, with Medicare expenditures actually decreasing in the six months ending March 31, 1999,[54] and private plans increasing premiums at double-digit rates.[55] Market-driven approaches assume that the short-term phenomenon of the early 1990s can be sustained into the future, despite the fact that recent trends have already moved in the opposite direction. Many analysts believe that the early cost savings associated with managed care were due primarily to the shift out of unmanaged fee-for-service plans and thus represented a one-time reduction only.[56]

The insurance industry itself has signaled doubt in its ability to achieve cost savings through competition in its response to Medicare's Competitive Pricing Demonstration project, also created by the BBA of 1997. This demonstration was intended to test the use of competitive bids by private Medicare+ Choice health plans in selected markets to establish what Medicare would pay them per beneficiary. However, the health plans in these markets vociferously protested the demonstration. Among their complaints was the fact that the markets chosen were those where managed care was already well established. The health plans claimed that competitive bidding in these markets would not be a fair test of potential savings from competitive bidding because there was less inefficiency to eliminate from the system. One health plan threatened that if competitive bidding were implemented, health plans would have to reduce benefits.[57] It should be noted that although administrative costs represent less than 2 percent of the public Medicare program's expenses,[58] private for-profit health plans spend an average of 14 percent on administration and profits.[59] Thus, a private health plan would have to decrease beneficiary medical costs by 12 percent before it could deliver any savings to the Medicare program. The response to the Competitive Pricing Demonstration suggests that private health plans may be less interested in true market competition than in a system that preserves their ability to obtain a guaranteed profit from the federal government.

If private sector managed care cannot demonstrate that it yields a permanent decrease in the rate of spending growth, then one crucial element of the premium support approach is undermined. Furthermore, the Medicare Commission staff acknowledged that even the savings forecast by Breaux-Thomas would not be sufficient to meet the Medicare program's need for additional resources to absorb the impact of the baby boom generation.[60]

Long-Term Solvency

If market competition alone cannot achieve long-term solvency for the Medicare program, how do premium support proponents plan to accomplish this goal? The answer lies in the definition of solvency. As discussed earlier, there are three sources of Medicare financing: the payroll tax funding Part A, and beneficiary premiums and general revenues supporting Part B. Payroll taxes and beneficiary premiums can be modified only by legislative action. The Part A Trust Fund is an accounting mechanism that allows the Medicare program to collect payroll taxes paid by workers and their employers and use them to fund current benefits without an explicit annual appropriation by Congress. It is technically insolvent when its reserves plus projected payroll tax collections fall below projected benefit obligations.

Declarations of insolvency have proven to be politically powerful tools for attempts to reform Medicare. However, solvency of the Part A Trust Fund does not accurately represent the financial requirements of the Medicare program overall. As medical care is increasingly provided in outpatient settings, Part B expenditures have created additional demands on the general fund (that is, general tax revenue). The existence of multiple funding streams has also led to accounting manipulation. In 1997, home health benefits were shifted from Part A to Part B, which improved Part A solvency but increased general fund obligations. Fiscal conservatives are concerned that over time, Medicare's current financing structure will create an open-ended demand on general revenue.

The real key to understanding premium support proposals is that they represent a strategy to limit the federal government's responsibility for Medicare costs, but not necessarily to control the overall growth in Medicare expenditures. The Breaux-Frist bill, for example, would cap general revenue expenditures at 40 percent of total Medicare costs.[61] This would be accomplished by converting Medicare from a program of *guaranteed benefits* to one of *defined contributions*, thereby placing beneficiaries at risk for the difference between the growth rate in the government's contribution and the growth rate in health care costs.

Beneficiary Costs

As discussed earlier in this chapter, the current Medicare program has imposed increasing financial burdens on beneficiaries. From a systemwide perspective, the impact of premium support on beneficiaries would depend on where the level of government support is set relative to the current Part B premium and average expenditures for Medigap premiums. Since a principal goal of the premium support approach is to limit the federal government's financial obligation, the federal contribution could be expected to decrease as a proportion of the total premium if health costs resume a high rate of growth. By definition, the financial burden on beneficiaries would increase.

All beneficiaries in traditional Medicare currently pay the same premium for Part B and face the same deductibles and coinsurance rates. Under premium support, health plans would be free to vary each of these factors. The financial impact on beneficiaries would differ depending on the premiums offered by health plans in their area and which plan they chose. In fact, this is the intent of premium support—to create a financial incentive for beneficiaries to select a lower-cost health plan. However, health plan premiums may not reflect true differences in efficiency and quality, but instead differences in health status that cannot be fully accounted for because of inadequate risk-adjustment mechanisms. Without adequate risk-adjusters, beneficiaries with severe disabilities or chronic illnesses may receive better care if they remain in the traditional program. In addition, not all beneficiaries live in markets with sufficient health plan competition, so beneficiaries in these markets could be subject to significantly higher costs. One study estimated out-of-pocket costs for traditional Medicare or a high-priced private plan could reach more than 39 percent of beneficiary income by 2025.[62]

There is probably no element more important to equitable implementation of a competitive market approach to Medicare reform than developing an adequate risk-adjustment mechanism. In a social insurance program such as traditional Medicare, risk is pooled so those beneficiaries with extensive health needs pay the same premium as do those who are healthy. Traditional FFS offers an incentive to provide additional services to those with the greatest need, even if this incentive results in overprovision of care. Medicare HMOs, however, receive a fixed amount per beneficiary, which creates an incentive to attract the healthiest members and to provide fewer services. As noted by one recent report, "[t]he more the Medicare beneficiary risk pool is split up, the greater the burden on the risk-adjustment mechanism to protect universal access."[63] In 1996, 5 percent of elderly Medicare beneficiaries accounted for 45 percent of program expenditures.[64] This means that a health plan could greatly improve its profits by avoiding enrollment of individuals with serious health problems, or encouraging their disenrollment by making specialist access difficult. In addition, beneficiary self-selection on the basis of risk is virtually inherent in a choice model, because healthier individuals are more willing to change providers and accept the primary care gatekeepers of HMO plans than are those with chronic illnesses.

In theory, risk adjustment of capitation rates according to beneficiary health status and expected expenditures could neutralize health plans' incentives to avoid enrollment of the sickest individuals. Unfortunately, the science of health care risk adjustment is still not advanced. The initial payment methodology for

Medicare+Choice led to significant overpayment of health plans.[65] HCFA estimated that the demographic adjusters used with its previous method for risk-adjusting capitation payments, the average adjusted per capita cost (AAPCC), explained only 1 percent of the variation in individuals' health care expenses. The risk-adjustment system mandated by the BBA of 1997, to be phased in over five years beginning in January 2000, is expected to explain 9 percent when fully implemented.[66] The new model is certainly an improvement over the previous method of paying Medicare HMOs, but it will be several years before there is any evidence regarding its effectiveness in reducing adverse selection. Some analysts believe that the only feasible means of minimizing both risk selection and underprovision of services is to use a system of partial capitation, in which some portion of health plan payments would be based on individuals' actual use of services.[67] However, the premium support proposals assume that an adequate risk-adjustment mechanism can be implemented.

Traditional Medicare Under Premium Support

Premium support proposals require that the traditional Medicare program administered by HCFA be financially self-supporting and compete with private health plans on the basis of price. However, there is a real risk that this approach would result in adverse selection significant enough to send the traditional Medicare program into a so-called death spiral. This occurs when persons with chronic health problems elect to stay in an FFS program while healthier individuals choose less-costly options. Average costs rise for those who remain in FFS, and premiums soon may become unaffordable for the group with the greatest health needs. All group plans that have attempted to maintain an FFS option within a range of choices have experienced this selection problem—including the FEHBP, the model for the premium support approach.[68]

Under premium support, it is likely that adverse selection would narrow the role of the traditional Medicare program to functioning as a safety net for the sickest and poorest beneficiaries. This could lead to erosion of its political support. The traditional program could be viewed as a welfare program rather than an entitlement for all beneficiaries, and its higher costs could easily be portrayed as an indicator of government inefficiency rather than a reflection of its risk pool. This would completely undermine the original social insurance motivation that led to the creation of Medicare. Premium support would also further erode the uniform benefits beneficiaries were entitled to under traditional Medicare, by allowing regional differences in benefits according to local market conditions and by fostering differences between traditional Medicare and Medicare managed care.

Impact of a Competitive Market on Access

A key feature of a competitive market is the free entry and exit of firms. When a Medicare HMO exits a market, elderly and disabled beneficiaries face two choices. They can enroll in another health plan, if one operates in their area, or return to traditional Medicare, which does not cover the supplementary benefits that are offered by most Medicare HMOs such as prescription drugs. This change of health plans may disrupt their continuity of care, requiring them to find a new physician and change their relationships with home health and other providers. The initial years of Medicare+Choice experience illustrate the potential impact of free market entry and exit.

In fall 1998, just prior to implementation of Medicare+Choice, ninety-nine health plans announced that they would withdraw from selected Medicare HMO markets or reduce the geographic area served by their plans, requiring 407,000 beneficiaries to choose a new health plan or return to FFS. These announcements took place after HCFA denied the HMOs' requests to modify their previously submitted plans by increasing premiums, raising co-payments, or reducing coverage of prescription drugs.

Some of the nation's largest managed care organizations participated in the pullout, including United Healthcare, Aetna, Prudential, and PacifiCare,[69] claiming that the proposed 2 percent increase in Medicare payments to HMOs was inadequate. When the General Accounting Office (GAO) investigated this development, it found that payment rates were indeed an issue; health plans withdrew from counties that had low AAPCC rates relative to other counties in the plan's service area.[70] However, more plans withdrew from high-payment markets than from low-payment areas. Health plans also withdrew from counties where they had limited Medicare experience, were unsuccessful in attracting a large number of members, faced competition from larger plans, or were unable to develop adequate provider networks.

HMOs' flight from Medicare+Choice has continued since 1999. Medicare HMOs dropped 327,000 beneficiaries in 2000. The Medicare HMO market is expected to become even more unstable in 2001, when HMO withdrawals are projected to affect approximately 934,000 beneficiaries. Over this three-year period, 27 percent of beneficiaries enrolled in Medicare HMOs were required to change health plans or return to FFS.[71]

Without explicit government regulation, health plans are free to withdraw from markets and to change benefits and cost sharing annually. Recent experience illustrates the instability inherent in relying on the market to maintain stable access to health care for seniors, for whom change is stressful and continuity of care is particularly important. Health plans generally withdrew from areas that are unprofitable. Society cannot, and should not, expect investor-owned insurers to put access and continuity of care before profits. Likewise, society should not place Medicare beneficiaries in the middle of the emerging political battle between managed care companies and Congress over the appropriate level for Medicare capitation rates.

Protecting Vulnerable Beneficiaries

Although the poverty rate among the elderly has dropped significantly since initiation of the Medicare program, many beneficiaries remain vulnerable in terms of income, health status, and other factors. In addition, racial and ethnic disparities persist. More than 30 percent have significant physical or cognitive impairments, or both.[72] As discussed previously, without adequate risk adjustment of payments, health plans have an incentive to avoid enrolling these individuals or to encourage their disenrollment through barriers to accessing services.

Another challenge facing a Medicare program based on private market competition is making available information on health plan choice in a way that elderly and disabled individuals can comprehend. A study conducted in areas of high Medicare HMO penetration found that only 11 percent of respondents had sufficient knowledge to be able to make an informed choice between Medicare HMOs and traditional Medicare, and 30 percent knew virtually nothing about HMOs.[73] The most common source of information for these beneficiaries was HMO advertisements.

The premium support proposal may also disadvantage rural residents. Rural areas face many challenges in giving their residents access to health services. Rural counties have both a higher proportion of elderly residents and higher rates of poverty than do metropolitan areas.[74] Under the traditional Medicare program, urban and rural residents alike receive Medicare Part A and pay the same premium for Part B. However, it is generally not in the business interests of HMOs to serve rural areas. These areas often rely on a single community hospital, meaning that health plans lack negotiating leverage to demand provider reimbursement cuts. Opportunities for meaningful competition are limited because rural areas do not have sufficient population or enough providers to support multiple managed care plans. There may even be insufficient population to justify the overhead costs of administering a single managed care plan. Because of the difficulty of operating managed care plans in rural areas, the majority of the counties from which Medicare HMOs withdrew in 1999 were rural.[75]

Quality

Because capitation creates incentives for health plans to reduce utilization and possibly to stint on needed services, increased attention has been focused on measuring quality of care and health plan performance. A review of the literature performed by Robert Miller and Harold Luft[76] showed mixed evidence regarding the quality of clinical care provided by managed care organizations in general. This should be unsurprising, since HMOs across the country differ greatly in the populations served, local market conditions, the amount of care delegated to physician organizations, and physician payment incentives. Overall, no significant differences were found in the clinical quality of care provided by HMOs and FFS health plans.

Their review did note several studies in which chronically ill and vulnerable patients had significantly worse outcomes when enrolled in an HMO in comparison with traditional Medicare. A Florida study showed that Medicare HMOs in the state enrolled beneficiaries who were healthier than those who stayed in traditional Medicare—and that health plan members were more likely to disenroll when they incurred higher utilization, that is, when they became sicker.[77] Evidence on member satisfaction is mixed as well.[78] Enrollees in FFS plans generally are more satisfied with the nonfinancial aspects of care, such as quality of physician interaction and access to specialists. HMO enrollees tend to be more satisfied with their cost of care in comparison with the out-of-pocket costs incurred by enrollees in an FFS plan. However, individuals with chronic illness enrolled in managed care plans report a significantly higher level of dissatisfaction than chronically ill persons in an FFS health plan.[79]

The Managed Care Backlash

Only a few years ago, managed care was hailed as the solution to the nation's rising health care costs. However, initial enrollees in managed care were healthy individuals who benefited from the coverage of preventive services and lower out-of-pocket costs, or those for whom group-model HMOs such as Kaiser were a long-established feature of their local health care system. As managed care became the major form of employer-sponsored health coverage, enrollment began to include individuals with chronic conditions and those whose employers no longer offered indemnity health plans.

This changing enrollment and other factors have led to a widespread managed care backlash. According to a survey conducted by health polling expert Robert Blendon, consumers rated managed care companies lower than telephone companies, banks, and oil companies in terms of customer service.[80] This dissatisfaction manifested itself in a flood of legislative efforts to protect consumers. As of 1998, more than a thousand managed care bills had been introduced in Congress and state legislatures.[81] Passage of a federal Patients' Bill of Rights was fiercely debated in 1999, including whether patients should be granted the right to sue their health plans. Facing the prospect of increased governmental regulation, a coalition of managed care organizations promised voluntary changes, including providing external review of service denial decisions, coverage of emergency room visits using a "prudent layperson" definition of *emergency*, and direct access to obstetrician-gynecologist services.[82] Some of the backlash has been fueled by anecdote or widely publicized horror stories; some by individuals' actual experiences, including those of some prominent advocates of managed care.[83] For a variety of reasons, consumer confidence in managed care has diminished.

Expanding Benefits

Policy makers agree that the Medicare benefits package should be updated to reflect changes in the needs of the elderly and in the practice of medicine. Yet past experience shows how difficult it is to devise a benefit that is not prohibitively expensive and is perceived by beneficiaries as meeting their needs. In June 1988, Congress passed the Medicare Catastrophic Coverage Act (MCCA); by November 1989 it was repealed. The MCCA expanded Part A benefits (reducing the beneficiary liability for hospital co-payments, increasing the SNF benefit, and expanding home health and hospice benefits), capped out-of-pocket expenses for Part B, and provided drug benefits (subject to a deductible and coinsurance).[84] Unlike existing Medicare benefits, however, it was designed to be budget-neutral for the federal government. Rather than increase the Social Security payroll tax, the MCCA was financed entirely by beneficiary premiums. Further departing from prior Medicare policies, the premium schedule was progressive, based on adjusted gross income. Following the principles of social insurance, the catastrophic coverage was compulsory, designed to provide the most protection for those with the greatest medical expenses and the lowest incomes.

The lobbying efforts to repeal this legislation stemmed from a number of factors, including its complexity and the resulting difficulty in communicating its benefits, pharmaceutical industry opposition, and lack of consumer understanding of the purpose and value of catastrophic coverage. Opposition was strong among the affluent elderly; they were satisfied with existing private Medigap policies and were least likely to need the protections of the new legislation.[85] At its founding in 1965, Medicare was established as a universal program. With the repeal of the MCCA, the public rejected a means-tested approach to expanding Medicare in which well-off beneficiaries would finance benefits for the vulnerable. This experience contained lessons for policy makers that apply to further expansion of Medicare benefits, including prescription drug coverage.

Beginning in 1999, rising awareness of the financial burden of drug costs on the elderly led to bipartisan support for a Medicare prescription drug benefit. The availability of prescription drug coverage was the reason many beneficiaries initially had enrolled in Medicare+Choice plans.[86] However, this coverage was not available to all enrollees, and its comprehensiveness eroded in the late 1990s as managed care plans experienced difficulty sustaining profitability in this line of business.

In 1998, 67 percent of Medicare+Choice plans offered a prescription drug benefit, and 84 percent of enrollees were covered.[87] In 1999, 21 percent of Medicare+Choice plans limited drug coverage to $500 or less, with this figure rising to 32 percent in 2000. In addition, health plans raised co-payments an average of 21 percent for brand-name drugs and 8 percent for generics.[88] The proportion of employers providing retiree coverage for Medigap or Medicare+Choice premiums also declined, from 40 percent in 1994 to 28 percent in 1999.[89] Individual Medigap plans that include prescription drug coverage are beyond the financial reach of most beneficiaries. As a result, almost half of Medicare beneficiaries lacked drug coverage for some or all of the year.[90]

The structure of proposals for a prescription benefit has reflected the overall debate regarding Medicare reforms. Conservatives in Congress would rely on enrollment in private health plans, while the Clinton administration sought to expand the benefits offered under traditional Medicare. All proposals afford financial protection for those with income below 135 percent of poverty. Relying on the private market to supply voluntary prescription drug coverage is problematic owing to the risk of adverse selection; even the Health Insurance Association of America expressed its skepticism.[91] The pharmaceutical industry is opposed to any government plan that would lead to regulation of drug prices or allow the federal government to use its position as a huge purchaser to negotiate low prices. Conservatives argue that a one-size-fits-all government plan is not what seniors want; liberals insist that relying on the private market cannot guarantee universal access to a specified benefit. The debate over prescription drugs thus represents a microcosm of the debate over the future of Medicare.

Conclusion

Medicare was implemented in 1965 as an incremental step toward national health insurance in the United States. Thirty-five years later, it survives as the country's second largest social insurance program and is likely to continue well into the twenty-first century as a separate program. The fundamental challenge facing the future of Medicare is whether it will continue to be a defined benefits program, or whether it will transition to a defined contribution program.

When Medicare was enacted, a founding principle was that it was supposed to reflect mainstream medicine, including mainstream delivery and payment methodologies. One obvious question regarding the future of Medicare is whether various reform proposals are consistent with this original principle. Despite the substantial movement during the past two decades toward defined contributions for pension benefits in the private sector, defined contributions for health benefits are still not common.[92] Before beginning a grand experiment with the future of Medicare, perhaps policy makers should wait until the private market fully embraces this reform.

In the meantime, incremental efforts to expand benefits and offer additional subsidies to low-income beneficiaries are likely to reduce existing disparities within the program and to improve the health and financial stability of those who are most vulnerable.

Notes

1. This section draws heavily upon Marmor, T. R. *The Politics of Medicare, 2nd edition.* New York: Aldine De Gruyter, 2000; and to a lesser extent upon Hirshfield, D. S. *The Lost Reform: The Campaign for Compulsory Health Insurance in the United States from 1932 to 1943.* Cambridge, Mass.: Harvard University Press, and Commonwealth Fund, 1970.
2. Dionne, E. J. "Medicare's Social Contract: Social Insurance Commentary." In R. D. Reischauer, S. Butler, and J. R. Lave (eds.), *Medicare: Preparing for the Challenges of the 21st Century.* Washington, D.C.: National Academy of Social Insurance, 1998.
3. Ball, R. M. "Medicare's Social Contract: Reflections on How Medicare Came About." In Reischauer, Butler, and Lave (1998).
4. Fishbein, M. "The Committee on the Costs of Medical Care." *Journal of the American Medical Association,* 1932, *99*, 1950–1952.
5. Marmor (2000).
6. Marmor (2000).
7. Ball (1998), p. 31.
8. An episode of care starts with an inpatient admission and ends sixty days after discharge from a hospital or skilled-nursing facility. Thus, beneficiaries can have multiple episodes per year.
9. Lifetime reserve days are a pool that can be used if a beneficiary has an inpatient episode that exceeds ninety days. Lifetime reserve days cannot be replaced once used.
10. For 2000, the Part A deductible was $776 per episode and coinsurance was $194 per day for the sixty-first through ninetieth days. SNF coinsurance was $97 per day for the twenty-first through the hundredth days. The Part B premium was $45.50 per month, and the deductible was $100 per year. See Health Care Financing Administration. "Medicare Deductible, Coinsurance, and Premium Amounts, 2000." Oct. 25, 1999. [http://www.hcfa.gov/stats/mdedco00.htm]

11. Health Care Financing Administration, Office of the Actuary. "National Health Expenditures, Aggregate, Per Capita, Percent Distribution, and Annual Percent Change by Source of Funds: Calendar Years 1960–98." n.d. [http://www.hcfa.gov/stats/nhe-oact/]

12. Health Care Financing Administration, Office of the Actuary.

13. Moon, M. *Medicare Now and in the Future.* Washington, D.C.: Urban Institute Press, 1996.

14. Carter, G. M., Jacobson, P. D., Kominski, G. F., and Perry, M. J. "Use of Diagnosis-Related Groups by Non-Medicare Payers." *Health Care Financing Review,* 1994, *16,* 127–158.

15. Pear, R. "'98 Medicare Growth Slowest Since Program Began in '65." *New York Times,* Jan. 12, 1999, p. A1.

16. Pear, R. "With Budget Cutting, Medicare Spending Fell Unexpectedly" *New York Times,* May 4, 1999, pp. A20, A24.

17. Moon, M. *Restructuring Medicare: Impacts on Beneficiaries.* Washington, D.C.: Urban Institute, 1999.

18. U.S. Census Bureau, Population Division. "National Population Projections." [http://www.census.gov/population/www/projections/natsum.html]

19. For further discussion of this topic, see Friedland, R. B., and Summer, L. *Demography Is Not Destiny.* Washington, D.C.: National Academy on an Aging Society, 1999.

20. Schmidley, A. D., and Gibson, C. U.S. Census Bureau, Current Population Reports. *Profile of the Foreign-Born Population in the United States: 1997.* (Series P23-195.) Washington, D.C.: U.S. Government Printing Office, 1999. [http://www.census.gov/prod/99pubs/p23–195.pdf]

21. Schmidley and Gibson (1999).

22. "Annual Report of the Board of Trustees of the Federal Hospital Insurance Trust Fund." (Corrected Apr. 20, 2000). [http://www.hcfa.gov/pubforms/tr/hi2000/toc.htm]

23. "2000 Annual Report of the Board of Trustees of the Federal Old-Age and Survivors Insurance and Disability Insurance Trust Funds, Table II.H.1." Apr. 7, 2000. [http://www.ssa.gov/OACT/TR/TR00/index.html]

24. White, J. "Uses and Abuses of Long-Term Medicare Cost Estimates." *Health Affairs,* Jan.–Feb. 1999, *18,* 63–79.

25. See Ikegami, N., and Campbell, J. C. "Health Care Reform in Japan: The Virtues of Muddling Through." *Health Affairs,* May–June 1999, *18,* 56–75; Anderson, G., and Poullier, J.-P. "Health Spending, Access, and Outcomes: Trends in Industrialized Countries." *Health Affairs,* May–June 1999, *18,* 178–192; and Reinhardt, U. "Perspective: 'Mangled Competition' and 'Managed Whatever.'" *Health Affairs,* May–June 1999, *18,* 92–94.

26. Fuchs, V. "Health Care for the Elderly: How Much? Who Will Pay for It?" *Health Affairs,* Jan.–Feb. 1999, *18,* 11–21.

27. Moon, M. *Growth in Medicare Spending: What Will Beneficiaries Pay?* Washington, D.C.: Urban Institute, 1999.

28. "Annual Report of the Board of Trustees of the Federal Hospital Insurance Trust Fund" (2000).

29. See Fuchs (1999); and Moon (1996).

30. Wolfe, J. R. *The Coming Health Crisis: Who Will Pay for Care for the Aged in the Twenty-First Century?* Chicago: University of Chicago Press, 1993.

31. White (1999).

32. Wolfe (1993).

33. Moon (1996).

34. "Annual Reports of the Board of Trustees of the Federal Hospital Insurance and Supplementary Medical Insurance Trust Funds." Mar. 30, 1999. [http://www.hcfa.gov/pubforms/tr/hi1999/HI2.htm]

35. "Annual Report of the Board of Trustees of the Federal Hospital Insurance Trust Fund" (2000).

36. Marmor (2000).

37. Health Care Financing Administration. *A Profile of Medicare: 1998 Chartbook*, Figure 31. Washington, D.C.: Health Care Financing Administration, 1998.

38. Health Care Financing Administration (1998), Figure 40.

39. Levit, K., and others. "Health Spending in 1998: Signals of Change." *Health Affairs*, Jan.–Feb. 2000, *18*, 124–132.

40. Health Care Financing Administration (1998).

41. Gibson, M. J., Brangan, N., Gross, D., and Caplan, C. *How Much Are Medicare Beneficiaries Paying Out-of-Pocket for Prescription Drugs?* Washington, D.C.: American Association of Retired Persons, 1999.

42. FamiliesUSA. *Cost Overdose: Growth in Drug Spending for the Elderly, 1992–2010*. Washington, D.C.: July 2000.

43. Dalaker, J. U.S. Census Bureau. *Current Population Reports. Poverty in the United States: 1998*, Table B-2. (Series P60-207.) Washington, D.C.: U.S. Government Printing Office, 1999. [http://www.census.gov/prod/99pubs/p60–207.pdf]

44. Moon (1999).

45. "Annual Report of the Board of Trustees of the Federal Hospital Insurance Trust Fund" (2000), p. 11.

46. Health Care Financing Administration. "Medicare Managed Care Market Penetration for All Medicare Plan Contractors—Quarterly State/County Data Files." Aug. 1, 2000. [http://www.hcfa.gov/medicare/mpsct1.htm]

47. Aaron, H. J., and Reischauer, R. D. "The Medicare Reform Debate: What Is the Next Step?" *Health Affairs*, Winter 1995, *14*, 8–30.

48. U.S. Congress. *Balanced Budget Act of 1997*. H.R. 2015, Sec. 4021.

49. Enthoven, A. C. "Consumer Choice Health Plan: A National Health Insurance Proposal Based on Regulated Competition in the Private Sector." *New England Journal of Medicine*, 1978, *298*, 709–720.

50. "Annual Reports of the Board of Trustees of the Federal Hospital Insurance and Supplementary Medical Insurance Trust Funds" (1999).

51. U.S. Congress. *Medicare Preservation and Improvement Act of 1999*. S. 1895, Nov. 9, 1999. [http://thomas.loc.gov/]

52. Cowan, C. A., and others. "National Health Expenditures, 1998." *Health Care Financing Review*, 1999, *21*, 165–210.

53. Health Care Financing Administration (1998), Figure 21.

54. Pear (1999).

55. As reported by American Health Line. "Federal Employees: Health Insurance Premiums Rise." September 14, 1998. [http://www.americanhealthline.com]; and "CalPERS to Let Health Rates Rise 9.7% in 2000." *Los Angeles Times*, May 19, 1999, p. 1. Medicare and private cost trends do not compare actuarially equivalent plans. Private health plans provide prescription drug coverage that is not included in traditional Medicare, while Medicare covers home health and long-term care benefits not typically found in private coverage.

56. Smith, S., Freeland, M., Heffler, S., and McKusick, D. "The Next Ten Years of Health Spending: What Does the Future Hold?" *Health Affairs*, Sept.–Oct. 1998, *17*, 128–140.

57. American Health Line. "Politics and Policy—Medicare+Choice: HMOs Warn AZ Pilot Has 'Big Problems.'" Apr. 1, 1999. [http://www.americanhealthline.com]

58. Health Care Financing Administration (1998).

59. Bodenheimer, T., and others. *Rebuilding Medicare for the 21st Century: A Challenge for the Medicare Commission and Congress*. San Francisco: National Campaign to Protect, Improve, and Expand Medicare, c/o Health Access, 1999.

60. National Bipartisan Commission on the Future of Medicare. "Building a Better Medicare for Today and Tomorrow." Mar. 16, 1999. [http://medicare.commission.gov/medicare]

61. *Medicare Preservation and Improvement Act of 1999*.

62. Moon (1999).

63. Urban Institute. *Can Competition Improve Medicare? A Look at Premium Support*. Washington, D.C.: Urban Institute, 1999, p. 16.

64. Health Care Financing Administration (1998), Figure 18.

65. Greenwald, L. M., Esposito, A., Ingber, M. J., and Levy, J. M. "Risk Adjustment for the Medicare Program: Lessons Learned From Research and Demonstrations." *Inquiry*, 1998, *35*, 193–209.

66. Health Care Financing Administration. *Report to Congress: Proposed Method of Incorporating Health Status Risk Adjusters into Medicare+Choice Payments*. Washington D.C.: Health Care Financing Administration, 1999.

67. Newhouse, J. P., Buntin, M. B., and Chapman, J. D. *Risk Adjustment and Medicare*. New York: Commonwealth Fund, 1999.

68. Serafini, M. W. "If It's Good Enough for Congressmen . . ." *National Journal*, 1999, *31*, 340.

69. Pear, R. "HMOs to Drop Thousands of Medicare Patients." *New York Times*, Oct. 2, 1998, pp. A17, A18.

70. U.S. General Accounting Office. *Medicare Managed Care Plans: Many Factors Contribute to Recent Withdrawals; Plan Interest Continues*. (GAO/HEHS-99-91.) Washington, D.C.: U.S. Government Printing Office, 1999.

71. Pear, R. "Estimate of Ousters by HMOs Is Raised." *New York Times*, July 25, 2000, pp. A20, A22.

72. Moon, M. "Will the Care Be There? Vulnerable Beneficiaries and Medicare Reform." *Health Affairs*, Jan.–Feb. 1999, *18*, 107–117.

73. Hibbard, J. H., Jewett, J. J., Engelmann, S., and Tusler, M. "Can Medicare Beneficiaries Make Informed Choices?" In J. K. Iglehart (ed.), *Medicare and Managed Care: A Primer from Health Affairs and the California HealthCare Foundation*. Millwood, Va.: Project HOPE, 1999.

74. In 1990, 15 percent of the population living outside metropolitan areas was elderly, compared with 12 percent within metropolitan areas. See U.S. Bureau of the Census, Current Population Reports, Special Studies. *65+ in the United States*. (P23-190.) Washington, D.C.: U.S. Government Printing Office, 1996; [http://www.census.gov/prod/1/pop/p23–190/p23–190.html] Poverty rates were 14.4 and 12.3 percent, respectively, in 1998 (U.S. Bureau of the Census. *Poverty in the United States 1998*, p. x.)

75. FamiliesUSA. "The Breaux-Frist Bill Puts Rural Residents at Risk." Mar. 2000. [http://www.familiesusa.org/pubs/fumed5.htm]

76. Miller, R. H., and Luft, H. S. "Does Managed Care Lead to Better or Worse Quality of Care?" *Health Affairs*, Sept.–Oct. 1997, *16*, 7–25.

77. Morgan, R. O., Virnig, B. A., DeVito, C. A., and Persily, N. A. "The Medicare-HMO Revolving Door—The Healthy Go in and the Sick Go out." *New England Journal of Medicine,* 1997, *337,* 169–175.

78. Dudley, R. A., Miller, R. H., Korenbrot, T. Y., and Luft, H. S. "The Impact of Financial Incentives on Quality of Health Care." *Milbank Quarterly,* 1998, *76,* 649–686; and Tudor, C. G., Riley, G., and Ingber, M. "Satisfaction with Care: Do Medicare HMOs Make a Difference?" *Health Affairs,* Mar.–Apr. 1998, *17,* 165–176.

79. Druss, B. A., Schlesinger, M., Thomas, T., and Allen, H. "Chronic Illness and Plan Satisfaction Under Managed Care." *Health Affairs,* Jan.–Feb. 2000, *19,* 203–209.

80. Blendon, R. J., and others. "Understanding the Managed Care Backlash." *Health Affairs,* July–Aug. 1998, *17,* 80–94.

81. Blendon and others (1998).

82. Bernstein, S. "Under Pressure, Health Plans Pledge Reforms." *Los Angeles Times,* July 19, 2000.

83. Singer, S. J. "What's Not to Like About HMOs: A Managed Care Maven Struggles with an HMO Runaround at a Vulnerable Time." *Health Affairs,* July–Aug. 2000, *19,* 206–209.

84. Moon (1996).

85. Moon (1996).

86. Schoen, C., and others. *Medicare Beneficiaries: A Population at Risk.* New York: Commonwealth Fund, 1998. [http://www.cmwf.org/programs/medfutur/medicare_survey97_308.asp]

87. Gold, M., Smith, A., Cook, A., and Defilippes, P. *Medicare Managed Care: Preliminary Analysis of Trends in Benefits and Premiums, 1997–1999.* Washington, D.C.: Mathematica Policy Research, 1999.

88. Pear, R. "Medicare HMOs to End Free Drugs, Report Says." *New York Times,* Sept. 22, 1999, pp. A18, A22.

89. Pollack, R. F., and Families USA. "Testimony Before the Commerce Committee of the House of Representatives." June 14, 2000.

90. Pollack (2000).

91. Toner, R. "Political Battle Lines Are Clearly Drawn in Fight over Medicare Drug Coverage." *New York Times,* July 24, 2000, p. A12.

92. Marquis, M. S., and Long, S. H. "Trends in Managed Care and Managed Competition, 1993–1997." *Health Affairs,* Nov.–Dec. 1999, *18,* 75–88.

CHAPTER SEVENTEEN

THE ROLE OF PREVENTION

Charles Lewis

For those looking for challenging health policy issues, prevention is currently a gold mine—but it was not always so.

Greek mythology has it that Chiron, a centaur, taught Aesculapius, a son of Apollo, the art of healing. Aesculapius has become well known, but few are aware of his mythical fate. As his healing powers became more renowned, so did the challenges presented to him. Finally, he restored life to the dead, and for this interference with fate, he was struck dead by a thunderbolt from Zeus.[1] (One need not expand on this as a parable for modern technology and the medical profession.)

Aesculapius had several children, including two daughters, Panacea (about whom little is known) and Hygia, the goddess of health. In early drawings and friezes, Hygia and Aesculapius are often pictured together. Only recently has the separateness, or political coolness, between curative medicine and hygiene—or health promotion and disease prevention—become apparent.[2]

With time and the growth of the science and technology base in each area, they have been recognized as relatives, and frequently competitors, for resources. Resolving unnecessary competition between them and prescribing a balance of the two present both challenges and opportunities to frame comprehensive preventive services and health care policy for the United States.

This chapter focuses on the answers to three questions. First, what is preventable? In well-designed studies, what interventions have been shown to work? These data lead to our present (2001) recommendations for preventive care services.

Second, what are the problems associated with applying our knowledge to the care of individuals and populations in the real world? We may know the risk factors for a condition and the biological changes that must be reversed or terminated, yet we may not be able to prevent the condition. We know more than we are able to do, because many of our treatments require major changes in human behavior or in society. Scholars have created theoretical models for these changes, enumerating key independent variables.[3] However, skilled practitioners concerned with behavioral changes may find these models less-than-helpful. Also, some potentially effective treatments are not currently acceptable to society as a whole.

The third and final group of questions is: What value does society place on prevention? What are we, as a nation, willing to do to eliminate certain causative agents or change our environment? How much are we willing to invest in something so that it will never occur? We may know what to do to prevent X, and how to do it, but lack the collective will to take the actions necessary to prevent X, even though the consequences of this inaction are obvious.

The future-oriented and value-laden nature of prevention must be recognized by those who would teach, promote, or practice it. From a cognitive developmental perspective, this requires that the recipient be in a *formal stage of operation*.[4] That is, the target must be able to recognize the causal relationship between actions taken today and their delayed preventive effects tomorrow (or believe unquestioningly in the recommendations). Individuals, therefore, must believe in tomorrow and place a value on their future, however short or long.

Those professionals who are prepared to provide preventive services certainly are able to understand the causal chain of events and have reason to be future-oriented. However, practicing prevention requires the ability to forgo the satisfaction of doing something that has immediate and visible effect (even if it is untoward) and to imagine the consequences of failure to prevent. A successful day in the practice of prevention could be seen as a series of zeros, or investments in the future, with nothing tangible to show for today's work.[5]

Recent History

Pioneers in public health, many of whom were concerned with environmental hygiene, lent statistical support to the maternal admonitions "always wash your hands" and "cleanliness is next to godliness." Florence Nightingale made sound recommendations to the British army, even though allegedly she never accepted the germ theory.[6] Still, scholarly inquiry occasionally helps us rewrite history. A recent biography by Hugh Small has explained some of the behavior attributed to her.[7] He has exposed a cover-up in which Nightingale was asked by the British army High Command to investigate the apparently unnecessary deaths of more than sixteen thousand soldiers in hospitals in the Crimea. She discovered that the problem was related to complete neglect of hospital hygiene, which had created, in essence, a "death camp." She subsequently pushed for the government to publish the evidence to mobilize opinion for public health reform. However, the government's refusal led, or contributed in a large measure, to her physical and mental breakdown.

Nightingale responded by leaking a report to the public that showed how the government had suppressed the vital evidence; she used this as a way of avenging the deaths of so many common soldiers. Small's published accounts of these episodes (and his discovery of the cover-up and its failure) indicate how important her contribution was to public health after the war, and that she had made use of the most scientific expertise of the day. Small goes ahead to note that Britain's urban death rate fell significantly after the war because public resistance to public health legislation regarding hygiene evaporated in the face of her careful arguments.

Apparently, after her death, her biographers tried to restore her reputation as the nurse with the lamp claiming that she had solved the hygiene problem at her wartime hospital, and reduced the death rate from 42 percent to 2 percent. In her notes, Nightingale indicates that the death rate rose from 8 percent to 42 percent in four months *after* her arrival, and that she was not responsible for the reduction. Small's book has swept away some of the myths and makes it possible to reevaluate her work. However, the enduring picture of the "lady with the lamp" may continue to put her in the camp of nursing, rather than environmental public health reform. The basics of public health are the tenets upon which the practice of prevention are based.

Over the past several years, the relative roles of the individual, the professions, and the government (in the form of public health activities) have changed. It has been accepted that individuals must bear responsibility for their health behaviors—thus our practice of blaming the victim. However, individuals have the right to expect that health care providers will recommend preventive services to them that are appropriate for their age and risk factors, and provide them when professional intervention is required (for example, immunizations and screening tests such as mammograms).

The role of public health agencies, though formerly limited to offering such services to special population groups, has grown from this role to providing leadership in terms of planning strategic objectives for prevention for the entire nation. In the process, public health practitioners have assumed a critical role in defining (answering) the questions posed.

The American Medical Association suggested the annual physical examination as a method for maintaining health in 1922. Despite growing awareness that preventive services on an annual basis were not clinically effective, the annual approach to the health examination was not revised by the AMA until 1983, in a policy statement that withdrew support for the annual physical examination and instead focused on an individualized periodic health visit.[8]

Despite the progress made in other fields of medical science, it was more than fifty years after the AMA's advocacy of annual preventive examinations that, in 1975, the La Londe Commission was established by the Canadian government to examine the scientific literature, and to bring forth a series of evidence-based recommendations for practicing clinical prevention.[9]

Shortly afterward, the most significant event in the history of prevention in the United States occurred. In 1977, the Department of Health, Education, and Welfare published *Healthy People: The Surgeon General's Report on Health Promotion and Disease Prevention*.[10] This landmark work spelled out the overall goals for five age groups; defined two examples for special focus within each; and defined four types of objective to be accomplished for each: public and professional awareness, surveillance and evaluation, service improvement, and risk reduction. It also named a federal public health agency to lead the work on each specific objective. Thus, it began to spell out the relationships among the private and public sectors, and it defined the players in the game of prevention. As suggested earlier, although the individual must be involved or feel empowered to take certain actions, these must be encouraged, recommended, and administered by health professionals. The public and the professions must know the threats to health and what is available to reduce the risks to an individual, and have the courage to ask questions that may embarrass the interviewee (such as "Are you sexually active?").

Primary prevention is obviously the prevention of choice. However, except under those circumstances in which immunizing agents have been developed, primary prevention involves the efforts of a variety of individuals to undo those learned lifestyle behaviors that are hazardous to one's health. As is evident in several studies, this is possible, but it requires considerable effort.

Subsequently, the federal government established the U.S. Preventive Services Task Force (USPSTF), which further contributed to our knowledge of what is worth doing.[11] The task force echoed the findings of the Canadian group, that many screening tests to detect disease at an early stage often produce a large number of false positive results, leading to unnecessary subsequent diagnostic assessments. The task force reiterated the fact that in examining proposals for secondary prevention (to be defined later in this chapter), screening tests—or those used to detect health problems early—must be accurate and reliable.

Here are some definitions that are fundamental to prevention through early detection.

Accuracy refers to the reliability, sensitivity, specificity, and positive predictive value of a test.

Reliability means the ability to produce the same result on repeated occasions (whether it is valid or not).

Sensitivity means the ability to detect individuals who have the condition targeted by the screening procedure. A test with low sensitivity will fail to detect a number of individuals with the condition, producing a high number of false negative values.

Specificity means the ability to differentiate individuals who have the condition targeted by the screening procedure from the rest of the population. A test with poor specificity results in a number of normal individuals being included in the group alleged to have the condition, producing a high number of false positive values.

Positive predictive value (PPV) means the ability of a test to produce reliable values for population screening rather than as part of a diagnostic workup. It is a function of the prevalence of the target condition in the population being tested as well as of the sensitivity and specificity of a test. The most important factor in determining the usefulness of the PPV is the prevalence of the target condition. A test with high sensitivity and specificity can still generate more false positives than true positives if it is used to screen for a relatively rare condition. Table 17.1 shows what happens when a test that is 99 percent sensitive and 99 percent specific is used to screen for a condition with a prevalence of 0.1 percent in a population of one hundred thousand individuals.

The PPV is the value that results from dividing the number of *true positive* individuals by the total number of those with positive test results. In this illustration,

TABLE 17.1. PREVALENCE, SENSITIVITY, AND SPECIFICITY IN HYPOTHETICAL TEST RESULTS.

Test Is:	Condition Is:		Totals
	Present	*Absent*	
Positive	99 (true positive)	999 (false positive)	1,098
Negative	1 (false negative)	98,901 (true negative)	98,902
Total	100	99,900	100,000

the 99 true positives represent 9.0 percent of the total of 1,098. If one is only concerned about the consequences of missing actual cases, this 99 percent sensitivity looks great. However, if one is concerned with the consequences of falsely labeling individuals—for example, telling healthy people they have human immunodeficiency virus (HIV) infection—the 9 percent PPV is unnerving. It indicates that roughly ten times as many persons are falsely labeled to have the condition in question as are truly identified. In addition to the psychological hardship thus imposed, a low PPV entails substantial additional expense for further evaluation and testing (necessary for all positive test results) of individuals who should have been properly identified initially.

Among the other critical issues considered by the task force was *lead time bias*, that is, whether or not early detection actually extends length of life or merely advances the diagnosis to an earlier date, with the patient dying at about the same time anyway. The gaps in evidence needed to answer the first question (What is worth doing?) were identified by the task force and suggested an enormous research agenda for preventive medicine.

Perhaps the most important contribution of the task force was creation of a rating guide by which all preventive practices could be graded.[12] The ratings are based on strength of recommendation as well as the quality of the evidence. Here is the grading system:

1. There is *good* evidence to support the recommendation that the condition be specifically considered in a periodic health examination.
2. There is *poor* evidence to support the recommendation that the condition be specifically considered in a periodic health examination.
3. There is *fair* evidence to support the recommendation that the condition be *excluded* from consideration.
4. There is *good* evidence to support the recommendation that the condition be *excluded* from consideration.

Good, fair, and *poor* are defined by examining the burden of suffering created by the condition, and the nature of the intervention (cost, simplicity, and so on). The *quality* of evidence is rated this way:

I.   Evidence is obtained from at least one properly designed, *randomized* clinical controlled trial (RCT).
II-1. Evidence is from at least one well-designed controlled trial, without randomization.
II-2. Evidence is from at least one well-designed, cohort-case controlled analytic study.

II-3. Evidence from a multiple time series design, with or without the intervention, in populations. All of the Type II evidence comes from quasi-experimental designs.

III.   Evidence is based upon opinions of respected authorities, their clinical experience, descriptive studies, and so on.

Thus, rating the recommendation for an annual mammogram in women over fifty years of age *IA* describes the quality of the evidence to support it (in this instance, good evidence from a randomized controlled trial).

Concepts Underlying Prevention

Before pursuing the health policy issues facing decision makers in the health care system of tomorrow, it is important for policy makers to understand certain terms or concepts drawn from epidemiology that underlie the practice of prevention.

The *natural history of a phenomenon* views a disease, illness, or threat to health as beginning at some point in time (often at birth) and increasing over time in terms of its degree of severity or impairment of functioning of a molecular system, an organ, or an individual. For example, at birth there is little evidence of the presence of atherosclerosis. With the passage of time, and depending on genetic influences, diet, physical activity, and other factors, there is subsequent narrowing of arterial vessels (such as the coronary arteries) because of the development of atheromata or lipid-laden plaques, until at some time in the history of this disorder the condition *breaks the clinical horizon*. That is, the individual ceases to be asymptomatic and the problem manifests itself in the form of physical evidence or symptoms (for example, chest pain on exertion or myocardial infarction).[13] This history may be relatively long, as in the case of coronary heart disease, or it may be relative short, as in the case of spousal violence.

The most important derivative of the natural history of a disease is that diseases or disorders are present at a *subclinical* stage, at which point they may be detected with appropriately sensitive and specific tests applied to those suspected of having the disease and for whom a test is clinically indicated. From this perspective, we derive definitions of the *level of prevention*.

Primary preventive services are those activities or procedures that maintain the health of the individual. *Secondary prevention* refers to early detection of a problem using a variety of screening techniques. This means identifying the presence of the problem before it breaks the clinical horizon or becomes symptomatic. In the case of coronary artery disease, data on some risk factors associated with the stage of the disease—a lipid profile, history of smoking, lack of exercise—may be obtained very easily. Such data can indicate the desirability of a more expensive test—a stress electrocardiogram—that may reveal diminished blood flow to the heart. When positive, this test lowers the clinical horizon and advances the point in time at which a diagnosis is made. Then, the question facing those concerned with prevention is, Can the individual be persuaded to alter those behaviors that lead to developing the condition?

Finally, although it may seem internally contradictory, *tertiary prevention* is defined as efforts to maintain the existing levels of functioning in an individual once afflicted with a problem (for example, maintaining residual musculoskeletal function after a cerebrovascular accident).

Host-agent interaction is a basic epidemiological concept that views phenomena threatening health in terms of the interactions among an *agent* (chemical, biological, or physical), a host (the individual), and the *environment* in which both exist. Both causes and means of prevention can be assessed in terms of these interactions.

The epidemiological basis for prevention is quite simple. Hosts can be altered; they can be changed immunologically through vaccination with biological agents, thus rendering them resistant to a specific agent in the environment. (There may be no general panaceas.) Host behavior that leads to increased risk of a disease (and there are many such behaviors) may be altered through counseling with regard to risk, and persuading individuals of the importance of behavior change. Clearly, the most effective prevention is accomplished when the host is completely passive in the prevention process (does not have to think or change), as with fluoridation of water. Unfortunately, such examples are rare.

With regard to causative agents, they may be eliminated, reduced in concentration, or altered. Smallpox has been eliminated from the globe, but handguns proliferate. Both India and Pakistan have detonated atomic weapons and have the means of settling a long-standing grudge permanently. A variety of public health measures make our water free of bacteria, and we have substituted less toxic materials for those that have been widely used in dwellings (for example, asbestos).

Changes in the environment can be accomplished by removing the agents, the hosts, or both, from a threatening environment, or affecting or attenuating their interactions. This may be done, for example, by laws associated with smog control, or in another arena by banning the sale of cigarettes from vending machines so as to prevent sales to underaged individuals (more theoretical than real)[14] or possibly eliminating the sale of attack weapons to the public. However, policy decisions leading to legislative changes that eliminate certain agents from the environment are often difficult to achieve. Many agents have very strong support from interest groups of their own; the National Rifle Association and certain political forces feel that society has seriously impaired the quality of their lives by limiting access to military assault weapons.

Policy Questions for Prevention

As suggested in the initial section, this chapter discusses issues related to prevention in our current health care system. First, What is worth doing? How do we know? A derivative of this question is, Who must be involved or responsible if prevention is to occur?

In the United States, other issues have clearly gained considerable policy importance. They relate to our concern with costs and overall resource allocation. One issue is, Who shall pay (and how much)? What is it worth (and to whom) to prevent X? As noted earlier, this is not a purely cognitive endeavor. Values are associated with prevention; thus the related question, Whose values shall prevail?

We pursue these questions not encyclopedically but by focusing on certain targets for prevention that illustrate the barriers faced by those concerned. These targets are pulmonary and cardiovascular disease associated with cigarette smoking, death due to firearms, and the AIDS epidemic. In each case, preventive procedures or maneuvers advocated for each are listed and potential barriers to their accomplishments reviewed. To do this, let's go back to the literature.

The Database: What Do We Know, and How Do We Know It?

The 1979 Surgeon General's Report listed one of the basic objectives as "surveillance and evaluation." Two years later, the Centers for Disease Control and Prevention (CDC), in collaboration with state health departments, initiated an ongoing system of telephone surveys designed to generate data on the prevalence of certain behaviors at the state level to track the progress of programs designed to affect health behaviors.

In 1982, twenty-five state health departments conducted telephone surveys using CDC training and standardization methods.[15] In 1984, these activities evolved into the Behavioral Risk Factor Surveillance System (BRFSS), which was also designed to support major public health initiatives in prevention, such as legislation concerning cigarette taxation and mandatory seat belts. The system employs the Waksberg method of using randomly chosen noninstitutionalized adults for telephone interviews. Two sets of questions are asked: a core set asked in all states, including standardized questions developed by the CDC; and questions developed by individual states to meet their specific objectives.

The BRFSS estimates a variety of important measures in the adult population, including the prevalence of being overweight, leading a sedentary lifestyle, smoking, or avoiding seat belts. For weight, the survey used the Body Mass

Index (BMI), defined as weight in kilograms divided by height in meters squared. In 1988, BRFSS data indicated 20.9 percent of the population exceeded the recommended BMI for their age). Sedentary lifestyle was defined as fewer than three sessions per week of twenty minutes or more of leisure physical activity; here the average was 58 percent. Cigarette smoking got a 24.7 yes rate, and seatbelt nonuse got 30.1 percent. Several other factors were also included, but not presented here.[16] Data are reported by age group and gender; those cited in this paragraph are for the entire adult population of the United States.

A considerable volume of literature exists on what should be done (and the evidence to support these recommendations). To examine this in one volume, the reader is referred to the *Guide to Clinical Preventive Services*.[17] This guide reviews the evidence on more than one hundred interventions to prevent sixty illnesses and conditions. The latter are grouped as in a traditional medically oriented systems review. There are also chapters on counseling and immunizations. Each chapter—for example, screening for lead toxicity—cites the relevant literature, available up to the time of publication, leading to a specific recommendation.

As indicated, the appointment of the task force was preceded by *Healthy People* (1979), which sets forth a litany of the health problems affecting the U.S. population. Subsequently, a series of similar reports (*Healthy People 1990* and *Healthy People 2000*) have marked our progress (or, in many cases, the lack of same) toward the goals. In each of these reports, voluminous literature is cited.[18]

The latest version of this prescriptive effort is part of an initiative, Put Prevention into Practice (PPIP), announced in the fall of 1994 by the secretary of Health and Human Services, Donna Shalala. The centerpiece of this effort is *The Clinician's Handbook of Preventive Services*.[19] It is divided into sections covering preventive services for children and adolescents, adults, and older adults, with appendices that include risk-factor tables. The PPIP kit includes the handbook *A Personal Health Guide*, designed to help patients work with their doctors and other health care providers. It has a reminder of recommended immunizations and screening tests, as well as spaces for recording the dates on which interventions are given. In addition, the PPIP kit includes reminder stickers for appointments, flow charts for office use, and other tools that have been shown to facilitate provision of preventive services.

In addition to the BRFSS data on self-reported risk factors, the National Health and Nutrition Examination Survey (NHANES) offers data on the prevalence of abnormal physical, mental, and social health disturbances, as determined by laboratory and clinical examination. NHANES collects data on hypertension, body mass, anthropomorphic measurements, and serum cholesterol, all done in the field. Extrapolating these data to the U.S. population requires that clinical and laboratory examination be performed (by a special team of examiners) on individuals carefully selected from the U.S. population in surveys designed by epidemiologists and statisticians. As suggested, both types of survey involve random samples of the U.S. population, stratified in such a way as to permit estimates with a stated limit of confidence.

The U.S. Public Health Service (USPHS) has a long history of disseminating such population-based data. Initially, this was done by the freestanding National Center of Health and Vital Statistics; it is now done by the same agency following its administrative transfer to the CDC.[20] This transfer has not diminished the quality of such efforts. Also, the *Morbidity and Mortality Weekly Reports (MMWR)* of the CDC are a rich source of summarized data from surveillance and evaluation activities conducted by the federal government.[21]

Community-Oriented Prevention

The majority of descriptive or analytical studies dealing with the efficacy of an intervention are based upon the study of *individuals*, where intervention X is done by professional Y. However, in the past two decades there has been an increase in the number of studies applying a public health model to prevention; that is, a *community* intervention as it relates to preventing specific diseases (or reducing risks in the population related to those diseases). In addition to offering mass screening or immunization campaigns, these make possible an intervention through the mass media and campaigns involving various civic and employer groups. These studies have, in general, shown some positive impact, but they have not produced the level of change anticipated.[22] As a result, they have begged the question for policy makers, How should we invest or divide our resources—through community efforts, or individualized clinical intervention? An editorial entitled "The Tribulations of Trials—Intervention in Communities" discussed the disappointing results of the Take Heart and COMMIT (smoking cessation) community trials.[23] The Take Heart effort produced no significant results; the COMMIT trial had one modest, positive outcome.

In addition to the efforts, already described, to provide preventive services in the public and private sectors, many private corporations have discovered the commercial benefits of organizing preventive services for their employees. Studies have shown such activities (exercise facilities at work, stress reduction classes, smoking cessation programs) result in reduced absenteeism, higher employee morale, and increased productivity.[24]

The process of reviewing scientific experimentation extends the frontiers of knowledge about prevention, but it is based on available studies. It is likely that certain studies that are important to policy makers will never be done because of the ethical consequences of randomizing populations (specifically the disadvantaged) to treatment and control groups and the costs of some longitudinal studies. An example of this was reported by Lewis and colleagues in a report of terminating a randomized controlled trial of asthma education for poor Latino children.[25]

Three Examples of Prevention

Here are three examples of preventive challenges, concerning smoking-related illness, mortality from gunshot wounds, and the HIV/AIDS epidemic.

In the first edition of this book, this section began with a discussion of preventing infectious disease in childhood. It chronicled achievements within the public arena in terms of increasing immunization levels among children for measles, rubella, diphtheria and tetanus (DPT), polio and hemophilus B, and influenza. Although some disparity in the level of immunization still exists among various racial and ethnic groups, the worldwide magnitude of the HIV/AIDS epidemic suggests that this is a more salient example to illustrate the obstacles to achieving the goals of prevention.

Example One: Cardiopulmonary Disease Attributable to Cigarette Smoking

The impact of cigarette smoking on health status is enormous. It is the primary cause of premature death in the United States.[26] Since the initial Surgeon General's report on smoking more than thirty years ago,[27] U.S. residents as a group have been gradually withdrawing from the addiction to nicotine produced by smoking. The CDC has developed software to estimate the smoking-attributable mortality of any population group and to project years of life lost thanks to smoking.[28]

A variety of efforts have been mounted over the past thirty years to reduce the prevalence of smoking. Something is working, but slowly. The prevalence of smoking has fallen 0.5 percent per year over the period 1965–1985 and more drastically, 1.1 percent per year, over the period 1986–1989. However, evidence suggests the prevalence of smoking among teenagers is increasing.[29]

Prevention efforts to reduce this unnecessary carnage have followed the four objectives originally defined in 1979:

1. Increase awareness. Recent studies indicate growing awareness of the risks associated with smoking, especially among physicians.[30]
2. Surveillance and evaluation systems are in place, including a Teenage Attitudes Toward Smoking system.[31]

3. Risk-factor reduction is occurring with the decreasing prevalence of smoking.
4. Service improvement is represented by increased attention to the problem in all health care settings.

About 25 percent of all adults are still addicted smokers. The prevalence of smoking is inversely associated with years of education. Among those with twelve or fewer years of education, 32 percent are smokers, versus 13.6 percent of those with sixteen or more years of education.[32]

A variety of programs have been designed to target the young, including legislation prohibiting sale of cigarettes to minors from vending machines in forty-four states. A growing number of public places and workplaces, such as restaurants, have been declared no-smoking zones by local or state ordinances. The number of places where one can conveniently light up is shrinking. Several U.S. airlines have designated all flights, including international ones, as nonsmoking.

Other proposed efforts, such as increasing taxes imposed on cigarettes, are gaining support. Manufacturers have been accused of spiking their cigarettes with extra nicotine to enhance their addictive capacity. If cigarettes were considered a drug because of the presence of nicotine, they would fall within the jurisdiction of the FDA and thus be subject to regulation. The U.S. Supreme Court has recently ruled, however, that the FDA does not have regulatory authority over tobacco.

Despite these consumer-oriented prevention programs, there have been few serious attempts to influence the providers or growers of the agent. The tobacco industry is large and powerful; growing the agent also represents the only means of economic survival for many farmers.

Given the slow reduction in the prevalence of smoking and the many programs designed to prevent teenagers from becoming addicted, the United States needs to address a major policy question. We seem to have reached a point where further reduction in tobacco consumption, especially among the young, is difficult to achieve. This begs the question, Should we continue to struggle to limit the growth of tobacco use while ignoring or even encouraging tobacco production? How much would it cost to buy out those commercial interests who help to maintain a cadre of nicotine-addicted individuals who suffer the morbidity and mortality associated with their habit? How do we compare the relative value of twenty-seven deaths from measles per year to four hundred thousand deaths per year from tobacco-related disease?

Example Two: Deaths from Gunshot Wounds

The magnitude of the problem of gunshot wounds has been described in many publications. Since 1960, more than half a million Americans have died from firearm injuries.[33] The term contains a heterogeneous group of specific problems;

all have one thing (agent) in common: the availability of a gun, usually a handgun. However, like the treatment of a medical symptom, such as a headache, it is necessary to establish a diagnosis (in this case, to define the problem clearly) before prescribing a treatment or preventive intervention. The total of more than thirty-one thousand deaths attributable to gunshot wounds that were reported in 1990 includes about nineteen thousand cases of suicide—or over 60 percent. Another two thousand were accidental deaths, mainly children who discover a loaded gun unsafely stored and kill themselves, and more than eleven thousand cases of homicide. Of the latter, most shootings (52 percent) were not done in the course of a crime, but by acquaintances or relatives of the victim as the result of escalating interpersonal conflict.[34]

As suggested, each occurs because of the availability of a gun, and each victim has his or her own group of survivors who seek to prevent another similar episode (no matter that the root causes may differ). One of the main problems faced by all these advocacy groups is that the use of guns has been associated in the media with crime, when in fact shootings associated with a felony represent only a fraction of all deaths from guns.[35]

The history of efforts to regulate guns in the United States is a comedy with tragic results. This includes federal initiatives (now under the purview of the Bureau of Alcohol, Tobacco, and Firearms) and a variety of community and state laws that have done little to stem the proliferation of handguns in the United States. It is estimated that there are currently two hundred million working firearms owned by U.S. citizens.[36]

A Comparison

The problems created by tobacco are secondary to the effects of inhaled smoke and development of a physical dependence because of addiction to nicotine. The problems associated with the existence of handguns are secondary to a psychological and cultural dependence fostered by popular myths about the so-called American way of life.

Both tobacco and handgun use are supported by large lobbying forces that have, to date, outsmarted governmental public health groups. For example, the California legislature passed five laws in 1994 specifically related to gun control. These laws prohibit gun sales to minors, prohibit sale of ammunition to anyone under eighteen years of age, require gun dealers to make records of their sales available to law enforcement officials, prohibit anyone under a restraining order for domestic violence from owning a gun while the order is in effect, and suspend a minor's driver's license if apprehended for a motor vehicle violation while carrying a concealed weapon.

All of these laws chip away at the central issue—the existence and ready availability of guns. All fail to recognize that the epidemic of homicide—the primary cause of death among African American young men—has grown with the availability of guns to this population. Those who have studied this subject feel these agents *must* be eliminated from the environment.[37] All existing laws (such as the Brady Bill) are primarily focused on changing the environment to make it more difficult to obtain a gun, not on removing a gun already in private hands. These existing laws could have some effect—a waiting period *may* reduce the number of suicides from gunshot wounds among those who do not have ready access to them at the peak of their depression—but barely address the main issue.

The popular image of the usefulness of guns in self-protection against criminals is furthered by the advertising practices of gun manufacturers. They clearly have recognized the importance of creating a new market by suggesting, in advertisements, how valuable a handgun is for a woman's self-protection. A study of trauma center workers in Alabama revealed that 74 percent of women (mostly nurses) employed in these centers owned a gun, and 45 percent carried a loaded gun in their car.[38]

What are the options for policy makers? Do they understand the epidemiology of firearm deaths? How will they limit the number of guns in the United States, in the face of a strong constituency that believes ownership of guns is a right protected by the Second Amendment to the Constitution? Perhaps in no other area of prevention are values so evident and so powerful. Our inaction suggests that we do not understand, or we do not care, or both. How can policy makers introduce rationality into this discussion?

Example Three: The AIDS Epidemic

This chapter began by posing a series of questions for public health professionals and policy makers concerned with prevention: What do we know? Who must be involved for prevention to occur? What are the barriers to applying what we know? What value does society place on prevention? The HIV/AIDS epidemic in Africa provides a compelling example of just how difficult it can be to address these questions. Worldwide, an estimated 36.1 million people are infected with human immunodeficiency virus (HIV). Seventy percent of these cases are in Sub-Saharan Africa, where the adult prevalence rate of 8.8 percent dwarfs the rates of 0.56 percent in South and Southeast Asia and 0.6 percent in North America.[39] Approximately fifty-five hundred people die of AIDS every day in Sub-Saharan Africa.[40] In South Africa, Botswana, and other Southern African countries with the highest rates of infection, it is estimated that more than one-third of today's teenagers will die of AIDS.[41]

What do we know? The first case of AIDS was identified in 1981; two years later, researchers isolated the HIV retrovirus. The scientific establishment in the developed world overwhelmingly accepts the research evidence showing that HIV is the agent that causes AIDS.[42] The virus is transmitted through sexual contact; through sharing of needles among infected users of injected drugs; by exposure to infected blood products; and from mother to infant during pregnancy, delivery, and possibly breast feeding. The primary prevention strategy for HIV/AIDS is education aimed at persuading individuals to modify high-risk behaviors. These education efforts must be multifaceted and employ targeted outreach because of the diverse population groups affected and the changing patterns of infection. In the United States, the virus spread initially mainly through men who have sex with men and through injected drug use. HIV infection is now increasingly associated with heterosexual contact, and women and racial and ethnic minorities represent an increasing proportion of cases. In Southern Africa, the dominant mode of transmission continues to be through heterosexual exposure. More than half of those infected are women;[43] in South Africa, it is estimated that more than 20 percent of pregnant women are HIV-infected. Secondary prevention involves treatment of those infected with HIV to delay the onset of AIDS, and to avoid the risk that infected mothers will transmit the virus to their babies *in utero* or at delivery. Considerable success has been achieved through the use of a "cocktail" of antiretroviral drugs. Like much of Western medicine, however, these remedies are costly. At an annual estimated cost of more than $10,000 per individual treated, the newest drug therapies are far beyond the means of the developing world.[44]

Even the question of what we know has become complicated. South African President Mbeki ignited an international controversy in 2000 when he argued that HIV does not cause AIDS, and that African leaders should not look to the developed countries for solutions to their unique pandemic.[45] Despite the evidence that antiretroviral drugs can reduce the risk of *in utero* transmission, Mbeki refused to allow these drugs to be given to HIV-infected pregnant women. He was reported to have told an African National Congress parliamentary caucus that "the United States and pharmaceutical companies have conspired to establish a false link between HIV and AIDS to promote the sale of antiretroviral drugs."[46] Here we see how prevention efforts can be complicated by beliefs and values developed through historical political struggles. Mbeki finally gave in to pressure from his allies at the end of 2000.

This leads us to the question of who should be involved in HIV/AIDS prevention. At the beginning of the epidemic, South Africa was absorbed in its struggle to end apartheid and in the challenge of creating a new democracy. The United States and the World Health Organization initially did little to intervene in the developing crisis. The *Washington Post* editorialized that Africa suffered from a "plague of denial."[47] The epidemic is having a devastating economic effect on the nations of Southern Africa. It is estimated that HIV/AIDS will reduce economic growth in South Africa by 17 percent between 2000 and 2010, the equivalent of $22 billion.[48] AIDS has decimated the ranks of teachers, deprived the economy of productive workers, and created millions of orphans. Accused of ignoring the problem until it threatened to affect their own self-interest, foreign nations recently have escalated the issue beyond the boundaries of Africa. In April 2000, the Clinton Administration took the unusual step of declaring AIDS to be a threat to national security, fearing that its spread could destabilize governments and undermine its efforts to support free-market democracies throughout the world.[49] Subsequently, several major pharmaceutical companies agreed to cut the prices of antiretroviral drugs sold in African countries, and the Export-Import Bank of the United States offered up to $1 billion in loans to purchase the drugs.[50] At a meeting of the World Bank and International Monetary Fund, the World Bank president identified AIDS as the most important development issue in Africa. Collaborating with UNAIDS (the Joint United Nations Programme on HIV/AIDS), the World Bank has established the Multisectoral AIDS Program for Africa, which will provide $500 million to support HIV/AIDS prevention and care.[51]

The increased international attention brings additional resources to bear on the AIDS epidemic, but it also brings a new set of players and potentially competing priorities. Even among the U.S. agencies involved, the National Security Council, the Office of the U.S. Trade Representative, and the CDC are not accustomed to collaborating with each other. A greater challenge for these diverse agencies is to recognize that the leadership for effective implementation of prevention programs must come from the African countries themselves. United Nations Secretary General Kofi Annan called for African leaders to make the AIDS epidemic their top priority in order to use these resources to greatest effect.[52]

Beyond the question of who should be involved in the prevention effort, the African countries must address behavioral, social, and economic factors that contribute to the spread of HIV infection. Efforts to educate young people about the dangers of casual sex and the importance of condom use are hampered as AIDS claims the lives of many teachers and increasing poverty leads youths to drop out of school. Male cultural attitudes result in multiple sexual partners and sexual relations between older men and young girls. When economic factors force workers to travel far from home to find work, they may spread the infection through a network of sexual partners. The low status of women limits their control over their partners' use of condoms. High rates of other sexually transmitted infections and low rates of male circumcision also contribute to an increase in HIV infection.[53]

In addition, suspicion of Western approaches to these problems is combined with a strong desire for self-determination. The African nations do not have the resources to fight AIDS alone, but they must take ownership of the prevention process.

Finally, what value does the world place on containing AIDS in Africa? Annan issued this challenge:

> The AIDS pandemic—unexpected, unexplained, unspeakably cruel—presents us with a tragedy we can barely comprehend, let alone manage. . . . AIDS leaves poor societies poorer still, and thus even more vulnerable to infection. It brings in its wake discrimination, prejudice, and often violations of human rights. It is taking away not only Africa's present, but also its future. . . . The challenge cannot be met without resources. But donors can and must do more than that. They must adopt policies and priorities that meet the needs of the countries most affected. And they must raise awareness in their own countries that AIDS is not over. That AIDS is far more than a medical problem, that AIDS is a threat to an entire generation—indeed, a threat to human civilization as a whole.[54]

Conclusion

Our three cases have one thing in common: all are due to agents—infectious, chemical, or physical. In the case of HIV/AIDS, science has yet to produce a preventive measure (vaccine), and the virus is spread by sexual contact and injected drug use. The other two cases are different: one is associated with chemical addiction to nicotine, and the other is a product of culture dependence. Both have powerful lobbies that have sought to confuse the public. One of these (smoking) is slowly being reduced at great public expense. Gun violence is still a symptom. One can only remember the Surgeon General's Report of 1979, noting that public and professional awareness, surveillance, and evaluation must precede reduction in risk factors and improvement of services.

Where should we invest? It seems clear that among these three cases, *values* (confounded with economic interests), not lack of knowledge, are the primary obstacles. Policy makers reviewing other targets for prevention listed in *Healthy People 2000* should count the number for which we know what to do but fail to do. Answers to the second question—What *can* we do?—reveal how many health problems are not preventable because of our inability to apply existing knowledge. In the end, when we examine our values, we find the cause of our limitations.

Notes

1. Schouten, J. (ed.). *The Rod and the Serpent of Aesculapius, Symbol of Medicine.* New York: Elsevier, 1969.
2. Susser, M. "The Bell Tolls for a School of Public Health—and for Thee?" *American Journal of Public Health*, 1993, *83*(11), 1524–1525.
3. Becker, M. H. (ed.). *The Health Belief Model and Personal Health Behavior.* Thorofare, N.J.: Slack, 1974.
4. Lupin, G., Magyar, J., and Poulsen, M. (eds.). *Proceedings of the Fourth Interdisciplinary Seminar: Piagetian Theory and the Helping Professionals.* Los Angeles: University of Southern California, Feb. 15, 1974.
5. Lewis, C. E. "The Untimely Death of Preventive Medicine: The 1988 Duncan Clark Lecture." *American Journal of Preventive Medicine*, 1988, *5*(1), 52–54.
6. Cook, E. *The Life of Florence Nightingale, Vol. 1.* London: Macmillan, 1913.
7. Small, H. *Florence Nightingale: Avenging Angel.* New York: St. Martin's Press, 1999.
8. Council on Scientific Affairs. "Medical Evaluations of Healthy Persons." *Journal of the American Medical Association*, 1983, *249*, 1626–1633.
9. La Londe Commission. *A New Perspective on the Health of Canadians.* Ottawa, Canada: Minister of Health and Welfare, 1975.
10. U.S. Department of Health, Education, and Welfare. *Healthy People: The Surgeon General's Report on Health Promotion and Disease Prevention.* DHEW-PHS, publication no. 79-55071. Washington, D.C.: Public Health Service, U.S. Department of Health, Education, and Welfare, 1979.
11. U.S. Preventive Services Task Force. *A Guide to Clinical Preventive Services: An Assessment of the Effectiveness of 169 Interventions.* Baltimore, Md.: Williams and Wilkins, 1989.
12. U.S. Preventive Services Task Force (1989).
13. Giorci, A. D., and Weisfeld, M. L. "Acute Myocardial Infarction." In A. M. Harvey and others (eds.), *The Principles and Practices of Medicine.* East Norwalk, Conn.: Appleton and Lange, 1988.
14. "Minors' Access to Cigarette Vending Machines—Texas." *Morbidity and Mortality Weekly Report*, Sept. 2, 1994, *43*, 625–626.
15. "Behavioral Risk Factor Surveillance, 1988." *Morbidity and Mortality Weekly Report*, June 1, 1990, *39*, 1–6.
16. "Behavioral Risk Factor Surveillance, 1988" (1990).
17. U.S. Preventive Services Tasks Force (1989).
18. U.S. Department of Health and Human Services. *Prevention, 1989–1990: Federal Programs in Progress.* (Public Health Service, Office of Disease Prevention and Health Promotion.) Washington, D.C.: U.S. Government Printing Office, 1990; U.S. Department of Health and Human Services. *Prevention, 1991–1992: Federal Programs in Progress.* (Public Health Service, Office of Disease Prevention and Health Promotion.) Washington, D.C.: U.S. Government Printing Office, 1992.
19. U.S. Department of Health and Human Services. *Clinician's Handbook of Preventive Services.* (Public Health Service, Office of Disease Prevention and Health Promotion.) Washington, D.C.: U.S. Government Printing Office, 1994.
20. "Centers for Disease Control: The Nation's Prevention Agency." *Morbidity and Mortality Weekly Report*, Nov, 6, 1992, *41*, 833.

21. Centers for Disease Control. *Mortality and Morbidity Weekly Reports.* These reports are available in print from the U.S. Government Printing Office and on the web at http://www.cdc.gov/mmwr.
22. Farquhar, J. W., and others. "Community Education for Cardiovascular Health." *Lancet,* 1977, *1*(8023) 1192–1195.
23. Susser, M. "The Tribulation of Trials—Intervention in Communities." *American Journal of Public Health,* 1995, *85*, 156–158.
24. Jones, R. C., Gly, J. L., and Richardson, J. E. "A Study of a Worksite Health Promotion Program and Absenteeism." *Journal of Occupational Medicine,* 1990, *32*, 95–99.
25. Lewis, M. A., and others. "The Termination of a Randomized Clinical Trial for Poor Hispanic Children." *Archives of Pediatric and Adolescent Medicine,* 1994, *148*, 365–367.
26. "Cigarette Smoking Among Adults—United States, 1991." *Morbidity and Mortality Weekly Report,* Apr. 12, 1993, *42*, 230–233.
27. U.S. Department of Health, Education, and Welfare. *Smoking and Health: Report of the Advisory Committee to the Surgeon General.* (Public Health Service report 641103.) Washington, D.C.: U.S. Government Printing Office, 1964.
28. "Cigarette Smoking . . ." (1993).
29. U.S. Department of Health and Human Services. *Health, United States, 1994.* Public Health Service, DHHS publication no. (PHS) 95-1232. Hyattsville, Md.: Public Health Service, Centers for Disease Control and Prevention, U.S. Department of Health and Human Services, 1995.
30. "Smoking Control Among Health Care Workers: World No-Tobacco Day." *Morbidity and Mortality Weekly Report,* May 21, 1993, *42*, 365–367.
31. "Changes in the Cigarette Brand Preferences of Adolescent Smokers—United States, 1989–1993." *Morbidity and Mortality Weekly Report,* Aug. 19, 1994, *43*, 577–581.
32. "Cigarette Smoking Among Adults in the United States—1992," and "Changes in the Definition of Current Cigarette Smoking." *Morbidity and Mortality Weekly Report,* May 20, 1995, *43*, 42–47.
33. Wintemute, G. J. "Firearms as a Cause of Death in the United States: 1920–1982." *Journal of Trauma,* 1987, *27*, 532–536.
34. Sugarman, J., and Rand, K. C. *Cease Fire: A Comprehensive Strategy to Reduce Firearms Violence.* Washington, D.C.: Violence Policy Center, 1994.
35. Sugarman and Rand (1994).
36. Wintemute, G. J. (ed.). *Ring of Fire: The Handgun Makers of Southern California.* Sacramento, Calif.: Violence Prevention Research Program, 1994.
37. Teret, S. P., and Wintemute, G. J. "Policies to Prevent Firearm Injuries." *Health Affairs,* 1993, *12*, 96–107.
38. Fargason, C. A., and Johnston, C. "Gun Safety Practices of Trauma Center Workers in a Southern City." *Southern Medical Journal,* 1994, *4*(87), 964–970.
39. UNAIDS. "AIDS Epidemic Update: December 2000." Geneva, Switzerland: Joint United Nations Programme on HIV/AIDS, World Health Organization, 2000.
40. "HIV Facts." *Washington Post* online. [http://www.washingtonpost.com/wp-srv/world/daily/july00/aidsgraphic4.htm.] Accessed Dec. 7, 2000.
41. UNAIDS (2000).
42. National Institute of Allergy and Infectious Diseases. "The Evidence That HIV Causes AIDS." Bethesda, Md.: Office of Communications and Public Liaison, National Institutes of Health. [http://www.niaid.nih.gov/factsheets/evidhiv.htm.] Nov. 29, 2000.

43. UNAIDS (2000).

44. Gellman, B. "S. African President Escalates AIDS Feud." *Washington Post,* Apr. 19, 2000, p. A1.

45. Gellman (2000).

46. Jeter, J. "South Africans Criticize Leader's Views on AIDS." *Washington Post,* Oct. 12, 2000, p. A18.

47. "A Plague of Denial." *Washington Post,* July 9, 2000, p. B6.

48. UNAIDS (2000).

49. Gellman, B. "AIDS Is Declared Threat to Security." *Washington Post,* Apr. 30, 2000, p. A1.

50. Brubaker, B. "U.S. Offers Loans to Fight AIDS in Africa." *Washington Post,* July 20, 2000, p. A17.

51. "World Bank HIV/AIDS Activities." [www.worldbank.org/aids.] Nov. 2000.

52. Reuters. "U.N.'s Annan Demands War Against AIDS in Africa." *New York Times on the Web.* [http://www.nytimes.com/reuters/world/international-aids-an.html.] Dec. 7, 2000.

53. UNAIDS (2000).

54. UNAIDS. "The Progress Report on the International Partnership against AIDS in Africa." [http://www.unaids.org/africapartnership/whatis.html.] May 2000.

CHAPTER EIGHTEEN

PUBLIC HEALTH AND PERSONAL HEALTH SERVICES

Lester Breslow and Jonathan E. Fielding

In our current effort to reform the organization, delivery, and financing of health care, which is more aptly described as personal health services or medical care, the broad question of how providers of these services contribute to the public health goals for our country receives little consideration. Most of the debate about personal health services has focused on how to control the enormous and continually escalating costs of medical, hospital, and other services; and how to overcome the access barriers that arise from lack of health benefits, inadequate ability to receive needed care, discrimination, poor distribution of providers, and other problems. In deciding how these medical care system problems should be addressed, what is the role, if any, of public health agencies?

Neglect of this question probably derives from the common view that public health is concerned only with disease control by such means as epidemiological investigation, immunization, health education, and attention to safety hazards in the physical environment. Another common public perception is that public health's primary concern is the economically disadvantaged segment of the population. The purpose of this chapter is to delineate the appropriate roles for public health in the personal health services system.

A perspective on this role starts with public health's mission. According to the Institute of Medicine, National Academy of Sciences, the mission is "fulfilling society's interest in assuring conditions in which people can be healthy."[1] Public health thus concerns itself with the health of the entire population and how it may be enhanced by improving the health-related conditions in which people live. Public health efforts are directed at modifying three conditions that can contribute to population health: the physical environment, social and behavioral factors, and the system of delivery of personal health care services.

The environment, the physical aspects of people's surroundings, profoundly affects their health. The well-known impact of working conditions, food handling, and exposure to fluoride—among myriad other living circumstances—illustrates the point. Therefore, from its outset public health has directed substantial effort toward ensuring a safe physical environment, at first mainly focusing on microbial threats to health but increasingly aiming more broadly at the whole physical milieu.

With the twentieth-century transition from communicable to noncommunicable diseases as the predominant health problem, evidence has grown that people's behavior (for example, with respect to tobacco and alcohol) has a strong and often definitive influence on the disease mechanisms that cause death, related disability, and the timing of disease development and progression. The Public Health Service has estimated that half of the premature deaths in the United States are due to the choices that people make in their everyday activities.[2] In analyzing the underlying causes of death rather than the disease mechanisms involved, McGinnis and Foege found that almost two-fifths are attributable to tobacco, diet or activity patterns, and alcohol (Table 18.1).[3]

The broader social environment—including such factors as the strength of family and other social relationships, sense of shared responsibility for the quality of life in the community, and beliefs about acceptable and unacceptable behavior—also strongly influence patterns of health and ill health in the population.[4]

TABLE 18.1. ACTUAL CAUSES OF DEATH IN THE UNITED STATES, 1990.

Cause	Estimated Number	Percentage of Total Deaths
Tobacco	400,000	19
Diet and activity patterns	300,000	14
Alcohol	100,000	5
Toxic agents	60,000	3
Firearms	35,000	2
Sexual behavior	30,000	1
Motor vehicles	25,000	1
Illicit use of drugs	20,000	<1
Total	970,000	46

Source: McGinnis, J. M., and Foege, W. H. "Actual Causes of Death in the United States." *Journal of the American Medical Association*, 1993, *270*, 2207–2212.

The third major influence on the health of the population is the availability and quality of personal health services, particularly medical care. Extensive achievements in this field during recent decades—in biochemistry, pharmacology, noninvasive testing procedures, surgical techniques and other areas—have increased the possibility of longer and healthier lives. The dramatic impact that they sometimes make on the individual's situation, however, creates a tendency to overestimate their overall health significance. Bunker attributes only five years of the thirty-year increase in life expectancy of Americans during the twentieth century to the work of the medical care system.[5]

Public health has generally operated inconspicuously, identifying and implementing means to improve all three conditions that can advance health and incorporating those advances into the context of life. Credit is rarely given for what has been accomplished through public health initiatives, in part because their success is often measured by health problems that do not occur or whose impact is controlled. Thus, we take for granted that water from the tap is safe to drink; that individuals with tuberculosis are identified quickly and appropriately treated so they are not a threat to the public; and, more recently, that automobiles have seatbelts and public buildings are largely smoke-free.

Given public health's history and orientation, what are appropriate public health roles related to personal health services? To summarize the reasons for public health involvement in personal health services:

1. Personal health services are becoming increasingly effective as a means of improving health, and thus a concern of public health.

2. A substantial proportion of the population either does not have access to them under current arrangements or may lose access with change in government programs or in living circumstances such as a job move.

3. A considerable portion of the personal health services delivered suffer from deficiency in quality, often affecting health outcomes.

4. The recent spiral in medical care costs has absorbed a disproportionate share of social resources, limiting investment to reduce inequality in access to health care services and preventing investment in other sectors (transportation, social services, housing, environmental protection, and so forth) that could potentially yield higher dividends in health at the population level.

Thus, examination of the role of public health in personal health services is timely and important. Public health represents society's interest, but how should society's interests be advanced, and what are the leverage points to effect change?

Public Providers of Personal Health Services

Public health departments, of course, have long administered certain personal health services aimed toward health promotion and disease prevention, such as prenatal care and childhood immunization. They have often provided such services directly, particularly for those segments of the population that the private health care system seldom reaches effectively. In many locales, the health department has served as planner, convener, and facilitator, helping to mobilize community resources, especially clinicians, to provide services to the economically disadvantaged. Also, in many states and communities, public health departments have assumed responsibility for a broader array of personal health services for people with low income. For example, some local public health agencies carry responsibility for Medicaid and local indigent care programs.

These responsibilities are exercised in several forms. Some jurisdictions operate health plans for Medicaid and other low-income individuals, contracting with physicians, hospitals, and other providers and performing the other required functions of a managed care organization. Other jurisdictions have comprehensive personal health care delivery systems, including both inpatient and outpatient activities. In some jurisdictions, the local health agency has statutory responsibility for health care for the indigent. The responsibility to provide health care services to this large population without health benefits has become so burdensome in some jurisdictions that it jeopardizes the conduct of other activities with a potentially greater impact on health.

Historically, actual involvement in personal health services emerged initially as a critical aspect of public health's original task: communicable disease control. During the early part of the century, when the struggle against infectious diseases extended beyond environmental action to include developing personal immunity in individuals, health departments undertook mass smallpox vaccinations (and subsequently other immunizations). More substantial engagement in personal health services by public health expanded with maternal and child health during the 1920s, from the growing conviction that such services could reduce the excessively high maternal and infant death rates recognized as prevailing at that time. Then came certain diagnostic procedures, especially as technology for communicable disease control advanced. For example, tuberculin testing of tuberculosis patients' contacts and then x-raying positive reactors became an accepted public health practice. Further, health department laboratories offered communicable disease diagnostic services to physicians in their communities. Subsequently, these services expanded into other realms such as screening for diseases having congenital and environmental causes.

Advances in clinical science and corresponding improvements in medical care necessitate greater public health attention to them as means of improving health. Widespread recognition of the potential of these advances to protect and enhance health has led to establishing large-scale, public programs of medical care for people identified as having an unmet personal health service need, thus filling substantial gaps in the delivery system.[6] In other cases, this lack of availability of health care in a defined population has been met by making payment for personal health services to individuals meeting specific eligibility requirements, such as Medicaid programs. In addition, the government may create financial incentives for private organizations to finance or provide care to populations unable to afford it. The traditional tax-exempt status of nonprofit organizations and voluntary private hospitals was, in part, based on the assumption that these institutions would help to meet the needs of the poor through uncompensated care.

Direct Service Delivery

Direct delivery of personal health services by government in the United States goes back to the U.S. Marine Hospital Service, which was established to provide care for merchant seamen in support of the nation's entry into international commerce, as well as to the country's early military medical services. These two agencies, for merchant seamen and military forces, have evolved into the current U.S. Public Health Service and the Armed Forces Medical System.

Over the years the federal government has assumed responsibility for directly providing medical services to other substantial segments of the population. The Department of Veterans Affairs operates an array of medical centers, nursing units, domiciliary care units, and outpatient clinics for its beneficiaries, many of which are affiliated with academic medical centers, both to enhance the quality of care and to give training opportunities to young physicians.[7] The Indian Health Service operates (or funds the operation by Indian tribal government of) hospitals, health centers and other types of ambulatory care unit on tribal lands throughout the country.[8]

State governments have historically provided hospital services not for such specific segments of the population but rather for people suffering from particular conditions, such as mental illness and tuberculosis. Beds for these purposes have declined substantially over the last quarter century as TB cases have fallen and also been treated increasingly on an ambulatory basis, and as state hospitalization for mentally ill patients has been curtailed with the notion that they would be better served in community centers. Unfortunately, the latter have not materialized to the extent needed.

County and city governments have provided both in-patient and out-patient general hospital services for the indigent, and emergency and some other medical services, often with financial support from state and federal sources. These have tended to be uneven, reflecting the lack of nationally assured services in the United States.

Since 1975, the total number of hospitals in the United States has dropped 15 percent and the number of beds almost 30 percent, but the proportion of beds under federal governmental auspices has fallen relatively more, from 10 to 6 percent (Table 18.2). The proportion of beds operated by state and local governments has remained quite steady, about one-seventh of the total. Meanwhile community nonprofit hospitals have expanded their proportion of beds, now well over half the total, and community for-profit hospitals have doubled their share, from 5 to 11 percent. The former increase largely reflects services of community hospitals that were previously undertaken by specialized rather than general hospitals.

TABLE 18.2.   TRENDS IN HOSPITALS AND BEDS, BY OWNERSHIP, 1975–1997.

	Hospitals		
	1975	1985	1997
All hospitals	7,156	6,872	6,097
Federal government	382	343	285
State and local government[1]	1,761	1,578	1,260
Community nonprofit[1]	3,339	3,349	3,000
Community for-profit[1]	775	805	797
	Beds (Thousands)		
	1975	1985	1997
All hospitals	1,466	1,318	1,035
Federal government	132	112	62
State and local government[1]	210	189	148
Community nonprofit[1]	658	707	591
Community for-profit[1]	73	104	115

Note: (1) excluded are long-term hospitals and hospital units in institutions such as prisons and college dormitories, facilities for the mentally retarded, and alcoholism and chemical dependency hospitals.

Source: National Center for Health Statistics. Health, United States, 1999. Hyattsville Md.: National Center for Health Statistics, 1999.

Core Public Health Responsibilities

The public health care system delivers substantial amounts of medical care, particularly for the economically disadvantaged and the chronic severely mentally ill and developmentally impaired. But this role is not necessarily central to the broad public health mission. In fact, local fiscal authorities have often diverted what resources are appropriated for the traditional public health core functions into personal health services for the poor, usually secondary and tertiary services. This reflects the strain of forty-four million Americans being without health benefits, a number that has every likelihood of continued growth in the absence of national policy that health care should be the right of every citizen and in the wake of the failure of national health reform. However, the other consequence of allocating money to what appears to be the most pressing priority—sick people without other sources of emergency medical services—is that these funds are not available for community-oriented prevention activities. Thus public health has a diminished ability to respond to serious public health threats such as the resurgence of tuberculosis and measles—or HIV/AIDS, the greatest new health threat.

The growing perception that our nation had lost sight of its public health goals, allowing the public health infrastructure to fall into disarray, led to the previously cited Institute of Medicine recommendation that the public health mission be defined as "fulfilling society's interest in assuring conditions in which people can be healthy." Based on this mission, the report identified three principal core functions for public health: assessment, assurance, and policy development.

Assessment

An indispensable role for a public health agency is to assess the opportunities to improve the health of the population in its area. In so doing, the public health agency needs sophistication in assessing the contributions of the various determinants of health to the burden on the population posed by ill health. An essential initial step is to collect (directly or through analysis of external databases) a health-and-disease profile of the population. Traditionally, assessments have targeted the major causes of morbidity, mortality, and more recently disability. In addition, health can be measured as a set of positive attributes based upon the expansive definitions of health adopted by public health bodies nationally and internationally. In *Healthy People 2000: National Health Promotion and Disease Prevention Objectives,* this perspective on the meaning of health is well captured: "health is best measured by citizens' sense of well-being."[9]

At the state and local levels, an ideal assessment would be to array the major causes of morbidity, disability, mortality, and lack of well-being for major segments of the population defined by age, gender, and geography, and possibly also by race or ethnic identity. Traditionally, ill health has been arrayed according to disease (cancer, heart disease, arthritis, and so on). However, as McGinnis and Foege have proposed, a better way to consider health improvement opportunities might be to focus on the common factors that underlie many of the most burdensome health conditions (Table 18.1). At least seven of these factors have in common that they can be ameliorated through behavior change.

In analogous fashion, how might we judge the potential contribution of health services to potential health improvement in the overall population of a defined area and in population subgroups? The point of departure for such an exercise is to determine the percentage of the population variance in key health measures that is associated with health services. To take as a hypothetical example acquired heart disease, health services might be found to account for 10 percent of the variance in mortality and disability rates. The next step would be to determine the characteristics of health service systems that are reproducibly associated with the best and worst outcomes.

To the degree possible, differences between the best and worst outcomes would be partitioned into problems of access to services, overuse and underuse of appropriate services, poor coordination of care, and poor technical quality of services. Although developing databases that would permit this degree of problem definition is at an early stage for most health conditions, a substantial investment in quality indicators, practice guidelines, and outcomes measurement should in time produce sufficient tools for public health departments to assume leadership in assessing the problems in organizing and delivering personal health services by both private and public providers.

A related role is to identify the characteristics of populations that are not receiving adequate care by virtue of diminished access, poor quality, or lack of financial resources. Traditionally, public health organizations have taken the lead in pointing out that there is a substantial segment of our population (now more than forty million Americans, including ten million children) who do not have access to any organized source of continuing medical care or payment for such care.[10] They are largely dependent on so-called emergency services that state or local governments may provide or require other local institutions to offer. In addition, many millions work in precarious job situations where they are at risk of both job loss and loss of health benefits offered by or through their employer. Although individuals losing their jobs can now continue to receive the same health benefits under federal legislation for up to eighteen months if their employer had twenty or more employees, many cannot afford to bear the entire cost and allow it to lapse.

What is most striking is that during the 1990s, a period of unprecedented economic growth in the United States, the number of uninsured continued to grow and the percentage of Americans covered by employer-related health benefits declined. Public health agencies should become the most trusted source for information on unmet service needs, the nature of quality assurance practices used by providers, health outcomes, and health status of subpopulations within their territory. They should also systematically assess the degree of integration of health services with other governmental and private sector services, such as education, social services, and welfare.

Tools are available to help public health agencies in the overall assessment and planning process. APEX (Assessment Protocol for Excellence in Public Health) and PATCH (Planned Approach to Community Health) are among a growing number of stepwise guides to assessing community health needs. Neither of these focuses primarily on personal health services, but assessment of these needs can and should be built into an overall community assessment. APEX includes a three-stage process, with the last one, policy development and assurance activities, intended to ensure implementation of the organizational action plan.[11] PATCH, developed by the Centers for Disease Control and Prevention (CDC) as a community health promotion tool, also emphasizes community mobilization.[12] Many health departments are using *Healthy Communities 2000: Model Standards,* a guidebook to marrying the national objectives in *Healthy People 2000* with local needs and priorities.[13]

Assurance

The Institute of Medicine report stressed "assurance" to their constituents that services necessary to achieve agreed-upon goals are provided, whether by encouraging actions by other entities (private or public sector), by requiring such action through regulation, or by providing services directly. Public health agencies should involve key policy makers and the general public in determining a set of high-priority personal and communitywide health services that governments will guarantee to every member of the community. This guarantee should include subsidization or direct provision of high-priority personal health services for those unable to afford them.[14]

Health assurance is a central function of public health. In proposing plans to improve the health of its population, a department of public health should ensure that all groups have access to a minimum set of high-quality personal health care services. The plan should also set expectations for the performance of health care systems and health care providers.

Developing large managed care organizations with broad responsibility for the health care of a defined population of enrollees is a natural point of leverage in assuring adequate performance of the health care system. Large managed care organizations are developing clinical data systems that generate databases amenable to analysis of outcomes of care and of the types of service provided to individuals and groups defined by disease (for example, adult onset diabetes mellitus), age group (such as infants from zero to one year), income level, or geography. In addition, "quality" has become a basis for competition in the market for personal health services. Therefore, health department leadership should include helping to define the kinds of outcome an organization should be able to show based on best practices observed in the literature.

Health departments should have special expertise in setting expectations for outcomes in clinical preventive services—such as age-specific immunization rates, mammography rates by age, and so on—and in monitoring these rates. However, monitoring the results of services provided when a disease state is present is of equal importance. Thus, public health agencies should also participate in setting expectations for disease and procedure outcomes, such as mortality rates for cardiovascular disease, or complication rates for endoscopy or angioplasty. They may also suggest the specifications and dissemination plans for report cards that are increasingly required of health care providers, as these reports can identify problems with access and quality.

Currently, most health departments have no jurisdiction over the organizations delivering comprehensive care, except for licensing institutions and sometimes provider groups. In some areas, particularly large cities, the health department may also deliver clinical services—presenting a potential conflict of interest in setting standards or expectations for results. Nonetheless, there are existing levers that can be used to help assure good outcomes from delivering personal health care services. The health department can help to establish a local coalition of private and public health benefit purchasers that sets requirements for both services to be provided and the quality and service data that plans and providers must make available in a standard format. The health department can also take the lead in disseminating information on what should be a required core of preventive services, such as those developed by the U.S. Preventive Services Task Force.[15] The department can also publicize the practice guidelines being developed through public and private processes and can urge consumers to ask questions about outcomes, both in general and for conditions about which they are concerned, before selecting choices under an employer-sponsored health benefit plan.

Public health agencies should make it a central function to receive, analyze, and report on the results of quality assurance efforts in personal health services delivery. They can use their role as guardian of the public's health to publicize both problems and progress to the public, as well as to inform providers and professional organizations about opportunities for improvement in an effort to assure both access and quality. Assuring that the public has objective information on the performance of alternative managed care organizations and physician groups is increasing in importance as more employers adopt a passive purchaser role vis-à-vis health plans, giving employees a fixed amount of money and letting them choose among a number of locally available plans.

Public Policy

A number of assurance functions are accomplished through participating in the development of public policy. Some access, data, and quality-assessment requirements are being incorporated into laws or administrative regulations. Public health, as an agent of the public with the responsibility of "fulfilling society's interest in assuring conditions in which people can be healthy,"[16] should be proactive in suggesting where and what regulation is appropriate and in commenting on proposals advanced by others.

An important public policy role is to underscore the large number of uninsured and the continuing growth of this population. Policy makers need to be shown that the uninsured population is much less likely to receive preventive care, seek care for serious symptoms, have continuing sources of care, and have problems diagnosed at an early and treatable stage. They need to understand that providing health benefits to the uninsured is even more challenging as the ability of public systems to deliver health services dwindles under competition from the private sector, and as the same private sector competition reduces the availability of services for those who cannot afford to pay.

Identifying the opportunity to improve some health outcomes through broader health benefit coverage is part of a larger need to educate the public and policy makers on the key determinants of health, and on how policy options can affect these factors. In this context, almost all careful studies of determinants of health have found that personal health care services make a difference in health, but this difference accounts for a small fraction of the variance in health among populations—overall and for specific health conditions. Determinants with a generally larger contribution to variance include genetics, income distribution, social factors, environmental exposure, and health behavior.

Among these items, health habits have received the most attention in recent years, but the other contributors to common diseases often display strong effects. For example, in acquired cardiovascular disease, the degree of social isolation displays risk gradients and effects of about the same order of magnitude as behavioral risk factors.[17] For most disease categories, and certainly for quality of well-being, poverty is a quantitatively more important risk factor than access to health care services or the quality of those services in describing the difference in health between populations. In addition, economic, community, social, and political factors are the primary contributors to such major societal problems of ill health as child abuse, spousal abuse, other violence, and birth outcomes.

As part of this educational effort, public health departments can provide data showing that the current level of investment in health care services is disproportionate to the ability of those services to alter the population burden of ill health. Whether the argument is for additional resources or for reallocation of existing resources to address other causal factors, the rhetoric is not likely to strike a responsive chord unless the health department can make a convincing case for what type of investment is likely to achieve greater societal returns. For example, would after-school programs for youth in areas of high risk of school dropout and gang membership be a better investment than a higher density of MRI machines, or increasing the Medicare payment for erythropoietin? Would a uniform home prenatal and postnatal home visiting program for lower-income pregnant women yield a better health return than routinely offering amniocentesis as a covered health benefit? Would a social marketing campaign to encourage youths to drink nonalcoholic beverages have more impact on alcoholism than more or better rehabilitation facilities?

Although there are no unequivocal answers to most of these questions, showing the effects of well-evaluated model programs is a useful initial step in this educational process.

Expertise and Capacity

What is the interest and capacity of public health agencies at the state and local levels to assume the set of responsibilities we have outlined? The Institute of Medicine report and strong efforts by the CDC, the American Public Health Association, and national and local health officer associations to define core public health functions have raised consciousness of the role public health should play in health promotion at the community level. Barriers to assuming these central roles include restricted flexibility in use of funds (which are often channeled from categorical programs), mismatch of skills and interests between existing personnel and new priorities, and outsiders' perception that a more limited role for public health agencies is advisable. For example, a survey of thirty-two health departments and districts in Washington state found that the self-assessed strengths of most were program management and direct provision of service. They felt that the major deficiencies were assessment functions and use of data to guide community and program planning and policy.[18] If public health is to assure the health of populations, then establishing its expertise and credibility as the pathfinding organizer and lead planner in achieving this area of goals must be accorded a high priority.

Notes

1. Institute of Medicine. *The Future of Public Health*. Washington, D.C.: National Academy Press, 1988.
2. U.S. Department of Health and Human Services, Public Health Service. *For a Healthy Nation: Returns on Investment in Public Health*. Washington, D.C.: U.S. Government Printing Office, 1994.
3. McGinnis, J. M., and Foege, W. H. "Actual Cases of Death in the United States." *Journal of the American Medical Association*, 1993, *270*, 2207–2212.
4. Evans, R. G., Barer, M. L., and Marmor, T. R. *Why Are Some People Healthy and Others Not?* New York: Aldine de Gruyter, 1994.
5. Bunker, J. P., Frazier, H. S., and Mosteller, F. "Improving Health: Measuring Effects of Medical Care." *Milbank Quarterly*, 1994, *72*, 225–258.
6. Afifi, A. A., and Breslow, L. "The Maturing Paradigm of Public Health." *Annual Review of Public Health*, 1994, *15*, 223–235.
7. U. S. Department of Veterans Affairs. *Annual Report of the Secretary of Veterans Affairs/Department of Veterans*. Washington, D.C.: U.S. Government Printing Office, 1994.
8. U. S. Department of Health and Human Services, Public Health Service. *Trends in Indian Health*. Washington, D.C.: U.S. Government Printing Office, 1994.
9. U.S. Department of Health and Human Services. *Healthy People 2000: National Health Promotion and Disease Prevention Objectives*. (DHHS publication no. PHS 91-50212.) Washington, D.C.: U.S. Government Printing Office, 1990.
10. Trevino, F. M., and Jacobs, J. P. "Public Health and Health Care Reform: The American Public Health Association's Perspective." *Journal of Health Policy*, 1994, *15*, 397–406; U.S. Bureau of the Census. *Current Population Survey*. (March supplement.) Washington, D.C.: U.S. Government Printing Office, 1993.
11. National Association of County Health Officials. *Assessment Protocol for Excellence in Public Health (APEX/PH)*. Washington D.C.: National Association of County Health Officials, 1991.
12. U.S. Department of Health and Human Services, Centers for Disease Control and Prevention. *Planned Approach to Community Health (PATCH)*. Atlanta: Public Health Service, 1992.
13. American Public Health Association. *Healthy Communities 2000: Model Standard*. (3rd ed.) Washington, D.C.: American Public Health Association, 1991.
14. Institute of Medicine (1988).
15. U.S. Preventive Services Task Force. *Guide to Clinical Preventive Services: An Assessment of the Effectiveness of 169 Interventions*. Baltimore, Md.: Williams and Wilkins, 1989.
16. Institute of Medicine (1988).
17. Syme, S. L., and Berkman, L. F. "Social Class, Susceptibility, and Sickness." *American Journal of Epidemiology*, 1976, *104*, 1–8.
18. Oberle, M. W., Baker, E. L., and Magenheim, M. J. "Healthy People 2000 and Community Health Planning." *Annual Review of Public* Health, 1994, *15*, 259–275.

CHAPTER NINETEEN

THE CONTINUING ISSUE OF MEDICAL MALPRACTICE LIABILITY

Ruth Roemer

Part of the national debate on health care reform in 1994 involved the contentious issue of medical malpractice liability and the tort system for addressing it. Despite the failure of health care reform in the 103rd Congress, the issue of medical malpractice liability continues to provoke debate and alternative proposals for modifying the tort system for handling it.

Several reasons make this issue an aspect of any major change in the health system, whether brought about by legislative or voluntary action. First is the charge that high medical malpractice insurance premiums and defensive medicine are major contributors to escalating health care costs. Second is the concern about the right to sue managed care organizations (MCOs) for medical malpractice. Third is the long-standing dissatisfaction with the tort system's handling of medical malpractice, for its failure to compensate many victims of malpractice and to deter negligent practice.

Does Medical Malpractice Litigation Increase Costs?

With respect to the first allegation, the evidence does not support the charge that medical malpractice litigation is a major cause of the rising costs of health care. On average, physicians pay less than 4 percent of annual practice receipts for malpractice insurance. This represents less than 1 percent of total U.S. health expenditures and therefore cannot be a primary cause of the growth in expenditures.[1] With respect to the impact of defensive medicine, although some procedures may be unnecessary, others may be beneficial and part of cautious, conservative medical practice.[2] Moreover, some precautions may prevent mistakes, making the net economic impact of defensive medicine unclear.[3] The Office of Technology Assessment (OTA) concludes that "overall only a small percentage of diagnostic procedures—certainly less than 8 percent—is likely to be caused primarily by *conscious* concern about malpractice liability."[4] Much of the increased spending on health care can more reasonably be explained by expanding and proliferating medical technology rather than by the practice of defensive medicine.[5]

Should Malpractice Suits Against MCOs Be Allowed?

With respect to the second concern, a central issue in the growth of managed care is the question of the liability of MCOs for malpractice.

Concerns about malpractice in managed care organizations are associated with the shift to outpatient care, which increases the exposure of physicians and utilization review entities, and with reliance on screening by primary care physicians and use of gatekeepers, which possibly restricts referral to specialists.[6] Court interpretations of the Employee Retirement Income Security Act of 1974 (ERISA) have barred some malpractice suits against managed care plans on the ground that ERISA preempts state laws that relate to health benefits of self-insured plans. Plaintiffs denied care by such plans are limited to relief in federal courts of payment for only the costs of the medical care denied; they cannot recover damages available in state courts for injuries suffered as a result of the denial.[7] In recent years, the interpretation of the ERISA preemption has been somewhat narrowed to bar only suits for denial of care (benefits decisions) but allow suits relating to quality of care (medical decisions)—a difficult distinction to draw.[8] Many decisions are mixed benefits and medical or treatment decisions, and in one such case, *Pegram* v. *Herdrich*, the U.S. Supreme Court held in a unanimous decision in June 2000 that MCOs cannot be held liable as fiduciaries under ERISA for wrongful conduct in making such mixed decisions.[9]

Further restriction of the ERISA preemption occurred in 1995 in a unanimous decision of the U.S. Supreme Court, holding that a New York statute imposing surcharges on hospitals and HMO fees for some health care payers, including ERISA plans, in order to create a pool of funding to cover the uninsured was not preempted by ERISA because the statute had only an indirect economic effect.[10] In the view of a legal authority on ERISA, this case may "signal a change both in methods of statutory interpretation and in the Court's willingness to allow state regulation of some aspects of health care delivery that affect ERISA plans."[11]

Those seeking to retain the immunity from suit that ERISA has provided to self-insured plans contend that allowing such suits increases the costs of health care. Advocates for increased legal accountability of MCOs deny this contention but say that some increased cost would be acceptable to protect patients from substandard care.[12]

Texas was the first state to enact legislation creating a cause of action against health insurance carriers, HMOs, and other managed care entities for negligent treatment decisions, so that these entities have a statutory duty to exercise ordinary care in making decisions that determine when services are provided or affect the quality of diagnosis, care, or treatment.[13] The right to sue managed care organizations and health plans for denial of care or substandard care has been a central feature of the Congressional debate on a Patient's Bill of Rights.

In view of the fact that 140 million workers and their families receive their health care through plans sponsored by employers and covered by ERISA,[14] it is a serious matter of equity to afford them access to the courts for medical malpractice. The recent changes in judicial interpretation of the ERISA preemption indicate that the time may be ripe to remedy this inequity in the law spawned by ERISA, to allow malpractice suits against MCOs for medical injuries—just as they are allowed against hospitals.[15]

Is the Tort System of Compensation Fair and Equitable?

The third concern is dissatisfaction with the tort system on the grounds that it costs too much; is an erratic, unpredictable, and inefficient method of compensating persons injured by substandard care; and fails to deter negligent practice.[16] Despite extensive state legislation designed to curb malpractice suits, the question is still unresolved as to whether the present tort system of handling medical malpractice liability meets the objectives of, first, fairly and adequately compensating persons injured by substandard care and, second, deterring negligent practice.

To examine the options available for addressing the issues concerning the medical malpractice liability system, it may be helpful first to review the medical malpractice insurance crises of the 1970s and 1980s and their sequelae—the causes, the state legislative responses that ensued, and evaluations of these legislative actions. Then we may turn to alternative proposals that have been advanced. Finally, some comments are offered on how best to compensate victims of substandard medical care and how best to deter negligent medical practice—a question that may become urgent with legislative or voluntary reform of the health system.

The Malpractice Insurance Crises of the 1970s and 1980s

In the 1960s and early 1970s, the frequency and severity of medical malpractice claims increased dramatically. Claim frequency increased nationally at an average annual rate of 12.1 percent, and paid claim severity (cost per claim, including awards and out-of-court settlements) increased at the rate of 10.2 percent. In some states, the increases were even greater. In California, both the frequency and severity increased between 1969 and 1974 at an average annual rate of nearly 20 percent.[17] Throughout the 1970s, awards rose at a rate in excess of the general rate of inflation and of the cost of medical care. Between 1970 and 1975, the average malpractice award increased from $11,518 to $26,565—an average annual rate increase of 18 percent. By 1978 the average award had increased to $45,187, representing a cumulative increase of 70 percent for the three years 1976–1978.[18]

Because of this escalation in the number of malpractice claims filed and in the size of awards, the premiums for malpractice liability insurance rose astronomically, by as much as 500 percent in some states.[19] In 1974, several important insurers withdrew from the market.[20] Thus, the crisis of the 1970s was not because a large number of patients were injured but because of the breakdown in the malpractice insurance market.[21]

As a result, many physicians without adequate insurance coverage avoided high-risk cases, limited their practices in other ways (as with obstetrician-gynecologists limiting their practices to office gynecology), withdrew from emergency service or from practice altogether, or practiced without insurance coverage or with lowered coverage.[22]

The problems with availability and affordability of malpractice insurance led to formation of compulsory pooling arrangements—joint underwriting associations—to compel insurers to provide insurance for malpractice as a condition of writing other insurance.[23] These joint underwriting associations were formed to ensure insurance coverage for physicians who could not obtain insurance, by requiring insurance companies offering property and casualty insurance to underwrite insurance for a physician who could not obtain liability insurance. Patient compensation funds, funded by a surcharge on all insurers, were established in nine states to settle catastrophic claims up to a certain limit. Some physicians formed their own insurance companies. These physician-owned firms insure about 60 percent of U.S. physicians and are represented by the Physicians Insurers Association of America.[24]

In response to this crisis, many states formed commissions to investigate and report on the medical malpractice insurance crisis in their states. In nearly every state, new statutes were enacted to restrain medical malpractice suits by restricting the scope of liability, limiting the size of awards, reducing the statute of limitations, limiting contingent fees of attorneys, and introducing pretrial screening panels or arbitration to discourage "frivolous" suits.[25] These measures are discussed later in this chapter.

After 1976, the frequency of claims leveled off, but the severity of awards continued to increase.[26] By 1985, however, when the second malpractice insurance crisis occurred, malpractice insurance premiums were again rising. From 1981 to 1986, malpractice insurance premiums rose 75 percent, according to the 1983 Physicians' Practice Costs and Income Survey and the 1986 Physicians' Practice Follow-Up Survey.[27] Claim frequency was rising by more than 12 percent after the increase in the 1970s that led to the 1975 crisis. Between 1975 and 1984, average medical malpractice verdicts increased at nearly twice the rate of the Consumer Price Index. These events prompted a leading authority on medical malpractice to say, "the fact that claim frequency and severity have continued to rise tends to confirm the fact that the response to the last crisis did not radically change the malpractice system."[28]

The medical malpractice insurance crises have been ascribed to medical factors, legal factors, and insurance practices. The medical factors include greater use of health services because of the enactment of Medicare and Medicaid and the growth of voluntary insurance; increased use of advanced medical technology entailing greater risk; and the fact that the practice of medicine is inherently a high-risk undertaking with a certain number of adverse outcomes, regardless of negligence. Also contributing to malpractice claims are heightened expectations on the part of consumers (the "every couple expects a perfect baby" syndrome) and changes in the doctor-patient relationship as medicine has become more highly specialized and technical, with resulting depersonalization of health services.[29]

Legal factors have also contributed to the increase in claims. Abolition or modification of the locality rule, making the acceptable standard of practice a state or national standard, tends to increase claims and make expert witnesses more available. Abolishing the charitable immunity rule that formerly insulated voluntary hospitals from suits was a factor that favored plaintiffs' suits. Another contributing factor was expanding the scope of informed consent, requiring a subjective scope of disclosure of the risks of a procedure as needed by a particular patient rather than the objective scope of disclosure afforded by what a reasonably prudent physician practicing in the same or similar circumstances would disclose. Similarly, expansion of the doctrine of *respondeat superior,* which imposes responsibility on an employer for an employee's wrongdoing, contributed to claim increases. States that abolished or expanded the locality rule, abolished charitable immunity, and adopted broadened informed consent and *respondeat superior* doctrines were found to have claim costs twice as high as states that made none of these changes.[30]

Insurance experience and practice also contributed to the crisis. In the mid-1970s a decline in the stock market reduced capital and earnings on the investments of the insurance companies. Since most companies wrote "occurrence" policies—the insurance company would be responsible for future claims as long as the incident on which the claim was based occurred in a year for which the insurance was purchased—insurance companies had to maintain large reserves to cover the "long tail" of future claims (the period from the occurrence of the incident to the eventual claim and its disposition).

After the 1975 crisis, insurance companies generally wrote "claims made" policies, in which the physician was covered for the year for which the policy was written, leaving a long tail of uninsured liability for the physician.[31] To cover a claim made after a claims-made policy has expired, the health care provider can purchase insurance known as "tail" coverage.[32] As a result of these experiences and practices, although insurance was available in the 1980s, it was more expensive and less coverage was provided, largely because of increasing loss payments, declining interest rates, tightening of the reinsurance market, and also because of increasing awards and uncertainty about the tort system.[33]

The medical malpractice insurance crises created problems in the medical, legal, and insurance sectors of society, but the main losers were consumers. The major part of the cost of these premium increases was paid neither by physicians nor hospitals but instead was passed on to third-party payers as part of the cost of medical and hospital service.[34]

State Legislative Reforms

Following the medical malpractice insurance crisis of the 1970s, most states enacted various laws to restrain malpractice suits. These changed laws have been grouped as relating to (1) filing claims, (2) defining standards of medical care or burden of proof, (3) determining the amount recoverable, and (4) alternatives to court resolution of claims.[35]

Filing Claims

In this category are a number of types of statute.

Ad Damnum Clause Reform. This legislation prohibits the plaintiff from stating the amount sought to be recovered, as is traditional in the pleadings, although some statutes permit the plaintiff's attorney to request a specific sum at the trial. The justification for this reform is the belief that publication of large claims is prejudicial to defendants and inappropriately influences juries.

Limitation on Attorneys' Fees. Most commonly, attorneys in medical liability cases are paid a fee contingent on the outcome of the case (35–50 percent of any award made to the plaintiff plus the expenses of litigation) rather than an hourly rate. Legislative reforms establish a sliding scale (the percentage declining with the size of the award) or set a reasonable amount as approved by the court.[36]

Contingent fees are supported on the ground that they constitute an incentive for lawyers to take cases that have a reasonable likelihood of success and to refuse those in which the plaintiff is unlikely to prove that the doctor was negligent. Theoretically, contingent fees allow recourse to the courts for low-income persons, but in reality lawyers will not take a case unless a substantial award is likely.[37] Thus, the contingent-fee system tends to screen out frivolous cases, but it also denies recourse for minor injuries or for injuries to the elderly, two types that do not promise large awards. The exclusion of small cases from the court system, however, may be due to high fixed costs of suit, including the costs of expert witnesses, not to contingent fees.[38]

Contingent fees are prohibited in England and Canada, which have historically had a lower rate of malpractice litigation than the United States, although the frequency of litigation has been increasing in these countries recently.

In the United States, the Federal Tort Claims Act limits contingent fees to 25 percent, and state workers' compensation laws also regulate contingent fees. Opposition to contingent fees is urged on the ground that they stimulate excessive litigation, create a conflict of interest between attorney and client, and impede settlement of claims.[39] About half the states specify a limit on attorneys' fees or authorize the courts to set fees.[40] From a public policy point of view, limitation of the plaintiff's attorney's fee is prejudicial to claimants when defendants (physicians, hospitals, and insurers) may spend unlimited amounts for the most skilled defense. In a dissenting opinion in a case holding constitutional the California Medical Injury Compensation Reform Act (MICRA), which prescribes a sliding scale of contingency fees, Chief Justice Rose Bird of the California Supreme Court stated that the act "prohibits severely injured victims of medical negligence from paying the general market rate for legal services, while permitting defendants to pay whatever is necessary to obtain high quality representation."[41]

Preventing Frivolous Suits. Legislation to discourage claims without legal merit requires the losing party in a malpractice case to reimburse the opposing party for costs if the suit is fraudulent or in bad faith. About fifteen states have such laws. Or a state may require a certificate of merit by way of an affidavit of an expert before a suit is filed.

Pretrial Screening Panels. Legislation to offer mandatory or voluntary screening of malpractice cases as a prerequisite to trial is intended to discourage nonmeritorious claims. The panel's decision is not binding and does not prevent the plaintiff from filing a lawsuit. The argument in favor of pretrial screening panels is that the number of claims going to trial is reduced. In opposition is the contention that these panels add an extra step in resolving claims and do not reduce the number of suits.[42] The OTA identified twenty-two states with some form of pretrial screening.[43]

The constitutionality of pretrial screening panels has been challenged as a violation of due process and equal protection, denial of a jury trial in violation of the Seventh Amendment to the Constitution, and improper delegation of judicial authority. Generally, the legislation has been upheld as a valid exercise of the police power of the state, but in six states such statutes have been declared unconstitutional.[44]

Statutes of Limitations. Many states have shortened the time within which a medical malpractice claim must be filed after an injury occurs or should have been discovered. States have also limited the latest age at which a child may bring an action, or they have specified that a statute would be suspended only until a child reached a certain age. California sets a limit of three years from the time of the injury or one year from discovery, whichever is earlier. For minors, the rule is three years or the eighth birthday, whichever is later. Longer deferred statutes of limitations are designed to protect victims of latent injuries, but some late claims may be suits to recover by retroactive application of new standards, adding to the costs of the tort system. Instead, an authority in this field recommends a short statute of limitations with additional time for discovery, as in California; to offset the incentive to conceal injuries, physicians should be required to pay an uninsurable fine for fraud or concealment of a negligent injury.[45]

Defining Standards of Care and Burden of Proof

In this category are five types of statute.

Standards of Care. Statutes specifying the applicable standard of care in a malpractice suit, whether community, state, or national, were passed as the old locality rule has been replaced by state or national standards. One of the reasons for changing the strict locality rule was the difficulty in finding physicians willing to testify against their local colleagues; expanding the locality rule enabled plaintiffs to engage national experts.[46]

Qualifications of Expert Witnesses. Some statutes specify the qualifications for an expert witness. For example, Ohio requires that an expert witness spend 75 percent of professional time in the active practice of his or her specialty.[47]

Clinical Practice Guidelines. Many specialty boards have developed clinical practice guidelines, and the Federal Agency for Health Care Policy and Research has supported the development of guidelines. Since such guidelines represent professional consensus on appropriate procedures, they may be applicable in medical malpractice cases, despite the possibility that courts may exclude them as evidence because of the rule against hearsay evidence or admit them only as part of expert testimony.

At least three states—Maine,[48] Minnesota, and Vermont—have passed legislation that permits guidelines to be used as a defense in malpractice litigation, under certain circumstances. Both Maine and Minnesota bar the plaintiff from introducing the guidelines as evidence that the physician failed to meet the standard of care. Vermont permits guidelines to be admitted in evidence by either the plaintiff or defendant in mandatory malpractice arbitration. Concern is expressed that guidelines may not reflect changes in medical practice promptly; that there is a potential for conflict among national, state, and institutional guidelines; and that these conflicts may hinder rather than help solve issues in medical liability.[49]

Informed Consent. The expansion in the 1970s of the doctrine of informed consent to a more patient-oriented standard, mentioned earlier, has led some states to enact legislation specifying what information must be given to the patient or specifying professional or customary standards of disclosure as a defense.[50]

Res Ipsa Loquitur. The legal doctrine of *res ipsa loquitur* ("the thing speaks for itself") was expanded in the 1970s from an inference of negligence to a presumption of negligence, which shifts the burden of proof from the plaintiff to the defendant and requires the defendant to show that the injury did not result from the defendant's negligence. This expanded application was found to place defendants at a disadvantage, with the result that some states have prohibited or limited use of the doctrine.[51]

Determining Amounts Recoverable

This category comprises six types of statute.

Joint and Several Liability. About two-thirds of the states have modified the rule on joint and several liability, which allows the plaintiff to sue all defendants responsible and recover from each in proportion to fault (*joint liability*) or to sue any one defendant and recover the total amount, with that defendant able to recover from the other defendants for their shares (*several liability*). In some states several liability was abolished. More commonly, the statutes limit several liability depending on the degree of the defendant's or plaintiff's fault or the ability of other defendants to pay the claim. For example, in Iowa, if the defendant is less than 50 percent responsible for all damages, he or she is liable only for his or her proportion of the damages; but if the responsibility is more than 50 percent, the defendant can be held severally liable for the entire amount of the damages.[52]

Collateral Source Offsets. The collateral source rule is a rule of evidence that prevents introducing evidence that the plaintiff has health or disability insurance covering the same injury. This rule originated at a time when individuals privately provided such coverage; the view was that the prudent person should not be penalized and the wrongdoer should not be relieved of liability because this would negate the deterrent effect of the penalty. The rule is opposed on the ground that recovery from multiple sources produces a windfall for the plaintiff (although in reality most health and disability policies require the plaintiff to reimburse the insurer for any payments received from the tort system).

At least thirty states have modified the collateral source rule, either to require juries to be informed about payment from other sources or to mandate an offset from the award for all or some of the collateral benefits. Also, a statute may be an exception to modification of the collateral source rule, allowing exclusion of collateral source benefits where the health care insurer has the right of *subrogation,* that is, the right to recover payment from an award in a tort action.[53]

Itemized Jury Verdicts. Requiring juries to itemize the various components of an award for damages instead of issuing a lump-sum figure is designed to promote objective and realistic awards by juries and to permit subsequent analysis of verdicts.[54] Thus, with itemized jury verdicts, the economic components of an award (past and future medical expenses, past and future income loss) and noneconomic components (pain and suffering, bereavement, loss of consortium, loss of parental or filial support, and punitive damages) are clearly set forth.

Caps on Damages. Caps on damages may set a limit on noneconomic damages only (such as pain and suffering), or put a total cap on both economic and noneconomic damages.

A number of states place some limit on noneconomic damage awards. These limits range from $250,000 to $1 million. Some states specify exceptions; the

Michigan cap does not apply to cases in which the patient has an injury to the reproductive system or has lost a bodily function.[55] Since no clear guidelines exist for assessing compensation for pain and suffering, proposals have been made to establish specific guidelines based on the age of the victim and the severity of the injury.

Only eight states have a cap on total damages, both economic and noneconomic. Permitted damages in these states range from $500,000 to $1 million. Four of these states have patient compensation funds.[56]

Statutory limits on damage awards are the subject of controversy and constitutional challenge. As of 1993, supreme courts in fifteen states had held caps on damages unconstitutional as a denial of due process or equal protection.[57]

A recent wave of decisions has invalidated caps on damages as a violation of provisions of the state constitution, most commonly as a violation of the right to a jury trial.[58] For example, in holding unconstitutional the $500,000 cap on noneconomic damages in the Oregon Tort Claims Act, the Supreme Court of Oregon stated that the cap "violates the injured party's right to receive an award that reflects the jury's factual determination of the amount of the damages as will fully compensate (plaintiffs) for all loss and injury to them."[59]

The supreme courts of Illinois, Kentucky, and New Hampshire have made similar decisions, and on Aug. 16, 1999, the Ohio Supreme Court, in a four-to-three decision, held unconstitutional a broad 1996 law designed to limit damage suits by capping damages, shortening the statute of limitations in certain suits, and otherwise curtailing damage suits.[60] In many states, these decisions have fomented a struggle between the legislature and the courts on change in the civil justice system, with business groups calling for limitation on liability lawsuits and the courts invalidating them on state constitutional grounds.

Other states, however, have upheld limits on noneconomic damages.[61] In a 1985 California case upholding the $250,000 limit on noneconomic damages in MICRA, on the ground that the limit is rationally related to the state's interest in reducing malpractice costs, mentioned earlier, Chief Justice Bird issued a stinging dissent, stating that victims of severe medical injury have been singled out to bear the bulk of relief in the medical malpractice insurance crisis, and the $250,000 limit on noneconomic damages cannot withstand any meaningful level of judicial scrutiny.[62]

Punitive Damages. Punitive damages may be imposed in a case of intentional, gross, or egregious negligence. Those who favor punitive damages in a malpractice action emphasize their deterrent effect; those who oppose punitive damages state that allegations of gross negligence are used for bargaining in settlement negotiations and that such conduct is more appropriately regulated by licensing bodies, institutional review committees, or the criminal justice system.[63] Some reformed statutes abolish punitive damages in any suit for compensation for negligence; others limit punitive damages in various ways (limiting the amount, paying the punitive damage award to the state instead of permitting a windfall to the plaintiff, restricting the contingency fee on a punitive damage award to reduce the incentive for pursuing such claims).[64]

Periodic Payments. By 1987, twenty-one states had enacted provisions requiring or allowing periodic payments of an award.[65] Periodic payments benefit the defendant and the insurer by reducing the cost of a large award and permitting modification of the award in the event the injured person dies, thus eliminating a windfall to the beneficiaries. Periodic payments benefit the injured person by ensuring availability of funds and avoiding the risk of mismanagement of a large lump sum.

Evaluations of State Legislative Reforms

To the ordinary observer, the increase in frequency and severity of medical malpractice claims in the 1980s, after the malpractice insurance crisis of the 1970s and the state legislative reforms that followed, would seem to indicate that these reforms were not effective. But one does not have to rely on this crude observation.

A number of studies have examined the effects of the various reforms described in the previous section. Of these, the OTA selected six principal empirical studies that examined the impact of tort reform in two or more states to ascertain whether these reforms reduced the frequency of medical malpractice claims, the size of awards or payments, or the level of medical malpractice insurance premiums, all of these collectively called "malpractice cost and indicators."[66]

OTA has performed a valuable service in excerpting from its meta-analysis the principal lessons for policy makers. Here we summarize the OTA evaluation of the various reforms, based on the six empirical studies in its meta-analysis:

• Only caps on damage awards and collateral source offsets reduced one or more of the malpractice cost indicators.

• Damage caps were found to reduce payment per claim paid in three studies. OTA concluded that caps on damages are effective in lowering payment per paid claim and therefore malpractice insurance premiums.

• With respect to collateral source offsets, the studies differed. Two studies found that mandatory collateral offsets had no effect on claim frequency. Danzon, however, examined discretionary and mandatory offsets and found a significant reduction in claim frequency and in amount of payment per paid claim.[67]

• Limit on attorneys' fees had no significant effect on frequency of claim, payment per claim paid, or insurance premiums.

• With respect to voluntary, binding arbitration, the findings differed. Danzon found that arbitration increased frequency and reduced payment per claim paid.[68] By contrast, Zuckerman, Bovbjerg, and Sloan found no significant impact of a preinjury arbitration agreement on frequency, amount paid, or level of insurance premium.[69]

• No significant effect of restricting the use of the *res ipsa loquitur* doctrine was found.

• One study found a greater number of malpractice claims from using the expanded, patient-oriented standard of informed consent. Another study found that statutory limits on the type of information that must be disclosed to the patient did not have a significant impact on payment per paid claim or on the probability that a claim would result in payment.

• Two studies found no significant impact of mandatory or discretionary periodic payments on payment per paid claim, and one study found no impact on malpractice insurance premiums.

The OTA concluded that two reforms significantly reduced one or more of the malpractice cost indicators: caps on damage awards, and mandatory collateral source offsets. No significant impact was found in three reforms: limits on attorneys' fees, mandatory or discretionary periodic payments, and restricting the use of *res ipsa loquitur*. Other reforms that were found to have mixed (some positive findings and some negative) or isolated effects (only one significant result) are restricting statutes of limitation, establishing pretrial screening panels, limiting the doctrine of informed consent, and allowing costs awardable in frivolous suits.

Since methods of alternative dispute resolution (ADR) have not been used extensively, no evaluation of the impact of these methods (neutral evaluation, court-annexed arbitration, summary jury trials, and mediation) was made. OTA comments that the reluctance to use ADR when it is voluntary and questions about its constitutionality when it is mandatory indicate that binding ADR is unlikely to have much impact on malpractice costs.[70]

Regarding use of practice guidelines as the standard of care, OTA predicts that practice guidelines may not be appropriate as a means of tort reform but that their development may be important in determining the standard of care under the existing tort system.

In its 1994 report on defensive medicine, the OTA offers further evaluation of various strategies in malpractice reform, particularly with respect to their impact on practicing defensive medicine. OTA concludes that tort reforms that tinker with the current system retaining personal liability of the physician are likely to be more successful in limiting the direct costs of malpractice—claim frequency, payment per paid claim, and insurance premiums—than in altering physician behavior. Use of practice guidelines is not a panacea, OTA states, but they may reduce defensive medicine because they offer guidance for the courts on standard of care.

ADR has the advantages of making available greater technical expertise in malpractice than a lay jury, and the process may be quicker—but it may also increase the number of claims and strengthen the link between malpractice claims and professional licensing.

Enterprise liability offers the advantages of reducing administrative costs associated with multiple defendants, of ensuring better quality control systems, and of removing the personal liability of the physician; but the physician is still likely to be called as a witness if the case goes to trial.

Selective no-fault, an administrative system compensating patients who experience an *accelerated compensation event*—an injury that is generally avoidable in good medical care—may limit physicians' involvement in the claims process, but the idea of personal responsibility may remain and thus may make unlikely any change in practicing defensive medicine.[71]

An earlier review of four published studies evaluating the effectiveness of tort reform in reducing claim frequency and severity concluded that piecemeal reforms have varied widely in measurable effects.[72] After summarizing the findings of these studies, Halley refers to Sylvia Law's characterization of tort reform as "consumer hostile."[73] Pointing out that these piecemeal measures make recovery by an injured person more difficult and restrict the awards obtained, Halley writes:

> In this view, tort reform compounds the other undesirable features of the tort approach: the lottery effect, yielding overcompensation to a few injured patients, and under compensation or no compensation to a larger number; long delays for those finally obtaining compensation; great system expense, since attorneys for the plaintiffs and the defense and insurers receive the major share of the premium dollar; and the increasing hardships of adversarial tort litigation [footnote omitted]. As a consequence, there has been considerable interest in new approaches, although none of these has obtained widespread support, and the level of such interest has always been crisis-driven.[74]

Criticisms of the Tort System

An important criticism of the tort system of handling medical malpractice is the small fraction of the premium dollar that reaches the injured person. In 1976, a landmark report of the Special Advisory Panel on Medical Malpractice in New

York state found that of total medical malpractice premiums only 25–40 percent goes to the claimant, and most of this payout goes to claimants with large claims.[75] In 1977, Munch (later Danzon) estimated that only forty to fifty cents of the premium dollar reaches the injured person—much less than the sixty-two cents for workers' compensation and eighty cents for first-party health insurance.[76]

Another criticism is the small proportion of injured patients who are compensated. In 1985, Danzon reported that the incidence of malpractice is much greater than the frequency of claims.[77] In 1991, the Harvard Medical Practice Study found that not more than 6.25 percent and possibly fewer than 1 percent of those injured receive compensation for medical injuries. Most victims of relatively minor injuries, and most victims of even severe injuries who are over sixty-five, receive no compensation.[78] The universe of injuries includes those due to adverse outcomes of the disease or medical procedures and those due to negligence. For those due to negligence, only a small proportion of patients injured sue; of those who sue, a smaller proportion receives any compensation. Figure 19.1, adapted by the OTA from J. R. Posner's work, depicts this experience.[79]

Despite the inequities and even injustices of the tort system for handling medical malpractice, it has persisted, with only the piecemeal changes we have described, because, as consumer advocates point out, it is "often the only practical means available to patients for exposing, punishing, and deterring substandard medical practice."[80]

FIGURE 19.1.   MEDICAL INJURIES, NEGLIGENT CONDUCT, AND MALPRACTICE CLAIMS.

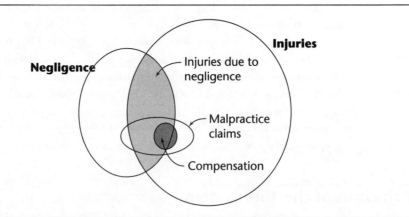

Source: Office of Technology Assessment. *Impact of Legal Reforms on Medical Malpractice Costs.* (OTA-BP-H-19.) Washington, D.C.: U.S. Government Printing Office, Oct. 1993, p. 9. Adapted from Posner, J. R. "Trends in Medical Malpractice Insurance, 1970–1985." *Law and Contemporary Problems,* 1986, *49*(2), 37.

Alternatives to the Tort System

Various alternatives have been proposed. The four main types (the first three of which have been briefly mentioned) can be summarized as (1) alternative dispute resolution (ADR), which includes conciliation, mediation, and arbitration; (2) enterprise liability; (3) no-fault insurance, which includes medical adversity insurance and "neo–no-fault" insurance; and (4) the Model Medical Accident Compensation System, patterned after the workers' compensation system.

Alternative Dispute Resolution

ADR is a nonjudicial process that includes conciliation (bringing the parties together), mediation (bringing the parties together and suggesting possible solutions),[81] and arbitration (holding a hearing at which the parties present their cases and an award is made). The most important of these is arbitration, which may be voluntary or mandatory, binding or nonbinding, an independent proceeding, or related to a court case.

Arguments in favor of arbitration are that it resolves claims quickly, reduces costs, permits greater access for small claims, and reduces the burden on the courts.

Arguments against arbitration are that it may favor providers if a provider is a member of the arbitration panel, it may not compensate the injured person adequately, it may reduce the provider's incentive to lower the incidence of malpractice because the private arbitration process avoids the stigma of a court suit, agreements to arbitrate may not be fully understood by the patient and thus may give an unfair advantage to the provider, and the informality of arbitration hearings may violate the due process rights of the parties.[82]

Experience with alternative dispute resolution is still limited. The courts have encouraged its use. Some state statutes allow binding, irrevocable arbitration agreements in medical malpractice cases, or, as in California, private agreements may lead to arbitration. In 1981, authorities in the field pointed out that arbitration has the advantages of accommodating all types of cases; offering various arbitration arrangements; and being expeditious, economical, and generally acceptable, so that it should be considered "not alone as a procedural alternative to litigation but as a substantive contribution to resolution of medical issues."[83]

Despite these alleged advantages of arbitration, concern has arisen that delay in the arbitration process and the ability of providers to select favorable arbitrators may prejudice injured patients. For example, in *Engalla* v. *Kaiser Permanente Medical Group*,[84] a mandatory arbitration case involving excessive delays in appointing an arbitrator, the California Supreme Court held that Kaiser

Permanente's failure to comply with the time requirements of the arbitration agreement would allow this case to be heard in court, but the California Supreme Court did not invalidate the mandatory arbitration system generally. In accordance with recommendations of a blue ribbon advisory panel appointed by Kaiser Permanente following this decision, Kaiser Permanente has reformed its arbitration process to include an independent administrator, use of a single neutral arbitrator, early mediation, explicit deadlines, and a broad advisory panel.[85] The increasing popularity of new strategies for conflict resolution may impel a resurgence of alternative dispute resolution of medical liability.

Enterprise Liability

Related to alternative dispute resolution is the concept of enterprise liability, which allows patients, providers, and health care institutions to enter into a contract placing all liability for the physician's action on the health care institution.

Those favoring contracting for enterprise liability argue that it encourages health care institutions to strengthen their quality control measures, reduces the cost of liability insurance and improves the physician-patient relationship by eliminating the threat of suit, reduces the need for defensive medicine, promotes early and more certain awards, and reduces insurers' administrative costs by reducing the number of individual policies and claims.

Against contracting for enterprise liability are the arguments that it does not cover all patients, the courts may look unfavorably on the contracts as an unfair limitation on the tort rights of patients, and consumers are not sufficiently informed or sufficiently powerful to protect their interests in contract negotiations.[86]

Enterprise liability may be a realistic possibility because of its compatibility with managed competition.[87] Even in the absence of managed competition, enterprise liability may gain acceptance because 80 percent of malpractice claims arise from hospital care, and the hospital would be the enterprise responsible for this care. HMOs that employ physicians directly are legally responsible for actions of their staff physicians. Hospitals are similarly responsible for care provided by interns and residents. *Darling* v. *Charleston Community Memorial Hospital*[88] established the legal obligation of the hospital for the quality of care it provides.

The growth of integrated health care delivery systems in which an organizational unit bears the insurance risk and also provides clinical services has fueled new support for replacing the current system of medical malpractice liability with a system of enterprise medical liability.[89]

There are several arguments advanced for enterprise liability.[90] First, the current system suffers from the well-known deficiencies of failing to compensate many injured patients and failing to deter negligence. Moreover, certain practices of malpractice insurers, such as not basing premiums on individual experience but rather on location and specialty, minimize incentives for quality improvement.[91] Second, the organizational unit that is ultimately responsible for efficient health care should also bear financial liability for malpractice so that it can include the cost of patient harm in its calculations. Third, placing liability for malpractice in the high policy-making level of the organizational unit tends to decrease defensive medicine, which has been estimated to cost about 8 percent of diagnostic procedures.[92]

Fourth, imposing liability at the high level of the organizational unit may also promote equity by encouraging policies that benefit the many with cost-effective procedures rather than the few with expensive procedures.[93] Fifth, imposing liability on health plans follows from a capitated payment system, since health plans must bear the cost of future medical care from the present payment, and enterprise liability would require plans to incorporate the cost of malpractice awards in their calculations.[94] Sixth, health plans are in a position to reduce the incidence of malpractice through organizational and managerial strategies. Finally, an integrated delivery system may have the capacity to arrange for sharing liability among numerous units in a health plan network.

Proponents of enterprise liability contend that such a system promotes quality by improving relations between health plans and health care professionals, promoting teamwork, and relieving physicians to some extent of the extremely negative experience of malpractice suits.

Despite the apparent cogency of these arguments, many questions are unanswered. Is enterprise liability feasible in the absence of comprehensive health care reform? Which enterprise should be responsible: the health plan, or the hospital or other enterprise directly involved in delivering health care?[95] What inequities result from the operation of different health plans? In a mixed health care system—part managed care and part traditional practice—how is malpractice liability handled fairly? Notwithstanding the theoretical appeal of many of the arguments for enterprise medical liability, can such a system realistically be implemented? Can it withstand legal challenge? Does it prejudice the injured patient by shifting liability to a powerful and invisible defendant? The growth of managed care and the national debate on managed care liability have given new life to the concept of enterprise liability.

No-Fault Compensation

The essence of the no-fault approach is that it is a compensation system that eliminates proof of negligence as a basis for collecting damages. As Grad points out, a no-fault system would recognize the fact that the risk of medical injury is inherent in modern medicine and would permit compensation for all such injuries, irrespective of negligence.[96]

In 1976–77, the California Medical Association and the California Hospital Association sponsored the Medical Insurance Feasibility Study in California to determine the economic feasibility of a pure no-fault system. This study is important for showing that adverse outcomes of medical care, although numerous, are finite and can be identified. The study found that 82 percent of adverse outcomes were class I adverse outcomes, involving complications of treatment (including giving drugs to patients). Class II adverse outcomes—the effects of incomplete or delayed diagnosis or treatment—accounted for only 15 percent of adverse outcomes.[97] Most no-fault systems now in use around the world cover only class I adverse outcomes and not class II outcomes. It is therefore suggested that since class I injuries account for 82 percent of total adverse outcomes, a no-fault system applicable to that 82 percent might be worthwhile, leaving class II outcomes in a residual fault-based liability system.[98]

In support of a no-fault insurance system, it would extend compensation to more injured persons, deliver compensation more promptly, avoid the substantial cost of proving negligence, make similar compensation available to patients with similar injuries, and create incentives for improving the quality of care by defining the causes of untoward outcomes and means of avoiding them and by basing insurance premiums on each provider's experience rating.

Those against a no-fault insurance system urge consideration that it may cost more than the current system because more people will be compensated; although the question of negligence is eliminated, the question of causation remains; it requires work to define the compensable events and the compensation schedule; the system covers only economic damages, not pain and suffering, although the compensation schedule might reflect some elements of pain and suffering; it removes a deterrent to substandard care; it may cause some providers to refuse to accept high-risk patients; and it may be complex in resolving claims involving multiple providers.[99]

Next we turn to two forms of limited no-fault insurance: medical adversity insurance and neo–no-fault insurance.

Medical Adversity Insurance. In 1973, Havighurst and Tancredi proposed a no-fault approach that they called "medical adversity insurance."[100] The proposal would identify those injuries that deserve compensation, calling them "designated compensable events." The proposal aimed to improve the quality of care by defining categories of untoward outcomes and the means for avoiding them. Although this system has not been implemented, benefits claimed for it are the impact on the quality of medical care (it generates a listing, specialty by specialty, of potential adverse effects of various procedures), administrative savings derived by avoiding court suits, and reduction of emotional stress and stigma for all parties.[101]

Neo–No-Fault Insurance. Another variation on the no-fault system is neo–no-fault.[102] The essence of this proposal is to encourage early out-of-court settlement for the actual economic losses and use the money that would have been spent on litigation and pain and suffering to pay for adequate injury compensation. This proposal differs from pure no-fault because the tort system is retained as an alternative.[103]

Under this proposal, a provider facing a malpractice claim has the option of offering the claimant, within 180 days after the claim is filed, periodic payment or a lump sum approved by the court as compensation for economic losses, including medical expenses, rehabilitation, and lost wages not covered by other insurance. Certain disincentives to sue would prevail: recovery is allowed only for wanton conduct; the standard of proof required is higher (not the usual standard in civil cases of preponderance of the evidence, but rather proof by clear and convincing evidence); limitation of noneconomic damages; and a penalty on the plaintiff of having to pay the defendant's costs if the claimant is awarded less than the noneconomic loss offered by the defendant.

The advantage of this proposal is that it produces prompt payment for economic loss in return for giving up the right to sue. But in egregious cases with great pain and suffering, the claimant would be permitted to bring a tort action.

Examples of U.S. No-Fault Systems. Three examples of limited no-fault systems exist in the United States.

In 1986, Congress enacted the National Childhood Vaccine Injury Act of 1986, with its no-fault compensation system for children injured as a result of side effects of immunization against childhood diseases. The legislation was designed to encourage vaccine manufacturers to increase their production of vaccines, which had declined dangerously because of the industry's fear of malpractice suits. Compensation is payable by the federal government on the basis of strict liability, that is, without regard to fault or negligence by the manufacturer or the administering physician.[104]

Two states, Virginia and Florida, have enacted no-fault compensation systems for birth-related neurological injuries. The Virginia Birth-Related Neurological Injury Compensation Act of 1987 was designed to make liability insurance for obstetrician-gynecologists affordable and available by taking claims for certain catastrophically injured newborns out of the tort system, thus permitting quicker compensation and increasing access to obstetrical care.[105]

Compensation is awarded only for those infants who meet a narrow statutory definition of injury to the spinal cord or brain—caused by deprivation of oxygen or mechanical injury in the course of labor, delivery, or resuscitation in the immediate postdelivery period in a hospital—that rendered the infant permanently "motorically disabled" and developmentally or cognitively disabled such that assistance in all activities of daily living is required, and that was not caused by congenital or genetic factors, degenerative neurological disease, or maternal substance abuse. The injury must have been caused by a physician who was participating in the program or at a participating hospital.

The program is funded by an annual assessment of $250 per licensed physician, voluntary assessments of $5,000 per participating physician, and $50 per delivery for participating hospitals, not to exceed $150,000 in any twelve-month period.[106]

The procedure is as follows. The claimant files a claim with the Workers' Compensation Commission and serves a petition on the fund that administers the program and determines whether the claim falls within the definition of the statute. If the fund finds that the injury is compensable, the commission issues an order without a hearing and sends the case to a medical review panel of three qualified and impartial physicians, which makes a recommendation to the commission as to whether the case is covered by the act. If the fund determines that the case does not fall within the definition, then the commission holds a hearing at which the panel's recommendation is given considerable but not determinative weight.[107] Awards are made according to statutory provisions.

The plaintiff has no option of an alternative remedy if the delivery was performed by a participating hospital, but final appeal may be made to the Virginia Court of Appeals. By the end of 1992, only four claims had been filed under this program.

The Florida Birth-Related Neurological Injury Compensation Act was passed in 1988 and is similar to that of Virginia but differs in several respects. The claim must be filed within five years, instead of ten; it is not required that the infant need assistance in all activities. A hospital is protected from liability only if the delivery is done by a participating physician, so hospitals either require their physicians to participate or pay the physician's assessment. Thus, about 90 percent of obstetricians in Florida participate.[108]

A thorough study of the experience under these no-fault, birth-injury statutes found that the number of cases is small, perhaps because of lack of outreach and the option remaining of choosing to sue in tort. The study also found that no-fault cases are resolved more quickly than tort suits, and that no-fault's low administrative costs are related to using only a few expert hearing officers and medical consultants.[109] The study concluded that no-fault programs are feasible and produce major gains in efficiency. In the opinion of the authors of the study, a broader no-fault injury program covering more eligible cases would improve both compensation and deterrence, though this outcome depends on the details of implementation of the statutes.[110]

Experience with No-Fault Insurance in Other Countries. Three countries have adopted systems of no-fault compensation for personal injury: New Zealand, Sweden, and Finland.

Since 1974, New Zealand has had a comprehensive system of compensation for all personal injuries, whether they occur at work, on the highway, in the home, in the hospital, or anywhere else. The scheme was introduced because of varying results for people with equal problems and equal needs, because many people received no compensation for injuries, and because extravagant and drawn-out adversary techniques reduced compensation to claimants.[111]

The intent of the scheme is to compensate all instances of physical or mental harm caused by accident but excluding those arising from illness or old age. The scope of the scheme is broad, but excluded are (1) the effects of a cardiovascular or cerebrovascular episode unless it is work-related and the result of undue strain, or unless the episode results from an injury by accident; and (2) physical or mental damage caused exclusively by disease, infection, or the aging process.[112]

Administered by a nonprofit, autonomous governmental organization (the Accident Compensation Corporation), the New Zealand program, as of 1989, compensated for total disability, in periodic payments, at a level of 80 percent of earnings up to a ceiling of $976 per week (N.Z. $1 = U.S. $0.62 as of Feb. 15, 1989). Proportionate adjustments are made for partial disability. The benefit level is fixed at 80 percent to create an incentive for rehabilitation. Payments are made for disability, adjusted for inflation, until age sixty-five, when pensions take over.

In addition to payment for loss of earnings, reasonable costs of medical and dental treatment are covered, as well as reasonable costs of transport to the doctor or hospital for initial treatment and for further rehabilitative treatment, rehabilitation, and retraining assistance; payment for reasonable cost of necessary constant personal attention of the injured person following the accident; lump sum for permanent physical disability; lump sum for pain and suffering; lump sum to dependent spouse and dependent children; and other benefits.[113]

The program is financed by contributions from employers and employees and the self-employed, together with payments from owners of motor vehicles (in 1989, $100 a year for a private car!) and a small supplement from general taxation. The New Zealand physician or surgeon in 1989 paid a levy based on income at the rate of 1.45 percent, or $920 up to the maximum levied income of $63,458 (subsequently raised to $104,000, with the annual levy raised to $2,600). These payments cover the physician for his or her own incapacity and also release the physician entirely from all risk of claims for damages from others.[114]

The New Zealand system has enjoyed wide public support for the years that it has been in operation. New Zealand has not experienced the growth in defensive medicine or the harm to the doctor-patient relationship associated with malpractice suits. As for the effect on the quality of medical practice, the Right Honorable Sir Owen Woodhouse, who is largely responsible for introducing and promoting the New Zealand compensation system, said that "it is a strange argument that physicians need to be made fearful of court actions in order to maintain those professional standards upon which their whole livelihood will depend. Certainly there are no signs in New Zealand that medical standards have deteriorated in the 15 years during which the comprehensive scheme has been operating."[115]

On January 1, 1975, Sweden introduced a voluntary patient insurance scheme administered by a consortium of insurers headed by Scandia Life. The scheme is funded and paid by the county councils on a per capita basis, costing about U.S. $1.76 per year. Injured patients may elect to bring an action in tort or may receive compensation under the patient compensation program without having to prove fault.[116] The program was not enacted by the Swedish government but is the result of an agreement between the Federation of County Councils and a consortium of Swedish insurers. Although the program is generally described as no-fault, it is not strictly so because error underlies most payments: "Such an error, however, does not have to be proved negligent; error may be assumed where the outcome is unusual."[117]

In January 1978, Sweden introduced a pharmaceutical scheme, which is also a voluntary, nonstatutory system covering injuries from vaccination and blood products. Impelled by the threat of legislation, the program is paid for by the drug industry, and premiums are based on each company's market share.

Five types of injury are covered under the Swedish compensation system: (1) treatments, (2) timing and accuracy of diagnosis, (3) accidents, (4) infections, and (5) injuries caused by diagnostic procedures. To be compensated, an individual must have reported sick for a minimum of fourteen days or been hospitalized for at least ten days, or have suffered permanent injury, or died. Compensation is paid for loss of income and for medical care, with indemnities for pain and suffering and permanent disfigurement.

The philosophy of the Swedish system is based on the principles of tort law in that injuries, complications, or undesired results as an unavoidable consequence of the illness or necessary treatment are not covered. Compensation is paid whether or not the error of judgment or clinical practice was negligent; therefore doctors and nurses are willing to admit errors and encourage patients to file claims.[118]

The claims process is simple, inexpensive, and easy to administer. The patient has the right to take an appeal to a claims panel, which meets for a day about twelve times a year. If the claims panel rejects the appeal, the patient's final resort is to submit the claim to arbitration.

Finland has introduced comprehensive pharmaceutical and treatment injury insurance modeled after the Swedish system. The Patient Injury Act of 1986 permits payments for loss of earnings, loss of amenities, and pain and suffering. Ninety-three percent of all medical care is provided by the State. Compensation is payable for any injury that has arisen from examination, treatment, or any similar action, or neglect of the same; that has been caused by an infection connected with examination or treatment; or that has been caused by accident connected with examination or treatment, occurring during ambulance transport, or resulting from a defect in medical equipment.

The scheme is financed through insurance, which doctors and other health providers must obtain. The Patient Insurance Association issues policies and handles claims and settlements. Failure to carry insurance makes the uninsured provider liable for ten times the normal premium. If a provider is uninsured, the Patient Insurance Association pays the patient and then collects the increased premium.[119]

In Finland, the Patient Injury Act of 1986 has eliminated the need to prove negligence entirely. In Sweden, negligence need be proved only if the injured person elects to sue in tort instead of seeking compensation through the patient insurance program. But, since the damages paid under the insurance program are the same as those recoverable in tort, there is little incentive to sue.[120]

The Model Medical Accident Compensation Act

Finally, we turn to the proposal for a system of medical accident compensation that applies the principles of workers' compensation to medical injury compensation.[121] In the belief that administrative or agency compensation is theoretically and realistically the solution for the medical professional liability dilemma, Halley and colleagues have advanced a model statute authored by Bryce B. Moore, former director of the Kansas workers' compensation program, and supported by extensive research by the Midwest Institute for Health Care and Law.

Like workers' compensation, the Model Medical Accident Compensation System involves a trade-off: it extends benefits to a larger number of injured individuals than are compensated currently in exchange for restricting the tort system. The administrative process is designed for prompt, limited, and certain compensation for an increased number of injured individuals, avoiding the delay, costs, and uncertainties of court procedures. A greater proportion of the premium dollar would go to the injured person than occurs under the adversarial process. Attorneys may represent claimants and providers in the administrative process.

Definition of the medical injury or compensable event is not through a schedule of compensable events but rather through review of individual cases, applying the standard of reasonable care. Proof of negligence is not required, but the concept of medical error or "fault" (responsibility for an outcome) is retained to distinguish compensable events from progression of the disease or unavoidable consequences of treatment. Administrative determination by the Medical Accident Compensation Board replaces adversarial tort litigation and the jury. The determination of compensable events is made by the Medical Accident Compensation Board, assisted by an expert review panel.

Payment of all compensation claims is guaranteed through requirements that health care providers carry insurance and through a Recovery Guarantee Fund. There are three methods of funding: (1) purchase of an insurance policy by an individual provider; (2) provider self-insurance (usually for an institution); and (3) membership in a group-funded self-insurance pool (a less-expensive method than individual purchase of insurance).

The Recovery Guarantee Fund is established in the state treasury to ensure payment of compensation in the event a provider is uninsured or unable to pay the benefits under the act. Payments from the fund are not expected to be large, since health care providers generally carry the required insurance, just as most employers carry the appropriate workers' compensation insurance.

Benefits are based on economic loss with equivalent compensation for claimants without ascertainable earnings, such as housewives, homemakers, retired persons, and children. Benefits include those for medical care and rehabilitation, temporary and permanent personal disability, death benefits, and burial expenses. Calculation of permanent personal injury benefits is based on the highest of three percentages: loss of the claimant's earning ability, overall reduction in the claimant's health level, and functional disability to the body as a whole.

The cost of an administrative system is an important concern because of the anticipated increase in the number of compensated injuries. These increased payments may be offset by the greater efficiency of the system and by cost controls built into the system: maximum limits on liability, a two-year statute of limitations on filing a claim, credit for duplicate payments (no windfall to the claimant from collateral sources), limitation on attorneys' fees, and so on.

The act allows appeal to the courts from a decision of the board. As in workers' compensation, appeals are based on the record of proceedings before the board. The courts have jurisdiction to determine whether the board has made a correct finding under the act.

Most important are provisions built into the model act to promote acceptable quality of health care. Separate from the compensation provisions are others for strengthened state agencies that conduct surveillance of medical practice, institutional review procedures, and other peer review mechanisms. Quality assurance is linked to the data-collection functions of the board, which are connected to state and national data banks.

Medical Malpractice Reform in the U.S. Context

The many proposals for change in the tort system of handling medical malpractice liability break down into three main types: (1) piecemeal reforms, or tinkering with the tort system; (2) no-fault compensation systems; and (3) an administrative program of compensation modeled on the workers' compensation system.

Twenty years' experience with piecemeal reforms has made only minor improvements in the tort system, which fails to compensate many injured persons; pays only 25–40 percent of total premium cost to injured persons; and is fraught with delays, high costs, and inequities among injured persons suffering from the same or similar injuries. Careful evaluation of the effects of piecemeal reform has confirmed their minimal benefits. The recurrence in the 1980s of the medical malpractice insurance crisis of the 1970s attests to the need for an alternative approach.

No-fault compensation systems are currently operating in the federal vaccine compensation program and in two states for compensation for birth-related neurological injuries. Examples of the no-fault approach exist in automobile insurance. Although the compensable event is clearly defined in automobile accidents, definition of potentially compensable medical events requires more work. The Medical Insurance Feasibility Study, sponsored by the California Medical Association and the California Hospital Association in the late 1970s, showed that it is possible to define potentially compensable events and that a no-fault system of medical injury compensation is feasible.[122] From a policy point of view, the well-documented report of New York's Special Advisory Panel on Medical Malpractice in 1976 strongly recommended a compensation system that does not pay damages for injuries caused by malpractice but rather compensates for bad medical results.[123]

The experience of New Zealand, Sweden, and Finland with their differing no-fault systems of medical injury compensation shows the rationality, equity, and public acceptance of no-fault systems. The systems of health insurance and social security benefits in these countries, however, are much more all-encompassing than in the United States.

Despite the soundness of the no-fault approach and the appeal of neo–no-fault in retaining the option of a suit in tort, political realities seem to militate against adoption of this alternative. Objections to the no-fault approach have been detailed earlier in this chapter, but the principal countervailing force lies in the power of the special interests that would be affected by adopting this approach (mainly the insurance companies and the trial lawyers).

In view of these realities, a feasible and rational alternative is the Model Medical Accident Compensation Act, patterned after the workers' compensation program and designed to be an administrative system for reasonable and rapid compensation for medical injuries. Even though workers' compensation may be in need of some modernization itself, such as increased benefits and strengthened rehabilitation provisions, few people would dream of ever returning to the tort system for redress of occupational injuries and diseases. Administrative law is increasingly the means in the United States for handling technical problems requiring expertise and prompt resolution. It is an appropriate vehicle for solving the problem of medical injury compensation. Extensive research and investigation have explored the economic, constitutional, and medical features of such a system, and precedents exist in other administrative law programs.

Regardless of when and how medical malpractice liability reform should be undertaken, the fundamental issue is quality of care. No system of medical care can eliminate all adverse outcomes, a certain number of which are inevitable in high-technology medicine, and no system can eliminate all bad actors and all substandard performance; but strategies can be adopted to monitor and continually improve the quality of care. The Model Medical Accident Compensation Act contains provisions on data collection and surveillance of care that can strengthen current protections of the quality of care.

Enacting national health insurance that ensures universal coverage of the total population may reduce the propensity to sue, since all medical care, including that needed because of adverse outcomes of earlier care, will be covered. Patient anger with the health care system—a necessary ingredient for a lawsuit—may be reduced by universal coverage.[124] Malpractice suits may also be restrained as health maintenance organizations and third-party administrators (such as Kaiser Permanente's Report Card on Quality of Care) introduce quality control measures to strengthen the existing quality system of state licensure, disciplinary actions, and peer review processes.

In 1986, an authority on medical malpractice called the current system not a compensation system but a liability system, pointing out that (1) our current system fails as a compensation system, (2) evidence is lacking that it has any deterrent effects, and (3) the costs of liability coverage and administration are too high.[125] More than a decade later, with health care reform still on the national agenda, the climate of opinion may indeed be favorable for rationalizing our handling of medical injury compensation by adopting an administrative system that is more equitable and less costly than the tort system.

Notes

1. Starr, P. *The Logic of Health Care Reform.* Knoxville, Tenn.: Whittle Books, Grand Rounds Press, 1992; U.S. Congress, Office of Technology Assessment. *Impact of Legal Reforms on Medical Malpractice Costs.* OTA-BP-H-19. Washington, D.C.: U.S. Government Printing Office, 1993.

2. Aaron, H. J. *Serious and Unstable Condition: Financing America's Health Care.* Washington, D.C.: Brookings Institution, 1991. The OTA states that "most defensive medicine is not of zero benefit." U.S. Congress, Office of Technology Assessment. *Defensive Medicine and Medical Malpractice.* OTA-H-602. Washington, D.C.: U.S. Government Printing Office, 1994.

3. Starr (1992).

4. Office of Technology Assessment (1994), p. l.

5. Aaron (1991).

6. Sage, W. M. "Enterprise Liability and the Emerging Health Care System." *Law and Contemporary Problems,* 1997, *60*(2), 159–210.

7. Rosenblatt, R. E., Law, S. A., and Rosenbaum, S. *Law and the American Health Care System.* Westbury, N.Y.: Foundation Press, 1997. See *Corcoran* v. *United Healthcare, Inc.,* 965 F. 2d 1321 (5th Cir. 1992), cert. denied 506 U.S. 1033 (1992).

8. See, for example, *Dukes* v. *U.S. Healthcare, Inc.,* 57 F. 3rd 350 (3rd Cir. 1995), cert. denied 116 S. Ct. 564 (1995); Sage (1997); Pear, R. "Series of Rulings Eases Constraints on Suing HMOs." *New York Times,* Aug. 15, 1999, pp. 1, 19; Jacobson, P. D., and Pomfret, S. D. "ERISA Litigation and Physician Autonomy." *Journal of the American Medical Association,* 2000, *283*(7), 921–926.

9. 120 S.Ct. 2143 (June 12, 2000). See Mariner, W. K. "What Recourse?—Liability for Managed-Care Decisions and the Employee Retirement Income Security Act." *New England Journal of Medicine,* 2000, *343*(8), 592–596.

10. *New York State Conference of Blue Cross and Blue Shield Plans* v. *Travelers Ins. Co.,* 115 S. Ct. 1671 (1995).

11. Rosenblatt, Law, and Rosenbaum (1997), p. 195.

12. Geyelin, M. "Courts Pierce HMO's Shield Against Lawsuits." *Wall Street Journal,* Apr. 30, 1999, pp. B1, B4.

13. *Tex. Civ. Prac. & Rem. Code,* ch. 88. See discussion of Texas law and legislative action in other states in Sage (1997), p. 178.

14. Rosenbaum, S., Frankford, D. M., and Moore, B. "Who Should Determine When Health Care Is Medically Necessary?" *New England Journal of Medicine,* 1999, *340*(3), 229–232. But see Butler, P. *ERISA Preemption Manual for State Health Policy Makers.* Washington, D.C.: Alpha Center and National Academy for State Health Policy, 2000, p. 8, for estimate that about 53 million of the 123 million American workers receiving coverage through the workplace in 1997 were not covered by state regulation.

15. *Darling* v. *Charleston Community Memorial Hospital,* 33 Ill. 2d326, 211 N.E. 2d 253 (1965).

16. U.S. General Accounting Office. "Medical Malpractice: No Agreement on the Problems or Solutions." (Report to Congressional Requesters; GAO/HRD 86-50.) Washington, D.C.:

U.S. General Accounting Office, 1986; Harvard Medical Practice Study. *Patients, Doctors and Lawyers: Medical Injury Malpractice Litigation and Patient Compensation in New York: The Report of the Harvard Medical Practice Study to the State of New York.* New York: New York Health Department, 1990; Sage (1997), pp.160–161.

17. Danzon, P. M. *The Frequency and Severity of Medical Malpractice Claims.* (RAND publication R-2870-ICJ/HCFA.) Santa Monica, Calif.: Institute for Civil Justice, RAND, 1982).

18. Danzon, P. M. *Medical Malpractice: Theory, Evidence, and Public Policy.* Cambridge, Mass.: Harvard University Press, 1985; Jacobson, P. D. "Medical Malpractice and the Tort System." *Journal of the American Medical Association,* Dec. 15, 1989, *262*(23), 3320–3327.

19. Danzon (1985).

20. Grad, F. P. "Medical Malpractice and Its Implications for Public Health." In R. Roemer and G. McKray (eds.), *Legal Aspects of Health Policy: Issues and Trends.* Westport, Conn.: Greenwood Press, 1980.

21. Danzon (1985).

22. Halley, M. M. "Tort Law Impact on Health Care." In M. M. Halley, R. J. Fowks, E. C. Bigler, and D. L. Ryan (eds.), *Medical Malpractice Solutions: Systems and Proposals for Injury Compensation.* Springfield, Ill.: Charles C. Thomas, 1989.

23. Danzon (1985).

24. Bigler, E. C. "Medical Professional Liability in the United States." In Halley, Fowks, Bigler, and Ryan (1989).

25. Danzon (1985).

26. Danzon (1982).

27. Rosenbach, M. L., and Stone, A. G. "Malpractice Insurance Costs and Physician Practice, 1981–1986." *Health Affairs,* Winter 1990, 176–185.

28. Danzon (1985), Preface.

29. Grad (1980); Danzon (1982).

30. Danzon (1982); Jacobson (1989).

31. Bigler (1989).

32. U.S. General Accounting Office (1986).

33. Halley, "Tort Law Impact . . ." (1989).

34. Grad (1980).

35. Halley, M. M. "Tort Reform: The Response to Crisis." In Halley, Fowks, Bigler, and Ryan (1989).

36. U.S. General Accounting Office (1986).

37. Law, S., and Polan, S. *Pain and Profit: The Politics of Malpractice.* New York: HarperCollins, 1978.

38. Danzon, P. M. *Contingent Fees for Personal Injury Litigation.* (Prepared for Health Care Financing Administration.) Santa Monica, Calif.: U.S. Department of Health, Education, and Welfare, and RAND, 1980.

39. Danzon (1985).

40. Office of Technology Assessment (1993).

41. *Roa* v. *Lodi Medical Group,* 37 Cal. 3d 920, 211 Cal. Rptr. 77, 695 P. 2d 164 (1985).

42. Halley, "Tort Reform . . ." (1989).

43. Office of Technology Assessment (1993).

44. Danzon (1985); Office of Technology Assessment (1993).

45. Danzon (1985).

46. Office of Technology Assessment (1993).

47. U.S. General Accounting Office (1986).

48. In incorporating into state law twenty practice guidelines for four specialties (anesthesiology, emergency medicine, obstetrics and gynecology, and radiology), the Maine legislature sought to resolve malpractice claims by eliminating the need to establish the standard of practice and hoped to control health care costs by reducing the incentive to perform unnecessary tests and procedures. See U.S. General Accounting Office. *Medical Malpractice: Maine's Use of Practice Guidelines to Reduce Costs.* GAO/HRD-94-80. Washington, D.C.: U.S. General Accounting Office, 1993.

49. Office of Technology Assessment (1993).

50. Office of Technology Assessment (1993).

51. Halley, "Tort Reform . . ." (1989).

52. Office of Technology Assessment (1993); Halley, "Tort Reform . . ." (1989).

53. Office of Technology Assessment (1993); Halley, "Tort Reform . . ." (1989).

54. Halley, "Tort Reform . . . (1989).

55. Office of Technology Assessment (1993).

56. Office of Technology Assessment (1993).

57. Office of Technology Assessment (1993); see also note 20.

58. Glaberson, W. "State Courts Sweeping away Laws Curbing Suits for Injury." *New York Times,* July 16, 1999, pp. 1, 13; Glaberson, W. "Looking for Attention with a Billion-Dollar Message." *New York Times,* July 18, 1999, Week in Review, p. 3. See, for example, *Sofie* v. *Fiberboard Corp.,* 112 Wash. 2d 636, 771 P. 2d 711 (Wash. 1989); *Moore* v. *Mobile Infirmary Assign,* 592 So. 2d 156 (Ala. 1991); *Bolton* v. *Deveau,* 1999 N.H. Lexis 338 (New Hampshire Apr. 21, 1999).

59. *Lakin* v. *Senco Products,* 1999 WL 498088, *10,29 (Or., July 15, 1999).

60. Glaberson, W. "Ohio Supreme Court Voids Legal Limits on Damage Suits." *New York Times,* Aug. 17, 1999, p. A9.

61. Office of Technology Assessment (1993); see also note 21. See, for example, *Pulliam* v. *Coastal Emergency Services of Richmond,* 357 Va. 1, 509 S.E.2d 307 (1999).

62. *Fein* v. *Permanente Medical Group,* 38 Cal. 3d 137, 695 P. 2d 665, 687 (1985).

63. Halley, "Tort Reform . . ." (1989).

64. Halley, "Tort Reform . . ." (1989).

65. Halley, "Tort Reform . . ." (1989); Office of Technology Assessment (1993).

66. Office of Technology Assessment (1993). The six studies analyzed are Adams, E. K., and Zuckerman, S. "Variation in the Growth and Incidence of Medical Malpractice Claims." *Journal of Health Politics. Policy and Law,* 1984, *9*(3), 475–488; Barker, D. K. "The Effects of Tort Reform on Medical Malpractice Insurance Markets: An Empirical Analysis." *Journal of Health Politics. Policy and Law,* 1992, *17*(1), 143–161; Blackmon, G., and Zeckhauser, R. "State Tort Reform Legislation: Assessing Our Control of Risks." In P. H. Schuck (ed.), *Tort Law and the Public Interest.* New York: Norton, 1991); Danzon, P. M. "The Frequency and Severity of Medical Malpractice Claims: New Evidence." *Law and Contemporary Problems,* 1986, *49*(2), 57–84; Sloan, F. A., Mergenhagen, P. M., and Bovbjerg, R. R. "Effects of Tort Reforms on the Value of Closed Medical Malpractice Claims: A Microanalysis." *Journal of Health Politics. Policy and Law,* 1989, *14*(4), 663–689; Zuckerman, S., Bovbjerg, R. R., and Sloan, F. "Effects of Tort Reforms and Other Factors on Medical Malpractice Insurance Premiums." *Inquiry,* 1990, *27*(2), 167–182.

67. Office of Technology Assessment (1993).

68. Office of Technology Assessment (1993).

69. Office of Technology Assessment (1993).

70. Office of Technology Assessment (1993).
71. Office of Technology Assessment (1994).
72. Halley, "Tort Reform . . ." (1989).
73. Halley, "Tort Reform . . ." (1989), p. 77; Law, S. A. "A Consumer Perspective on Medical Malpractice." *Law and Contemporary Problems,* 1986, *49*(2), 306–320.
74. Halley, "Tort Reform . . ." (1989), p. 77.
75. *Report of the Special Advisory Panel on Medical Malpractice* (Jan. 1976), discussed at length in Grad (1980).
76. Danzon (1985).
77. Danzon (1985).
78. Harvard Medical Practice Study (1990).
79. Office of Technology Assessment (1993), figure adapted from Posner, J. R. "Trends in Medical Malpractice Insurance, 1970–1985." *Law and Contemporary Problems,* 1986, *49*(2), 37.
80. Law and Polan (1978), p. 155.
81. See Metzloff, T. B., Peeples, R. A., and Harris, C. T. "Empirical Perspectives on Mediation and Malpractice." *Law and Contemporary Problems,* 1997, *60*(1), 107; Dauger, E. A., and Marcus, L. J. "Adapting Mediation to Link Resolution of Medical Malpractice Disputes with Health Care Quality Improvement." *Law and Contemporary Problems,* 1997, *60*(1), 185.
82. U.S. General Accounting Office (1986); Fowks, R. J. "Arbitration." In Halley, Fowks, Bigler, and Ryan (1989).
83. Ladimer, I., Solomon, J. C., and Mulvihill, M. "Experience in Medical Malpractice Arbitration." *Journal of Legal Medicine,* 1981, *2*(4), 433–470; quote on p. 452.
84. *Engalla* v. *Kaiser Permanente Medical Group,* 938 P. 2d 903 (Cal. 1997).
85. Sage (1997), pp. 190–191 and note 158 in that work.
86. Havighurst, C. C. "Malpractice Reform: Getting There by Private Vehicle." In Halley, Fowks, Bigler, and Ryan (1989).
87. Office of Technology Assessment (1993).
88. *Darling* v. *Charleston Community Memorial Hospital* (1965).
89. Sage, W. M. "Enterprise Liability and the Emerging Managed Health Care System." *Law and Contemporary Problems,* 1997, *60*(2), 159; Sage, W. M., Hastings, K. E., and Berenson, R. A. "Enterprise Liability for Medical Malpractice and Health Care Quality Improvement." *American Journal of Law and Medicine,* 1994, *20*(1 and 2), 1–28; Abraham, K. S., and Weiler, P. S. "Enterprise Medical Liability and the Choice of the Responsible Enterprise." *American Journal of Law and Medicine,* 1994, *20*(1 and 2), 29–36.
90. These arguments are drawn from Sage, Hastings, and Berenson (1994).
91. Sage, Hastings, and Berenson (1994), p. 3, citing Danzon (1985) and Darling, L. L. (Note.) "The Applicability of Experience Rating to Medical Malpractice Insurance." *Case Western Reserve Law Review,* 1987–88, *38*, 255, 261–265.
92. U.S. Congress, Office of Technology Assessment. *Defensive Medicine and Medical Malpractice.* OTA-H-602. Washington, D.C.: U.S. Government Printing Office, 1994. See also Sage, Hastings, and Berenson (1994), p. 9, citing a 1992 study by Lewin-VHI, Inc., estimating that malpractice reform might save $25–76 billion in unnecessary tests and procedures over a five-year period. Rubin, R., and Mendelsohn, D. *Estimating the Costs of Defensive Medicine.* Lewin-VHI, Oct. 21, 1992.
93. Sage, Hastings, and Berenson (1994).

94. Sage, W. M. "Enterprise Liability and the Emerging Managed Health Care System." *Law and Contemporary Problems*, 1997, *60*(2), 159–210.

95. Abraham and Weiler (1994).

96. Grad (1980).

97. Mills, D. H. "The Case for and Against Pure No-Fault." In Halley, Fowks, Bigler, and Ryan (1989). The original study is *Report on the Medical Insurance Feasibility Study*, sponsored by California Medical Association and California Hospital Association (D. H. Mills, administrator, editor, and contractor). San Francisco: Sutter, 1977.

98. Mills (1989).

99. Office of Technology Assessment (1993); Danzon (1985).

100. Havighurst, C. C., and Tancredi, L. E. "'Medical Adversity Insurance'—a No-Fault Approach to Medical Malpractice and Quality Assurance." *Insurance Law Journal*, Feb. 1974, *613*, 69–97.

101. Tancredi, L. R. "Designated Compensable Events." In Halley, Fowks, Bigler, and Ryan (1989).

102. O'Connell, J. "Neo No-Fault Remedies for Medical Injuries: Coordinated Statutory and Contractual Alternatives." *Law and Contemporary Problems*, 1986, *49*(2), 125–141.

103. O'Connell, J. "Neo No-Fault: Settling for Economic Losses." In Halley, Fowks, Bigler, and Ryan (1989).

104. National Childhood Vaccine Injury Act, P.L. no. 99–660, sec. 311, 100 Stat. 3755, 1986; Grad, F. P. *The Public Health Law Manual.* (2nd ed.) Washington, D.C.: American Public Health Association, 1990.

105. Virginia Birth-Related Neurological Injury Compensation Act of 1987, Va. Code Ann., Sec. 38.2-5000-5021 (1993); Institute of Medicine. *Medical Professional Liability and the Delivery of Obstetrical Care.* Vol. I and Vol. II: "An Interdisciplinary Review." V. P. Rostow and R. J. Bulger (eds.). (Division of Health Promotion and Disease Prevention, Committee to Study Medical Professional Liability and the Delivery of Obstetrical Care.) Washington, D.C.: National Academy Press, 1989).

106. Institute of Medicine (1989).

107. Office of Technology Assessment (1993).

108. Florida Birth-Related Neurological Injury Compensation Act of 1988, Fla. Stat., sec. 766. 303–315 (1994); Office of Technology Assessment (1993).

109. Bovbjerg, R. R., Sloan, F. A., and Rankin, P. J. "Administrative Performance of "No-Fault" Compensation for Medical Injury." *Law and Contemporary Problems*, 1997, *60*(2), 71.

110. Bovbjerg, R. R., and Sloan, F. A. "No-Fault for Medical Injury: Theory and Evidence." *University of Cincinnati Law Review*, 1998, *67*(1), 55, 123.

111. Woodhouse, Sir O. "The New Zealand Experience." In Halley, Fowks, Bigler, and Ryan (1989).

112. Woodhouse (1989).

113. U.S. General Accounting Office (1986).

114. Woodhouse (1989).

115. Woodhouse (1989), p. 179.

116. Brahams, D. "The Swedish and Finnish Patient Insurance Schemes." In Halley, Fowks, Bigler, and Ryan (1989); GAO (1986).

117. Brahams (1989), p. 186.

118. Brahams (1989).

119. Brahams (1989). See also Kokkonen, P. "No-Fault Liability and Patient Insurance: The Finnish Patient Injury Law of 1986." *International Digest of Health Legislation*, 1989, *40*(1), 241–246.

120. Brahams (1989), p. 200.

121. This section is based on four chapters in Halley (1989).

122. Mills (1989). In Halley, Fowks, Bigler, and Ryan (1989).

123. Grad (1980).

124. Lander, L. *Defective Medicine: Risk, Anger, and the Malpractice Crisis.* New York: Farrar, Straus & Giroux, 1978.

125. Bovbjerg, R. R. "Medical Malpractice on Trial: Quality of Care Is the Important Standard." *Law and Contemporary Problems*, 1986, *49*, 321–347.

CHAPTER TWENTY

ETHICAL ISSUES IN PUBLIC HEALTH AND HEALTH SERVICES

Pauline Vaillancourt Rosenau and Ruth Roemer

T he cardinal principles of medical ethics[1]—autonomy, beneficence, and justice—apply in public health ethics but in somewhat altered form. Personal autonomy and respect for autonomy are guiding principles of public health practice as well as of medical practice. In medical ethics, the concern is with the privacy, individual liberty, freedom of choice, and self-control of the individual. From this principle flows the doctrine of informed consent. In public health ethics, autonomy, the right of privacy, and freedom of action are recognized insofar as they do not result in harm to others. Thus, from a public health perspective, autonomy may be subordinated to the welfare of others or of society as a whole.[2]

Beneficence, which includes doing no harm, promoting the welfare of others, and doing good, is a principle of medical ethics. In the public health context, beneficence is the overall goal of public health policy and practice. It must be interpreted broadly, in light of societal needs, rather than narrowly, in terms of individual rights.

Justice—whether defined as equality of opportunity, equity of access, or equity in benefits—is the core of public health. Serving the total population, public health is concerned with equity among various social groups, with protecting vulnerable populations, with compensating persons for suffering disadvantage in

We would like to thank our research assistant, Jessica Neal, for her enormous help in preparing this chapter. Her competence and diligence made this project possible.

health and health care, and with surveillance of the total health care system. As expressed in the now-classic phrase of Dr. William H. Foege, "Public health is social justice."[3]

This chapter concerns public health ethics as distinguished from medical ethics. Of course, some overlap exists between public health ethics and medical ethics, but public health ethics, like public health itself, applies generally to issues affecting populations, whereas medical ethics, like medicine itself, applies to individuals. Public health involves a perspective that is population-based, a view of conditions and problems that gives preeminence to the needs of the whole society rather than exclusively to the interests of single individuals.

Public health ethics evokes a number of dilemmas, many of which may be resolved in several ways, depending on one's standards and values—that is, one's normative choices. Ours are indicated. Data and evidence are relevant to the normative choices involved in public health ethics. We refer the reader to health services research wherever appropriate.

To illustrate the concept of public health ethics, we raise several general questions to be considered in different contexts in this chapter[4]:

- What tensions exist between protection of the public health and protection of individual rights?
- How should scarce resources be allocated and used?
- What should the balance be between expenditures and quality of life in the case of chronic and terminal illness?
- What are appropriate limits on using expensive medical technology?
- What obligations do health care insurers and health care providers have in meeting the right-to-know of patients as consumers?
- What responsibility exists for the young to finance health care for older persons?
- What obligation exists for government to protect the most vulnerable sectors of society?

We cannot give a clear, definitive answer that is universally applicable to any of these questions. Context and circumstance sometimes require qualifying even the most straightforward response. In some cases, differences among groups and individuals may be so great and conditions in society so diverse and complex that no single answer to a question is possible. In other instances, a balance grounded in a public health point of view is viable. Sometimes there is no ethical conflict at all because one solution is optimal for all concerned: for the individual, the practitioner, the payer, and society. For example, few practitioners would want to perform an expensive, painful medical act that was without benefit and might do damage. Few patients would demand it, and even fewer payers would reimburse for it.

A likely societal consensus would suggest that public health is better served if scarce health resources are used for better purposes.[5] But in other circumstances, competition for resources poses a dilemma, as with a new, effective, but expensive drug of help to only a few, on the one hand; and use of a less-expensive but less-effective drug for a larger number of persons, on the other. The necessity for a democratic, open, public debate about rationing in the future seems inevitable; seven countries in the Organization for Economic Cooperation and Development (OECD) have already implemented such plans.[6]

Even in the absence of agreement on ethical assumptions, and facing diversity and complexity that prohibit easy compromises, we suggest mechanisms for resolving the ethical dilemmas in health care that do exist. We explore these in the concluding section of this chapter.

A word of caution: space is short and our topic complex. We cannot explore every dimension of every relevant topic to the satisfaction of all readers. We offer here, instead, an introduction whose goal is to awaken readers—be they practitioners, researchers, students, patients, or consumers—to the ethical dimension of public health. We hope to remind them of the ethical assumptions that underlie their own public health care choices. This chapter, then, is limited to considering selected ethical issues in public health and the provision of personal health services. We shall examine our topic by way of components of the health system: (1) development of health resources, (2) economic support, (3) organization of services, (4) management of services, (5) delivery of care, and (6) assurance of the quality of care.[7]

Overarching Public Health Principles: Our Assumptions

We argue for these general assumptions of a public health ethic:

- Provision of care on the basis of health need, without regard to race, religion, gender, sexual orientation, or ability to pay
- Equity in distribution of resources, giving due regard to vulnerable groups in the population (ethnic minorities, migrants, children, pregnant women, the poor, the handicapped, and others)
- Respect for human rights—including autonomy, privacy, liberty, health, and well-being—keeping in mind social justice considerations

Central to the solution of ethical problems in health services is the role of law, which sets forth the legislative, regulatory, and judicial controls of society. The development of law in a particular field narrows the discretion of providers in making ethical judgments. At the same time, law sets guidelines for determining policy on specific issues or in individual cases.[8]

Ethical Issues in Developing Resources

When we talk about developing *resources*, we mean health—personnel, facilities, drugs and equipment, and knowledge. Choices among the kinds of personnel trained, the facilities made available, and the commodities produced are not neutral. Producing and acquiring each of these involves ethical assumptions, and they in turn have public health consequences.

The numbers and kinds of personnel required and their distribution are critical to public health. We need to have an adequate supply of personnel and facilities for a given population in order to meet the ethical requirements of providing health care without discrimination or bias. The proper balance of primary care physicians and specialists is essential to the ethical value of beneficence so as to maximize health status.[9] The ethical imperative of justice requires special measures to protect the economically disadvantaged, such as primary care physicians working in health centers. The imperfect free market mechanisms employed in the United States to date have resulted in far too many specialists relative to generalists. Canada has achieved some balance, but this has involved closely controlling medical school enrollments and residency programs.

At the same time, the ethical principle of autonomy urges that resource development also be diverse enough to permit consumers some choice of providers and facilities. Absence of choice is a form of coercion. It also reflects an inadequate supply. But it results, as well, from the absence of a range of personnel. Patients should have some—though not unlimited—freedom to choose the type of care they prefer. Midwives, chiropractors, and other effective and proven practitioners should be available if health resources permit it without sacrificing other ethical considerations. The ethical principle of autonomy here might conflict with that of equity, which would limit general access to specialists in the interest of better distribution of health care access to the whole population. The need for ample public health personnel is another ethical priority, necessary for the freedom of all individuals to enjoy a healthful, disease-free environment.

Physician assistants and nurses are needed, and they may serve an expanded role, substituting for primary care providers in some instances to alleviate the shortage of primary care physicians, especially in underserved areas.[10] But too great a reliance on these providers might diminish quality of care if they are required to substitute entirely for physicians, particularly with respect to differential diagnosis.[11] The point of service is also a significant consideration. For example, more effective and expanded health care and dental care for children could be achieved by employing the school as a geographic point for monitoring and providing selected services.[12]

Health personnel are not passive commodities, and freedom of individual career choice may conflict with public health needs. Here autonomy of the individual must be balanced with social justice and beneficence. In the past, the individual's decision to become a medical specialist took precedence over society's need for more generalists. A public health ethic appeals to the social justice involved and considers the impact on the population. A balance between individual choice and society's needs is being achieved today by restructuring financial compensation for primary care providers.

Similarly, in the United States an individual medical provider's free choice as to where to practice medicine has resulted in underserved areas, and ways to develop and train health personnel for rural and central city areas are a public health priority.[13] About 20 percent of the U.S. population lives in rural communities, and four in ten do not have adequate access to health care. Progress has been made in the complex problem of assuring rural health clinics. The Health Resources and Services Administration's Rural Hospitals Flexibility Program, which grants funding to improve services, is a step in the right direction, but more needs to be done.[14] For example, one option is to increase funds for the National Health Service Corps.[15] If needs and preferences of the NHSC doctors and their families are taken into consideration, they remain at their posts longer and have better morale.[16] A second option is to develop and apply quality standards that are appropriate to rural areas and that are practical, useful, and affordable.[17]

An important issue in educating health professionals is the need to assure racial and ethnic diversity in both the training and practice of health professionals. In several cases, the U.S. Supreme Court has invalidated affirmative action programs (as in the *Bakke* case in 1978[18] and *Hopwood* in 1996).[19] Nevertheless, there are several grounds for a strong legal and ethical case for restoring affirmative action programs in education for the health professions. Writing about affirmative action in medical education, De Ville points out that three facts may constitute compelling state interest justifying diversity: (1) that diversity increases the number of physicians in underserved areas and in primary care, (2) that it promotes an effective exchange of ideas in medical education, and (3) that it results in improved care for minority patients.[20]

Similar ethical public health dilemmas are confronted with respect to health facilities. From a public health point of view, the need for equitable access to quality institutions and for fair distribution of health care facilities takes priority over an individual real estate developer's ends or the preferences of for-profit hospital owners. Offering a range of facilities to maximize choice suggests the need for both public and private hospitals, community clinics and health centers, and inpatient and outpatient mental health facilities, as well as long-term care facilities and hospices. At the same time, not-for-profit providers seem to do a better job than the for-profit institutions, at least to date. They have lower disenrollment rates,[21] offer more community benefits,[22] feature more preventive services,[23] and provide hospital care at lower cost[24] and better overall quality.[25] How long this can continue to be the case in the highly competitive health care market is unknown because not-for-profits must adopt for-profit business practices to survive.[26]

The financial crisis facing public hospitals throughout the nation poses an ethical problem of major proportions.[27] At stake is the survival of facilities that handle an enormous volume of care for the poor, that train large numbers of physicians and other health personnel, and that make available specialized services—trauma care, burn units, and others—for the total urban and rural populations they serve.

Research serves a public health purpose too. It has advanced medical technology, and its benefits in new and improved products should be accessible to all members of society. Public health ethics also focuses on the importance of research in assessing health system performance, including equity of access and medical outcomes. Only if what works and is medically effective can be distinguished from what does not and is medically ineffective are public health interests best served. Health care resources need to be used wisely and not wasted. Health services research can help assure this goal. This is especially important in an era in which market competition appears, directly or indirectly, to be having a negative influence on research capacity.[28]

Research is central to developing public health resources. Equity mandates a fair distribution of research resources among the various diseases that affect the public's health because research is costly, resources are limited, and choices have to be made.[29] Research needs both basic and applied orientation to assure quality.[30] There is a need for research on matters that have been neglected in the past,[31] as has been recognized in the field of women's health.[32] Correction of other gross inequities in allocating research funds is urgent. Recent reports indicate that younger scientists are not sufficiently consulted in the peer review process, and they do not receive their share of research funds. Ethical implications involving privacy, informed consent, and equity affect targeted research grants for AIDS, breast cancer, and other special diseases. The legal and ethical issues in the human genome project involve matters of such broad scope—wide use of genetic screening, information control, privacy, and possible manipulation of human characteristics—that Annas has called for "taking ethics seriously."[33] The orphan drug law, through tax exemption, focuses enormous resources on diseases that affect a very few individuals.[34] This law may be an instance of society assuming that beneficence takes precedence over equity and social justice. Apparent exaggerations in pricing and profitability have led to regulatory efforts to limit abuse.[35] By contrast, in some instances discoveries made while researching diseases that have an effect on only a few individuals, as with basic research, can lead to findings that benefit broader populations.

Federal law in the United States governs conduct of biomedical research involving human subjects. Ethical issues are handled by ethics advisory boards, convened to advise the Department of Health and Human Services on the ethics of biomedical or behavioral research projects, and by institutional review boards of research institutions seeking funding of research proposals. Both kinds of board are charged with responsibility for reviewing clinical research proposals and for ensuring that the legal and ethical rights of human subjects are protected.[36] Among the principal concerns of these boards is assurance of fully informed and unencumbered consent, by patients competent to give it, in order to assure the autonomy of subjects. They are also concerned with protecting the privacy of human subjects and the confidentiality of their relation to the project. An important legal and ethical duty of researchers, in the event that a randomized clinical trial proves beneficial to health, is to terminate the trial immediately and make the benefits available to the control group and to the treated group alike.

The ethical principles that should govern biomedical research involving human subjects are a high priority, but criticism has been leveled at the operation of some institutional review boards as lacking objectivity and as being overly identified with the interests of the researcher and the institution.[37] Recommendations to correct this type of problem include appointing patient and consumer advocates to review boards, in addition to physicians and others affiliated with the institution and along with the sole lawyer who is generally a member of the review board; having advocates involved early in drawing up protocols for the research; having third parties interview patients after they have given their consent to make sure that they understood the research and their choices; requiring the institution to include research in its quality assurance monitoring; and establishing a national human experimentation board to oversee the four thousand institutional review boards in the country.[38]

Correction of fraud in science and the rights of subjects are important ethical considerations in developing knowledge. Ethical conflict between the role of the physician as caregiver and as researcher is not uncommon inasmuch as what is good for the research project is not always what is good for the patient. Certainly, in some instances society stands to benefit at the expense of the research subject, but respect for the basic worth of the individual means that he or she has a right to be informed before agreeing to participate in an experiment. Only when consent is informed, clear, and freely given can altruism, for the sake of advancing science and humanity, be authentic. Still, exceptions to informed consent are sometimes justified. For example, because of the need for medically trained emergency personnel, a convincing case can be made for using deceased patients to teach resuscitation procedures. There is "no risk to the dead person, and families could not realistically be expected to discuss consent at such a difficult time."[39]

Policy makers concerned with developing resources for health care thus confront tensions between protecting public health and protecting the rights of individual patients and providers. They face issues concerning allocation of scarce resources and use of expensive medical technology. We trust that in resolving these issues their decisions are guided by principles of autonomy, beneficence, and justice as applied to the health of populations.

Ethical Issues in Economic Support

Nowhere is the public health ethical perspective clearer than on issues of economic support. Personal autonomy and respect for privacy remain essential, as does beneficence. But a public health orientation suggests that the welfare of society merits close regard for justice. It is imperative that everyone in the population have equitable access to health care services with dignity, so as not to discourage necessary utilization; in most cases, this means universal health insurance coverage.[40] Forty-four million Americans lack health insurance, which makes for poorer medical outcomes even though individuals without health insurance do receive care in hospital emergency rooms and community clinics.[41] Most of the forty-four million are workers in small enterprises whose employers do not offer health insurance for their workers or dependents.[42]

From a public health perspective, financial barriers to essential health care are inappropriate. Yet they exist to a surprising degree.[43] If each and every human being is to develop to his or her full potential, to participate fully as a productive citizen in our democratic society, then preventive health services and alleviation of pain and suffering[44] due to health conditions that can be effectively treated must be available without financial barriers. Removing economic barriers to health services does not mean that the difference in health status between rich and poor will disappear. But it is a necessary, if not sufficient, condition for this goal.

Economic disparity in society is a public health ethical issue related to justice. Increasing evidence suggests that inequality in terms of income differences between the rich and the poor has a large impact on a population's health.[45] This may be due to psychosocial factors,[46] or a weakened societal social fabric,[47] or loss of social capital,[48] or a range of other factors.[49] Whatever the cause, "income inequality together with limited access to health care has serious consequences for the working poor."[50]

From a public health point of view, the economic resources to support health services should be fair and equitable. Any individual's contribution should be progressive, based on ability to pay. This is especially important because the rise of managed care has made it increasingly difficult to provide charity care.[51] This may be because of funding restrictions for a defined population. Although some individual contribution is appropriate—no matter how small—as a gesture of commitment to the larger community, it is also ethically befitting for the nation to take responsibility for a portion of the cost. The exact proportion may vary across nation and time, depending on the country's wealth and the public priority attributed to health services.[52]

Similarly, justice and equity suggest the importance of the ethical principle of social solidarity in any number of forms.[53] By definition, social insurance means that there is wisdom in assigning responsibility for payment by those who are young and working to support the health care of children and older people no longer completely independent. A public health orientation suggests that social solidarity forward and backward in time, across generations, is ethically persuasive. Those in the most productive stages of the life cycle today were once dependent children, and they are likely one day to be dependent older persons.

Institutions such as Social Security and Medicare play a moral role in a democracy. They were established to attain common aims and are fair in that they follow agreed-upon rules.[54] The alternatives to social solidarity between the young and the elderly are simply unacceptable. As members of a society made up of overlapping communities, our lives are intricately linked together. No man or woman is an island; not even the wealthiest or most "independent" can exist alone. The social pact that binds us to live in peace together requires cooperation of such a fundamental nature that we could not travel by car (assuming respect for traffic signals) to the grocery store to purchase food (or assume it is safe for consumption) without appealing to social solidarity. These lessons apply to health care as well.

In 1983, the President's Commission for the Study of Ethical Problems in Medicine and Biomedical and Behavioral Research made as its first and principal recommendation on ethics in medicine that society has an obligation to assure equitable access to health care for all its citizens.[55] Equitable access, the commission said, requires that all citizens be able to secure an adequate level of care without excessive burden. Implementation of this principle as an ethical imperative is even more urgent all these years later, as an increasing number of people become uninsured and as the prices of pharmaceuticals dramatically increase.[56]

Ethical Issues in Organization of Services

The principal ethical imperative in organization of health services is that services be organized and distributed in accordance with health needs and the ability to benefit. The problem with rationing on the basis of ability to pay is that it encourages the opposite.[57] The issues of geographic and cultural access also illustrate this ethical principle.

To be fair and just, a health system must minimize geographic inequity in distributing care. Rural areas are underserved, as are inner cities. Any number of solutions have been proposed and tried to bring better access in health services to underserved areas, be they rural or inner-city. They include mandating a period of service for medical graduates as a condition of licensure, loan forgiveness and expansion of the National Health Service Corps, rural preceptorships, creating economic incentives for establishing a practice in a rural area, and employing physician assistants and nurse practitioners.[58] Telemedicine may make the best medical consultants available to rural areas in the near future,[59] but the technology involves initial start-up costs that are not trivial. Higher Medicare payments to rural hospitals also ensure that they will remain open.[60]

Similarly, the principles of autonomy and beneficence require health services to be culturally relevant to the populations they are designed to serve.[61] This means that medical care professionals need to be able to communicate in the language of those they serve and to understand the cultural preferences of those for whom they seek to provide care.[62] The probability of success is enhanced if needed health professionals are from the same cultural background as those they serve. This suggests that schools of medicine, nursing, dentistry, and public health should intensify their efforts to reach out and extend educational and training opportunities to qualified and interested members of such populations. To carry out such programs, however, these schools must have the economic resources required to offer fellowships and teaching assistant positions.

The development of various forms of managed care—health maintenance organizations, prepaid group practices, preferred provider organizations, and independent practice associations—raises another set of ethical questions. As experienced in the United States in recent years, managed care is designed more to minimize costs than to ensure that health care is efficient and effective. If managed care ends up constraining costs by depriving individuals of needed medical attention (reducing medically appropriate access to specialists, for instance), then it violates the ethical principle of beneficence because such management interferes with doing good for the patient.[63] If managed care is employed as a cost-containment scheme for Medicaid and Medicare without regard to quality of care, it risks increasing inequity. It could even contribute to a two-tiered health care system in which those who can avoid various forms of managed care by paying privately for their personal health services will obtain higher-quality care.

Historically, the advantages of staff-model managed care are clear: team practice, emphasis on primary care, generous use of diagnostic and therapeutic outpatient services, and prudent use of hospitalization. All contribute to cost containment. At the same time, managed care systems have the disadvantage of restricted choice of provider. Today's for-profit managed care companies run the risk of underserving; they may achieve cost containment through cost shifting and risk selection.[64]

The ethical issues in the relationships among physicians, patients, and managed care organizations include denial of care, restricted referral to specialists, and gag rules that bar physicians from telling patients about alternative treatments (which may not be covered by the plan) or from discussing financial arrangements between the physician and the plan (which may include incentives for cost containment).[65] Requiring public disclosure of information about these matters has been proposed as a solution,[66] but there is little evidence that disclosure helps the poor and illiterate choose a better health plan or a less-conflicted health care provider.

The ethical issues in managed care are illustrated most sharply by the question of who decides what is medically necessary: the physician or others, the disease management program,[67] the insurer, the employer, or the state legislature.[68] This question is not unique to managed care; it has also arisen with respect to insurance companies and Medicaid.[69] On the one hand, the physician has a legal and ethical duty to provide the standard of care that a reasonable physician in the same or similar circumstances would. On the other hand, insurers have traditionally specified what is covered or not covered as medically necessary in insurance contracts. The courts have sometimes reached different results, depending on the facts of the case, the character of the treatment sought (whether generally accepted or experimental), and the interpretation of medical necessity.[70] With the rise of managed care, the problem becomes even more of an ethical dilemma because, as even those highly favorable to managed care agree, there is a risk of too little health care.[71]

In the past, malpractice suits against managed care organizations in self-insured plans have been barred by the provision in the Employee Retirement Income Security Act that preempts or supersedes "any and all state laws insofar as they may now or hereafter relate to any employee benefit plan."[72] As a result of the preemption, employees covered by such plans have been limited to the relief provided by ERISA—only the cost of medical care denied—with no compensation for lost wages and pain and suffering.[73] Self-insured health insurance plans that cause injury by denying care or providing substandard care have had *de facto* immunity from suit because of legal interpretation of ERISA, but the situation appears to be changing.

In recent years, the interpretation of the ERISA preemption has been somewhat narrowed to bar only suits for denial of care but to allow suits relating to quality of care.[74] In 1995, further restriction of the ERISA preemption occurred in a unanimous decision of the U.S. Supreme Court holding that a New York statute imposing surcharges on hospitals and HMO fees for some health care payers, including ERISA plans, in order to create a pool of funding to cover the uninsured, was not preempted by ERISA because the statute had only an indirect economic effect.[75] This decision may signal a change in the legal climate of opinion on the right of employees in self-insured plans to sue their plans for denial of care.

In view of the fact that 140 million people receive their health care through plans sponsored by employers and covered by ERISA, it is a serious matter of equity to allow them access to the courts for medical malpractice.[76] In fact, several states have recently adopted legislation that permits patients to hold managed care companies responsible for health care decisions imposed by the plan.[77] Experience suggests that according patients the right to hold their HMO liable generates little additional cost.[78] Federal courts appear to be moving in this direction as well.[79]

But in June 2000, the U.S. Supreme Court held that a patient cannot sue a health maintenance organization under ERISA for giving physicians a financial incentive to cut treatment costs.[80] "No H.M.O. organization could survive without some incentive connecting physician reward with treatment rationing," Justice Souter wrote. The Court held that mixed treatment-eligibility decisions by physicians are not fiduciary acts within the meaning of ERISA, which stipulates that fiduciaries shall discharge their duties solely in the interest of the participants and beneficiaries. In absolving the HMO of liability for breach of fiduciary responsibility, the Court left open the question of whether a decision on eligibility, as distinguished from a treatment decision, is a fiduciary matter for which the HMO would be liable, and it suggested that a health maintenance organization might be liable under ERISA for failure to disclose financial incentives to physicians.

This decision denying relief under ERISA emphasizes the urgency of state legislation granting patients the right to sue their HMOs for malpractice. Any state legislation, however, needs to guarantee the opportunity to sue a managed care organization for denied or delayed care. Such legislation will compel the courts to address issues thus far ignored.

As more and more integrated health care delivery systems are formed, as more mergers of managed care organizations occur, as pressure for cost containment increases, ethical issues concerning conflict of interest, quality of care choices, and patients' rights attain increasing importance. The principles of autonomy, beneficence, and justice are severely tested in resolving the ethical problems facing a complex, corporate health care system.

If medicine is "for-profit," as seems to be the case today and for the near future in the United States, then the ethical dilemma between patients' interests and profits will be a continuing problem.[81] Sometimes the two can both be served, but it is unlikely to be the case in all instances. Surveys of business "executives admit and point out the presence of numerous generally accepted practices in their industry which they consider unethical."[82] As Fisher and Welch conclude, "Stakeholders in the increasingly market-driven U.S. health care system have few incentives to explore the harms of the technologies from which they stand to profit."[83] That both consumers and employers are concerned about quality of care is clear from Paul Ellwood's statement expressing disappointment in the evolution of HMOs because "they tend to place too much emphasis on saving money and not enough on improving quality—and we now have the technical skill to do that."[84]

Ethical Issues in Management of Health Services

Management involves planning, administration, regulation, and legislation. The style of management depends on the values and norms of the population. Planning involves determining the population's health needs (with surveys and research, for example) and then ensuring that programs are in place to provide these services. A public health perspective suggests that planning is appropriate to the extent that it provides efficient, appropriate health care (beneficence) to all who seek it (equity and justice). Planning may avoid waste and contribute to rational use of health services. But it is also important that planning not be so invasive as to be coercive and deny the individual any say in his or her health care unless such intervention is necessary to protect public health interests. The ethical principle of autonomy preserves the right of the individual to refuse care, to determine his or her own destiny, especially when the welfare of others is not involved. A balance between individual autonomy and public health intervention that affords benefit to the society is not easy to achieve. But in some cases the resolution of such a dilemma is clear, as in the case for mandatory immunization programs. Equity and beneficence demand that the social burdens and benefits of living in a disease-free environment be shared. Therefore, for example, immunization requirements should cover all those potentially affected.

Health administration has ethical consequences that may be overlooked because they appear ethically neutral: organization, staffing, budgeting, supervision, consultation, procurement, logistics, records and reporting, coordination, and evaluation.[85] But all these activities involve ethical choices. Faced with a profit squeeze, the managed care industry is pressuring providers to reduce costs and services.[86] The result has been downsizing, which means more unlicensed personnel are hired to substitute for nurses.[87] California is the first state to mandate nurse-to-patient staffing ratios.[88] Surveys of doctors suggest patients do not always get needed care from HMOs.[89] Denial of appropriate needed health care is an ethical problem related to beneficence. In addition, the importance of privacy in record keeping (to take an example) raises once again the necessity to balance the ethical principles of autonomy and individual rights with social justice and the protection of society.[90]

Distribution of scarce health resources is another subject of debate. The principle of first come, first served may initially seem equitable. But it also incorporates the "rule of rescue," whereby a few lives are saved at great cost, and this policy results in the "invisible" loss of many more lives. The cost-benefit or cost-effectiveness analysis of health economics attempts to apply hard data to administrative decisions. This approach, however, does not escape ethical dilemmas because the act of assigning numbers to years of life, for example, is itself value-laden. If administrative allocation is determined on the basis of the number of years of life saved, then the younger are favored over the older, which may or may not be equitable. If one factors into such an analysis the idea of "quality" years of life, other normative assumptions must be made as to how important quality is and what constitutes quality. Some efforts have been made to assign a dollar value to a year of life as a tool for administering health resources. But here, too, we encounter worrisome normative problems. Does ability to pay deform such calculations?[91]

Crucial to management of health services are legal tools—legislation, regulations, and sometimes litigation—necessary for fair administration of programs. Legislation and regulations are essential for authorizing health programs; they also serve to remedy inequities and to introduce innovations in a health service system. Effective legislation depends on a sound scientific base, and ethical questions are especially troubling when the scientific evidence is uncertain.

For example, in a landmark decision in 1976, the Court of Appeals for the District of Columbia upheld a regulation of the Environmental Protection Agency restricting the amount of lead additives in gasoline based largely on epidemiological evidence.[92] Analysis of this case and of the scope of judicial review of the regulatory action of an agency charged by Congress with regulating substances harmful to health underlines the dilemma the court faced: the need of judges trained in the law, not in science, to evaluate the scientific and epidemiological evidence on which the regulatory agency based its ruling.[93] The majority of the court based its upholding of the agency's decision on its own review of the evidence. By contrast, Judge David Bazelon urged an alternative approach: "In cases of great technological complexity, the best way for courts to guard against unreasonable or erroneous administrative decisions is not for the judges themselves to scrutinize the technical merits of each decision. Rather, it is to establish a decision making process that assures a reasoned decision that can be held up to the scrutiny of the scientific community and the public."[94]

The dilemma of conflicting scientific evidence is a persistent ethical minefield, as reflected by a 1993 decision of the U.S. Supreme Court involving the question of how widely accepted a scientific process or theory must be before it qualifies as admissible evidence in a lawsuit. The case involved the issue of whether a drug prescribed for nausea during pregnancy, Bendectin, causes birth defects. Rejecting the test of "general acceptance" of scientific evidence as the absolute prerequisite for admissibility, as applied in the past, the Court ruled that trial judges serve as gatekeepers to ensure that pertinent scientific evidence is not only relevant but reliable. The Court also suggested various factors that might bear on such determinations.[95]

It is significant for the determination of ethical issues in cases where the scientific evidence is uncertain that epidemiological evidence, which is the core of public health, is increasingly recognized as helpful in legal suits.[96] Of course, it should be noted that a court's refusal (or an agency's) to act because of uncertain scientific evidence is in itself a decision with ethical implications.

Enactment of legislation and issuance of regulations are important for management of a just health care system, but these strategies are useless if they are not enforced. For example, state legislation has long banned the sale of cigarettes to minors, but only recently have efforts been made to enforce these statutes rigorously through publicity, "stings" (arranged purchases by minors), penalties on sellers, threats of license revocation, and banning cigarette sales from vending machines.[97] A novel case of enforcement involves a Baltimore ordinance prohibiting billboards promoting cigarettes in areas where children live, recreate, and go to school, enacted in order to enforce the minors' access law banning tobacco sales to minors.[98]

Thus, management of health services involves issues of allocating scarce resources, evaluating scientific evidence, measuring quality of life, and imposing mandates by legislation and regulations. Although a seemingly neutral function, management of health services must rely on principles of autonomy, beneficence, and justice in its decision-making process.

Ethical Issues in Delivery of Care

Delivery of health services—actual provision of health care services—is the end point of all the other dimensions just discussed. The ethical considerations of only a few of the many issues pertinent to delivery of care are explored here.

Resource allocation in a time of cost containment inevitably involves rationing. At first blush, rationing by ability to pay may appear natural, neutral, and inevitable, but the ethical dimensions for delivery of care may be overlooked. If ability to pay is recognized as a form of rationing, the question of its justice is immediately apparent. The Oregon Medicaid program is another example. It is equitable by design and grounded in good part in the efficacy of the medical procedure in question, thus respecting the principle of ethical beneficence. It is structured to extend benefits to a wider population of poor people than those entitled to care under Medicaid. The plan does not qualify as equitable and fair, however, because it does not apply to the whole population of Oregon, but only to those on Medicaid. It denies services to some persons on Medicaid in order to widen the pool of beneficiaries. It presents significant ethical problems in this respect.[99]

Rationing medical care is not always ethically dubious; rather, it may conform to a public health ethic. In some cases, too much medical care is counterproductive and may produce more harm than good. Canada, Sweden, the United Kingdom, and the state of Oregon, among others, have rationing of one sort or another.[100] For example, Canada rations health care, pays one-third less per person than the United States, and offers universal coverage; yet health status indicators do not suggest that Canadians suffer. In fact, on several performance indicators Canada surpasses the United States.[101] If there were better information about medical outcomes and the efficacy of many medical procedures, rationing would actually benefit patients if it discouraged the unneeded and inappropriate treatment that plagues the U.S. health system.[102]

Rationing organ transplants, similarly, is a matter of significant ethical debate. The number of organs available for transplant is less than the need. Rationing, therefore, must be used to determine who is given a transplant. Employing tissue match makes medical sense and also seems ethically acceptable. But to the extent that ability to pay is a criterion, ethical conflict is inevitable. It may, in fact, go against scientific opinion and public health ethics if someone who can pay receives a transplant even though the tissue match is not so good as it would be for a patient who is also in need of a transplant but unable to pay the cost. Rationing on this basis seems ethically unfair and medically ill advised.[103]

One solution would be to make more organs available through mandatory donation from fatal automobile accidents, without explicit consent of individuals and families. A number of societies have adopted this policy because the public health interest of society and the seriousness of the consequences are so great for those in need of a transplant that it is possible to justify ignoring the individual autonomy (preferences) of the accident victim's friends and relatives. Spain leads other nations regarding organ donation by interpreting an absence of prohibition to constitute a near-death patient's implicit authorization for organ transplantation.[104] This has not been the case in the United States to date.[105]

Delivery of services raises conflict-of-interest questions for providers that are of substantial public health importance. Criminal prosecution of fraud in the health care sector increased threefold between 1993 and 1997.[106] In today's market-driven health system, about half of all doctors report that they have "exaggerated the severity of a patient's condition to get them care they think is medically necessary."[107] Hospitals pressed by competitive forces strain to survive and in some cases do so only by less-than-honest cost shifting—and even direct fraud. A recent survey of hospital bills found that more than 99 percent included "mistakes" that favored the hospital.[108]

Class action suits claim that HMOs are guilty of deceiving patients because they refuse to reveal financial incentives in physician payment structures.[109] Physicians have been found to refer patients to laboratories and medical testing facilities that they co-own to a far greater extent than can be medically justified.[110] As the trend to make medicine a business develops, the AMA's Council on Ethical and Judicial Affairs has adopted guidelines for the sale of nonprescription, health-related products in physicians' offices. The purpose is to "help protect patients and maintain physicians' professionalism."[111] The public health ethic of benefi-cence is called into question by unnecessary products and inappropriate medical tests.

The practice of medicine and public health screening presents serious ethical dilemmas. Screening for diseases for which there is no treatment, except where such information can be used to postpone onset or prevent widespread popula-tion infection, is difficult to justify unless the information is explicitly desired by the patient for personal reasons (life planning and reproduction). In a similar case, screening without provision to treat those discovered to be in need of treatment is unethical. Public health providers need to be sure in advance that they can offer the health services required to provide care for those found to be affected. These are the ethical principles of beneficence and social justice.

The tragic epidemic of HIV/AIDS has raised serious ethical questions concerning testing, reporting, and partner notification. The great weight of authority favors voluntary and confidential testing, so as to encourage people to come forward for testing, counseling, and behavior change.[112] All states require confidential reporting of AIDS cases by name. The need to improve the track-ing of the epidemic caused twenty-eight states, as of January 1998, to adopt confidential names-based reporting of HIV as well.[113] A study by the U.S. Centers for Disease Control and Prevention (CDC) concludes that confidential names-based reporting of HIV has not deterred testing and treatment.[114] Nevertheless, concern about violation of privacy and possible deterrence of testing and treatment with confidential names-based reporting of HIV persists. In California, it led to an agreement between the California Medical Association and AIDS advocacy groups to support a unique identifier system, that is, using a number to link the test and the patient.[115]

This issue raises sharply the ethical conflict between the individual's right to confidentiality and the needs of public health. Some guidance for resolving ethical questions in this difficult sphere is presented by Stephen Joseph, former commissioner of health for New York City, who states that the AIDS epidemic is a public health emergency involving extraordinary civil liberties issues—not a civil liberties emergency involving extraordinary public health issues.[116]

Partner notification was at first generally disapproved on grounds of non-feasibility and protection of privacy, but in accordance with CDC guidelines, some states have enacted legislation permitting a physician or public health department to notify a partner that a patient is HIV-positive if the physician believes that the patient will not inform the partner.[117]

With the finding that administration of AZT during pregnancy to an HIV-positive woman reduces the risk of transmission of the virus to the infant (from approximately 25 percent to 8 percent if administered in the later stages of pregnancy and during labor and to infants in the first six weeks of life), CDC recommends that all pregnant women be offered HIV testing as early in pregnancy as possible because of the available treatments for reducing the likelihood of perinatal transmission and maintaining the health of the woman. CDC also recommends that women should be counseled about their options regarding pregnancy by a method similar to genetic counseling.[118]

The field of reproductive health is a major public health concern, affecting women in their reproductive years. Here the principles of autonomy, beneficence, and justice apply to providing contraceptive services, including long-acting means of contraception, surgical abortion, medical abortion made possible by development of Mifepristone, sterilization, and use of noncoital technologies for reproduction. The debate on these issues has been wide, abrasive, and divisive. Twenty-two years after abortion was legalized by the U.S. Supreme Court's decision in *Roe* v. *Wade*,[119] protests against abortion clinics have escalated. Violence against clinics and murders of abortion providers threaten access to abortion services and put the legal right to choose to terminate an unwanted pregnancy in jeopardy. The shortage of abortion providers in some states and in many rural areas restricts reproductive health services. The mergers of Catholic hospitals with secular institutions and the insistence that the merged hospital be governed by the Ethical and Religious Directives for Catholic Health Care Services means that not only abortion services are eliminated but also other contraceptive and counseling services, sterilization procedures, infertility treatments, and emergency postcoital contraception (even for rape victims).[120]

We state our position as strongly favoring the pro-choice point of view in order to ensure the autonomy of women, beneficence for women and their families faced with unwanted pregnancy, and justice in society. In the highly charged debate on teenage pregnancy, we believe that social realities, the well-being of young women and their children, and the welfare of society mandate access to contraception and abortion and respect for the autonomy of young people. The ethics of parental consent and notification laws, which often stand as a barrier to abortions needed and wanted by adolescents, is highly questionable.[121]

Many other important ethical issues in delivering health care have not been discussed extensively in this chapter because of space limitations. There are three such issues that we want to mention briefly.

First, the death debate is generally considered a matter of medical ethics involving the patient, his or her family, and the physician. But this issue is also a matter of public health ethics because services at the end of life entail administrative and financial dimensions that are part of public health and management of health services.[122]

Second, in the field of mental health, the conflict between the health needs and legal rights of patients on the one hand and the need for protection of society on the other illustrates sharply the ethical problems facing providers of mental health services. This conflict has been addressed most prominently by reform of state mental hospital admission laws to make involuntary admission to a mental hospital initially a medical matter, with immediate and periodic judicial review as to the propriety of hospitalization—review in which a patient advocate participates.[123] The *Tarasoff* case presents another problem in providing mental health services: the duty of a psychiatrist or psychologist to warn an identified person of a patient's intent to kill the person, despite the rule of confidentiality governing medical and psychiatric practice.[124] In both instances, a public health perspective favors protection of society as against the legal rights of individuals.

Third, basic to public health strategies and effective delivery of preventive and curative services are records and statistics. The moral and legal imperative of privacy to protect an individual's medical record gives way to public health statutes requiring reporting of gunshot wounds, communicable diseases, child abuse, and AIDS.[125] More generally, the right of persons to keep their medical records confidential conflicts with society's need for epidemiological information to monitor the incidence and prevalence of diseases in the community and to determine responses to this information.

At the same time, it is essential, for example, that an individual's medical records be protected from abuse by employers, marketers, etc.[126] A common resolution of this problem is to make statistics available without identifying information. Congress has promised medical privacy legislation but, as of this writing, has failed to act. The Department of Health and Human Services, under instructions from President Clinton, is preparing to issue federal rules to protect the privacy of medical records, but the extent of police access to medical records has become an issue.[127]

Ethical problems in delivering services will surely increase in number and kind in a period of great change in the health service system as private, fee-for-service, solo practice is being replaced by new ways of financing and providing health care. The most prominent problem is the question of who decides the appropriateness of services—the payer or the provider, the managed care plan or the physician—and what role the consumer has in the new system that is evolving.

Ethical Issues in Assuring Quality of Care

If a public health ethic requires fair and equitable distribution of medical care, then it is essential that waste and inefficiency be eliminated. Spending scarce resources on useless medical acts is a violation of a public health ethic.[128] To reach this public health goal, knowledge about what is useful and medically efficacious is essential.

As strategies for evaluating the quality of health care have become increasingly important, the ethical dimensions of peer review, practice guidelines, report cards, and malpractice suits—all methods of quality assurance—have come to the fore. Established in 1972 to monitor hospital services under Medicare to ensure that they were "medically necessary" and delivered in the most efficient manner, professional standards review organizations came under attack as overregulatory and too restrictive.[129] Congress ignored the criticism and in 1982 passed the Peer Review Improvement Act, which did not abolish outside review but consolidated the local peer review agencies, replaced them with statewide bodies, and increased their responsibility.[130] In 1986, Congress passed the Health Care Quality Improvement Act, which established national standards for peer review at the state and hospital levels for all practitioners regardless of source of payment.[131] The act also established a national data bank on the qualifications of physicians and provided immunity from suit for reviewing physicians acting in good faith.

The functions of peer review organizations (PROs) in reviewing the adequacy and quality of care necessarily involve some invasion of the patient's privacy and the physician's confidential relationship with his or her patient. Yet beneficence and justice in an ethical system of medical care mandate a process that controls the cost and quality of care. Finding an accommodation between protection of privacy and confidentiality on the one hand and necessary but limited disclosure on the other has furthered the work of PROs. Physicians whose work is being reviewed are afforded the right to a hearing at which the patient is not present, and patients are afforded the protection of outside review in accordance with national standards.

Practice guidelines developed by professional associations, health maintenance organizations and other organized providers, third-party payers, and governmental agencies are designed to evaluate the appropriateness of procedures. Three states—Maine, Minnesota, and Vermont—have passed legislation permitting practice guidelines to be used as a defense in malpractice actions under certain circumstances.[132] Defense lawyers are reluctant to use this legislation, however, because they fear their case will be caught up in a lengthy constitutional appeal. Such a simplistic solution, however, avoids the question of fairness: whose guidelines should prevail in the face of multiple sets of guidelines issued by different bodies, and how should accommodation be made to evolving and changing standards of practice?[133]

Beneficence and justice are involved in full disclosure of information about quality to patients. Health plan report cards aim to fulfill this role.[134] Employers, too, could use report cards to choose health plans for their employees, though some studies suggest that many employers are interested far more in cost than quality.[135] How well reports actually measure quality is itself subject to debate.[136] There are major problems with those that currently exist.[137]

Malpractice suits constitute one method of regulating the quality of care, although an erratic and expensive system. The subject is fully discussed elsewhere in this volume. Here we raise only the ethical issue of the right of the injured patient to compensation for the injury and the need of society for a system of compensation that is more equitable and more efficient than the current system.

The various mechanisms for ensuring quality of care all pose ethical issues. Peer review requires some invasion of privacy and confidentiality to conduct surveillance of quality, although safeguards have been devised. Practice guidelines involve some interference with physician autonomy but in return afford protection for both the patient and the provider. Malpractice suits raise questions of equity, since many injured patients are not compensated. In the process of developing and improving strategies for quality control, the public health perspective justifies social intervention to protect the population.

Mechanisms for Resolving Ethical Issues in Health Care

Even in the absence of agreement on ethical assumptions, and in the face of diversity and complexity that prohibit easy compromise, mechanisms for resolving ethical dilemmas in public health do exist. Among these are ombudsmen, institutional review boards, ethics committees, standards set by professional associations, practice guidelines, financing mechanisms, and courts of law. Some of these mechanisms are voluntary. Others are legal. None is perfect. Some, such as financing mechanisms, are particularly worrisome.

Although ethics deals with values and morals, the law has been very much intertwined with ethical issues. In fact, the more that statutes, regulations, and court cases decide ethical issues, the narrower is the scope of ethical decision making by providers of health care.[138] For example, because the *Cruzan* case defines the conditions for terminating life support for persons in a persistent vegetative state (clear and cogent evidence of a prior statement by the patient, when competent, of her desire not to be kept alive by artificial means in a persistent vegetative state), the scope of decision making by physicians and families is constrained.[139] A court of law, therefore, is an important mechanism for resolving ethical issues.

The law deals with many substantive issues in numerous fields, including that of health care. It also has made important procedural contributions to resolving disputes by authorizing, establishing, and monitoring mechanisms or processes for handling claims and disputes. Such mechanisms are particularly useful for resolving ethical issues in health care because they are generally informal and flexible and often involve the participation of all the parties. Administrative mechanisms are much less expensive than litigation and in this respect potentially more equitable.

Ombudsmen in health care institutions are a means of providing patient representation and advocacy. They may serve as channels for expression of ethical concerns of patients and their families.

Ethics committees in hospitals and managed care organizations operate to resolve ethical issues involving specific cases in the institution. They may be composed solely of the institution's staff, or they may include an ethicist specialized in handling such problems.

Institutional review boards, discussed earlier, are required to evaluate research proposals for their scientific and ethical integrity.

Practice guidelines, also discussed earlier, offer standards for ethical conduct and encourage professional behavior that conforms to procedural norms generally recognized by experts in the field.

Finally, financing mechanisms that create incentives for certain procedures and practices have the economic power to encourage ethical conduct. At the same time, they may function to encourage the opposite behavior.[140]

As the health care system continues to deal with budget cuts, greater numbers of uninsured persons, and restructuring into managed care and integrated delivery systems, ethical questions loom large. Perhaps their impact can be softened by imaginative and rational strategies to finance, organize, and deliver health care in accordance with the ethical principles of autonomy, beneficence, and justice.

Ethical issues in public health and health services management are likely to become increasingly complex in the future. New technology and advances in medical knowledge challenge us and raise ethical dilemmas. In the future they will need to be evaluated and applied in a public health context and submitted to a public health ethical analysis. Few of these developments are likely to be entirely new and without precedent, however. Already, current discussions, such as that presented here, may inform these new developments.

Notes

1. Beauchamp, T. L., and Childress, J. F. *Principles of Biomedical Ethics.* New York: Oxford University Press, 1989, especially chapters three, four, and five); Beauchamp, T. L., and Walters, L. *Contemporary Issues in Bioethics.* Belmont, Calif.: Wadsworth, 1999 (chapter one).

2. Burris, S. "The Invisibility of Public Health: Population-Level Measures in a Politics of Market Individualism." *American Journal of Public Health,* 1997, *87*(10), 1607–1610.

3. Foege, W. H. "Public Health: Moving from Debt to Legacy. 1986 Presidential Address." *American Journal of Public Health,* 1987, *77*(10), 1276–1278.

4. Another public health question is how threats to the environment should be reconciled with the need for employment. We acknowledge that issues in environmental control have an enormous impact on public health. Here, however, our focus is on the ethical issues in policy and management of personal health services. For a discussion of equity and environmental matters, see Paehlke, R., and Vaillancourt Rosenau, P. "Environment/ Equality: Tensions in North American Politics." *Policy Studies Journal,* 1993, *21*(4), 672–686.

5. See Eddy, D. "Rationing Resources While Improving Quality." *Journal of the American Medical Association,* 1994, *272,* 818–820, for some examples.

6. Maynard, A., and Bloor, K. "Our Certain Fate: Rationing in Health Care." (ISBN 1 899040 70U6.) London: Office of Health Economics, 1998.

7. This outline is taken from Roemer, M. I. *National Health Systems of the World. Vol. 1: The Countries.* New York: Oxford University Press, 1991. Financial resources are treated later in the section on economic support.

8. For an example of the symbiotic relationship between ethics and law, see Annas, G. J. *Some Choice: Law, Medicine, and the Market.* New York: Oxford University Press, 1998. The work analyzes ethical issues in public health by weaving together the ethical, legal, and health service aspects of each problem discussed.

9. Cooper, R. A. "Seeking a Balanced Physician Workforce for the 21st Century." *Journal of the American Medical Association,* 1994, *272*(9), 680–687. Quality of care declines where specialists are not available. See Ayanian, J., and others. "Knowledge and Practices of Generalist and Specialist Physicians Regarding Drug Therapy for Acute Myocardial Infarction." *New England Journal of Medicine,* Oct. 27, 1994, p. 1136.

10. State regulation has a significant impact on the success of such programs. See Sekscenski, E., and others. "State Practice Environments and the Supply of Physician Assistants, Nurse

Practitioners, and Certified Nurse-Midwives." *New England Journal of Medicine*, Nov. 10, 1994, p. 1266.

11. Roemer, M. I. "Primary Care and Physician Extenders in Affluent Countries." *International Journal of Health Services*, 1977, *7*(4), 545–555.

12. U.S. General Accounting Office. *Health Care: School-Based Health Centers Can Expand Access for Children.* GAO/HEHS-95-35. Washington D.C.: General Accounting Office, 1994.

13. Braden, J. *Health Status and Access to Care of Rural and Urban Populations.* Rockville, Md.: U.S. Department of Health and Human Services, 1994; and Helms, D. *Delivering Essential Health Care Services in Rural Areas.* Rockville, Md.: U.S. Department of Health and Human Services, 1991.

14. Anonymous. "Rural Hospitals Receive Means to Improve Care." *Nation's Health*, Oct. 1999, p. 24. Fogel, L. A., and MacQuarrie, C. "Benefits and Operational Concerns of Rural Health Clinics." *Healthcare Financial Management*, Nov. 1994, 40–46.

15. Wolfe, L. "From the Congressional Office of Technology Assessment: The National Health Service Corps: Improving on Past Experience." *Journal of the American Medical Association*, Nov. 27, 1991, *266*, 2808.

16. Pathman, D. Konrad, T., and Ricketts, T. "The National Health Service Corps Experience for Rural Physicians in the Late 1980s." *Journal of the American Medical Association*, Nov. 2, 1994, *272*, 1341.

17. Moscovice, I., and Rosenblatt, R. "Quality of Care Challenges for Rural Health." Published by Rural Health Research Centers at University of Minnesota and University of Washington. [http://www.hsr.umn.edu/centers/rhrc/rhrc.html] Accessed Oct. 17, 1999.

18. *Regents of University of California* v. *Bakke*, 438 U.S. 265, 1978.

19. *University of Texas* v. *Hopwood*, 78 F.3d 932 (5th Cir. 1996), cert. denied, 116 S.Ct. 2581, 1996.

20. De Ville, K. "Defending Diversity: Affirmative Action and Medical Education." *American Journal of Public Health*, 1999, *89*(8), 1256, 1258.

21. Dallek, G., and Swirsky, L. *Comparing Medicare HMOs: Do They Keep Their Members?* Washington, D.C.: Families USA Foundation, 1997.

22. Claxton, G., Feder, J., Shactman, D., and Altman, S. "Public Policy Issues in Nonprofit Conversions: An Overview." *Health Affairs*, 1997, *16*(2), 9–27.

23. Himmelstein, D. U., Woolhandler, S., Hellander, I., and Wolfe, S. M. "Quality of Care in Investor-Owned vs. Not-for-Profit HMOs." *Journal of the American Medical Association*, 1999, *282*(2), 159–163.

24. Silverman, E., Skinner, J., and Fisher, E. "The Association Between For-Profit Hospital Ownership and Increased Medicare Spending." *New England Journal of Medicine*, 1999, *341*(6), 420–426; Woolhandler, S., and Himmelstein, D. U. "Costs of Care and Administration at For-Profit and Other Hospitals in the United States." *New England Journal of Medicine*, 1997, *336*(11), 769–774.

25. Himmelstein, Woolhandler, Hellander, and Wolfe (1999); Taylor, D. H., Jr., Whellan, D. J., and Sloan, F. A. "Effects of Admission to a Teaching Hospital on the Cost and Quality of Care for Medicare Beneficiaries." *New England Journal of Medicine*, 1999, *340*(4), 293–299; Born, P., and Geckler, C. "HMO Quality and Financial Performance: Is There a Connection?" *Journal of Health Care Finance*, 1998, *24*(2), 65–77; Woolhandler, S., and Himmelstein, D. U. "When Money Is the Mission—The High Costs of Investor-Owned Care." *New England Journal of Medicine*, 1999, *341*(6), 444–446.

26. Melnick, G., Keeler, E., and Zwanziger, J. "Market Power and Hospital Pricing: Are Nonprofits Different?" *Health Affairs*, 1999, *18*(3), 167–173.

27. Sack, K. "Public Hospitals Around Country Cut Basic Service." *New York Times*, Aug. 20, 1995, p. Al.

28. Moy, E., and others. "Relationship Between National Institutes of Health Research Awards to US Medical Schools and Managed Care Market Penetration." *Journal of the American Medical Association*, 1997, *278*(3), 217–221.

29. Pear, R. "Health Agency Is Urged to Re-evaluate Spending Priorities," *New York Times*, July 9, 1998; Varmus, H. "Evaluating the Burden of Disease and Spending the Research Dollars of the National Institutes of Health." *New England Journal of Medicine*, June 17, 1999, *340*, 1914–1915; Dionne, E. J., Jr. "44 Million Uninsured and Counting." *Washington Post*, Aug. 13, 1999, p. A25. Light, D. W. "Good Managed Care Needs Universal Health Insurance." *Annals of Internal Medicine*, Apr. 20, 1999, *130*, 686–689.

30. Comroe, J. H., Jr., and Dripps, R. D. "Scientific Basis for the Support of Biomedical Science." *Science*, 1976, *192*, 105–111.

31. Gross, C. P., Anderson, G. F., and Powe, N. R. "The Relation Between Funding by the National Institutes of Health and the Burden of Disease." *New England Journal of Medicine*, June 17, 1999, *340*, 1881–1887; Varmus, H. "Evaluating the Burden of Disease and Spending the Research Dollars of the National Institutes of Health." *New England Journal of Medicine*, June 17, 1999, *340*, 1914–1915.

32. Hafner-Eaton, C. "When the Phoenix Rises, Where Will She Go? The Women's Health Agenda." In Vaillancourt, P. Rosenau (ed.), *Health Care Reform in the Nineties*. Thousand Oaks, Calif.: Sage, 1994; Council on Ethical and Judicial Affairs, American Medical Association. "Gender Disparities in Clinical Decision Making." *Journal of the American Medical Association*, 1991, *266*, 559–562; U.S. Public Health Service. *Women's Health: Report of the Public Health Service Task Force on Women's Health Issues*. Washington, D.C.: U.S. Department of Health and Human Services, 1985.

33. Annas, G. J. "Who's Afraid of the Human Genome?" *Hastings Center Report*, 1989, *19*(4), 19–21.

34. See special issue of the *International Journal of Technology Assessment in Health Care* on orphan technologies, J. Wagner guest editor, 1992, *8*(4).

35. Coster, J. M. "Recombinant Erythropoietin, Orphan Product with a Silver Spoon." *International Journal of Technology Assessment in Health Care*, 1992, *8*, 635, 644–646.

36. 422 USCS Secs. 289,289a-1–6, 1994), 21 CFR Secs. 56–58, 1994. See Ladimer, I., and Newman, R. W. (eds.). *Clinical Investigation in Medicine: Legal, Ethical and Moral Aspects, An Anthology and Bibliography*. Boston: Law-Medicine Research Institute, Boston University, 1963.

37. Annas, G. J. "Ethics Committees: From Ethical Comfort to Ethical Cover." *Hastings Center Report*, May-June 1991, 18–21. At the same time U.S. institutional review boards would object to studies carried out in Europe on the ground that they are not adequately protective of subjects. See Patriarca, P. A. "A Randomized Controlled Trial of Influenza Vaccine in the Elderly: Scientific Scrutiny and Ethical Responsibility." *Journal of the American Medical Association*, Dec. 7, 1994, *272*, 1700.

38. Hilts, P. J. "Conference Is Unable to Agree on Ethical Limits of Research: Psychiatric Experiment Helped Fuel Debate." *New York Times*, Jan. 15, 1995, p. 12.

39. Burns, J., Reardon, F., and Truog, R. "Using Newly Deceased Patients to Teach Resuscitation Procedures." *New England Journal of Medicine*, Dec. 15, 1994, *331*, 1653. See also Orlowski, J. P., Kanoti, G. A., and Mehlman, J. J. "The Ethics of Using Newly Dead

Patients for Teaching and Practicing Intubation Techniques." *New England Journal of Medicine*, 1988, *319*, 439–441.

40. Light, D. W. "Good Managed Care Needs Universal Health Insurance." *Annals of Internal Medicine*, Apr. 20, 1999, *130*, 686–689.

41. Dionne (1999); Weissman, J. S., and Epstein, A. M. *Falling Through the Safety Net: Insurance Status and Access to Health Care*. Baltimore: Johns Hopkins University Press, 1994; Braveman, P. A., and others. "Insurance-Related Differences in the Risk of Ruptured Appendix." *New England Journal of Medicine*, Aug. 18, 1994, 444–449; Haas, J., Udvarhelyi, S., and Epstein, A. "The Effect of Health Coverage for Uninsured Pregnant Women on Maternal Health and the Use of Cesarean Section." *Journal of the American Medical Association*, 1993, *270*(1), 61–64.

42. Schauffler, H. H., Brown, E. R., and Rice, T. "The State of Health Insurance in California, 1996." Los Angeles: Health Insurance Policy Program, University of California Berkeley School of Public Health, and UCLA Center for Health Policy Research, 1997.

43. Flores, G., Bauchner, H., Feinstein, A. R., and Nguyen, U. S. "The Impact of Ethnicity, Family Income, and Parental Education on Children's Health and Use of Health Services." *American Journal of Public Health*, 1999, *89*(7), 1066–1071; Brown, E. R., Wyn, R., and Ojeda, V. "Noncitizen Children's Rising Uninsured Rates Threaten Access to Health Care." Los Angeles: Center for Health Policy Research, UCLA, June 1999. [http://www.healthpolicy.ucla.edu]

44. The state medical boards are only now coming to sanction doctors who undertreat pain. Foubister, V. "Oregon Doctor Cited for Negligence for Undertreating Pain." *American Medical News*, Sept. 27, 1999. [http://www.ama-assn.org/sci-pubs/amnews/pick_99/prfa0927.htm] In addition, underuse of preventive services is increasingly a public health problem; see Center for the Evaluative Clinical Services. "The Quality of Medical Care in the United States." *Dartmouth Atlas of Health Care*, 1999.

45. Wilkinson, R. G. *Unhealthy Societies: The Afflictions of Inequality*. London: Routledge, 1996.

46. Kawachi, I., Kennedy, B. P., Lochner, K. and Prothrow-Stith, D. "Social Capital, Income Inequality, and Mortality." *American Journal of Public Health*, 1997, *87*, 1491–1498. Kawachi, I., and Kennedy, B. P. "Income Inequality and Health: Pathways and Mechanisms." *Health Services Research*, 1999, *34*(1), 215–228.

47. Wilkinson (1996).

48. Putnam, R. D. "Bowling Alone: America's Declining Social Capital." *Journal of Democracy*, 1995, *6*(1), 65–78.

49. Evans, R. G., Barer, M. L., and Marmor, T. R. *Why Are Some People Healthy and Others Not? The Determinants of Health of Populations*. Hawthorne, N.Y.: Aldine de Gruyter, 1994.

50. Lynch, J. W., Kaplan, G. A., and Shema, S. J. "Cumulative Impact of Sustained Economic Hardship on Physical, Cognitive, Psychological, and Social Functioning." *New England Journal of Medicine*, 1997, *337*(26), 1889–1895.

51. Winslow, R. "Rise in Health-Care Competition Saps Medical-Research Funds, Charity Care." *Wall Street Journal*, Mar. 24, 1999, p. B6; Cunningham, P. J., Grossman, J. M., St. Peter, R. F., and Lesser, C. S. "Managed Care and Physicians' Provision of Charity Care." *Journal of the American Medical Association*, 1999, *281*(12), 1087–1092. Preston, J. "Hospitals Look on Charity Care as Unaffordable Option of Past." *New York Times*, Apr. 14, 1996, pp. A1 and A15.

52. Roemer (1991).

53. For an explanation of the communitarian form of social solidarity, see "The Responsive Communitarian Platform: Rights and Responsibilities: A Platform." *Responsive*

Community, Winter 1991/1992, 4–20. Robert Bellah, Richard Madsen, William Sullivan, Ann Swindler, and Steven Tipton take a similar view in *Habits of the Heart* (New York: HarperCollins, 1985). See also Minkler, M. "Intergenerational Equity: Divergent Perspectives." (Paper presented at the annual meeting of the American Public Health Association, Washington, D.C., Nov. 1994); also Minkler, M., and Robertson, A. "Generational Equity and Public Health Policy: A Critique of 'Age/Race War' Thinking." *Journal of Public Health Policy,* 1991, *12*(3), 324–344.

54. Bellah, R., and others. *The Good Society.* New York: Knopf, 1991.

55. President's Commission for the Study of Ethical Problems in Medicine and Biomedical and Behavioral Research (A. M. Capron, exec. dir.). *Securing Access to Health Care: The Ethical Implications of Differences in the Availability of Health Services, Vol. 1.* Washington, D.C.: U.S. Government Printing Office, 1983.

56. Soumerai, S. B., and Ross-Degnan, D. "Inadequate Prescription-Drug Coverage for Medicare Enrollees—A Call to Action." *New England Journal of Medicine,* Mar. 4, 1999, *340,* 722–728; Freudenheim, M. "Patients Are Facing Sharp Rise in Costs for Drug Purchases." *New York Times,* Jan. 25, 1999, pp. A11, A18.

57. Maynard and Bloor (1998).

58. Lewis, C. E., Fein, R., and Mechanic, D. *The Right to Health: The Problem of Access to Primary Medical Care.* New York: Wiley, 1976.

59. Wheeler, S. V. "TeleMedicine." *BioPhotonics,* Fall 1994, 34–40; and Smothers, R. "150 Miles Away, the Doctor Is Examining Your Tonsils." *New York Times,* Sept. 16, 1992 (Late Edition Final), p. C14.

60. Moscovice, I., Wellever, A., and Stensland, J. "Rural Hospitals: Accomplishments and Present Challenges, July 1999." Rural Health Research Center, School of Public Health, University of Minnesota, July 1999. [www.hsr.umn.edu/centers/rhrc/rhrc.html] Accessed Oct. 18, 1999.

61. Marin, G., and VanOss Marin, B. *Research with Hispanic Populations.* Thousand Oaks, Calif.: Sage, 1991, chapter three. See, for example, Orlandi, M. (ed.). *Cultural Competence for Evaluators.* Rockville, Md.: U.S. Department of Health and Human Services, 1992.

62. Rafuse, J. "Multicultural Medicine." *Canadian Medical Association Journal,* 1993, *148,* 282–284; Maher, J. "Medical Education in a Multilingual and Multicultural World." *Medical Education,* 1993, *27,* 3–5.

63. There is no evidence that HMOs, prior to 1992, offered reduced quality of care. Miller, R. H., and Luft, H. S. "Does Managed Care Lead to Better or Worse Quality of Care?" *Health Affairs,* 1997, *16*(5), 7–25. The evidence on HMOs and quality of care in the context of today's market competition is still out. The not-for-profit HMOs seem to provide better quality than do the for-profit HMOs. "How Good Is Your Health Plan?" *Consumer Reports,* Aug., 1996, pp. 40–44; Kuttner, R. "Must Good HMOs Go Bad? The Commercialization of Prepaid Group Health Care." *New England Journal of Medicine,* 1998, *338*(21), 1558–1563; Kuttner, R. "Must Good HMOs Go Bad? The Search for Checks and Balances." *New England Journal of Medicine,* 1998, *338*(22), 1635–1639; Himmelstein, Woolhandler, Hellander, and Wolfe (1999).

64. Rice, T. *The Economics of Health Reconsidered.* Chicago: Health Administration Press, 1998; Luft, H. S. *Health Maintenance Organizations: Dimensions of Performance.* New York: Wiley, 1981.

65. Miller, T. E., and Sage, W. M. "Disclosing Physician Financial Incentives." *Journal of the American Medical Association,* 1999, *281*(15), 1424–1430.

66. Miller and Sage (1999).

67. Bodenheimer, T. "Disease Management: Promises and Pitfalls." *New England Journal of Medicine*, 1999, *340*(15), 1202–1205.

68. Mariner, W. K. "Patients' Rights After Health Care Reform: Who Decides What Is Medically Necessary?" *American Journal of Public Health*, 1994, *84*(9), 1515–1519; Rosenbaum, S., Frankford, D. M., Moore, B., and Borzi, P. "Who Should Determine When Health Care Is Medically Necessary?" *New England Journal of Medicine*, Jan. 21, 1999, *340*, 229–232. *Fox v. Health Net of California*, California Superior Court, no. 219692, Dec. 23 and 28, 1993.

69. *Pinneke v. Preisser*, 623 F.2d 546 (8th Cir. 1980); *Bush v. Barham*, 625 F.2d 1150 (5th Cir. 1980).

70. Mariner (1994).

71. Danzon, P. M. "Tort Liability: A Minefield for Managed Care?" (Part 2.) Journal of Legal Studies, 1997, *26*(2), 491–519.

72. 29 U.S.C. sec. 1144 (a)-(b), 1994.

73. *Shaw v. Delta Airlines*, 463 U.S. 85, 1983; *Corcoran v. United Healthcare, Inc.*, 965 F.2d 1321 (5th Cir.), cert. denied 506 U.S. 1033, 1992. See Kilcullen, J. K. "Groping for the Reins: ERISA, HMO Malpractice, and Enterprise Liability." *American Journal of Law and Medicine*, 1996, *22*(1), 7.

74. See, for example, *Dukes v. U.S. Healthcare Inc.*, 57 F.3d 350 (3rd Cir. 1995), cert. denied 116 S. Ct. 564, 1995.

75. *New York State Conference of Blue Cross and Blue Shield Plans v. Travelers Ins. Co.*, 115 S. Ct. 1671, 1995.

76. Rosenbaum, Frankford, Moore, and Borzi (1999).

77. Rundle, R. L. "California's Managed-Care Legislation Generally Draws Industry's Support." *Wall Street Journal*, Sept. 13, 1999; Ingram, C., and Morain, D. "Ambitious Plan to Reform HMOs Nears Completion." *Los Angeles Times*, Sept. 10, 1999; Sterngold, J. "California Law to Let Patients Sue HMO's." *New York Times*, Sept. 28, 1999, pp. A1, A18; Johnson, D. "Illinois Court Lets Patients Sue HMO's." *New York Times*, Oct. 2, 1999, p. A7. See Tex. Civ. Proc. & Rem. Code, Chapter 88; Marquis, J., Rubin, A. J., and Ingram, C. "Broad Health Care Reform Package Signed into Law." *Los Angeles Times*, Sept. 28, 1999, pp. 1, 18.

78. Page, L. "Texas Law on HMO Liability Generates Little Cost—So Far." *American Medical News*, Oct. 18, 1999, p. 13.

79. Pear, R. "Series of Rulings Eases Constraints on Suing HMO's." *New York Times*, Aug. 15, 1999, pp. 1, 19.

80. *Pegram v. Herdrich*, U.S. 29 S. Ct. 2143 (2000).

81. Emanuel, E. J. "Choice and Representation in Health Care." *Medical Care Research and Review*, 1999, *56*(1), 113–140.

82. Baumhart, R. C. "How Ethical Are Businessmen?" *Harvard Business Review*, July/Aug. 1961, pp. 6–19, 156–176.

83. Fisher, E. S., and Welch, H. G. "Avoiding the Unintended Consequences of Growth in Medical Care: How Might More Be Worse?" *Journal of the American Medical Association*, 1999, *281*(5), 452; Deyo, R. A., and others. "The Messenger Under Attack: Intimidation of Researchers by Special-Interest Groups." *New England Journal of Medicine*, 1997, *336*(16), 1176–1180.

84. Ellwood quoted in Noble, H. B. "Quality Is Focus for Health Plans." *New York Times*, July 3, 1995, pp. 1, 7. For discussion of problems in business ethics, see Cederblom, J., and Dougherty, C. J. *Ethics at Work*. Belmont, Calif.: Wadsworth, 1990; Iannone, A. P. (ed.).

Contemporary Moral Controversies in Business. New York: Oxford University Press, 1989; Bayles, M. D. *Professional Ethics.* (2nd ed.) Belmont, Calif.: Wadsworth, 1989; Callahan, J. C. *Ethical Issues in Professional Life.* New York: Oxford University Press, 1988.

85. Roemer (1991).

86. Kuttner, R. "The American Health Care System: Wall Street and Health Care." *New England Journal of Medicine,* Feb. 25, 1999, *340,* 664–668.

87. Shindul-Rothschild, J., Berry, D., and Long-Middleton, E. "Where Have All the Nurses Gone? Final Results of Our Patient Care Survey." *American Journal of Nursing,* Nov. 1996, *96,* 25–39.

88. Rundle, R. L. "California Is the First State to Require Hospital-Wide Nurse-to-Patient Ratios." *Wall Street Journal,* Oct. 12, 1999, p. B6.

89. Kaiser Family Foundation and Harvard University School of Public Health. *Survey of Physicians and Nurses: Randomly Selected Verbatim Descriptions from Physicians and Nurses of Health Plan Decisions Resulting in Declines in Patients' Health Status.* Menlo Park, Calif.: Kaiser Family Foundation, July 1999.

90. See, for example, *Whalen* v. *Roe,* 429 U.S. 589, 1977, upholding the constitutionality of a state law requiring that patients receiving legitimate prescriptions for drugs with potential for abuse have name, address, age, and other information reported to the state department of health.

91. Hillman, A. L., and others. "Avoiding Bias in the Conduct and Reporting of Cost-Effectiveness Research Sponsored by Pharmaceutical Companies." *New England Journal of Medicine,* 1991, *324,* 1362–1365.

92. *Ethyl Corporation* v. *Environmental Protection Agency,* 541 F.2d 1, 1976.

93. Silver, L. "An Agency Dilemma: Regulating to Protect the Public Health in Light of Scientific Uncertainty." In R. Roemer and G. McKray (eds.), *Legal Aspects of Health Policy: Issues and Trends.* Westport, Conn.: Greenwood Press, 1980.

94. Silver (1980), p. 81, quoting this passage from Judge Bazelon's concurring opinion in *International Harvester Company* v. *Ruckelshaus,* 478 F.2d 615, 652, 1973.

95. *Daubert* v. *Merrell Dow Pharmaceuticals, Inc.,* 509 U.S. 579, 113 S. Ct. 2786, 125 L.Ed. 2d 469, 1993.

96. Ginzburg, H. M. "Use and Misuse of Epidemiologic Data in the Courtroom: Defining the Limits of Inferential and Particularistic Evidence in Mass Tort Litigation." *American Journal of Law and Medicine,* 1986, *12*(3 and 4), 423–439.

97. Roemer, R. *Legislative Action to Combat the World Tobacco Epidemic.* (2nd ed.) Geneva, Switzerland: World Health Organization, 1993; U.S. Department of Health and Human Services. *Reducing the Health Consequences of Smoking: 25 Years of Progress. A Report of the Surgeon General.* (DHHS publication no. CDC 89-8411.) Washington, D.C.: Office on Smoking and Health, Center for Chronic Disease Prevention and Health Promotion, Centers for Disease Control, Public Health Service, U.S. Department of Health and Human Services, 1989.

98. *Penn Advertising of Baltimore, Inc.* v. *Mayor of Baltimore,* 63 F.3d 1318 (4th Cir. 1995) aff'g 862 F. Supp. 1402 (D. Md. 1994), discussed by Garner, D. W. "Banning Tobacco Billboards: The Case for Municipal Action." *Journal of the American Medical Association,* 1996, *275*(16), 1263–1269. On Sept. 1, 1999, the U.S. Court of Appeals for the 7th Circuit ruled that Chicago's cigarette and alcohol sign ordinance was not federally preempted. If the ordinance is found not in violation of the First Amendment (as the 4th Circuit determined for a similar ordinance), the way will be open for local boards of health to regulate tobacco

advertising. *Federation of Advertising Industry Representatives, Inc.* v. *City of Chicago,* nos. 98–3191, 99–1115, and 99–1516, 1999.

99. Annas, G. J. *The Standard of Care: The Law of American Bioethics.* New York: Oxford University Press, 1993; Rosenbaum, S. "Mothers and Children Last: The Oregon Medicaid Experiment." *American Journal of Law and Medicine,* 1992, *18*(1 and 2), 97–126.

100. Maynard and Bloor (1998).

101. Anderson, G. F., and Poullier, J. P. "Health Spending, Access, and Outcomes: Trends in Industrialized Countries." *Health Affairs,* 1999, *18*(3), 178–182.

102. Greenberg, D. S. "Snapshots of Substandard Health Care." *Washington Post,* Sept. 1, 1999, p. A23; Schuster, M. A., McGlynn, E. A., and Brook, R. H. "How Good Is the Quality of Health Care in the United States?" *Milbank Quarterly,* 1999, *76*(4), 517ff.

103. Sale of organs is unethical as well as scientifically unsound as a means of rationing, and yet it exists and persists. See Fox, R., and Swazey, J. *Spare Parts: Organ Replacement in American Society.* Oxford University Press, 1992; U.S. General Accounting Office. *Organ Transplants: Increased Effort Needed to Boost Supply and Ensure Equitable Distribution of Organs.* (GAO/HRD-93-56.) Washington D.C.: General Accounting Office, 1993.

104. Bosch, X. "Spain Leads World in Organ Donation and Transplantation." *Journal of the American Medical Association,* July 7, 1999, *282,* 17–18.

105. Roels, L., and others. "Three Years of Experience with a 'Presumed Consent' Legislation in Belgium: Its Impact on Multiorgan Donation in Comparison with Other European Countries." *Transplantation Procedures,* 1991, *23,* 903–904; Associated Press. "Bill Would Allow Automatic Donation." *American Medical News,* Mar. 22–29, 1993, p. 10.

106. Defino, T. "Mediscare." *Healthcare Business,* 1999, *2*(3), 60–70.

107. Kaiser Family Foundation, pp. 7, 16.

108. The GAO estimate quoted is in Rosenthal, E. "Confusion and Error Are Rife in Hospital Billing Practices." *New York Times,* Jan. 27, 1993; see also Kerr, P. "Glossing over Health Care Fraud." *New York Times,* Apr. 5, 1992, p. F17; U.S. General Accounting Office. *Health Insurance: Remedies Needed to Reduce Losses from Fraud and Abuse—Testimony.* (GAO/T-HRD-9308.) Washington, D.C.: General Accounting Office, Mar. 8, 1993. Alan Hillman, director of the Center for Health Policy at the University of Pennsylvania, suggests that hospital records are so deformed and manipulated for billing and reimbursement purposes that they are no longer of any use for outcomes research (quoted in *New York Times,* Aug. 9, 1994, p. A11.)

109. Pear, R. "Stung by Defeat in House, HMO's Seek Compromise." *New York Times,* Oct. 9, 1999, p. A9.

110. Hillman, B., and others. "Physicians' Utilization and Charges for Outpatient Diagnostic Imaging in a Medicare Population." *Journal of the American Medical Association,* Oct. 21, 1992, *268,* 2050–2054; Mitchell, J., and Scott, E. "Physician Ownership of Physical Therapy Services: Effects on Charges, Utilization, Profits, and Service Characteristics." *Journal of the American Medical Association,* Oct. 21, 1992, *268,* 2055–2059; Kolata, G. "Pharmacists Help Drug Promotions; Pharmacists Paid by Companies to Recommend Their Drugs." *New York Times,* July 29, 1994, pp. Al, D2; Hilts, P. J. "FDA Seeks Disclosures by Scientists: Financial Interests in Drugs Are at Issue." *New York Times,* Sept. 24, 1994, p. 7; Winslow, R. "Drug Company's PR Firm Made Offer to Pay for Editorial, Professor Says." *Wall Street Journal,* Sept. 8, 1994, p. B12; U.S. General Accounting Office. *Medicare: Referrals to Physician-Owned Imaging Facilities Warrant HCFA's Scrutiny.* (GAO/HEHS-95-2.) Washington, D.C.: General Accounting Office, 1994.

111. Prager, L. O. "Selling Products OK—But Not for Profit." *American Medical News,* July 12, 1999, p. 1.

112. *WHO Consultation on Testing and Counseling for HIV Infection.* (WHO/GPA/NF/93.2.) Geneva, Switzerland: Global Programme on AIDS, World Health Organization, 1993; Field, M. A. "Testing for AIDS: Uses and Abuses." *American Journal of Law and Medicine, 16*(1 and 2), 33–106; Fluss, S. S., and Zeegers, D. "AIDS, HIV, and Health Care Workers: Some International Perspectives." *Maryland Law Review,* 1989, *48*(1), 77–92.

113. Centers for Disease Control and Prevention. *HIV/AIDS Surveillance Report.* (Vol. 32, report no. 9.) Atlanta: Centers for Disease Control and Prevention, 1997.

114. Nakashima, A. K., and others. "Effect of HIV Reporting by Name on Use of HIV Testing in Publicly Funded Counseling and Testing Programs." *Journal of the American Medical Association,* 1998, *280*(16), 1421.

115. Marquis, J. "Use of Names Won't Lessen HIV Testing, Study Says." *Los Angeles Times,* Oct. 28, 1998, pp. A3, A14.

116. Joseph, S. C. *Dragon Within the Gates: The Once and Future AIDS Epidemic.* New York: Carroll and Graf, 1992.

117. "1998 Guidelines for Treatment of Sexually Transmitted Diseases." *Morbidity and Mortality Weekly Report,* Jan. 23, 1998, *47*(RR-1), 16. See California Health and Safety Code, sec. 199.25 (1990) and the insightful analysis of Bayer, R. "HIV Prevention and the Two Faces of Partner Notification." *American Journal of Public Health,* Aug. 9, 1992, *82,* 1156–1164.

118. "1998 Guidelines . . ." (1998); "Public Health Service Task Force Recommendations for the Use of Antiretroviral Drugs in Pregnant Women Infected with HIV-1 for Maternal Health and for Reducing Perinatal HIV-1 Transmission in the United States." *Morbidity and Mortality Weekly Report,* Jan. 30, 1998, *47*(RR-2).

119. 410 U.S. 113, 1973.

120. Lagnado, L. "Their Role Growing, Catholic Hospitals Juggle Doctrine and Medicine." *Wall Street Journal,* Feb. 4, 1999, pp. 1, 8; Dressler, T. "Rise of Religious Hospitals Seen as Threat to Reproductive Rights." *Los Angeles Daily Journal,* Feb. 5, 1999, pp. 1, 8; O'Donnell, J. "Catholic Hospital Deals Limit Access, Activists Say." *USA Today,* Apr. 8, 1999, pp. B1, B2.

121. See "Abortion Denied: Shattering Young Women's Lives." (Video.) Feminist Majority Foundation, 8105 W. 3rd St., Los Angeles, CA 90048, 1990.

122. Scitovsky, A. A. "Medical Care in the Last Twelve Months of Life: The Relation between Age, Functional Status, and Medical Care Expenditures." *Milbank Memorial Fund Quarterly,* 1988, *66*(4), 640–660; Temkin-Greener, H., Meiners, M. S., Petty, E. A., and Szydlowski, J. S. "The Use and Cost of Health Services Prior to Death: A Comparison of the Medicare-only and the Medicare-Medicaid Elderly Populations." *Milbank Quarterly,* 1992, *70*(4), 679–701. For an insightful analysis of how a society's cultural beliefs, concept of autonomy, and informed consent laws influence resource allocation at the end of life, see Annas, G. J., and Miller, F. H. "The Empire of Death: How Culture and Economics Affect Informed Consent in the U.S., the U.K., and Japan." *American Journal of Law and Medicine,* 1994, *20*(4), 359–394.

123. See, for example, N.Y. Mental Hygiene Law, Article 9, Secs 9.01–9.59, 1988 and Supp. 1995); Special Committee to Study Commitment Procedures of the Association of the Bar of the City of New York, in cooperation with the Cornell Law School. *Mental Illness and Due Process: Report and Recommendations on Admission to Mental Hospitals Under New York Law.* Ithaca, N.Y.: Cornell University Press, 1962.

124. *Tarasoff* v. *Regents of the University of California*, 17 Cal. 3d 425, 551 P. 2d 334, 131 Cal. Rptr. 14, 1976.

125. Grad, F. P. *The Public Health Law Manual.* (2nd ed.) Washington, D.C.: American Public Health Association, 1990.

126. Starr, P. "Health and the Right to Privacy." *American Journal of Law and Medicine*, 1999, *25*(2 and 3), 193–201.

127. Murray, S. "Clinton Pushes Lawmakers to Approve Medical Privacy Legislation This Fall." *Wall Street Journal*, Sept. 9, 1999, p. A10; Murray, S. "On Medical-Privacy Issue, the Doctor Finally May Be in." *Wall Street Journal*, Aug. 20, 1999, p. A12.

128. McGlynn, E. A., and Brook, R. H. "Ensuring Quality of Care." In R. M. Andersen, T. H. Rice, and G. F. Kominski (eds.), *Changing the U.S. Health Care System.* San Francisco: Jossey-Bass, 1996; Chassin, M. R., and Galvin, R. W. "The Urgent Need to Improve Health Care Quality: Institute of Medicine National Roundtable on Health Care Quality." *Journal of the American Medical Association*, 1998, *280*(11), 1000–1005; Detsky, A. S. "Regional Variation in Medical Care." *New England Journal of Medicine*, 1995, *333*(9), 589–590; Leape, L. L. "Error in Medicine." *Journal of the American Medical Association*, 1994, *272*, 1851–1857.

129. For a thoughtful discussion of peer review organizations under the law as it existed in November 1979, see Price, S. J. "Health Systems Agencies and Peer Review Organizations: Experiments in Regulating the Delivery of Health Care." In Roemer and McKray (1980). For a more recent analysis, see Luce, G. M. "The Use of Peer Review Organizations to Control Medicare Costs." *ALI-ABA Course Materials-Journal*, 1986, *10*, 111–120; Pear, R. "Clinton to Unveil Rules to Protect Medical Privacy." *New York Times*, Oct. 27, 1999, p. A1.

130. 42 U.S.C. Sec. 1320c et seq.

131. 42 U.S.C. Sec. 11101 et seq.

132. U.S. Congress, Office of Technology Assessment. *Impact of Legal Reform on Medical Malpractice Costs.* (OTA-BP-H-19.) Washington, D.C.: U.S. Government Printing Office, 1993.

133. For analysis of various aspects of practice guidelines, see Capron, A. M. "Practice Guidelines: How Good Are Medicine's New Recipes?" *Journal of Law, Medicine and Ethics*, 1995, *23*(1), 47–56; Parker, C. W. "Practice Guidelines and Private Insurers." *Journal of Law, Medicine and Ethics*, 1995, *23*(1), 57–61; Kane, R. L. "Creating Practice Guidelines: The Dangers of Over-Reliance on Expert Judgment." *Journal of Law, Medicine and Ethics*, 1995, *23*(1), 62–64; Pauly, M. V. "Practice Guidelines: Can They Save Money? Should They?" *Journal of Law, Medicine and Ethics*, 1995, *23*(1), 65–74; Halpern, J. "Can the Development of Practice Guidelines Safeguard Patient Values?" *Journal of Law, Medicine and Ethics*, 1995, *23*(1), 75–81.

134. The Joint Commission on Accreditation of Healthcare Organizations is going to make available to consumers information about provider performance or outcomes. The National Committee on Quality Assurance, a national agency located in Washington, D.C., will undertake similar activities. See http://www.ncqa.org/Pages/Main/index.htm. *Consumer Reports, Newsweek,* and *U.S. News & World Report* publish HMO assessments from time to time.

135. McLaughlin, C. G., and Ginsburg, P. B. "Competition, Quality of Care, and the Role of the Consumer." *Milbank Quarterly*, 1998, *76*(4), 737–743; Weinstein, M. M. "Economic Scene: The Grading May Be Too Easy on Health Plans' Report Cards." *New York Times*, Aug. 19, 1999, p. C2.

136. Hofer, T. P., and others. "The Unreliability of Individual Physician 'Report Cards' for Assessing the Costs and Quality of Care of a Chronic Disease." *Journal of the American Medical Association,* 1999, *281*(22), 2098–2105.

137. Poole, W. "The Rating Game." *California Medicine,* June 1997, pp. 18ff.

138. Grad, F. P. "Medical Ethics and the Law." *Annals of the American Academy of Political and Social Science,* May 1978, *437,* 19–36.

139. *Cruzan* v. *Missouri Department of Health,* 497 U.S. 261, 1990.

140. See the references in note 110 on conflict of interest and referral.

Name Index

Subject Index

A

AAPCC (average adjusted per capita cost), 425

AAPI. *See* Asian Americans; Pacific Islanders

Accelerated compensation event, 483

ACCESS (Access to Community Care and Effective Services and Supports Program), 360–361, 365–366, 369

Access to care: areas for research on, 26; conceptual framework for, 4, 6–10; conceptualizing and measuring, 3, 53n.2; defining/improving dimensions of, 10–15; HIV/AIDS and, 231–234; by homeless population, 343–344; impact of Medicare reform on, 426–427; policy purposes of measuring, 11*f*; public health ethics and, 507–508; trends in, 15–25

Access to care conceptual framework: on contextual enabling characteristics, 6; on contextual need characteristics, 6–7; on contextual predisposing characteristics, 4, 6; on health behaviors, 8–9; on individual need characteristics, 8; on individual predisposing characteristics, 7; on outcomes, 9–10

Access to care trends: equitable access, 19–22; realized access (utilization over time), 15, 18–19

Accountability, 277–279

Accuracy, 440

Ad damnum clause reform, 476

ADAP (AIDS Drug Assistance Program), 247

Adolescents: AIDS and special needs of, 248–249; homelessness among, 341–342; mental illness/suicide by, 304. *See also* Children

ADR (alternative dispute resolution), 482, 483, 485–486

Adverse events, 172–173, 175–176

Advertising (DTC), 119

Aetna Life Insurance, 410

AFDC (Aid to Families with Dependent Children), 39–40, 41, 324

Affirmative action programs, 507

African Americans: access to insurance by female, 322; HIV/AIDS access to care by, 233; as home care workers, 216; homicide of young men among, 450; hospital admission rates for, 20*t*, 21–22; use of long-term care by, 212; Medicare access by, 38, 39; mental illness and, 304; need for services by elderly, 211; personal health care use by, 20*t*; physician and dental visits by, 20*t*, 22; uninsured among, 33. *See also* Race/ethnic groups

Agency for Healthcare Research and Quality, 90–91, 143

AHCPR (Agency for Health Care Policy and Research), 23

AHQR (Agency for Health Quality Research), 246

AHRQ (Agency for Healthcare Research and Quality), 23, 162, 163

AHSR (Association for Health Services Research), 277